THE ENCYCLOPEDIA OF

THE DIGESTIVE SYSTEM
AND DIGESTIVE DISORDERS

Second Edition

THE ENCYCLOPEDIA OF

THE DIGESTIVE SYSTEM
AND DIGESTIVE DISORDERS

Second Edition

Anil Minocha, M.D.
Christine Adamec

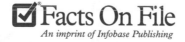

An imprint of Infobase Publishing

The Encyclopedia of the Digestive System and Digestive Disorders, Second Edition

Facts On File
An imprint of Infobase Publishing, Inc.
132 West 31st Street
New York NY 10001

Library of Congress Cataloging-in-Publication

Minocha, Anil.
The encyclopedia of the digestive system and digestive disorders / Anil Minocha, Christine Adamec. — 2nd ed.
p. ; cm. — (Facts on File library of health and living)
Includes bibliographical references and index.
ISBN-13: 978-0-8160-7661-1 (hardcover : alk. paper)
ISBN-10: 0-8160-7661-8 (hardcover : alk. paper) 1. Gastrointestinal system—Encyclopedias. 2. Digestive organs—Encyclopedias. 3. Gastrointestinal system—Diseases—Encyclopedias. 4. Digestive organs—Diseases—Encyclopedias. I. Adamec, Christine A., 1949–   II. Title. III. Series: Facts on File library of health and living.
[DNLM: 1. Digestive System—Encyclopedias—English. 2. Digestive System Diseases—Encyclopedias—English. WI 13]
RC802.M567 2010
616.3003—dc22   2010028790

Facts On File books are available at special discounts when purchased in bulk quantities for businesses, associations, institutions, or sales promotions. Please call our Special Sales Department in New York at (212) 967-8800 or (800) 322-8755.

You can find Facts On File on the World Wide Web at http://www.factsonfile.com

Text design by Annie O'Donnell
Composition by Hermitage Publishing Services
Cover printed by Sheridan Books, Ann Arbor, Mich.
Book printed and bound by Sheridan Books, Ann Arbor, Mich.
Date printed: November 2010

Printed in the United States of America

10 9 8 7 6 5 4 3 2 1

This book is printed on acid-free paper.

Dr. Minocha would like to dedicate this book to his loving parents, Ram. S. Minocha and Kamla Devi Minocha, and to his daughter, Geeta P. Minocha.

Christine Adamec would like to dedicate this book to her husband, John Adamec, in grateful appreciation of his continued support throughout this project.

CONTENTS

FOREWORD

I am a practicing gastroenterologist and a medical school professor, as well as the author of numerous articles for medical journals and self-help books for the general public, such as *How to Stop Heartburn* and *Natural Stomach Care*, in addition to books written specifically for physicians. My different roles give me a broad and current overview of both common and rare diseases and disorders of the digestive system. From these perspectives, I see significant advances as well as some disturbing trends. For example, I have seen overweight and obesity rates escalate dramatically in the United States. The majority (two-thirds) of all Americans are known to be either overweight or obese. As a result, they are at risk for many disorders, such as diabetes mellitus, gallbladder disease, hypertension, and the third-most common form of cancer, colorectal cancer, as well as cancers of the stomach and the liver. I urge and challenge readers with a weight problem to lose weight to decrease their risk for these diseases. Even a loss of 10 pounds can make a dramatic difference.

Another issue affecting public health is the rapidly aging population in the United States, with the first of the baby boomers (born between 1946 and 1964) reaching age 65 in 2011, and many more to follow. Older people are more prone to many digestive disorders ranging from gastroesophageal reflux disease and ulcers to cancers of the digestive system. Many elderly people also suffer from chronic constipation and other daily digestive annoyances. These topics are all thoroughly covered in this second edition.

In addition, my coauthor and I discuss alternative remedies for digestive disorders as well as the broad range of medications used to treat digestive diseases. This new edition covers concerns that have recently come to light, such as the risks of nonsteroidal anti-inflammatory drugs (NSAIDs) along with withdrawal of COX-2 inhibitors. In fact, some organizations, such as the American Geriatrics Society, are so concerned about the effects of NSAIDs that in 2009 they urged their members to prescribe opiates to elderly patients rather than NSAIDs.

The new edition also covers the latest technology used to diagnose and treat digestive diseases and disorders; for example, wireless endoscopy enables physicians using a noninvasive means to visualize regions of the small bowel that are not easily within the reach of standard endoscopy, thus increasing the likelihood of pinpointing the causes of obscure gastrointestinal bleeding and other digestive problems. At the same time, double-balloon enteroscopy enables physicians to evaluate most of the length of the small bowel, regions formerly difficult to explore.

The effects of bacteria have been known for more than a hundred years, but despite this knowledge, many patients worldwide have died of bacterial and parasitic infections that were transmitted through contaminated food and water. This new edition provides recent data on both common and less common bacterial infestations that affect the digestive system, such as cholera, *Clostridium*, and *Cryptosporidium*. However, many digestive enigmas remain unresolved. There remains much to learn, and important research continues. For example, many forms of cancer are still rapid killers, such as pancreatic cancer or esophageal cancer, frequently causing no symptoms or signs until the disease is far advanced. Other diseases and disorders, such as Crohn's disease or irritable bowel syndrome, although they usually do not kill patients, can cause misery for years or even decades. However, because of medical advances, instead of wearing a colostomy bag after the removal of the colon for ulcerative colitis, patients may now choose newer surgeries that enable continent bowel function through the anal canal.

Other health problems directly or indirectly lead to digestive diseases or disorders; for example, alcoholism leads to numerous diseases, including heart disease, pancreatitis, and vitamin and mineral deficiencies; some alcoholics suffer from the damage and destruction of the liver (liver cirrhosis), for which the only cure may be a liver transplantation.

For about one-fourth of all Americans cigarette smoking contributes to many digestive diseases. Smoking is the one preventable cause of death in about 400,000 cases each year. Patients who have Crohn's disease worsen with continued smoking, as do individuals who have gastroparesis (slow stomach emptying). Paradoxically, smoking is protective against ulcerative colitis.

In this volume, I provide a comprehensive overview of the major as well as the less well known digestive diseases and disorders, including the symptoms and the diagnosis of each disease and what is known about its causes. I also provide information on the epidemiological characteristics of the disease or disorder, which identify the people most likely at risk. I also discuss the treatments for each disease and disorder.

In addition, my coauthor and I explain the lab and diagnostic tests that determine the presence of the disease and methods of ruling out other diseases. We also provide information on available treatments for diseases. In many cases, patients can take preventive actions to improve their condition: changing diet, losing weight, avoiding certain activities, increasing exercise level, requesting specific laboratory tests, and so forth. Raising the level of the head end of the bed or using a reflux wedge, though seemingly minor, can provide significant pain relief to many patients with chronic heartburn. Similarly, raising the head end of the bed for tube-fed patients reduces the risk of aspiration pneumonia.

This second edition of *The Encyclopedia of the Digestive System and Digestive Disorders* provides an overview of digestive illnesses so nonphysician readers can be better educated about illnesses they may face with knowledge of key questions to ask their physicians. Knowing that I could not describe all of the information on every possible digestive disease, I have selected the major illnesses that may occur as well as some rare diseases that may interest readers. I hope that readers find this encyclopedia helpful and informative.

—Anil Minocha, M.D.

INTRODUCTION:
A History of Digestive Diseases and Disorders

The digestion of food is necessary to sustain life. This fact is as true today, in the 21st-century era of high technology and a dazzling array of newly approved medications and therapeutic medical devices, as it was millennia ago when humans actively hunted or farmed for the basic food that they needed in order to survive. Modern computerized equipment—even the most remarkable medical discoveries—cannot change one unalterable fact: Everyone needs to eat and to digest food in order to stay alive; the only options are tubes or intravenous feeding, both of which may cause complications.

The Wall Street genius, the street child, and the retired person in a nursing home all need to eat to survive, although the components of their diet and even the way they eat may vary considerably. The gourmet delicacies taken for granted by the wealthy are very different from the garbage scraps that homeless people subsist on. These types of food are also very different from the nutrition that is directly placed into the FEEDING TUBE or the intravenous line of the severely ill in nursing homes or hospitals. But in the digestive system, whether it is oysters and chocolate or leftover fast food from a trash can, all food is basically the same: It must be processed and used, and its waste material eliminated, for the primary purpose of keeping the individual alive and as healthy as possible.

The need for nutrition occurs even before birth. The fetus is nourished in the mother's womb through the umbilical cord. After the baby is born, whether the child is fed with mother's breast milk or with infant formula, the infant's digestive system actively works to extract everything needed for its continued life as well to propel the child forward on a course of active growth and development. This need for food and the necessity to digest the food will continue until death.

Sometimes the digestive system malfunctions and does *not* properly digest the food that is ingested. According to the National Commission on Digestive Diseases in their 2009 report, at least 60 to 70 million Americans suffer from digestive diseases each year, at an estimated annual medical cost of more than $100 billion. In addition, 10 to 15 percent of all inpatient hospitalizations occur as a result of digestive diseases and disorders.

Medications for treating digestive diseases are used daily by many people; for example, the drugs that are prescribed for GASTROESOPHAGEAL REFLUX DISEASE are among the most commonly prescribed medications in the United States, according to the National Commission on Digestive Diseases.

A broad array of problems can occur in the digestive system. They range from transient and easily correctable illnesses that can be managed without medical assistance, such as a minor stomachache or temporary DIARRHEA caused by a minor infection, upward to chronic and/or severe problems that must be treated by physicians. According to the National Center for Health Statistics, in 2006, 16 million doctor visits were related to complaints of ABDOMINAL PAIN or distress, cramps, and spasms and this category was among the 20 top reasons why patients saw their doctors.

In most cases, doctors can diagnose the problem, make recommendations, and order efficacious medications and treatments to completely resolve or at least improve the broad array of digestive diseases and disorders. In other cases, routine screening enables physicians to identify serious diseases, such as COLORECTAL CANCER, which can often be detected, treated, and even cured in its early stages (or in precancerous stages, as with precancerous POLYPS) with a colonoscopy.

Yet when all is well, it is very easy to take the digestive system for granted, and most people do so until a peptic ULCER, CROHN'S DISEASE, gastroesophageal reflux disease, or another troubling digestive ailment develops. Then emergency treatment is often urgently sought.

A Marvel of Cooperation: The Digestive System

Digestion is an amazingly complicated process. The digestive system manages a marvelous process that no machine could possibly duplicate in its myriad of interactive tasks, both with other organs and with the blood, the bones and nerves, and other systems of the body.

The food that is so necessary to sustain life must be completely broken down with special enzymes and digestive juices and then absorbed and assimilated by the body in a complex symphony of cooperation among many different organs. In the digestive system—which includes the oral cavity, the ESOPHAGUS (the food tube that connects to the stomach), the stomach, the PANCREAS, the LIVER, the GALLBLADDER, the small intestine, and the colon—these organs play critically important roles in managing the complex process of digestion and absorption. (See illustration on page xiii.)

The digestion process begins when a person takes the first bite of food, and it continues until there is no further use for what is left, and that material is excreted from the body, transformed into fecal matter.

Rather than a start-stop type of operation, the digestive system is nearly a "24–7" operation that rarely shuts down altogether. Often while breakfast and a midmorning snack are being processed and assimilated, a person may be eating lunch, and, thus, the stomach, the small intestine, and the colon are all involved in various processes of breaking down and absorbing the water and nutrients from food and ultimately in excreting what is not needed into fecal material. No factory on Earth could sustain such a continuous operation for 75 or more years of life, and it is not surprising that minor and major problems in the digestive system will develop in the course of an individual's life.

To understand digestive diseases and disorders, it is important to have a basic understanding of the gastrointestinal system and the organs that it comprises as well as to have an understanding of the digestive process. Digestion actually begins at the mouth, where individuals produce the saliva that helps to break down the food even before it enters the esophagus (the food tube) and begins its passage downward through the gastrointestinal system.

The gastrointestinal system is primarily composed of a series of connecting hollow and looping tubes. This system processes the food and moves it along, breaking down some of the food for fuel and eliminating what is not needed as waste products.

From the mouth and throat, and proceeding on to the gut, the digestive system continues through the stomach and small intestine, where the absorption of most water and nutrients occurs. It ends at the colon, also known as the large intestine, where the unused excrement is eliminated via the rectum and through the anus.

Other important parts of the digestive system are actively involved in digestion as well. The gallbladder, the pancreas, and the liver are all intimately involved in providing special digestive juices containing enzymes and other substances that are essential in order to break down and absorb food, transforming it into usable energy to fuel the body.

The gallbladder, pancreas, and liver can also malfunction—become infected, inflamed, or cancerous—as well as experience other medical prob-

The Digestive System

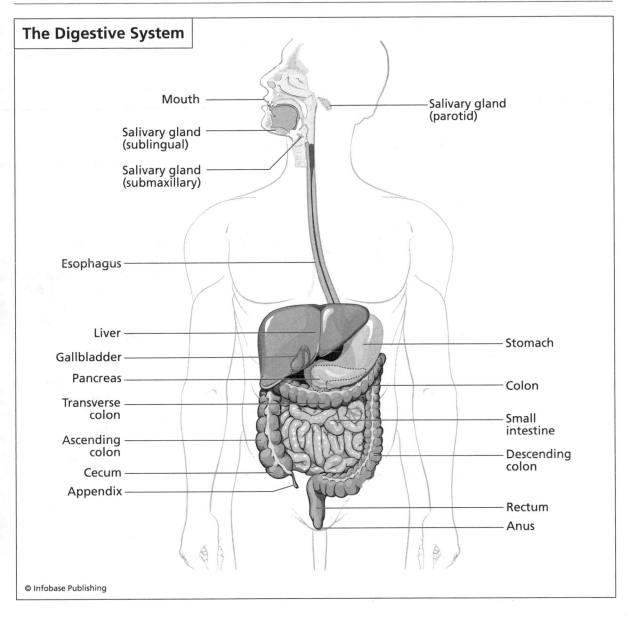

Mouth

Salivary gland (sublingual)

Salivary gland (submaxillary)

Salivary gland (parotid)

Esophagus

Liver

Gallbladder

Pancreas

Transverse colon

Ascending colon

Cecum

Appendix

Stomach

Colon

Small intestine

Descending colon

Rectum

Anus

© Infobase Publishing

lems. For example, the body may store too much iron (HEMOCHROMATOSIS), causing damage to the liver, the pancreas, and the heart, or it may store too much copper (WILSON'S DISEASE), causing an overload of metal that can become dangerous or toxic to the liver and the brain. Occasionally, the first manifestation of Wilson's disease may be a life-threatening, fulminant hepatic (liver) failure, which necessitates LIVER TRANSPLANTATION. The gallbladder may develop GALLSTONES that have potential for complications such as CHOLECYSTITIS and PANCREATITIS. However, most gallstones remain asymptomatic, and their mere presence does not usually indicate the need for a cholecystectomy. The liver or pancreas may become inflamed due to various causes.

When the Digestive System Goes Awry

Problems with digestion can arise from internal or external factors. In most cases, the body successfully rids itself of excessive or disagreeable food or illness, and the symptoms of disease disappear, too.

At other times, an individual's digestive system malfunctions in a far more serious way, leading to cancerous growths, inflammatory diseases, or other severe and possibly life-threatening chronic medical problems, such as digestive ULCERS, DIABETES MELLITUS, CIRRHOSIS (the dangerous scarring of the liver), or other serious digestive diseases and disorders. According to the National Center for Health Statistics in 2007, 8 percent of all adults ages 18 years and older had ever received a diagnosis of diabetes, while 6 percent had ever been diagnosed with an ulcer. In addition, 1 percent had been told in the past 12 months that they had liver disease.

Emergency Situations   When pain from a digestive disorder becomes extreme, most individuals call their physician or they head for the nearest hospital emergency room. APPENDICITIS is an example of a painful inflammation of the appendix that leads an individual to actively seek help, and cholecystitis (gallbladder inflammation) is another such EMERGENCY DIGESTIVE PROBLEM. If the intestines are acutely obstructed or they become perforated, the individual will likely experience severe pain and will urgently need medical assistance.

Untreated ulcer disease can accelerate further, causing blood loss, ANEMIA, and other medical complications, including perforation of the stomach or the small intestine, potentially resulting in a life-threatening illness. Untreated bacterial, viral, or PARASITIC INFECTIONS can spiral out of control and become life-threatening.

Lifestyle Choices Causing or Contributing to Digestive Problems

In some cases, the individual's own lifestyle contributes to (or sometimes causes) digestive problems. For example, OBESITY is the major cause of type 2 diabetes in the United States, and excess weight can also increase risk for the development of some cancers, such as ESOPHAGEAL CANCER. Two-thirds of all adults in the United States are either overweight or obese, making this problem and the accompanying health risks common. ALCOHOL ABUSE also leads to an array of digestive problems, including VITAMIN DEFICIENCIES, liver disease, and cirrhosis of the liver. SMOKING worsens many digestive problems as well as shortens the life of the smoker.

A lack of EXERCISE is another lifestyle issue that contributes to digestive problems such as obesity, gastroesophageal reflux disease, and CONSTIPATION. According to the National Center for Health Statistics, 39 percent of all U.S. adults said that they were inactive in 2007, while about 30 percent had some leisure-time physical activity, and only about 31 percent reported that they exercised on a regular basis. In general, men are more likely to exercise than women, as are individuals ages 18 to 44 years old and those with a bachelor's degree or higher. Inactivity is also directly linked to family income, and about half (50.4 percent) of those with family incomes less than $35,000 are inactive, compared to only 22.3 percent of those with a family income of $100,000 or greater. Married people are more likely to exercise than unmarried or widowed people. (See Table 1 for further details.)

Both HEREDITY AND ENVIRONMENT are important issues for those with digestive disorders, and many digestive disorders have a hereditary component, such as with diabetes and hypertension. In addition, many forms of cancer have a familial component, such as colorectal cancer and esophageal cancer. Many other diseases also have a familial genetic basis, and if a parent or sibling is diagnosed with a digestive disorder, such as precancerous POLYPS in the colon or cancer, the health risk for the development of the illness is increased for other family members.

Genetic risks are found with many digestive diseases, including celiac disease, Crohn's disease, hemochromatosis, CELIAC SPRUE, diabetes, most forms of cancer, and many other digestive diseases

TABLE 1: PERCENT OF INDIVIDUALS AND LEISURE-TIME PHYSICAL ACTIVITY AMONG ADULTS AGES 18 AND OLDER, BY SELECTED CHARACTERISTICS, UNITED STATES, 2007

Selected characteristic	Total	Inactive	Some leisure-time activity	Regular leisure-time activity
Total	100.0	39.1	30.1	30.8
Gender				
Male	100.0	37.0	30.1	32.9
Female	100.0	41.0	30.1	29.0
Age				
18–44 years	100.0	34.4	31.3	34.3
45–64 years	100.0	38.0	31.1	30.0
65–74 years	100.0	48.1	27.2	24.7
75 years and older	100.0	60.9	21.2	17.9
Race and ethnicity				
One race	100.0	39.2	30.0	30.8
White	100.0	37.4	30.4	32.1
Black or African American	100.0	51.0	26.0	23.0
American Indian or Alaska Native	100.0	39.8	37.6	22.6
Asian	100.0	38.9	31.0	30.1
Native Hawaiian or Other Pacific Islander	100.0	34.2	29.3	36.5
Two or more races	100.0	37.5	32.1	30.4
Black or African American and white	100.0	42.0	28.1	29.9
American Indian or Alaska Native and white	100.0	36.5	31.2	32.3
Hispanic or Latino origin and race				
Hispanic or Latino	100.0	51.3	25.0	23.7
Mexican or Mexican American	100.0	51.9	25.4	22.7
Not Hispanic or Latino	100.0	37.1	30.8	32.0
White, single race	100.0	34.7	31.4	33.9
Black or African American, single race	100.0	50.8	26.2	23.0
Education				
Less than a high school diploma	100.0	63.8	21.3	14.9
High school diploma or GED	100.0	49.1	29.2	21.7
Some college	100.0	35.0	32.9	32.0
Bachelor's degree or higher	100.0	23.1	33.6	43.3
Family income				
Less than $35,000	100.0	50.4	26.3	23.3
$35,000 or more	100.0	32.2	32.9	34.9
$35,000–$49,999	100.0	43.2	28.7	28.1
$50,000–$74,999	100.0	34.7	33.6	31.8
$75,000–$99,999	100.0	30.2	35.8	34.0
$100,000 or more	100.0	22.3	33.4	44.3

(Table continues)

(Table continued)

Selected characteristic	Total	Inactive	Some leisure-time activity	Regular leisure-time activity
Marital status				
Married	100.0	37.8	31.5	30.8
Widowed	100.0	64.1	18.6	17.4
Divorced or separated	100.0	44.9	26.9	28.3
Never married	100.0	39.0	27.9	33.1
Living with a partner	100.0	40.6	29.8	29.6
Region				
Northeast	100.0	37.5	31.4	31.1
Midwest	100.0	34.2	33.5	32.3
South	100.0	45.9	26.7	27.4
West	100.0	34.3	30.9	34.8
Gender and ethnicity				
Hispanic or Latino, male	100.0	47.5	26.5	26.0
Hispanic or Latina, female	100.0	54.8	23.4	21.8
Not Hispanic or Latino:				
White, single race, male	100.0	33.3	30.9	35.8
White, single race, female	100.0	35.8	32.0	32.2
Black or African American, single race, male	100.0	45.7	26.2	28.0
Black or African American, single race, female	100.0	54.7	26.2	19.1

Adapted from Pleis, J. R. and J. W. Lucas. *Summary Health Statistics for U.S. Adults: National Health Interview Survey, 2007.* Washington, D.C.: National Center for Health Statistics, 2009, 80–81.

and disorders. Of course, the diagnosis of an illness in a relative does *not* mean that everyone in the family is inevitably doomed to the development of the disease as well. It does mean, however, that often the risk is increased among family members for the development of the disease, and, thus, it is important for patients to report such a family history to physicians so they can attempt to monitor possible symptoms that may arise. For example, if a parent develops PANCREATIC CANCER, physicians should look for signs and symptoms of this form of cancer in the person's children.

Infectious Diseases

The gastrointestinal tract is colonized with thousands of microorganisms from birth, and many of these microbes are yet to be identified by researchers. In most cases, these microbes either facilitate digestion or they are neutral, rather than causing any harm. However, sometimes bacteria, viruses, and other microbes impair or harm the digestive system. They may cause temporary or persistent diarrhea.

Diarrhea caused by an infection is often only a temporary inconvenience, but in some cases, subsets of such microbes as ESCHERICHIA COLI *(E. coli)*, or enteroaggregative *E. coli* (EAEC), have been linked to persistent childhood diarrhea, traveler's diarrhea, and even to emergency room visits due to the severe persistent nature of the disorder.

Infections may directly or indirectly cause such digestive diseases as IRRITABLE BOWEL SYNDROME, according to the National Commission on Digestive Diseases. Some common bacteria, such as HELICOBACTER PYLORI, have been directly linked to the development of peptic ulcers and gastritis, and patients with such disorders need ANTIBIOTICS as well as medications to calm and soothe the agitated stomach lining.

Digestive problems can also be caused by influences from outside the body. Often, illness is caused by the ingesting of bacteria or other microbes that are transmitted in some contaminated food prepared by individuals who failed to wash their hands *after* using the toilet and before preparing food. Sometimes, bacteria are passed on to others in contaminated water.

People who believe they have never had a digestive ailment that was caused by CONTAMINATED FOOD OR WATER may be right; however, most infected people experience relatively mild symptoms such as diarrhea, nausea, and/or a mild fever, and they or their physicians assume the problem was caused by an unknown virus said to be "going around."

Only if the individual's stools were analyzed and checked by a laboratory, a process not routinely performed because of the vast numbers of possible microbes that could be present, could anyone determine whether or not a digestive illness was caused by food, or waterborne bacteria, parasites, or viruses. Even after exhaustive testing in an expert laboratory, some offending pathogens may not be identified.

Many different forms of digestive infections found in the United States include *AMEBIASIS*, *GIARDIA*, *CLOSTRIDIUM*, *CRYPTOSPORIDIUM*, *HELICOBACTER PYLORI* (HP), and *LISTERIOSIS*.

Infection with HP also increases the risk for other diseases, particularly peptic ulcer disease (PUD). According to the National Commission on Digestive Diseases in their 2009 report, 9 percent of women and 12 percent of men experience a lifetime prevalence of PUD. HP also increases the risk for the development of STOMACH CANCER if it continues untreated.

The risk for infection is also increased in individuals with weakened immune systems as well as among those who suffer from digestive diseases. An invasion of the wall of the appendix can be very dangerous and can lead to inflammation, perforation, and even gangrene.

In general, the specific microbes that are involved in appendicitis are often found among the species of *E. coli*, *Peptostreptococcus*, *B. Fragilis*, and *Pseudomonas*, according to research reported in *Opportunities and Challenges in Digestive Diseases Research: Recommendations of the National Commission on Digestive Diseases* in 2009. However, if an emergency appendectomy is performed as needed, and the person is treated with adequate antibiotics, in most cases, affected people will make a complete recovery. (See EMERGENCY ISSUES IN DIGESTIVE DISEASES.)

Although much rarer in the United States than in other countries, infectious diseases such as CHOLERA and TUBERCULOSIS can be devastating. In the United States, the majority of individuals infected with tuberculosis were born in another country. Parasitic infections are also more common outside the United States, although they can be a problem in the United States as well.

Inflammation

Some digestive diseases and disorders either stem from or cause inflammation. In general, any disease that ends with the suffix "itis" refers to an inflammation of the organ, as with pancreatitis (inflammation of the pancreas), hepatitis (inflammation of the liver), or appendicitis (inflammation of the appendix). DIVERTICULITIS is an inflammation of the colon caused by a microperforation in the diverticulum. This microperforation usually seals itself, and the condition can usually be treated by antibiotics. However, a perforated diverticulum may present as an acute emergency and require drainage by a radiologist or surgeon.

Inflammation of an organ may have many different possible causes; for example, acute pancreatitis is often caused by the presence of gallstones that inflame the pancreas by blocking drainage into the duodenum. Alcoholism may also lead to the development of pancreatitis. In addition, pancreatitis may be caused by genetic mutations affecting the pancreas, such as in the cystic fibrosis transmembrane conductance regulator (CFTR) gene. (See CYSTIC FIBROSIS)

Medications Can Cause Digestive Diseases

Most medications are processed by either the liver or the kidneys. If a medication is taken by mouth, it has the potential of causing harm to the stomach, especially when used on a chronic or excessive basis.

Medications can cause many short- or long-term digestive problems, often as a side effect; for example, NONSTEROIDAL ANTI-INFLAMMATORY DRUGS (NSAIDs) that are taken to alleviate the severe and chronic pain of arthritis or other illnesses can be harmful to the stomach when used on a chronic basis, and their excessive use has led to the development of peptic ulcers in thousands of patients. In fact, NSAIDs (including aspirin) can cause ulcers to develop in the small intestine as well as in the large intestine (colon).

The use of acetaminophen (Tylenol) in high doses can harm the liver, especially among individuals with alcoholism. Many other medications that are prescribed for a broad array of illnesses, including simple antibiotics that are prescribed for respiratory infection, may cause the side effects of nausea, vomiting, diarrhea, constipation, heartburn, and other distressing side effects.

Sometimes narcotics that are prescribed to treat chronic and severe pain can lead to digestive problems, such as severe constipation, NARCOTIC BOWEL SYNDROME, and even FECAL IMPACTION. Whenever possible, patients need to work with their doctors to taper off the narcotic gradually, as well as to take LAXATIVES as needed and to consume plenty of fluids to keep their bowels working well.

Antibiotics that are given to treat common infections may alter the balance of the normal flora of the gastrointestinal system, leading to infections with CANDIDA (yeast) and to problems such as diarrhea and colitis.

Cancers of the Digestive System

Digestive system cancers are common problems in the United States and other parts of the world. An estimated 270,000 Americans developed a form of a digestive cancer in 2008 according to the National Commission on Digestive Diseases, and about half of them will die from these cancers. (See Table 2.)

The most commonly occurring digestive cancer in the United States is colorectal cancer, and the lifetime risk for colorectal cancer in the United States is 5 to 6 percent. However, colorectal cancer can be screened for and detected in many cases with the use of the colonoscopy. Some cases of colorectal cancer are also found with the SIGMOID-OSCOPY, a test that visualizes only the lower part of the colon. Other forms of cancer are more difficult to screen for in the early stages, such as pancreatic cancer or esophageal cancer.

Some Groups Are Prone to Digestive Diseases

Some groups are at significant risk for developing digestive diseases; for example, the ELDERLY are at risk for many digestive disorders, including

TABLE 2: INCIDENCE AND DEATHS FROM GASTROINTESTINAL CANCERS IN THE U.S. (2008 ESTIMATED)					
Cancer Site	Overall incidence	Male incidence	Female Incidence	Deaths	Annual Number of Deaths Divided by Incidence (Percentage)
Pancreas	37,680	18,770	18,910	34,290	91%
Esophagus	16,470	12,970	3,500	14,280	87%
Liver and intrahepatic duct	21,370	15,190	6,180	18,410	86%
Stomach	21,500	13,190	8,310	10,880	51%
Other digestive organs	4,760	1,470	3,290	2,180	46%
Gallbladder and biliary ducts	9,520	4,500	5,020	2,340	35%
Colon and rectum	148,810	77,250	71,560	49,960	34%
Small intestine	6,110	3,200	2,910	1,110	18%
Anus and anorectum	5,070	2,020	3,050	680	13%
Totals	**271,290**	**148,560**	**122,730**	**135,130**	**50%**

Source: Adapted from: U.S. Department of Health and Human Services. *Opportunities and Challenges in Digestive Diseases Research: Recommendations of the National Commission on Digestive Diseases.* Bethesda, Md.: National Institutes of Health. March, 2009, 82.

chronic problems such as constipation as well as serious COMPLICATIONS OF DIGESTIVE DISORDERS, such as the complications related to diverticulosis, e.g. diverticulitis and diverticular bleeding. In addition, the elderly are more likely to take medications that may cause side effects or even harm to the digestive system. The elderly often have a more impaired immune system than do younger people and thus, are more likely to become very ill from infections derived from contaminated food or water. In contrast, younger people are more likely to develop such problems as appendicitis.

A Combination of Causes May Exist

The body can be affected by *both* internal and external influences, and these forces are constantly working on individuals, such as children who contract an illness at the day-care center or school and then cough the germs on all their family members at home. In another example, the excessive and chronic consumption of alcohol can lead to diseases of the liver and the pancreas. The ailing, scarred, and weakened liver or pancreas may then cause increased risk for the development of cancerous tumors or other internal problems.

Often it is a combination of causes that may result in digestive diseases; for example, when people consume a diet that is heavy in caffeine, fatty foods, and alcohol, if they also have a genetic propensity for the development of diseases such as gastroesophageal reflux disease (GERD) as well as other digestive disorders, then this combination of environment and heredity substantially increases the risk for developing these diseases.

It is also true that some medical problems are associated with a risk of development of a digestive disease; for example, infection with HEPATITIS C, if it leads to liver cirrhosis, can increase the risk of the development of liver cancer. Patients with diabetes mellitus are often at risk for development of GASTROPARESIS (slow stomach emptying). Individuals with the HUMAN IMMUNODEFICIENCY VIRUS (HIV) have an increased risk for developing many infections, as do many patients with active tuberculosis.

Nontreatment of an existing disease such as GERD can result in a precancerous condition such as BARRETT'S ESOPHAGUS, which eventually may lead to esophageal cancer, a difficult form of cancer.

Severe Symptoms Do Not Always Indicate the Presence of Severe Diseases

Although pain is often an indicator of a problem, the presence of extreme pain is not always an indicator of a severe digestive problem, just as the *absence* of pain does not mean that a disorder is a minor one. Some relatively minor and correctable digestive diseases, such as the early stages of chronic ACID REFLUX (gastroesophageal reflux disease), may cause far more discomfort than is seen in some cases of cancerous tumors of the digestive system. For this reason, individuals should discuss recurrent digestive problems with their physicians, and individuals should also have regular physical examinations and investigations as needed (for example, screening for colon cancer) to help detect any underlying medical problems.

Differences among People Who Have Digestive Diseases and Disorders

Incidences of digestive disorders vary by age, gender, and many other factors. (See DEMOGRAPHIC FACTORS AND DIGESTIVE DISEASES.) The prevalence of diseases themselves have changed over time; for example, in developed countries, the prevalence of peptic ulcer disease has changed over the second half of the 20th century from being a disease predominant in males to one with a nearly comparable prevalence in both sexes.

Often, middle-aged and older people are more likely to have digestive diseases; however, in some cases, younger people are more likely to be diagnosed with specific diseases. For example, most people who are diagnosed with Crohn's disease, a severe inflammatory disease of the gastrointestinal tract (especially the small intestine and/or colon), are between ages of 10 and 30 years. Older people are more likely to suffer from most cancers than are younger or middle-aged people.

Racial and ethnic differences are found among people suffering from digestive diseases; for example, blacks are more than three times more likely than whites to have SARCOIDOSIS, a systemic disease that can harm the digestive system, just as they are much more likely to be diagnosed with hepatocellular carcinoma, a severe form of liver cancer. In addition, blacks are more likely to suffer from the adverse consequences of hepatitis C, whereas whites are more likely to suffer from Barrett's esophagus and its related esophageal cancer (adenocarcinoma).

Combined risk factors may increase the odds of development of a digestive disease or disorder; for example, in considering both gender and age, women between the ages of 20 and 60 years have from double to triple the risk of the development of gallstones than men of the same age. In considering race and gender, Native American women are more likely than others to have gallstones, while black women have a higher risk than others for the development of type 2 diabetes.

Alternative Medicine and Digestive Diseases

Sometimes doctors are unable to determine an effective treatment for a disorder, particularly a chronic medical problem such as BACK PAIN or arthritis, and as a result, many people turn to ALTERNATIVE MEDICINE for help. According to the National Center for Complementary and Alternative Medicine (NCCAM), consumers spend billions of dollars on supplements, herbal remedies, and homeopathic treatment, as well as receiving treatment in the form of acupuncture, massage therapy, hypnosis, and other forms of alternative treatments. In most cases, insurance companies do not pay for these remedies or treatments, so they are generally used by well-educated individuals of comfortable means. However, some carriers do provide coverage for chiropractic, acupuncture, and so forth, depending on the company and the patient's primary medical complaint.

Ignorance Is Not Bliss: It May be Harmful or Even Deadly

Many people are ignorant of the basics of digestive diseases; for example, most people have no idea that at least 50 to 90 percent of all peptic (stomach and duodenal) ulcers are caused by bacteria known as *Helicobacter pylori*. Most of the rest of ulcers are caused by nonsteroidal anti-inflammatory drugs (NSAIDs). A few of the non-*H. pylori*, non-NSAID ulcers may be caused by other mechanisms such as viral infection, drugs other than NSAIDs (e.g. bisphosphonates, tumors like gastrinoma or even another *Helicobacter* bacteria, *Helicobacter heilmanii*).

Most people continue to believe mistakenly that if they alleviate stress in their life as much as possible and eat a healthful diet, then they will stay healthy and avoid such disorders as ulcers. The reality is that only antibiotics can cure an ulcer that was caused by bacteria and prevent it from recurring. Acid blocking medications can temporarily heal an ulcer, but an ulcer due to *H. pylori* infection is likely to return unless the patient takes an appropriate "cocktail" of medications, including antibiotics, to eradicate the bacteria and calm the stomach. Similarly, patients at risk for NSAID-induced ulcers may generally reduce their risk for ulcers by using CYCLOOXYGENASE-2 (COX-2) INHIBITORS instead of NSAIDs. Several COX-2 inhibitors have recently been withdrawn because of serious toxicities, resulting in multiple class-action law suits.

Another option would be to institute NSAID prophylaxis with another medication (such as a medication in the PROTON PUMP INHIBITOR class) to combat the ulcerogenic effect of the NSAID.

Knowledge of digestive diseases can help patients and their physicians counteract the impact of the disease or disorder. Information and education cannot eradicate all digestive diseases, but they can help people to obtain diagnoses in the early stages of diseases, when they are usually easier to treat, and to avoid behavior that harms the digestive system, such as smoking, overeating, failing to exercise, and drinking to excess.

Looking Back in Time and Viewing Past Remedies

People have suffered from many different types of digestive diseases throughout recorded time, as well as before written records were ever kept. Hunters and gatherers faced death from bacterial diseases such as tuberculosis and cholera and some parasitic diseases (some of which still exist today) such as hookworm and TRICHINOSIS.

The Pilgrims favored regular enemas as a key to a healthy digestive system. In the 18th and 19th centuries, antimony, arsenic, and mercury were remedies for ulcerlike symptoms. Remedies to treat the common diseases of the time as well as the more exotic ailments of the digestive organs ranged from medications that were copiously laced with opium or alcohol to treatments such as bleeding or purging with emetics that caused vomiting.

In considering food products alone, conditions have come a long way from a past, when dairy products were not pure because Louis Pasteur had not yet developed PASTEURIZATION. Without the Food and Drug Administration (FDA) in the United States, there was no regulation or oversight of foods or drugs. Horrific abuses in the meat packing industry came to light in Upton Sinclair's popular novel *The Jungle* (1906); this book caused such an intense furor that Congress passed the Meat Inspection Act of 1906. In that same year, a law regulating foods and drugs was also passed.

In addition, many medications such as penicillin had not yet been discovered. Also, it was not until 1921 that the Canadian physicians Banting and Best discovered that insulin could be used to treat type 1 diabetes. Before their discovery, everyone who had that form of diabetes died at a young age, and it was usually a slow and agonizing death. (At that time, type 2 diabetes was unknown because very few people were obese or overweight.)

Sailors and others who made long voyages in the past often became extremely ill with scurvy, a vitamin C deficiency. Scurvy causes easy bruising, apathy, bleeding gums, swollen legs, and other symptoms. It can also cause death, and according to the researcher Jeremy Hugh Baron, a Dutch East Indies Fleet sailed in 1595 with 249 men but returned with only 88, presumably largely because of deaths from scurvy. Then in 1598, the ship left with lemon juice and also grew horseradish and scurvy grass and lost only 15 men. (According to Baron, scurvy grass is *Cochlearia officinalis*, and it contains as much ascorbic acid as orange juice.) Baron also writes that 50 of the 102 passengers of the *Mayflower* (the ship that landed at Plym-outh Rock in the New World) died, mostly from scurvy.

Some seamen in the 16th century had discovered on their own that the disease could be prevented or cured with oranges or lemons; however, the medical establishment of the time scoffed at such a theory, relying instead on bleeding, purging (causing patients to vomit), and drugs. Then in 1754, *Treatise of the Scurvy* was published by James Lind, and based on his recommendations the British Navy provided fresh lemons and oranges to sailors. According to Baron, scurvy returned when lime juice (an ineffective antiscorbutic substance) was substituted in about 1860, especially among those who went on polar expeditions.

Today, the diet of most sailors is replete with vitamin C and other needed vitamins and minerals, and scurvy is a problem of the past; however, for many poor children in developing countries, it continues to cause harm.

Past Remedies for Digestive Complaints

Treatments for digestive ailments through the ages have ranged from the possibly efficacious to the ridiculous and dangerous. Doctors in past years often did not have a basic knowledge of microbiology, of the importance of sanitation, or even of the basic anatomy of the internal organs. In addition, many doctors in previous centuries received little or no training other than an apprenticeship to an existing physician.

Knowledge (and ignorance) about medicine was passed from generation to generation. However, some past remedies were actually useful, such as senna (an ingredient in some modern laxatives) for constipation, ipecac (to treat some poisoning cases), and opium (narcotics that are used in many painkilling drugs and anesthetics), are still used today.

In early America, Dover's powder, invented by Thomas Dover in 1740, was a popular medication for digestive disorders such as DYSPEPSIA or DYSENTERY. This concoction was composed of 10 percent ipecac, 10 percent opium, and 80 percent potassium sulfate. Such a concoction could not kill the bacteria, viruses, or other organisms that undoubtedly infected many people; however, some people eventually recovered probably because their immune system had destroyed the infection. However, they mistakenly attributed their improved health to the drug.

Some remedies for digestive ailments were quite bizarre; for example, the fifth-century physician Anthimus considered bacon a cure for intestinal parasites, and he also believed that partridge flesh that was cooked in goat's milk was a good remedy for dysentery (an infectious diarrhea).

Some ancient physicians did have a basic understanding of some diseases, but obviously they did not have access to the modern medications and treatments of the 21st century. For example, the great physician Hippocrates believed that patients who were suffering from tuberculosis (once called "consumption" or the "white plague" because of the customary pallor it caused) should leave the city for the country, rest, and eat nutritious foods. (Rest was the only valid remedy, although it was no cure.) The famed Greek physician Galen also recommended that patients with tuberculosis travel to warmer climates where they should rest. He also noted that people who slept in the same bed and who shared clothes with an infected person often contracted tuberculosis.

From ancient times until the early 20th century, digestive diseases were treated with narcotics and/or alcoholic drinks. In medieval Russia, scurvy was treated with gold in the form of gold leaf on bread. It was not until the 18th century that many doctors and the general public finally realized that lemon juice was actually the appropriate treatment for scurvy.

Some past remedies for illness were truly bizarre. For example, according to Christine El Mahdy in her book *Mummies, Myth and Magic in Ancient Egypt*, from the 14th to the 16th centuries, wealthy Europeans believed that Egyptian mummies had amazing health properties, and they were convinced that drinking a concoction composed of ground-up mummy dust would help to resolve many disparate medical problems. They were wrong, and this remedy invariably failed. In fact, the mummy dust treatment reportedly (and not surprisingly) made the consumers who actually tried this concoction feel much worse.

According to the French physician Ambroise Pare, in decrying the mummy dust remedy as a treatment, "It causes great pain in their stomachs, gives them evil smelling breath and brings about serious vomiting." But for a while, this remedy was so popular that Egyptian mummy dust sellers ran out of old mummies, and the demand for the mummy dust created what amounted to almost a production line of new mummies to satisfy the intense demand for the alleged mummy dust cure.

A popular remedy in England for a wide variety of diseases was the belief that the laying on of hands by particular people such as members of royalty was curative. To be touched by a king was considered particularly healthful by many people. According to Benjamin Lee Gordon in his book *Medieval and Renaissance Medicine*, so many people surged forward in their eagerness to receive the "king's touch" from Charles II that seven people were actually trampled to death in the rush. King Charles's touch apparently had very little therapeutic properties, and many people who touched him nevertheless died from scrofula, then a prevalent form of tuberculosis. According to Gordon, "It is of interest to note that more people died of scrofula during the time of Charles II than at any other period in English history."

For centuries, medical knowledge of the digestive system was either lacking or mostly wrong. For example, physicians believed that tickling a patient's abdomen with leeches would somehow take out the "bad blood." Bloodletting was also used to treat indigestion, constipation, and many other ailments. An excessive loss of blood likely caused illness and even death.

However, not all past medical recommendations were nonsensical. The 18th-century inventor, author, and political leader Benjamin Franklin, although he was not a physician, had some recommendations that doctors today would consider valid. According to Kirsner in *The Early Days of American Gastroenterology*, "Franklin's rules of health included a vegetarian diet, exercise, and the avoidance of tobacco."

Many digestive remedies that were available in the late 19th and early 20th centuries were liberally laced with alcohol, opium, or cocaine. These drugs were sold directly to consumers, who often had no idea of the ingredients in their "medicine," since there were no labeling laws at the time and there was no Food and Drug Administration (FDA) in the United States. These so-called medications were often referred to as "patent medicines," although they were not patented and no one except the manufacturer and possibly the sales staff really knew what was in them.

Even temperance-minded individuals sometimes unknowingly imbibed concoctions heavily laced with alcohol. Such remedies were also given to teething babies and individuals of all ages, regardless of the source of their pain.

In the past, even the fashions of the day actually caused digestive ailments. For example, very tight corsets, usually worn by women, that constricted the stomach and abdomen could make the smooth functioning of the digestive system difficult. However, people who sneer at such fashions of the past should consider their own modern fashions; for example, in the 21st-century tight-fitting jeans could have the same effect on the abdomen as did the Victorian corset.

Medical Breakthroughs of the Nineteenth and Twentieth Centuries

A variety of medical discoveries made in the 19th and 20th centuries, and now accepted as commonplace, have become invaluable to physicians and to patients with digestive diseases as well as other disorders. Manuel Garcia invented the laryngoscope (the precursor to the gastrointestinal endoscope) in 1855, and X-rays were discovered by W. K. Roentgen in 1895. Joseph Lister first wrote about the effect of bacteria on wounds in 1867; unfortunately, it was years before his work demonstrating the necessity for sterile conditions was actually heeded by surgeons and other physicians. In fact, some experts believe that sterile conditions existing today in hospitals could be improved even further with basic sanitary measures, such as more frequent hand washings by staff members and physicians.

It was also in the 19th century that Robert Koch discovered both the tuberculosis and the anthrax bacteria (1882), and it was when August Gartner in Germany first isolated SALMONELLA bacteria in a case of food poisoning. In 1928, Sir Alexander Fleming discovered penicillin; however, its practical use was delayed considerably because it was not used as a drug to treat humans with bacterial infections until the drug was first tried on soldiers in 1940. In 1944, Selman Waksman at Rutgers University discovered streptomycin, and physicians began using the drug as an effective antibiotic. After this point, doctors began using antibiotics to treat infections on a large scale, both in the United States and in other countries.

Surgery was an agonizing procedure in past centuries, and it was rarely performed because it was so often fatal. The only available anesthetic drug for surgical patients was opium before Sir Humphry Davy discovered nitrous oxide in 1798 and J. C. Warren and then W. Morton developed ether in 1846. Since then, many anesthetics that allow virtually pain-free surgery have been developed by researchers.

Breakthroughs in medical procedures occurred as well in the 19th and 20th centuries; for example, the first cholecystectomy (removal of the gallbladder) in the United States was performed in 1867. However, at that time (and in many cases, for years afterward), many people with digestive disorders requiring surgery did not have the surgery, and they either recovered from their illness or they died. Instead of cholecystectomy with a large abdominal incision, today it is mostly performed by laparoscopy requiring tiny abdominal incisions and with a rapid healing time.

Medical devices and therapeutic techniques improved considerably throughout the 20th century; for example, the semiflexible gastroscope, a device invented by Rudolf Schindler in 1932, preceded the flexible endoscope that was later developed by Basil Hirschowitz in 1957. Endoscopic ultrasonography, an ULTRASOUND method of imaging the internal organs through an endoscope placed into the gut lumen, was first developed in the 1980s.

The time is not too far off when surgeries like the removal of the appendix and the gallbladder shall be done through an endoscope, such that no abdominal incision is required. The first such appendectomy was performed by Dr. Reddy in India. Since then, some centers have removed the gallbladder, done tubal ligation, and performed other procedures using the same technique. As of this writing, these techniques remain experimental.

The development of ultrasound technology further advanced the ability of physicians to diagnose many different digestive diseases and disorders; for example, studies have shown that the use of ultrasound imaging of the gallbladder can provide physicians with an accurate diagnosis of gallstones in the majority of cases.

Better diagnostic tests were created for diagnosing disease, such as the Schilling test developed in 1953 to detect the presence of both PERNICIOUS ANEMIA and vitamin B_{12} malabsorption. Breath tests were created in the late 20th century to detect the presence of the *Helicobacter pylori* bacteria that cause the majority of peptic ulcers. Today, BREATH TESTS can also be used to detect LACTOSE INTOLERANCE as well as small bowel bacterial overgrowth

Physicians have discovered illnesses that had previously not been identified and diagnosed, such as IRRITABLE BOWEL SYNDROME. (Note that there were individuals with this disorder, but their illness was not diagnosed prior to the understanding of IBS.) Researchers and doctors have increasingly recognized and treated this common gastroenterological problem.

The formation of the American Gastroenterological Association in 1897 and of subsequent professional organizations such as the American College of Gastroenterology and the American Society for Gastrointestinal Endoscopy have further advanced the state of knowledge of digestive diseases and disorders. However, gastroenterology as a medical specialty did not actually take off until the 1950s and the 1960s, according to the medical historian Joseph B. Kirsner.

Other medical advances, including some truly amazing developments, occurred in the 20th century, such as the ability to perform liver transplantation. The first liver transplantations, performed in 1967 as heroic lifesaving measures, kept patients alive briefly; for example, a one-and-a-half-year-old child lived for 400 days after a liver transplantation. Then in 1979, the antirejection drug cyclosporine came on the market, causing a paradigm shift in organ transplantations. Other more sophisticated antirejection drugs have been developed to help transplant patients.

According to the physician Thomas E. Starzl in *The Growth of Gastroenterologic Knowledge during the Twentieth Century,* "Of our first 12 liver recipients treated with cyclosporine and prednisone in the first 8 months of 1980, 11 lived for more than a year and 7 are still alive more than 12 years later." Since Starzl's success with liver transplantations, some medical facilities have been successful with partial liver donations from living liver donors, usually for family members and friends.

Nutritional deficiencies that were not identified in the past, such as pernicious anemia and various vitamin and mineral deficiencies, were recognized by researchers and physicians, and treatments became available.

The Era of Health and Safety Regulations: The Nineteenth Century to Today   In the United States and other developed countries, it is generally taken for granted that meat to be sold to the public will first be inspected for parasites and bacteria and that restaurants will be periodically and randomly investigated by the local health department. It is also taken for granted that drug companies must perform massive clinical studies of new medications before physicians are allowed to prescribe these new drugs. Few people think about the existing government-dictated processes that sanitize the water or that sterilize dairy products in order to minimize the risk of harboring harmful pathogens that could be passed on to consumers.

Health and sanitation requirements that are assumed to be the norm today were completely unknown in past centuries when thousands of people died of diseases caused by infections spread through contaminated food or water. It is still true that in developing countries the major cause of death among INFANTS is diarrhea, which is usually caused by poor sanitation and a lack of medical treatment, such as simple drugs that are taken for granted in developed countries.

In 1906, President Theodore Roosevelt signed the Food and Drugs Act into law, which banned the interstate commerce of misbranded and adulterated foods and drinks. On the same day in 1906, the Meat Inspection Act, created because of revelations of extremely unsanitary conditions that had led to diseases, was also passed. In 1938, the Federal Food, Drug and Cosmetic Act was passed, initiating the regulation of drugs. This law also required factory inspections and a variety of other procedures planned for the public safety.

According to the Food and Drug Administration (FDA), its origin occurred in 1862, when President Lincoln appointed the chemist Charles M. Wetherill to the newly created Department of Agriculture, and the Bureau of Chemistry was created within the Department of Agriculture. In 1883, Dr. Harvey W. Wiley, the "father of the Food and Drugs Act," expanded the bureau's work on food adulteration.

In 1927, the Bureau of Chemistry was subdivided into the Food, Drug, and Insecticide Administration of the Bureau of Chemistry and Soils. Then in 1930, the name was changed to the Food and Drug Administration.

In 1962, on the heels of thousands of birth defects caused by the drug thalidomide, which had been introduced as a sleep remedy and also for the treatment of NAUSEA AND VOMITING in PREGNANCY, the Kefauver-Harris Drug Amendments were passed. They required pharmaceutical companies to prove to the FDA that their products were safe before they were allowed to sell them. In 1973, the U.S. Supreme Court upheld the challenged 1962 law.

In response to deaths caused by adulterated Tylenol in the early 1980s, in 1983 Congress passed the Tamper-Resistant Packaging regulations, making it a crime to tamper with packaged consumer products. In 1990, Congress passed the Nutrition Labeling and Education Act, requiring all packaged foods to provide nutritional information and also standardizing such terms as *low-fat* and *light*.

Because of the intense consumer interest in vitamin and mineral supplements, in 1994 Congress passed the Dietary Supplement Health and Education Act, which classifies dietary supplements as foods rather than drugs and does not require manufacturers to prove that their products are safe or effective. Instead, the FDA can remove such products from the market only if it finds that they are unsafe.

In 2004, the Food Allergy Labeling and Consumer Protection Act was passed, which requires the labeling of any food that contains a protein derived from any one of the following foods that, as a group, account for the vast majority of food allergies: peanuts, soybeans, cow's milk, eggs, fish, crustacean shellfish, tree nuts, and wheat.

In 2009, President Barack Obama signed the Family Smoking Prevention and Tobacco Control Act, which grants the FDA the authority to regulate tobacco products. According to the FDA, some key provisions of the law are as follows:

- By October 2009, cigarettes were prohibited from having candy, fruit, and spice flavors as their characterizing flavors.

- By January 2010, tobacco manufacturers and importers would submit information to the FDA about ingredients and additives in tobacco products.

- By April 2010, the FDA would reissue the 1996 regulation aimed at reducing young people's access to tobacco products and curbing the appeal of tobacco to the young.

- By July 2010, tobacco manufacturers could no longer use the terms *light*, *low*, and *mild* on tobacco products without an FDA order in effect.

- By July 2010, warning labels for smokeless tobacco products would be revised and strengthened.

- By October 2012, warning labels for cigarettes will be revised and strengthened.

In August 2009, the FDA launched its new Center for Tobacco Products to provide information to the public on tobacco. It is located in Silver Spring, Maryland, at 10903 New Hampshire Avenue.

Looking to the Future Many exciting advances lie ahead in the near future for patients with digestive diseases and disorders and the physicians who treat them. For example, with the use of the wireless capsule ENDOSCOPY, patients swallow a tiny camera that is about the size of a capsule. It then transmits imaging information to a cordless receiver worn by the patient. The data on the receiver set can then be downloaded to a computer so that the doctor can view the capsule in the gut lumen as it travels down through the patient's gastrointestinal system. If problems are detected, further diagnostic and therapeutic procedures and a standard endoscopy can then be performed on the patient.

As of this writing, several limitations to the wireless camera (also known as a pill or capsule camera) include its use primarily for visualization of areas that are hard to reach through an endoscopy, such as the small intestines.

Some experts are also using this pill camera for examination of the esophagus for screening for Barrett's esophagus and varices. The studies on examining the colon using this technique look promising, and this may one day become the procedure of choice for the screening of colon cancer.

The virtual colonoscopy or CT colography is also in use in many medical centers where radiologic imaging enables physicians to image the colon to determine whether polyps or other potential medical problems are present so that they can be treated. In addition, modern advances may allow patients to forgo bowel purging (medication that induces diarrhea to cleanse the bowel so it can be easily visualized) when they have a virtual colonoscopy. (This purging is still a requirement for the standard colonoscopy.) If problems are noted in the virtual colonoscopy, then patients will have a standard colonoscopy so that their physicians can remove any existing polyps, as well as take biopsy specimens or perform any other actions that are needed when disease is present.

The virtual colonoscopy has been investigated for its effectiveness in colorectal cancer screening, and it may be almost as good as real-time colonoscopy. Recent refinements of this technique have allowed it to be used as one of the recommended options for screening colonoscopy; however, therapeutics cannot be done, and if a lesion is found, the patient has to have a full colonoscopy. To date, however, the FDA has refused to accept the virtual colonoscopy as a substitute for the colonoscopy.

Major diagnostic tests that are available today using the endoscope and imaging and ultrasound technologies as well as combined technologies such as the endoscopic ultrasound can identify many diseases such as cancers, infections, and inflammatory conditions that were not detectable to physicians in past years.

Research actively continues on the genetic causes of diseases, and this information has the potential to be extremely helpful to doctors and patients. If doctors know that a patient has a family history of a disease that is largely or even partly hereditary, they can often test the patient for those diseases and therefore provide treatment early on in the course of the illness before any long-term ill effects will have occurred. Such testing is already commonly done for families with a medical history of familial adenomatous polyposis and hemochromatosis.

Researchers are also studying methods of treating serious illnesses such as inflammatory bowel disease, rheumatoid arthritis, cancer, and other diseases with the use of immunotherapy, to enable the body to better fight off disease. New medications for the treatment of inflammatory bowel disease have been introduced into the market.

Major colon cancer diagnostic breakthroughs are on the horizon; for example, early versions of stool tests to check for several genetic mutations in the tumor cells shed in stool are already available, and advanced stool testing for an expanded number of genetic mutations is under development as of this writing and should be available to the general public within several years. In addition, researchers are increasingly looking for a potentially increased role for chemoprophylaxis to treat Barrett's esophagus and also to prevent the recurrence of colon polyps.

Conclusion

Major and minor digestive diseases and disorders play a significant role in the lives of many people worldwide. Gone are the days when patients with digestive diseases were largely treated with opium, bloodletting, or enemas, and today many patients are fortunate to have their lives extended by major advances in diagnosis and treatment that often was built on the research that was performed in the past and which continues on into the present. The future looks even brighter.

At the same time, doctors cannot do everything for patients, and it is increasingly clear as time passes that, just as Benjamin Franklin believed in the 18th century, patients who desire good digestive health need to eat fruits and vegetables, lose weight if they are overweight, stop smoking, and to exercise and maintain (or to adopt) healthful lifestyle habits. These behaviors cannot offer a person immortality, which is an option that is available to no one. But they often can extend an individual's life for many years.

Ackerknecht, Erwin H., M.D. *A Short History of Medicine.* Rev. ed. Baltimore: Johns Hopkins University Press, 1982.

Ahmed, Nessar, et al. *Biology of Disease.* New York: Taylor & Francis Group, 2007.

Baron, Jeremy Hugh. "Sailors' Scurvy Before and After James Lind—A Reassessment." *Nutrition Reviews* 67, no. 6 (2009): 315–322.

Cherry, Donald K., et al. "National Ambulatory Medical Care Survey: 2006 Summary." National Health Statistics Reports 3 (August 6, 2008). Hyattsville, Md.: National Center for Health Statistics.

El Mahdy, Christine. *Mummies, Myth and Magic in Ancient Egypt.* New York: Thames & Hudson, 1989.

Everhart, James E., M.D. *The Burden of Digestive Diseases in the United States.* Washington, D.C.: National Institute of Diabetes and Digestive and Kidney Diseases, 2008.

Food and Drug Administration, "About FDA: Significant Dates in U.S. Food and Drug Law History." Available online. URL: http://www.fda.gov/AboutFDA/ WhatWeDo/History/Milestones/ucm128305.htm. Accessed August 28, 2009.

Food and Drug Administration. "Background." Available online. URL: http://www.fda.gov/AboutFDA/What WeDo/History/ResearchTools/Background/default. htm. Accessed August 28, 2009.

Gordon, Benjamin Lee, M.D. *Medieval and Renaissance Medicine.* New York: Philosophical Library, 1959.

Kirsner, Joseph B. *The Early Days of American Gastroenterology.* Cedar Knolls, N.J.: Lippincott-Raven Healthcare, 1996.

———. *The Growth of Gastroenterologic Knowledge during the Twentieth Century.* Philadelphia: Lea & Febiger, 1994.

Minocha, Anil, et al. "Detailed Characterization of Epidemiology of Uninvestigated Dyspepsia and Its Impact on Quality of Life among African Americans as Compared to Caucasians." *American Journal of Gastroenterology* 101, no. 2 (Feb 2006): 336–342.

Pleis, J. R. and J. W. Lucas. *Summary Health Statistics for U.S. Adults: National Health Interview Survey, 2007.* Hyattsville, Md.: National Center for Health Statistics, 2009.

Porter, Roy, ed. *Cambridge Illustrated History of Medicine.* Cambridge: Cambridge University Press, 1996.

Starzl, Thomas E. "The Contribution of Transplantation to Gastroenterologic Knowledge." In *The Growth of Gastroenterologic Knowledge during the Twentieth Century.* Philadelphia: Lea & Febiger, 1994.

U.S. Department of Health and Human Services. *Opportunities and Challenges in Digestive Diseases Research: Recommendations of the National Commission on Digestive Diseases.* Bethesda, Md.: National Institutes of Health, March 2009.

ENTRIES A TO Z

abdominal pain   Mild to severe discomfort that occurs in the midsection of the body. Abdominal pain may be caused by a variety of conditions, such as ULCERS, PANCREATITIS, CHOLECYSTITIS, biliary colic, CONSTIPATION, gastroenteritis, food-borne illnesses, infections, inflammation, menstrual cramps, gynecological conditions, or a reaction to a medication. The pain may be a temporary condition that lasts a few minutes to hours to a few days, or it may be chronic, lasting months to years. It may also be acute pain that is caused by APPENDICITIS or by other severe and acute life-threatening ailments that require medical or surgical treatment.

Sometimes abdominal pain is referred pain: the patient experiences pain at a site away from its actual source; for example, the pain of a gallbladder attack may be felt in the shoulder blade. Similarly the pain of a heart attack may be felt in the abdomen.

See also PAIN.

achalasia   An uncommon digestive disorder of the esophagus, in which the lower esophageal sphincter (the opening that allows food to move from the ESOPHAGUS into the stomach) does not relax to allow the food to pass from the esophagus to the stomach. In addition, peristalsis, which is the wavelike muscular movement that helps to propel the food downward, does not occur in the smooth muscles of the esophagus. Achalasia stems from the inflammatory degeneration of the nerve cells of the myenteric plexus in the esophagus. The cause of this disorder is unknown, but it is speculated to be an autoimmune disorder. Chronic viral infections as a cause have also been postulated.

Achalasia-like abnormalities in the esophagus may be mimicked by malignancies, CHAGAS'

DISEASE, AMYLOIDOSIS, SARCOIDOSIS, neurofibromatosis, EOSINOPHILIC GASTROENTERITIS, juvenile Sjögren's syndrome, and chronic idiopathic intestinal pseudo-obstruction. It should also be noted that patients with achalasia are at an increased risk for developing esophageal cancer over the long term. (See ESOPHAGEAL CANCER.)

Symptoms and Diagnostic Path

The major indicator of achalasia is DYSPHAGIA (trouble with swallowing). Most patients have difficulty swallowing both liquids and solids. In addition, the majority of patients have difficulty with BELCHING, although most patients must be specifically asked about this by their doctors, since it does not occur to them that having difficulty belching is a symptom of disease.

Other symptoms that may occur are as follows:

- CHEST PAIN
- HEARTBURN
- unintended weight loss, although profound weight loss is uncommon
- regurgitation of food from the esophagus, such as undigested food ingested several hours or a day earlier
- chronic hiccups

Many patients have achalasia almost five years or more before they are diagnosed. Often they are treated for GASTROESOPHAGEAL REFLUX DISEASE or other digestive disorders before achalasia is diagnosed.

Diagnostic tests for achalasia include the barium swallow test, which is nearly 95 percent accurate in diagnosing this condition. To confirm the presence of achalasia, doctors also usually order MANOMETRY to assess esophageal motility. This test measures pressures in the esophagus and the lower esophageal sphincter and also shows the relaxation pattern of the lower esophageal sphincter (LES). In addition, an ENDOSCOPY can be useful in diagnosis, especially to exclude any other diseases, such as cancer that mimics achalasia.

Treatment Options and Outlook

Achalasia cannot be cured, but it can be improved. Medications in the calcium channel blocker class and nitrates can help to relax the lower esophageal sphincter, although they may be effective over the short term only in some patients. They have significant side effects and are generally not recommended except in those patients who are either unwilling or unable to tolerate other more effective treatments. Patients take these drugs sublingually (under the tongue) 10 to 15 minutes before eating meals.

Other treatments for achalasia include botulinum toxin (Botox) injections given through an endoscope to relax the lower esophageal sphincter and also pneumatic balloon dilation. Botulinum injections have been highly effective in some patients; however, the effect usually lasts only a few months and is reserved for patients who have other severe illnesses that preclude surgery as an option. In addition, the long-term efficacy and safety of Botox remains uncertain; as such it is used in those who are either too sick or unwilling to undergo more invasive techniques.

Usually either a pneumatic dilation of the LES via an endoscopy or a surgical myotomy is performed to improve achalasia. The dilators used for achalasia are much bigger in size than those used for stretching the esophageal strictures. Surgical myotomy can be performed by laparoscopic technique. Since myotomy predisposes the patient to increased ACID REFLUX, some surgeons perform an antireflux procedure along with the myotomy.

Risk Factors and Preventive Measures

Achalasia occurs in about one in 100,000 people, and men and women are affected equally. Although it may occur at any age, the disorder usually occurs in adulthood, in individuals who are between 25 and 60 years old. Patients with achalasia are at an increased risk for developing esophageal cancer over the long term.

There are no known preventive measures for achalasia.

acid blocking agents Prescribed or over-the-counter medications that prevent acid formation in the stomach. Prescribed medications are generally but not always stronger and of longer duration than are over-the-counter medications. In fact many of the formerly prescription medications are now available as over-the-counter medications. Generic versions are also available. Intravenous formulations are available for use in sick, hospitalized patients, especially in those individuals who have high-risk bleeding ulcers. Both kinds of medications may be taken by people with chronic heartburn, which is also known as GASTROESOPHE-GEAL REFLUX DISEASE. These medications also heal peptic ulcers.

See also ACID REFLUX; HEARTBURN; HISTAMINE-2 BLOCKERS; PROTON PUMP INHIBITORS.

acid reflux A backward flow, in an upward direction, of stomach contents including acidified food (up from the stomach toward the mouth, rather than downward and toward the intestines). Acid reflux is also sometimes referred to as heartburn. Some degree of acid reflux is normal in relation to meals. When acid reflux becomes excessive, and it causes symptoms enough to affect quality of life or causes complications, it is then called GASTRO-ESOPHAGEAL REFLUX DISEASE (GERD).

Although heartburn is usually due to GERD, this symptom can occur in the absence of any reflux. In addition to heartburn, chronic acid reflux may cause chest pain, asthma, hoarseness, loss of dental enamel, and bad breath. Long-standing acid reflux can cause a precancerous condition of the esophagus that is known as BARRETT'S ESOPHAGUS.

Excessive acid reflux or GERD can be treated with medications, such as over-the-counter (OTC) medications and prescribed ACID BLOCKING AGENTS, including ranitidine (Zantac), cimetidine (Tagamet), famotidine (Pepcid), omeprazole (Prilosec), omeprazole plus sodium bicarbonate (Zegerid

OTC™), lansoprazole (Prevacid), pantoprazole (Protonix), rabeprazole (Aciphex), dexlansoprazole (Kapidex), and esomeprazole (Nexium).

GERD may also be treated with lifestyle recommendations, such as smoking cessation, avoiding alcohol, not eating for at least two to four hours before bedtime, patients avoiding eating heavy meals at night, and patients sleeping with the head of the bed tilted upward. Patients who have chronic acid reflux should be evaluated by physicians if they have heartburn more than once a week, before their condition worsens further. Long-term acid reflux can lead to complications, including cancer.

See also HISTAMINE-2 BLOCKERS; PROTON PUMP INHIBITORS; ULCERS, PEPTIC.

Minocha, Anil, M.D., and Christine Adamec. *How to Stop Heartburn: Simple Ways to Heal Heartburn and Acid Reflux.* New York: John Wiley & Sons, 2001.

activated charcoal   A remedy for a drug overdose. The charcoal is highly refined into very small particles to give it a very large surface area to which the poison or drug can attach, thus preventing the poison from becoming absorbed from the digestive tract and into the bloodstream. Use of activated charcoal has also been advocated for excessive GAS, although its efficacy is controversial.

Activated charcoal is the preferred method for ridding the gut of poisons and toxins and is superior to syrup of ipecac as well as gastric lavage for gastric decontamination. It is an insoluble, nonabsorbable, inert, fine carbon powder. It has numerous interconnecting pores that adsorb the poison (binding and trapping chemicals). Thus, the absorption and the subsequent toxicity of the poison can be prevented. Its efficacy depends upon its adsorptive capacity and depends upon numerous physico-chemical factors such as molecular size, dissolution of ingested drug, and the surface area of the activated charcoal used.

Usually, activated charcoal has a surface area of 950 to 2000 m2 per gram and can adsorb between a few mg and 1 g of intoxicant per gram of activated charcoal. Usually, 10 times the dose of charcoal is needed relative to the dose of poison ingested, and it should be administered as soon as possible after ingestion of poison. Maximal efficacy is assured if given within one hour of ingestion. However, charcoal cannot adsorb small, highly ionized chemicals such as metals, electrolytes, acids, and alkali. Examples include lithium, iron, and caustics like antifreeze.

Activated charcoal must not be administered to those with bowel obstruction or perforation.

Complications include NAUSEA AND VOMITING, abdominal cramps, and DIARRHEA, especially when the drug is used with sorbitol. CONSTIPATION may occur especially in high doses. Aspiration may cause pneumonia.

Minocha, Anil, D. A Herold, D. E. Bruns, and D. A. Spyker, "Effect of Activated Charcoal in 70% Sorbitol in Healthy Individuals." *Clinical Toxicology* 22, no. 6 (1985): 529–536.

Minocha, Anil, D. A. Herold, J. T. Barth, D. G. Roberson, and D. A. Spyker "Activated Charcoal and Ethanol Absorption: Lack of Effect in Humans." *Clinical Toxicology* 24, no.3 (1986): 225-234.

acute abdomen   A condition of sudden and severe ABDOMINAL PAIN. There are many different possible causes for acute abdomen, including an inflammation or rupture of the appendix, an obstruction such as a gallstone that is blocking the cystic duct and causing inflammation of the gallbladder (acute CHOLECYSTITIS), a stone in the ureter (ureteric colic), or an inflammation that is caused by either PANCREATITIS or DIVERTICULITIS. The medical problem may also be a systemic one, stemming from a Herpes zoster infection, a heart attack, or heavy metal poisoning. These are only a few of the many possibilities that physicians must consider when determining the cause of acute abdomen.

Symptoms and Diagnostic Path
The condition is sometimes accompanied by NAUSEA AND VOMITING, abdominal distention, failure of passage of the stools, or loose stools. Physicians take into account the location and severity of the pain as well as the patient's medical history and other symptoms and signs in order to make a diagnosis and determine the treatment that is needed.

Some patients do not present with typical signs and symptoms, especially the elderly and the immune compromised, such as those who have DIABETES MELLITUS and acquired immunodeficiency syndrome (AIDS).

In addition to taking a medical history from the patient (or from others if the patient is unable to provide sufficient details), the doctor performs a physical examination to ascertain where the pain is most severe and what its effects are on the adjacent structures and the rest of the body. Gentle pressure may reveal that an organ is enlarged or that a mass is present. A gentle tapping of the abdomen may reveal to the physician that there is a source of inflammation in the abdomen.

Physicians usually also order laboratory tests, such as a complete blood count. In cases of acute abdomen, whatever the cause, the white blood cell count is often higher than normal, especially when the cause is an infection or an inflammation. An elevation of the serum amylase level usually indicates the presence of PANCREATITIS, but an elevation may also occur with intestinal perforation.

An elevated level of serum bilirubin may indicate an overproduction of bilirubin due to a breakdown of red blood cells. This overproduction of bilirubin is seen with conditions such as a sickle cell crisis. A blockage of flow of bile through the bile duct system may also cause an elevated bilirubin, e.g. with gallstones causing pancreatitis. Acute or chronic liver disease may also cause increased bilirubin levels manifesting clinically as jaundice.

A plain X-ray of the abdomen is done to look for any intestinal obstruction or perforation. A computed tomography (CT) scan may reveal some evidence of the source of the pain, showing existing conditions such as pancreatitis, cholecystitis, and APPENDICITIS. A CT scan may also indicate further complications, such as an abscess or perforation.

For patients who have ASCITES (fluid-filled abdomen), physicians may perform a diagnostic PARACENTESIS, in which fluid is withdrawn for laboratory analysis.

Treatment Options and Outlook

The treatment for acute abdomen is directly linked to the diagnosis. Treatment may be medical, as in

most cases of pancreatitis. In some cases of acute abdomen, exploratory surgery may be indicated, such as in an emergency or when APPENDICITIS is suspected; in other cases, the patients may be observed to see whether the condition improves or worsens. If the condition does not improve over the course of 24 to 48 hours, the physician may decide that exploratory surgery cannot be avoided.

Risk Factors and Preventive Measures

There are no particular risk factors or preventive measures.   See also ABDOMINAL PAIN.

adaptations to daily living and lifestyle factors

Chronic digestive diseases and disorders can profoundly affect an individual's daily life. Making regular or periodic adaptations to the disorder as well as working on coping with the common emotional reactions on a regular daily basis, usually help people with such diseases considerably.

Taking these daily actions cannot *cure* the chronic disease, but instead they may often ease both the pain and distress of the individual's symptoms. For example, limiting or altogether avoiding some types of foods are important for individuals with some diseases and doing so can often decrease symptomatic pain. This is the case for the person with DIABETES MELLITUS (DM), who needs to restrict (although not to totally eliminate) the daily intake of carbohydrates. Diabetes also requires daily adaptations, such as testing the blood sugar level at least once per day, depending on the recommendation of the individual's physician. The individual must then take the appropriate action based on the findings of the blood test, should the results show problematic high or low levels of blood glucose.

In another example, the person with DIARRHEA-predominant IRRITABLE BOWEL SYNDROME (IBS) needs to remember to bring (or to purchase) prescribed or over-the-counter (OTC) antidiarrheal medications on every trip away from his or her home city (and sometimes on every outing). He or she may also need to plan ahead so that there will be an opportunity to visit a restroom in the event of an emergency need to stop. The individual with ULCERATIVE COLITIS and CROHN'S DISEASE may

DOS AND DON'TS: ADAPTATION ADVICE FOR PATIENTS WITH CHRONIC OR SERIOUS DIGESTIVE DISEASES

Do	Do Not Do or Think This
After receiving a diagnosis of a serious digestive disorder, write down questions for your doctor. Call and ask the nurse urgent questions and save other questions for your next visit.	Use your cell phone or your e-mail to contact all your friends or relatives about what they would do if they had your illness. Do whatever is the most popular choice among them all.
Ask your doctor if there are any alternative remedies which may give you some relief.	Ask the clerk at the local health food store what herbs or other remedies she would recommend that you use for your illness. Don't ask her what qualifies her to give you medical advice, just take it on faith that she knows what she is talking about.
If you think that you may be clinically depressed because of your condition (eating much more or less, losing interest in activities you normally like and crying a lot), ask your doctor if you may need an antidepressant. Consider consulting with a psychiatrist. Most psychiatrists treat normal people suffering from life's problems, which may cause anxiety or depression.	Assume that everybody who receives a serious diagnosis gets upset and just soldier on without asking for any help. Antidepressants are for sissies or babies and psychiatrists are for crazy people.
Ask your doctor for practical tips and suggestions that may help you deal better with the symptoms of your digestive disease. Also, check reliable sources such as the National Center for Complementary and Alternative Medicine (NCCAM).	Try to find the answer to your problem on the Internet on Web sites/boards where people write in to talk about their illnesses and discuss various remedies that they have tried. Assume they know what they are talking about and that they all are honest.
If weight loss would improve your condition, ask your doctor to help you make a plan to lose the weight. Lose the weight at a sensible rate of no more than a few pounds a week. Crash diets can be very dangerous and you don't want to become ill from a sudden weight loss. (Risking gallstones, electrolyte imbalances, and other health risks.)	Buy the latest weight loss drug that is advertised on cable television or the newest best-selling book written by a celebrity on how to lose weight really fast. Follow the plan even if it sounds like it might be dangerous or make you sicker than you already are. The speed of your weight loss is very important, and it should be as fast as possible.
If a medication causes minor side effects, continue taking it; however, if it causes serious problems that affect your ability to work or function, call the doctor. The side effects of many medications will wear off in a few days and the doctor may wish you to continue to try the medication. She may also wish you to end the medication. You won't know until you ask the doctor.	Try a medication that the doctor has recommended for you for a day or two, and if it does not seem to help, then just stop taking it. Do not tell the doctor that you stopped taking the medication because he might yell at you.
If you are a religious person, ask people in your faith group to pray for you. At the same time, continue to follow the advice of your physician, assuming that he or she is the expert in the medical field.	Assume that if God wanted you to get better, then He would make you better without you having to do anything about it. Avoid medical treatments recommended by your physician and rely on prayer alone.
Realize that digestive diseases are common and usually not your fault, and do what you can do to manage your symptoms.	Try to figure out what you have done in the past that has led to your being punished by suffering from this disease.
If your problem is obesity, don't concentrate on blaming yourself. Blame leads to guilt and shame as well as feelings of hopelessness, and that often increases overeating. Instead, work with your doctor to find a means get rid of the weight and become healthier.	Tell yourself that you're fat because of what you put in your mouth. Other people aren't fat.
	Alternatively, tell yourself that there's nothing you can do about your weight. Some people are just born to be fat and you are one of them.

become familiar with the location of all the bathrooms in the local supermarkets, pharmacies, convenience stores, and other locations because of past bathroom emergencies.

Individuals who are diagnosed with FOOD ALLERGIES or with food intolerances, such as CELIAC DISEASE (an intolerance to gluten, found in many breads and other substances) or with LACTOSE INTOLERANCE (an inability to digest dairy products, such as milk) often must make daily adjustments to avoid extreme discomfort if they fail to plan ahead their daily food intake. Individuals with cancer probably have to make the greatest adaptations of all, dealing with not only the shock and fear of a cancer diagnosis, but also with coping with the tests, procedures, and therapies that are recommended and which sometimes may be painful and distressing.

Cancer

When cancer is diagnosed, whether it is a condition that is identified in the early stages and one that is readily treatable or it is one that will require the individual to receive extensive treatment and different types of therapies for months or longer, then the individual must make emotional daily living adaptations to this personally cataclysmic new situation. Whether the patient has COLORECTAL CANCER, ORAL CANCER, STOMACH CANCER, or any one of the various forms of DIGESTIVE CANCERS (as well as one of the nondigestive forms of cancer), most people respond to the initial diagnosis with shock, fear, and panic, which may also be followed by anxiety and a state of depression.

Once the immediate distress of the diagnosis is over, individuals with cancer must then learn how to deal with many basic and yet often difficult questions related to adapting to their cancer. These include whether they will need to take time off from work and if so, how much time off will be needed, as well as how a person with cancer will manage to cope with the treatments and therapies that their physicians recommend. In addition, if the patient with cancer is currently responsible for others, such as a spouse with Alzheimer's disease or a minor child, then he or she must make a plan for who will care for that person if the cancer patient should become too weak or debilitated to provide the needed care. Even concern over a plan for pro-

viding necessary care for a beloved pet can become a matter of considerable distress to the individual who is diagnosed with cancer.

If the individual with cancer is elderly and/or disabled, then he or she may struggle with numerous practical matters, such as how to travel to treatment centers to obtain needed surgery, radiation treatments, chemotherapy, or other forms of treatment, at a time when he or she may feel very ill. Even if the individual is not elderly or disabled, such treatments can be debilitating for most people, who may need to learn to lean on others more than they normally would. It can be hard for an independent person to ask others for help. Sleep can become a major problem for patients with ileostomy, who may need to empty the ileostomy bag as many as eight to 12 times in 24 hours, including nights.

Many people who do not have cancer have no idea how to talk about cancer with a person who has been diagnosed with the disease. The individual with cancer may find that friends and family members either avoid the subject altogether or sometimes attempt to avoid the person completely, often afraid that they will say or do the wrong thing. Sadly, some people have an irrational fear that cancer is somehow contagious and thus, they do not want to "catch it" by associating with the ill person. These behaviors can compound the general anxiety and distress of the person with cancer.

Unfortunately, some individuals find that their friends and sometimes even their life partners, fiancés, or spouses may become unresponsive at this time of great emotional need. However, most people try to provide as much emotional and practical support as they can offer.

Chronic Constipation

Many people have issues with chronic constipation, especially ELDERLY people—although individuals of any age may develop a constipation problem. If common medical causes for constipation have been ruled out, such as hypothyroidism or a low-fiber diet, then some lifestyle changes and adaptations can often improve this situation. For example, exercising on a regular basis may help, and even as simple an activity as taking a daily walk can often improve regularity. Many people who are constipated also have an undiagnosed problem with mild dehydration, and this issue can be resolved by increasing their fluid intake, particularly of water. It is generally best for constipated individuals to avoid caffeinated beverages, which may tend to dehydrate and further constipate them.

The addition of two to three fruits per day to the daily diet can also give considerable help to many people with constipation. Adding at least two helpings of green vegetables per day should also help most people with chronic constipation. Some people also benefit from yogurt, which include probiotics, "friendly" microbes that can help with digestion and elimination. If an alternative remedy is sought, herbs such as goldenseal or minerals such as magnesium may help. Before using such herbs or minerals, it is always best to consult with a physician. (See ALTERNATIVE MEDICINE.)

Be aware that some constipated patients have a very slow gut. In such cases, fiber may actually cause more problems, and a low-residue diet and laxatives may be prescribed.

Diabetes Mellitus

Millions of people in the United States have diabetes mellitus, and most (about 95 percent) have type 2 diabetes. This is the form of diabetes that often develops in adulthood and which is frequently directly related to overweight or OBESITY. Older individuals also have an increased risk for the development of type 2 diabetes. In contrast, type 1 diabetes, formerly known as insulin-dependent diabetes, often presents in childhood, and the individual with untreated type 1 diabetes is usually slender. With type 1 diabetes, the pancreas makes very little or no insulin, and thus, the individual must receive insulin externally through injections or sometimes through an implanted insulin pump.

With type 2 diabetes, the pancreas may produce sufficient insulin, but the body is unable to use it all, which is known as *insulin resistance*. Type 2 diabetes is treated with a variety of oral medications. However, sometimes the individual with type 2 diabetes requires insulin, as when he or she becomes very ill and/or is hospitalized.

Individuals with diabetes often have high blood sugar levels, but sometimes they may develop unusually low sugar (hypoglycemia), and they will need to take some form of carbohydrate to raise their blood sugar levels.

Unfortunately, the daily adaptations needed by the person with diabetes are sometimes *not* taken, as when the patient is a child, adolescent, or an elderly person. This can occur despite a person knowing how to cope on a daily basis with their illness. Sometimes even a person who is normally very conscientious about taking medications and not eating excessive carbohydrates will throw caution to the wind. When this happens, the individual can become severely ill and, in the worst case, could develop a coma or even die.

If the noncompliance with the blood testing and the medication regimen recommended by the doctor continue, the person with diabetes may develop other severe health problems, such as hypertension, kidney failure, stroke, and so forth. In addition, many people with diabetes are at risk for blindness caused by diabetic retinopathy or leg and foot amputations caused by blood vessel damage.

Compliance involves advance planning. For example, the person who plans to be gone from home for the day and who needs to test her blood several times while away must remember to bring her blood test meter with her. It is also wise to bring some form of carbohydrate in the event that the blood sugar drops precipitously (as with hypoglycemia), as well as to bring medication should the blood sugar level rise excessively.

Children and adolescents with diabetes may have a particularly difficult time coping with their needed daily adaptations because many schools still make it difficult for children to bring their blood test equipment with them, and thus, they must go to the nurse's office to test their blood (or to have it tested by others). Children with type 1 diabetes may also feel embarrassed about giving themselves injections of insulin when needed, and they may suffer from the taunts of others who suggest that the child is injecting an illegal drug. In addition, the child who needs to consume carbohydrates because their blood sugar is low may find them unavailable in school, or they may be criticized or ridiculed if they suddenly eat a candy bar during a class. Yet to a large extent, parents, teachers, and the educational staff of the school can help improve such situations.

Adults with diabetes often also find it difficult to maintain their needed daily regimens. In addition, they may fear that if people see them injecting insulin at work or elsewhere, that others will mistakenly believe that they are illegal drug users. Adults with diabetes may also wish to avoid the curiosity and prying questions of others and try to keep information and awareness about their diabetes limited to only a select few. Yet, some people with diabetes are very open about their illness and what they need to do in order to maintain good glycemic levels as often as possible.

Gastroesophageal Reflux Disease (GERD)

Individuals with GASTROESOPHAGEAL REFLUX DISEASE (GERD), which is also often referred to as chronic heartburn, need to make basic and usually simple adjustments to their daily lives to deal more effectively with their pain and discomfort. For example, whenever possible, the person with GERD should avoid eating anything within two to four hours of going to bed. In addition, raising the head of the bed helps to decrease the discomfort of heartburn. Sometimes individuals with GERD use alternative medicine to obtain relief, such as herbs and homeopathic remedies to ease their daily symptoms.

Individuals suffering from chronic heartburn, as well as those who have frequent general bouts of indigestion and sour stomach (dyspepsia) that have not been diagnosed as GERD, should be sure to avoid consuming alcohol when they take medications, particularly such medications as nizatidine (Axid), metoclopramide (Reglan), cimetidine (Tagamet), or ranitidine (Zantac).

According to the National Institute on Alcohol Abuse and Alcoholism (NIAAA), alcohol directly interacts with these medications. Consequently, the combination of alcohol and one of these medications together can cause a rapid heartbeat as well as sudden changes in blood pressure (particularly with metoclopramide). There may also be an elevated alcoholic effect with these medications, leading to a more rapid intoxication. Likewise, the threshold for acetaminophen (Tylenol) toxicity is lowered in patients who consume alcohol. This is particularly true among elderly individuals with diabetes.

Some foods are specifically aggravating to individuals suffering from GERD, such as foods in the following categories: caffeinated drinks; foods that include onions, citrus fruits, and tomatoes. Orange juice may be particularly irritating to the person with GERD. Individuals with GERD should eliminate such foods from their diets for at least a month and observe if their condition improves.

Additional advice for the individual with GERD is to avoid taking some common and everyday actions, such as avoiding bending over after eating; for example, it is best to avoid eating and then going out and weeding the garden, which requires frequent bending motions. Individuals with GERD should not take a nap after eating a large dinner meal, such as a holiday meal at Thanksgiving, New Year's, or other holidays. (It is best to avoid overeating, but many people tend to eat more than usual during holidays.) Instead, the discomfort from excess eating can be eased by taking a leisurely walk.

It is very important for individuals with GERD to gain control over their condition because if the condition does not improve or if it worsens, then the individual is at risk for the development of BARRETT'S ESOPHAGUS, a precancerous condition that often leads to ESOPHAGEAL CANCER. According to research discussed by the National Institute of Diabetes & Digestive & Kidney Diseases (NIDDK) in their report issued in 2009, eating fruits and vegetables decreases the risk for Barrett's esophagus and is also likely to reduce the risk for the development of esophageal cancer. Fruits and vegetable contain antioxidants, which are natural cancer fighters.

Ulcerative Colitis

Some individuals have so much difficulty with their ULCERATIVE COLITIS and the bouts of sudden and very urgent needs to use the toilet that their doctors may advise them to take Imodium (an over-the-counter antidiarrheal medication). In the worst case, the individual with an attack has an "accident" in their underpants because he or she cannot make it to a toilet in sufficient time. This type of incident can be terribly embarrassing. Others who do not know better may think that the person is senile or mentally slow because of this toileting problem—or the person with ulcerative colitis may fear that others will have this attitude if they should find out about the "problem."

Some experts have suggested that various options that are available through alternative medicine can be very helpful; for example, some herbs and other combinations of medications have given relief to some patients with ulcerative colitis. Turmeric is effective in ulcerative colitis, and probiotics have been shown to be helpful in pouchitis. (See ALTERNATIVE MEDICINE.)

Chronic Peptic Ulcers

Most ulcers are caused by either *HELICOBACTER PYLORI* (*H. pylori*), a prolific type of bacterium, or by the excessive use of nonsteroidal anti-inflammatory drugs (NSAIDs.) Some people may develop ulcers as a result of both conditions: *H. pylori* is present in their gut, and they also frequently use NSAIDs to decrease their pain from other illnesses, such as arthritis, back pain, and so forth. In general, ending the use of NSAIDs and treating *H. pylori* with a regimen of appropriate antibiotics should resolve the problem; however, the cause of ulcers may not be apparent in some cases, and some people suffer from recurrent bouts with ulcers.

Esophagitis and/or Dysphagia

Esophagitis is the inflammation of the esophagus, which is also known as the food tube. Dysphagia, trouble swallowing, sometimes may stem from esophageal narrowing due to GERD or cancers as well as other conditions such as cancer in head and neck region. When one of these conditions becomes a severe and recurrent problem, then the individual requires treatment as soon as the condition is diagnosed. Patients with benign stricture may need to have the esophagus dilated during the course of an ENDOSCOPY; however treatment is needed irrespective of narrowing. Patients with cancer require surgery in addition to chemotherapy and radiation as determined by their doctor. Esophageal stents may be needed for palliative care in nonoperable esophageal cancer. This problem and this solution sometimes occurs among elderly individuals with higher frequency. (See MAJOR DIAGNOSTIC TESTS.)

For minor or moderate cases of esophagitis, there is an array of basic adaptations that the person can take to decrease the risk of pain. For example, it is a bad idea for a person with esophagitis (or even for a person who does *not* have esophagitis) to take large bites of hard food items and then attempt to swallow them before they are fully chewed up. Such an action risks that the food particle may become lodged in the esophagus, where it could cause a blockage and severe pain and distress, as the person chokes, changes skin color, and starts to panic.

Another recommendation is to eat small amounts of foods very slowly. It can be annoying to do so at first, and sometimes may make the person feel childlike to cut up his or her food into tiny little pieces and to take longer than everyone else to consume a meal; however, it is far more aggravating to eat "normally" and then choke on one's food, scare oneself and others, and experience extreme pain.

Food Allergies and Intolerances

Both food allergies and food intolerances are common digestive problems in the United States for both adults and children. It is important to note that a food allergy is very different from a food intolerance in that the person with a food allergy actually develops an allergic response involving the bodily production of histamines if he or she should consume the offending food. In the worst case, the allergic reaction can be so severe that it is life-threatening.

In contrast, in the case of food intolerances, there is no allergic reaction to the food, but instead the body has a painful and distressing reaction to certain foods that it cannot digest properly, often including such common foods as milk, wherein digestive system cannot easily handle the lactose present in milk. Thus, the person may suffer from pain in the abdomen. This is true for people with LACTOSE INTOLERANCE (in which the person cannot digest lactose containing milk products while lactose-free products may be okay) as well as with CELIAC DISEASE (in which case the person cannot digest gluten, a substance found in many foods).

Obviously the person with severe food allergies should avoid those particular foods, as should the person with an intolerance to a certain type of food. However, sometimes the problem food is ingested accidentally, as when an individual is visiting a friend or eating at a restaurant and is served the offending food. For this reason, it is best to tell friends and others which foods an individual absolutely cannot eat and also to make it clear that it is not a matter of simply disliking a food but rather that the food makes him or her very sick.

Hiatal Hernia

Many people have hiatal hernias (see HERNIA, HIATAL) with no symptoms, while others experience very painful symptoms with their hiatal hernias. As with those suffering from GERD, it is advisable for the individual with a hiatal hernia to elevate the head of the bed four to six few inches above the height of the feet. In addition, as with GERD patients, those with hiatal hernias should avoid eating within two to four hours of going to bed. In general, large meals should be altogether avoided.

In addition, individuals with hiatal hernias should avoid eating directly after exercising, to avoid exacerbating their condition.

Obesity

The patient who is obese faces many challenges, and the person who is morbidly obese (about 100 pounds overweight) faces even more challenges. Not only is he or she usually dismayed by their own excessive weight and experiencing (or soon to experience) many health consequences, but they may also be aware that others, sometimes including their own physicians, have an extremely negative view of them, largely because of their obesity. This is not paranoia: Studies bear out that many people feel negatively toward those who are obese or extremely obese.

In an analysis of studies by Rebecca M. Puhl and Chelsea A. Jeuer on the attitudes of physicians toward obese patients, reported in *Obesity* in 2009, the researchers found that more than half of the primary care doctors stated that they believed that their obese patients were ugly and awkward. Other studies that were analyzed by Puhl and Jeuer showed that significant numbers of doctors described their obese patients with such pejorative terms as *sloppy, weak, self-indulgent,* and

unmotivated. In addition, research has also indicated that obese people are often stereotyped as lazy and self-absorbed by medical professionals as well as by members of the general public.

Some people who are obese also have an eating disorder, such as bulimia or binge eating disorder. Others simply consume many more calories than their bodies need for their current lifestyle.

Weight loss can be extremely difficult and challenging. EXERCISE is one effective means of weight loss, yet most Americans exercise very little or not at all. Reducing the daily caloric intake is the other means to weight loss. Many people in the United States rely largely upon high-calorie fast foods rather than vegetables and salads. Because obesity is associated with an increased risk for hypertension, diabetes, cardiac disease, some forms of cancer, and many other ailments, it is important for doctors and others to avoid demonizing obese people and instead help them find ways to lose weight. Even a weight loss of five or 10 pounds can bring significant health benefits.

See also DEMOGRAPHIC FACTORS AND DIGESTIVE DISEASES; DIGESTIVE CANCERS; ELDERLY; MEDICATIONS FOR DIGESTIVE DISEASES.

Berkson, Lindsey. *Healthy Digestion the Natural Way: Preventing and Healing Heartburn, Constipation, Gas, Diarrhea, Inflammatory Bowel and Gallbladder Diseases, Ulcers, Irritable Bowel Syndrome, Food Allergies, and More.* New York: John Wiley & Sons, 2000.

Minocha, Anil, M.D., and Christine Adamec. *How to Stop Heartburn: Simple Ways to Heal Heartburn and Acid Reflux.* New York: John Wiley & Sons, 2001.

Minocha, Anil, M.D., with David Carroll. *Natural Stomach Care.* New York: Penguin Putnam, 2003.

National Institute of Diabetes & Digestive & Kidney Diseases (NIDDK). *Recent Advances & Emerging Opportunities.* Bethesda, Md.: National Institutes of Health. February, 2009.

Puhl, Rebecca M., and Chelsea L. Heuer. "The Stigma of Obesity: A Review and Update" *Obesity* 17, no. 5 (2009): 941–964.

albumin A protein that is synthesized by the liver and that circulates in the blood. Albumin performs many important functions in the body, such as maintenance of the plasma oncotic pressure. This pressure holds water inside the blood vessels. If the albumin level is low, water then leaks out of the vessels, causing edema. Albumin also helps to transport numerous substances in the body.

If the liver is damaged, the albumin levels in the blood are decreased. Sometimes albumin is found in the urine, and that presence may be an indicator of kidney disease. In some kidney diseases, the loss of protein in the urine is so severe that blood levels are low. Low serum albumin level may also be a sign of MALNUTRITION.

alcohol abuse and alcoholism Severe problem drinking, a disorder that may also cause serious heart as well as digestive diseases, such as cirrhosis of the liver, liver failure, and death. It also increases the risk for development of alcoholic HEPATITIS. This form of hepatitis is usually caused by heavy drinking rather than by an infectious illness. Severe alcoholic hepatitis may be fatal.

The difference between alcohol abuse and alcohol dependence is a matter of degree and depends on whether or not physical dependency is present. Both forms of excessive alcohol consumption are injurious to health; chronic alcohol dependence is the worse of the two types. Alcoholism includes both a psychological and a physical dependency, and it is an even more serious problem than is chronic alcohol abuse.

Many people who are heavy drinkers are also heavy smokers, and the combination of the two types of behavior can worsen any existing digestive problems or create new health problems; for example, people who drink and smoke are more prone to development of various forms of CANCER such as ESOPHAGEAL CANCER than are people who do not drink or smoke.

Experts disagree on the cause of alcoholism. It may be caused by a genetic factor or by biochemical abnormalities that predispose some individuals to the inability to limit their alcohol consumption.

Social pressure may play some role in alcohol abuse, although few cultures condone chronic alcohol abuse or alcoholism.

Both alcohol abuse and alcoholism can severely and permanently affect the digestive system (particularly the liver); although the effect on alcoholics is more profound, to the point that alcoholism may cause the patient's death from CIRRHOSIS of the liver or from other digestive diseases. Alcoholism is also linked to an increased risk of development of STOMACH CANCER, esophageal cancer, and COLORECTAL CANCER. It may cause ANEMIA, particularly among alcoholics who are eating very little food and who are obtaining most or all of their caloric intake from alcohol. Alcohol has poor nutritional value, although it has many calories.

Many alcoholics have VITAMIN DEFICIENCIES, which may be extremely severe. They may be particularly deficient in thiamine (vitamin B_1), and this deficiency may seriously damage the nerves, brain, and heart and may also cause memory and other intellectual problems.

Chronic heavy drinking can lead to alcoholic PANCREATITIS, an illness that causes severe abdominal pain and vomiting. Alcoholic men in their 40s have the greatest risk of development of alcoholic pancreatitis. This disease can cause death if it becomes severe. The person with an attack of alcoholic pancreatitis may need to be hospitalized and given intravenous painkillers. It can cause chronic abdominal pain with acute exacerbations as well as malabsorption syndrome. The individual must subsequently give up alcohol completely, to increase the interval between attacks. Surgery may be needed in some cases of alcoholic pancreatitis.

The alcoholic may also suffer from MALLORY-WEISS SYNDROME, a digestive disorder that is experienced by many alcoholics. This medical problem results in mild to heavy internal bleeding due to a tear in the area where the esophagus joins the stomach. It is usually caused by vomiting and retching, which are common actions among many people with severe alcohol problems.

Pregnant women who are heavy drinkers or alcoholics may cause their infant to suffer from fetal alcohol syndrome, a condition that is characterized by physical and intellectual deficits and birth defects.

Symptoms and Diagnostic Path

Alcohol dependence is characterized by alcohol use that is associated with three or more of the following indicators:

• tolerance

• withdrawal symptoms

- use of a substance in a larger quantity than was intended
- persistent desire to cut down or control the use of alcohol
- a significant time spent obtaining, using, or recovering from alcohol
- neglect of social, occupational, or recreational tasks
- continued use of alcohol despite physical and psychological problems

Physicians diagnose chronic alcohol abuse or alcoholism on the basis of behavior, information provided by family members, and laboratory tests of the blood and liver. Severe alcoholics may exhibit clearly visible symptoms of alcohol use, such as tremors (chronic shaking), bloodshot eyes, and difficulty in thinking. LIVER ENZYME/FUNCTION TESTS may be abnormal, and an imaging scan of the liver may show an enlarged or damaged liver.

If the individual is going through acute alcohol withdrawal, which in its severest form is also known as delirium tremens, he or she is clearly ill and may exhibit hallucinations, confusion, hyperactivity, and seizures. The patient may also be severely dehydrated. Withdrawal symptoms are precipitated by the complete lack of alcohol in an alcoholic person, and usually they commence about 12 to 48 hours after the last drink was taken. Delirium tremens generally occur 48 to 72 hours after withdrawal from alcohol, but they may also occur as late as seven days after the last drink. People in this condition require inpatient treatment in a hospital.

Treatment Options and Outlook

Residential treatment at a clinic is commonly used for long-term alcoholics, and there are many residential facilities in the United States, Canada, and other countries.

Some experts treat patients with medications. In the past, disulfuram (Antabuse) was the drug most commonly used to treat alcoholism. An alcoholic person who took Antabuse and later consumed even a small amount of alcohol became violently nauseated and sick. More recently, experts have found naltrexone (ReVia), a drug that blocks the pleasure centers of the brain to be helpful in treatment of alcohol dependence. It reduces pleasurable effects of alcohol, prevents the "high" from drug abuse, and reduces the craving for alcohol. If the alcoholic normally obtains a feeling of euphoria and well-being from drinking, such feelings do not occur with naltrexone. Patients on naltrexone are more likely to participate in other alcohol-related treatments like Alcoholics Anonymous (AA). It also reduces relapse and number of drinking days. Patients frequently go into relapse once naltrexone is discontinued.

Some alcoholics find success with self-help organizations, such as Alcoholics Anonymous (AA), which require complete abstinence from alcohol and offer considerable support in helping the alcoholic achieve that goal. AA does not charge dues, and the only membership requirement is a sincere commitment to drinking no alcohol (abstinence).

Risk Factors and Preventive Measures

Males are more typically problem drinkers or alcoholics than females, although women can experience these problems as well. Women who are alcoholics are more likely to deny and/or to minimize their alcohol problem. In considering heavy chronic drinking, men are about four times as likely to fit an alcoholic pattern as women. Even among younger people, such as teenagers, it is usually adolescent boys who are heavy drinkers rather than teenage girls.

See also ANEMIA; CIRRHOSIS; COLORECTAL CANCER; ESOPHAGEAL CANCER; LIVER; LIVER CANCER; LIVER FAILURE; LIVER TRANSPLANTATION; PANCREAS; PANCREATITIS; VITAMIN DEFICIENCIES; WERNICKE'S ENCEPHALOPATHY.

Gold, Mark, M.D., and Christine Adamec. *The Encyclopedia of Alcoholism and Alcohol Abuse.* New York: Facts On File, 2010.

alternative medicine Refers to the use of nontraditional remedies and treatments, also known as *complementary medicine.* Some individuals define alternative medicine as supplements or treatments that are used instead of standard medical therapy, while they view complementary medicine as therapy and treatments that are used in addition to medical therapy provided by physicians. However, most people use the general phrase "alternative medicine." In the scientific literature, it is frequently referred to as *complementary and alternative medicine* or CAM.

It is unknown what percentage of alternative remedies are used to treat most digestive disorders, but since conditions such as DYSPEPSIA, NAUSEA, and HEARTBURN are common problems, it is likely to represent a significant percentage. The use of alternative medicines such as botanicals (which include herbal medicines and other supplements that are derived from plants) as well as the use of massage therapy, tai chi, and many other additional options available under the auspices of alternative medicine, are very popular in the United States. According to the National Center for Health Statistics, Americans spent $33.9 billion on visits to alternative medicine practitioners as well as on purchases of products, classes, and materials in 2007. Both adults and children in the United States use alternative medicine.

Adults Who Use Alternative Medicine

In considering the demographics of individuals using alternative medicine, according to the National Center for Health Statistics, women were heavier users than men, and 42.8 percent of women used some form of alternative medicine in 2007 compared to 33.5 percent of men. (See Table 1 for more information.)

TABLE 1: PERCENTAGES OF ADULTS AGES 18 YEARS AND OLDER WHO USED SELECTIVE COMPLEMENTARY AND ALTERNATIVE MEDICINE IN THE PAST 12 MONTHS, BY SELECTED CHARACTERISTICS: UNITED STATES: 2007

Characteristic	All CAM	Biologically based therapies	Mind-body therapies	Alternative medical systems	Energy healing therapy	Manipulative and body-based therapies
Total	38.3	19.9	19.2	3.4	0.5	15.2
Gender						
Male	33.5	17.8	14.4	2.7	0.4	12.2
Female	42.8	21.9	23.8	4.2	0.7	18.1
Age						
18-29 years	36.3	15.9	21.3	3.2	0.3	15.1
30-39 years	39.6	19.8	19.9	3.6	0.5	17.2
40-49 years	40.1	20.4	19.7	4.8	0.8	17.4
50-59 years	44.1	24.2	22.9	4.9	1.0	17.3
60-69 years	41.0	25.4	17.3	2.8	0.5	13.8
70-84 years	32.1	19.3	11.9	1.8	Not available	9.9
85 years and older	24.2	13.7	9.8	1.9	Not available	7.0
Race and ethnicity						
Hispanic	23.7	11.8	10.6	3.0	0.1	6.7
Non-Hispanic white, single race	43.1	22.7	21.4	3.7	0.7	18.7
Non-Hispanic black or African American, single race	25.5	12.3	14.8	1.4	0.2	6.5
Non-Hispanic American Indian or Alaska Native, single race	50.3	23.7	23.3	13.2	Not available	13.4
Non-Hispanic Asian, single race	39.9	19.6	23.4	5.4	0.3	11.1
Non-Hispanic Native Hawaiian or Other Pacific Islander, single race	43.2	26.1	24.5	Not available	Not available	Not available

(Table continues)

(Table continued)

Characteristic	All CAM	Biologically based therapies	Mind-body therapies	Alternative medical systems	Energy healing therapy	Manipulative and body-based therapies
Hispanic or Latino origin						
Puerto Rican	29.7	14.2	16.8	2.4	Not available	7.6
Mexican	18.2	8.9	6.9	3.9	Not available	4.1
Mexican American	27.4	14.0	11.6	2.1	Not available	7.9
Cuban or Cuban American	22.9	11.2	14.1	Not available	Not available	8.5
Dominican (Republic)	28.2	12.3	18.5	Not available	Not available	5.3
Central or South American	23.4	12.8	10.0	3.5	Not available	7.4
Education						
Less than high school	20.8	9.8	7.6	2.1	Not available	6.4
High school graduation or GED recipient	31.0	16.3	12.1	2.0	0.4	11.5
Some college-no degree	45.0	24.4	22.0	4.3	0.7	18.0
Associate of Arts degree	47.2	24.9	24.3	3.6	0.5	18.2
Bachelor of Arts or Science degree	49.6	27.5	25.5	5.4	0.8	20.7
Master's, Doctorate, Professional Degree	55.4	30.1	34.2	6.1	1.2	23.6
Poverty status						
Poor	28.9	13.7	16.5	3.2	0.5	8.4
Near poor	30.9	15.6	16.0	2.6	0.5	10.1
Not poor	43.3	23.0	21.6	3.9	0.6	18.1
Region of the U.S.						
Northeast	38.0	18.2	21.1	3.8	0.8	15.0
Midwest	41.4	20.4	20.6	2.8	0.8	17.9
South	32.5	17.7	15.0	2.4	0.3	11.5
West	44.6	24.4	23.2	5.6	0.9	18.4
Leisure time physical activity						
Never or unable to engage in activity	23.6	11.5	9.8	2.2	0.2	8.5
Engage in some activity but less than regular	43.3	22.5	22.4	3.6	0.7	16.8
Engage in regular activity	51.5	28.1	27.5	4.8	0.8	21.7
Body weight status						
Underweight	31.4	16.7	17.0	3.4	Unavailable	8.6
Healthy weight	41.0	20.7	21.6	4.7	0.7	17.8
Overweight	37.3	19.0	18.4	2.7	0.5	14.6
Obese	37.6	21.2	17.8	2.9	0.5	13.3

Characteristic	All CAM	Biologically based therapies	Mind-body therapies	Alternative medical systems	Energy healing therapy	Manipulative and body-based therapies
Lifetime cigarette smoking status						
Current smoker	35.6	17.0	19.4	2.4	0.5	12.8
Former smoker	48.1	26.8	24.7	4.8	0.9	19.2
Never smoker	36.0	18.6	17.8	3.3	0.5	14.8
Lifetime alcohol drinking status						
Lifetime abstainer	23.5	11.1	11.0	2.2	0.3	7.5
Former drinker	37.6	19.3	19.8	3.2	0.4	12.8
Current infrequent or light drinker	44.6	23.7	23.0	4.0	0.7	18.3
Current moderate or heavy drinker	45.4	24.2	22.3	3.8	0.7	19.3
Hospitalized in the past year						
Yes	42.1	20.2	23.7	3.4	0.4	16.2
No	37.9	19.9	18.8	3.4	0.6	15.1
Number of health conditions						
0 conditions	21.3	10.0	9.8	1.4	0.1	7.5
1-2 conditions	33.3	16.5	16.2	2.2	0.2	12.5
3-5 conditions	42.3	22.8	19.5	3.9	0.7	18.1
6 or more conditions	53.8	28.4	30.6	5.7	1.1	22.1
Number of visits to a doctor in past 12 months						
0 visits	24.5	13.0	13.2	2.0	0.4	6.0
1 visit	32.3	16.8	14.7	2.7	0.3	10.7
2-3 visits	39.4	20.9	19.7	3.1	0.5	15.0
4-9 visits	47.2	25.1	23.8	4.2	0.7	20.6
10 or more visits	53.4	25.3	28.8	6.7	1.2	28.3

Source: Adapted from Barnes, Patricia M., and Barbara Bloom. "Complementary and Alternative Medicine Use Among Adults and Children: United States, 2007." *National Health Statistics Reports* 18 (December 10, 2008): 14–15.

Among different races and ethnicities, the greatest percentage of users of all types of alternative therapies were American Indian or Alaska Natives (50.3 percent), followed by Native Hawaiians or Other Pacific Islanders (43.2 percent), and then whites (43.1 percent). Hispanics (23.7 percent) and African Americans (25.5 percent) were the least likely to use alternative remedies.

Interestingly, highly educated people were the most likely to use alternative medicine, and 55.4 percent of those with a master's, doctorate, or a professional degree used some form of alternative medicine, compared to 49.6 percent of those with a bachelor's degree. Those with less than a high school education were the least likely to use some form of alternative medicine (20.8 percent). Perhaps more educated people have more confidence in their abilities to evaluate and use alternative medicine effectively. In addition, they are more likely to have the funds available to pay for such remedies, since most insurance companies do not pay for them.

In considering the age of individuals using alternative and complementary medicine, it is those who are between the ages 50–59 who were the most likely to use some form of alternative medicine (44.1 percent) in 2007, followed by those ages 60–69 (41.0 percent). In contrast, those age 85 years and older were the least likely to use alternative medicine (24.2 percent).

Not surprisingly, individuals with many health conditions were more likely to turn to alternative medicine; for example, among those with six or more health problems, the majority (53.8 percent) used some form of alternative medicine, while only 21.3 percent of those with no health problems used alternative medicine. See Table 1 for further details.

TABLE 2: FREQUENCIES AND PERCENTAGES OF ADULTS 18 YEARS AND OLDER WHO USED COMPLEMENTARY AND ALTERNATIVE MEDICINE IN THE PAST 12 MONTHS, BY SELECTED DISEASES AND CONDITIONS FOR WHICH IT WAS USED: UNITED STATES, 2007

Disease or Condition	Number in thousands	Percent
Back pain or problem	14,325	17.1
Neck pain or problem	5,031	5.9
Joint pain or stiffness or other joint condition	4,537	5.2
Arthritis	3,057	3.5
Anxiety	2,293	2.8
Cholesterol	1,827	2.1
Head or chest cold	1,693	2.0
Other musculoskeletal	1,498	1.8
Severe headache or migraine	1,359	1.6
Insomnia or trouble sleeping	1,191	1.4
Stress	1,124	1.3
Stomach or intestinal illness	974	1.2
Depression	962	1.2
Regular headaches	813	1.0
Hypertension	842	0.9
Fibromyalgia	755	0.8
Diabetes	650	0.7
Sprain or strain	605	0.7
Coronary heart disease	586	0.7

Source: Adapted from Barnes, Patricia M., and Barbara Bloom. "Complementary and Alternative Medicine Use Among Adults and Children: United States, 2007." *National Health Statistics Reports* 18 (December 10, 2008): 13.

It is also interesting to note the primary medical reasons for which alternative medicine was used, in adults. Table 2 provides this data. For example, the predominant reason for using CAM among adults in 2007 was back pain or back problem, used by 17.1 percent of those who used alternative medicine or more than 14 million people. Arthritic type pain, including back pain, neck pain, joint pain, or simply "arthritis" constituted a large number of users. However, nearly a million people reported using alternative remedies for their stomach pain or intestinal illnesses.

As can be seen from Table 3, more than 38 million people saw an alternative medicine practitioner in 2007, spending nearly $12 billion on this segment alone of alternative medicine. Most saw chiropractors (49.2 percent), followed by massage therapists (47.4 percent).

The Growth in the Popularity of Alternative Medicine

Alternative medicine has vastly grown in popularity from 2002 to 2007—and it is likely to be even more popular in the future and beyond. See Table 4 for information on the numbers and percentages of adults ages 18 and older using alternative medicine and therapies in both 2002 and 2007. As can be seen from the table, for nearly all categories, the numbers of users of alternative medicine therapies were significantly higher in 2007 than in 2002. For example, about 2.1 million adults used acupuncture in 2002, but that number increased to 3.1 million by 2007. In another example, about 3.4 million adults used homeopathic treatments in 2002, and this number increased to 3.9 million by 2007.

Dietary Supplements

Americans spent $23.7 billion on dietary supplements in 2007 alone, according to the General Accounting Office (GAO). A dietary supplement is defined by the federal government as a product that is intended for ingestion to supplement the diet, is labeled as a dietary supplement, and is not represented as a conventional food or an item of a meal. The most popular dietary supplements are multivitamins, sports nutrition powders and formulas, and calcium. Weight-loss products are

TABLE 3: FREQUENCIES AND PERCENTAGES OF PERSONS AGES 18 AND OLDER WHO SAW ALTERNATIVE MEDICINE PRACTITIONERS DURING THE PAST 12 MONTHS, TOTAL PRACTITIONER VISITS AND TOTAL OUT-OF-POCKET COSTS PER YEAR, BY TYPE OF THERAPY, UNITED STATES, 2007

Therapy	Total persons		Total visits per year		Total out-of-pocket costs per year (dollars)	
	Number (thousands)	Percent	Number (thousands)	Percent	Number (thousands)	Percent
Total	38,146	100.0	354,203	100.0	11,938,611	100.0
Alternative medical systems	4,965	13.1	27,734	7.8	1,392,508	11.7
Acupuncture	3,141	8.2	17,629	5.0	827,336	6.9
Ayurveda	214	0.6	1,068	Not provided	18,793	0.2
Homeopathic treatment	862	2.3	3,411	1.0	167,416	1.4
Naturopathy	729	1.9	3,180	0.9	275,863	2.3
Biologically based therapies	1,828	4.8	9,600	2.7	630,439	4.3
Chelation therapy	111	0.3	426	0.1	31,913	0.3
Nonvitamin, nonmineral, and natural products	1,488	3.9	8,273	2.3	566,650	4.7
Manipulative and body-based therapies	33,044	86.7	276,861	78.2	8,629,455	72.3
Chiropractic or osteopathic manipulation	18,740	49.2	151,220	42.7	3,901,894	32.7
Massage	18,068	47.4	95,296	26.9	4,175,124	35.0
Mind-body therapies	3,821	10.2	32,806	9.3	864,567	7.2
Biofeedback	362	1.0	1,991	0.6	83,542	Not provided
Relaxation techniques	3,131	8.3	28,882	8.2	707,175	5.9
Hypnosis	561	1.5	1,933	0.5	73,850	0.6
Energy healing therapy	1,216	3.2	7,203	2.0	421,602	3.5

Source: Adapted from Nahin, Richard L., et al. "Costs of Complementary and Alternative Medicine (CAM) and Frequency of Visits to CAM Practitioners: United States, 2007." *National Health Statistics Reports* 18 (July 30, 2009): 6.

also popular. Some supplements, including some which have been recalled by the Food and Drug Administration (FDA) because of adverse events (serious side effects that were reported to the federal government), are promoted to enhance male sexual performance.

In 1994, there were about 4,000 dietary supplements available to consumers; by 2008, there were an astonishing 76,000 dietary supplements that were available, according to the GAO.

The National Center for Health Statistics reports that in 2007, nearly 11 million adults used products that fit the categories of fish oil, omega 3, or DHA in the past 30 days. (See Table 5.) This was the most popular nonvitamin, nonmineral natural product included, and it was used by 37.4 percent of those who used such products. Note, however, that many adults used more than one product. The next most popular product was glucosamine, used by 6.1 million people or nearly 20 percent of those who used such products.

Botanical Remedies

Botanicals are plant-based remedies that include herbs as well as any other plants that are not specifically designated as herbs and which are

TABLE 4: FREQUENCIES AND PERCENTAGES OF ADULTS AGES 18 YEARS OF AGE AND OLDER WHO USED COMPLEMENTARY AND ALTERNATIVE MEDICINE IN THE PAST 12 MONTHS, BY TYPE OF THERAPY: UNITED STATES, 2002 AND 2007.

Therapy	2002		2007	
	Number in thousands	Percent	Number in thousands	Percent
Alternative medical systems				
Acupuncture	2,136	1.1	3,141	1.4
Ayurveda	154	0.1	214	0.1
Homeopathic treatment	3,433	1.7	3,909	1.8
Naturopathy	498	0.2	729	0.3
Biologically based therapies				
Nonvitamin, nonmineral, natural products	38,183	18.9	38,797	17.7[1]
Megavitamin therapy	5,739	2.8	Not provided	Not provided
Mind-body therapies				
Biofeedback	278	0.1	362	0.2
Meditation	15,336	7.6	20,541	9.4
Guided imagery	4,194	2.1	4,866	2.2
Progressive relaxation	6,185	3.0	6,454	2.9
Deep breathing exercises	23,457	11.6	27,794	12.7
Hypnosis	505	0.2	561	0.2
Yoga	10,386	5.1	13,172	6.1
Tai chi	2,565	1.3	2,267	1.0
Qui gong	527	0.3	625	0.3
Energy healing therapy/Reiki	1,080	0.5	1,216	0.5

1 According to the researchers, data for 2002 and 2007 in the category of nonvitamin, nonmineral natural products are not comparable because of the question order and the products covered in the separate years.

Source: Adapted from Barnes, Patricia M., and Barbara Bloom. "Complementary and Alternative Medicine Use Among Adults and Children: United States, 2007." *National Health Statistics Reports* 18 (December 10, 2008): 10.

used as alternative medicine. For example, ginger (*Zingiber officinale*) has been shown effective at treating minor stomach upsets, such as nausea, DIARRHEA, and stomachaches. Ginger is also commonly prescribed for the nausea and vomiting that are associated with pregnancy, even by mainstream physicians.

According to the National Center for Complementary and Alternative Medicine (NCCAM), many digestive and antinausea supplements include ginger root as an ingredient. Ginger is also used to improve osteoarthritis, rheumatoid arthritis, and joint and muscle pain. Ginger is found in tablets, capsules, fresh or dried root, or liquid extracts and teas. In addition to ginger, other herbs that are used to help people with digestive problems include chamomile, meadowsweet, and ginseng. For example, Iberogast®, is a patented combination of nine herbs that modulate gastric motility and provide relief in patients with functional dyspepsia.

Chamomile is an herb that is promoted for upset stomach, diarrhea, and gas, as well as for insomnia and anxiety. Chamomile is available in capsules, tablets, liquid extracts, or teas. According to the NCCAM, some early studies have indicated that chamomile may help with upset stomach and diarrhea in children. It may also be helpful for mouth ulcers and can be applied in cream form. Some people are allergic to chamomile, and those most at risk are individuals who are allergic to related plants, such as ragweed, chrysanthemums, marigolds, and daisies.

European elder is a tree from which a supplement is created, and it is commonly called European elder, black elder, or elderberry. Elderberry and the elder flower are used for constipation and sinus infections, as well as flu, colds, and fevers. There is no reliable information to support the use of any products made from the European elder tree, according to the NCCAM. The supplement may act as a diuretic and should not be used with medications that increase urination.

Turmeric is an herb that is related to ginger, and it has been used for individuals with heartburn, stomach ulcers, and gallstones. The stems of the turmeric plant are dried and made into a powder or used in capsules, liquid extracts, or teas. Several studies have documented its antitumor properties in laboratory studies. Human studies suggest that turmeric has beneficial effects in patients with ULCERATIVE COLITIS.

Licorice root (glycrrhiza) is used to treat stomach ulcers as well as bronchitis and sore throat. Licorice root is found in capsules, pills, and liquid extracts. Some research has indicated that licorice root might decrease complications suffered by patients with hepatitis C, although the NCCAM says further research is needed. Licorice root does have some possible and significant side effects, including high blood pressure, the retention of salt and water, and low potassium levels, which could lead to cardiac problems. Licorice root taken with DIURETICS could reduce the potassium levels of the body to dangerously low levels. Pregnant women should avoid using licorice as either a supplement or as a food because it could increase their risk for preterm labor. Commercial products are generally avoided because of potential side effects.

Peppermint oil (*Mentha x piperita*) is used to treat nausea and indigestion as well as IRRITABLE BOWEL SYNDROME and stomach pain. It is taken in very small dosages. According to the NCCAM, some studies have suggested that peppermint oil improves irritable bowel symptoms. In addition, some preliminary studies indicate that peppermint oil in combination with caraway oil helps to relieve indigestion.

Some research has found that pineapple extract may be useful in treating CROHN'S DISEASE and ulcerative colitis (together known as INFLAMMATORY BOWEL DISEASE), according to the NCCAM. A study funded by NCCAM was performed by Duke University researchers on 51 subjects, including eight controls, 20 subjects with ulcerative colitis, and 23 with Crohn's disease. This study was reported in 2008 in *Clinical Immunology*. The researchers used bromelain, an enzyme derived from pineapple stems, and they found that several pro-inflammatory cytokines were reduced in the treated subjects. The researchers concluded that bromelain could potentially benefit some patients, although further research is needed.

Milk thistle is a plant that has been used to treat liver disease and jaundice for centuries. It is also used by some people with liver disease in the United States. According to the NCCAM, milk thistle may protect and promote the growth of liver

TABLE 5: FREQUENCIES AND PERCENTAGES OF ADULTS 18 YEARS OF AGE AND OLDER WHO USED SELECTED TYPES OF NONVITAMIN, NONMINERAL NATURAL PRODUCTS FOR HEALTH REASONS IN THE PAST 30 DAYS, BY TYPE OF PRODUCT USED: UNITED STATES, 2007

Nonvitamin, nonmineral, natural products	Number in thousands	Percent
Fish oil or omega 3 or DHA	10,923	37.4
Glucosamine	6,132	19.9
Echinacea	4,848	19.8
Flaxseed oil or pills	4,416	15.9
Ginseng	3,345	14.1
Combination herb pill	3,446	13.0
Ginkgo biloba	2,977	11.3
Chondroitin	3,390	11.2
Garlic supplements	3,278	11.0
Coenzyme Q-10	2,691	8.7
Fiber or psyllium	1,791	6.6
Green tea pills	1,528	6.3
Cranberry (pills, gelcaps)	1,560	6.0
Saw palmetto	1,682	5.1
Soy supplements of isofavones	1,363	5.0
Melatonin	1,296	4.6
Grape seed extract	1,214	4.3
MSM (methylsufonylmethane)	1,312	4.1
Milk thistle	1,001	3.7
Lutein	1,047	3.4

Note that some respondents used more than one product.

Source: Adapted from Barnes, Patricia M., and Barbara Bloom. "Complementary and Alternative Medicine Use Among Adults and Children: United States, 2007." *National Health Statistics Reports* 18 (December 10, 2008): 12.

cells and inhibit inflammation, although the results of clinical studies have been mixed.

Homeopathic Treatment

Homeopathy is based on a system originally devised by Samuel Hahnemann, a 19th-century physician. He noted that large quantities of quinine made healthy individuals feverish and sick with malaria-like symptoms but smaller quantities of quinine made people who actually had malaria feel better. He developed his "law of similars," which is basically that large quantities of some substances may cause illnesses but much smaller quantities may provide relief; for example, belladonna is a poison, but it is used by homepaths in minute quantities to treat migraine headaches.

Many, but not all, of the independent reviews and placebo-controlled trials of homeopathy such as by Wayne B. Jonas and colleagues in 2003, have concluded that its benefits seem to be more than just a placebo effect.

In 2005, David Spence et al. published the results of their 6-year, university-hospital outpatient observational study of homeopathic treatment for chronic diseases, including gastrointestinal diseases. They found that 71 percent of the patients reported positive health changes, with 51 percent recording their improvement as better or much better.

Many physicians in the United States do not consider homeopathy to be a valid therapy, especially since the drug formulations are so highly diluted that many may contain little active drug at all. As such, it defies medical plausibility and continues to baffle scientists. On the other hand, this form of medicine is highly popular in many countries of Europe and Asia, including in the United Kingdom and India.

Probiotics

The use of probiotics has been found by many researchers to be beneficial in treating infectious diarrhea. According to the NCCAM, probiotics are live microorganisms (usually bacteria) that are similar to the microorganisms found in the healthy human gut. Probiotics are primarily found in dietary supplements or foods. According to the NCCAM, one widely used definition of probiotics is that they are "live microorganisms, which, when administered in adequate amounts, confer a health benefit on the host."

Many individuals use such products (available in yogurt as well as in capsules), including some people who have been taking a long course of antibiotics and who may try probiotics in an attempt to "restore" their healthy intestinal flora. Others may take probiotics to resolve such common gastrointestinal problems as CONSTIPATION, diarrhea, ulcerative colitis, Crohn's disease, or irritable bowel syndrome. The NCCAM says that limited evidence supports the use of probiotics, but further study is needed. For example, some evidence supports the following uses of probiotic products:

- to treat diarrhea, especially diarrhea caused by rotavirus
- to treat irritable bowel syndrome
- to prevent recurrent intestinal infection caused by *Clostridium difficile*
- to prevent POUCHITIS, a condition that may follow surgery removing the COLON
- to prevent and treat infections of the urinary tract or genitals in females
- to reduce the recurrence of bladder cancer
- to prevent and manage eczema in children

Probiotics may have mild side effects if used as directed, such as gas or bloating. They may also rarely cause infections in some people who are very sick. Anyone considering using a probiotic should first consult with his or her physician.

The Dietary Supplement Health and Education Act of 1994

The leading law that governs the use of alternative medicine in the United States is the Dietary Supplement Health and Education Act of 1994. On the basis of this legislation, herbal remedies and vitamin supplements were thereafter regulated differently from both over-the-counter (OTC) and prescribed medications. However, most consumers do not realize this, and they mistakenly assume that the same government protections that are established for prescribed and OTC drugs apply to herbs and supplements.

The FDA is allowed to ban supplements that are deemed to be a public health risk. For example, the FDA banned the sale of ephedra, a stimulant, in 2004. However, because of the way that the laws are written, it is more difficult to ban dietary supplements than it is to forbid the sale of prescribed medications or over-the-counter medications.

Sometimes it is difficult to determine whether a product is a dietary supplement or a food with added dietary ingredients; for example, a tea with herbal ingredients could be regarded as either a dietary supplement or a food product.

Children and Alternative Medicine

Many children of all ages under age 18 use alternative remedies; for example, in 2007, 524,000 children used echinacea, and 441,000 used fish oil, omega 3, or DHA. (See Table 6.) An estimated 11.8 percent of children younger than age 18 use some form of CAM, with the greatest percentage (4.7 percent) using biologically-based therapies, such as nonvitamin and nonmineral natural products or diet-based therapies. Yet few clinical studies have been performed on children using CAM.

TABLE 6: FREQUENCIES AND PERCENTAGES OF CHILDREN UNDER 18 YEARS OF AGE WHO USED SELECTED TYPES OF NONVITAMIN, NONMINERAL, NATURAL PRODUCTS FOR HEALTH REASONS IN THE PAST 30 DAYS, BY TYPE OF PRODUCT USED: UNITED STATES, 2007

Nonvitamin, nonmineral, natural products	Number in Thousands	Percent
Echninacea	524	37.2
Fish oil or omega 3 or DHA	441	30.5
Combination herb pill	296	17.9
Flaxseed oil or pills	233	16.7
Prebiotics or probiotics	199	13.6
Goldenseal	143	8.6
Garlic supplements	84	5.9
Melatonin	92	5.8

Source: Adapted from Barnes, Patricia M., and Barbara Bloom. "Complementary and Alternative Medicine Use Among Adults and Children: United States, 2007. *National Health Statistics Reports* 18 (December 10, 2008): 12.

One exception is with chamomile, according to Paula Gardner, M.D. in her article for *Pediatrics in Review*. According to Gardner, studies have found that a chamomile and pectin preparation was effective in treating diarrhea in children. Chamomile in combination with other herbs has also been used to treat colic and dyspepsia as well as pain from teething. Gardner says that in one study, 93 colicky babies were treated with a combination of chamomile, fennel, and lemon balm or placebo. The crying time was reduced in 85.4 percent of the infants given the herbal remedy and in 48.9 percent of the placebo group.

An estimated 4.3 percent of children used mind-body therapies in 2007, including such therapies as biofeedback, meditation, guided imagery, progressive relaxation, deep breathing exercises, hypnosis, yoga, tai chi, or qi gong.

Among children using alternative therapies in 2007, the largest percentage (16.4 percent) were ages 12–17 years, followed by children ages 5–11 years (10.7 percent) and then those 0–4 years (7.6 percent). As with adults, the sicker that the child is, the more likely that alternative medicine is used; for example, among children with no health conditions, 4.0 percent used alternative medicine. This percentage increased to 8.5 percent for children with one to two conditions then further to 14.1 percent among children with three to five health conditions, and among those with six or more health conditions, the percentage was 23.8 percent.

Children who used alternative remedies used them most frequently for back or neck pain (6.7 percent of children) or to treat anxiety and stress (4.8 percent). Some children were treated for attention deficit/hyperactivity disorder (ADHD) with alternative remedies (2.5 percent), possibly because their parents were fearful of the use of stimulant or nonstimulant medications prescribed to treat ADHD. (See Table 8 for further details.)

Children using alternative medicine were more likely to have a parent who also used alternative medicine; for example, 23.9 percent of children who used any form of alternative medicine had a parent who also used alternative medicine, compared to 5.1 percent of children using alternative medicine whose parents did not use alternative therapies.

TABLE 7: PERCENTAGES OF CHILDREN UNDER AGE 18 YEARS WHO USED SELECTIVE COMPLEMENTARY AND ALTERNATIVE MEDICINE CATEGORIES IN THE PAST 12 MONTHS, BY SELECTED CHARACTERISTICS: UNITED STATES, 2007.

Therapy	All children		Children Whose Parent Used Alternative Medicine	
	Number in thousands	Percent	Number in thousands	Percent
Alternative medical systems				
Acupuncture	150	0.2	27	0.2
Ayurveda	79	0.1	7	Not provided
Homeopathic treatment	907	1.3	354	2.8
Naturopathy	237	0.3	111	Not provided
Manipulative and body therapies				
Chiropractic	2,020	2.8	754	5.7
Massage therapy	743	1.0	297	2.2
Mind-body therapies				
Biofeedback	119	0.2	36	0.3
Meditation	725	1.0	400	3.0
Guided imagery	293	0.4	197	1.5
Progressive relaxation	329	0.5	164	1.3
Deep breathing exercises	1,558	2.2	704	5.4
Hypnosis	67	0.1	18	Not provided
Yoga	1,505	2.1	618	4.7
Tai chi	113	0.2	56	0.4
Qi gong	50	Not available	4	Not available
Energy healing therapy	161	0.2	52	0.4

Source: Adapted from Barnes, Patricia M., and Barbara Bloom. "Complementary and Alternative Medicine Use Among Adults and Children: United States, 2007." *National Health Statistics Reports* 18 (December 10, 2008): 11.

According to the NCCAM, parents should consider the following points before deciding on whether to use alternative remedies or treatments with their children:

- Ensure that the child has received a diagnosis from a licensed health care provider and also that alternative remedies do not replace or delay conventional medical care.
- If alternative medicine is used, do not increase the dose or length of treatment beyond what is recommended.
- If the child experiences an effect from the therapy that concerns the parent, then the child's health care provider should be contacted.
- Herbal and other dietary supplements should be stored out of reach of children. Do not assume that "childproof caps" are inevitably safe.

- Women who are breastfeeding or pregnant (see PREGNANCY) should know that some therapies may affect a fetus or nursing infant.

Types of Alternative Treatments

There are many different types of alternative treatments, including acupuncture, biofeedback, chiropractic, and so forth. This section covers several key treatments.

Acupuncture and Acupressure Acupuncture refers to the insertion of tiny needles, while acupressure is the noninvasive manipulation of specific trigger points. Acupuncture is more commonly used than acupressure. The most common use of acupuncture is for the treatment of back pain, joint pain, and headache. It is also used to treat FIBROMYALGIA. According to NCCAM, research on acupuncture has been mostly inconclusive. Human studies suggest that acupuncture is helpful in nausea and vomiting, and also promotes gastric emptying, thus helping in GASTROPARESIS.

Ayurvedic medicine   According to the NCCAM, more than 200,000 adults used Ayurvedic medicine in 2006 for many different medical problems. The underlying concept of Ayurvedic medicine, a system used in India for thousands of years, is that there is a universal connectedness between the constitution of the body (prakriti) and its life forces (doshas). The belief is that disease arises when a person is out of harmony with the universe.

The life forces, or *doshas*, control body activities, and each person has its one combination of doshas, although one dosha usually dominates. The most powerful dosha is the vata dosha, which controls movement of the gut, respiration, cardiac functions, waste discharge, and the mind. The vata is aggravated by fear and grief as well as by staying up too late or eating before the prior meal had a chance to be digested. Individuals whose vata is their prominent dosha are said to be at risk for neurological and skin conditions as well as heart disease, rheumatoid arthritis, anxiety, and insomnia.

The second of the three doshas is the pitta dosha, which represents fire and water and controls the digestive juices. The person with a pitta imbalance may suffer from heartburn within two to three hours of eating. The person with a dominant pitta dosha gets out of balance by consuming spicy or sour food or becoming fatigued. These individuals are believed to be at risk for Crohn's disease as well as hypertension, heart disease, and infectious diseases.

Last is the kapha dosha, believed by adherents to represent the elements of water and the earth. The person with a dominant kapha may eat too many sweet foods, continue eating after being satiated, and drink and eat foods with too much salt and water. Individuals whose pitta dosha dominates are said to be at risk for diabetes, obesity, cancer, and asthma.

Sickness occurs when the body and the doshas are in disharmony. The Ayurvedic practitioner determines the patient's dosha and then seeks to create balance by modifying the life style as well as diet (foods to eat and foods to avoid) in addition to medications.

Biofeedback   With biofeedback, the individual is trained to observe measurable changes of his or her bodily function such as pulse, heart rate, and other body measures that are related to stress. These readings are observable to the individual, often on a computer screen, and the person is then trained to lower these rates with relaxation. As the vital signs slow down, so does the pressure and tension in the body as well. Biofeedback may be helpful with individuals who have high levels of stress and anxiety. Biofeedback is very helpful in patients with chronic constipation especially those with pelvic dyssynergia or dyssynergic defecation.

Chiropractic Manipulation   Chiropractic is the manipulation of the spine and is largely used to treat back pain, neck pain, and headache. Chiropractors may also provide counseling about diet, dietary supplements, and weight loss. Many Americans rely upon chiropractors; for example, in 2007, 18.7 million American adults had chiropractic treatments. Chiropractic practitioners earn a doctor of chiropractic (DC) from a college that is accredited by the Council on Chiropractic Education. Each state has its own laws on the regulation of chiropractic therapy.

TABLE 8: FREQUENCIES AND PERCENTAGES OF CHILDREN YOUNGER THAN 18 YEARS OF AGE WHO USED COMPLEMENTARY AND ALTERNATIVE MEDICINE IN THE PAST 12 MONTHS BY SELECTED DISEASES AND CONDITIONS FOR WHICH IT WAS USED: UNITED STATES, 2007

Disease or Condition	Number in thousands	Percent
Back or neck pain	705	6.7
Anxiety or stress	427	4.8
Other musculoskeletal	378	4.2
ADHD/ADD	237	2.5
Insomnia or trouble sleeping	158	1.8
Asthma	137	1.6
Sinusitis	117	1.5
Depression	110	1.0
Abdominal pain	75	0.8

Source: Adapted from Barnes, Patricia M., and Barbara Bloom. "Complementary and Alternative Medicine Use Among Adults and Children: United States, 2007." *National Health Statistics Reports* 18 (December 10, 2008): 13.

Hypnosis Hypnosis, also known as hypnotherapy, places the individual in a voluntary trancelike state in which he or she is suggestible to making changes, such as giving up smoking or eating less so that they can lose weight. Sometimes hypnosis is used for minor surgery or procedures as well. There are many practitioners of hypnosis, ranging from physicians to individuals with lesser degrees and credentials. About 561,000 American adults used hypnotherapy in 2007. It has been used with some benefit in patients with functional dyspepsia as well as for the prevention of recurrences in patients with healed duodenal ulcer. Gut-oriented hypnosis accelerates gastric emptying in dyspeptic as well as healthy subjects

Massage Therapy Massage therapy is provided by licensed practitioners, generally for pain relief. It may also be used to alleviate stress, increase relaxation and rehabilitate individuals with sports injuries. There are different types of massage, including Swedish massage, in which the therapist uses deep circular movements, vibration, kneading, and tapping. Trigger point massage, in contrast, concentrates on painful muscle points. Reflexology is massage applied to the feet, hands, or ears to promote healing and relaxation.

According to the NCCAM, the following cautions should be observed by those considering massage therapy:

- Vigorous massage should be avoided by individuals with bleeding disorders, low blood platelet counts, or those taking blood thinning medications such as warfarin (Coumadin).

- Massage should be avoided in any areas with fractures, open wounds, blood clots, or bones weakened from osteoporosis or cancer as well as any part of the body that has recently been treated surgically.

- Cancer patients should consult with their oncologists before receiving deep massage. They should not receive massage pressure over any area that includes a tumor.

- Pregnant women should discuss whether massage therapy is advisable for them.

Progressive Relaxation Progressive relaxation is a form of therapy in which the individual is taught to relax groups of muscles throughout the body, often starting at one end of the body and working through to the opposite end. For example, the person is told to relax the muscles of the head and face, letting go of the tension and stress of the day. The neck may be the next area that is addressed, as many people carry tension in their neck. Relaxation exercises can reduce the number of episodes of gastroesophageal reflux and the symptoms of heartburn in patients with GERD.

Problems and Risks of Alternative Medicine

One problem with alternative remedies is that many patients assume if a drug is "natural," such as virtually any herbal remedy or mineral supplement that they purchase in a health food store or in a pharmacy, then it must be completely safe. This is an erroneous belief, because some herbal remedies or supplements, just as with other medications, can be harmful to some individuals. Just because a substance is natural does not mean it is safe: poison ivy is a natural substance as is snake venom, and both are harmful to humans. For example, the herb *Ginkgo biloba* is a blood thinner, and if the patient is already taking a blood-thinning medication such as warfarin (Coumadin), the addition of the *Ginkgo biloba* could contribute to internal bleeding and, in rare instances, even to death.

For this reason, it is crucially important that patients who are taking herbal remedies or supplements (or who even seriously think about taking them) should first check with their doctor to make sure that the herb or supplement will not be harmful to them and also that it will not interact with any other medications they are taking. At the least, the drug should not be harmful. It would also be helpful if the drug provided the relief that patients seek, although the federal law does not require any scientific confirmation that the remedy is efficacious.

It is also extremely important for parents considering alternative remedies for their children to consult with the child's pediatrician first before beginning the therapy. Sicker children are more likely to be given alternative remedies, but such children may be taking prescribed or over-the-counter medications that could interact with herbs, supplements, or natural remedies. Children are not small adults; instead, they are growing individuals who can be greatly affected by the use of drugs, whether they are prescribed, over-the-counter, or remedies purchased in a health food store or online.

Benefits of Alternative Remedies

Despite some problems with alternative remedies, it is clear that there are also many benefits that people may gain from their use. Some herbal remedies can improve digestion, constipation, and other digestive and health problems. Patients with chronic medical problems should be sure to see their physician to make sure that there are no serious medical risks. In addition, some alternative treatments can considerably reduce the physical pain and distress that is caused by a wide variety of ailments, including digestive diseases and disorders.

See also FISH OIL; INFLAMMATORY BOWEL DISEASE; IRON; MAGNESIUM; SELENIUM; VITAMIN DEFICIENCIES/EXCESSES.

Barnes, Patricia M., and Barbara Bloom. "Complementary and Alternative Medicine Use Among Adults and Children: United States, 2007." *National Health Statistics Reports* 18 (December 10, 2008):1–24.

Gardner, Paula. "Complementary, Holistic, and Integrative Medicine: Chamomile." *Pediatrics in Review* 28, no. 4 (2007): 16–18.

General Accounting Office. *Dietary Supplements: FDA Should Take Further Actions to Improve Oversight and Consumer Understanding. Report to Congressional Requesters.* Washington, D.C.: General Accounting Office, January 2009.

Jonas, Wayne B., M.D., Ted J. Kaptchuk, and Klaus Linde, M.D. "A Critical Overview of Homeopathy." Annals of Internal Medicine 138, no. 5 (2003): 393–399.

Minocha, Anil, M.D., with David Carroll. *Natural Stomach Care.* New York: Penguin Putnam, 2003.

Minocha, Anil, M.D., and Christine Adamec. *How to Stop Heartburn: Simple Ways to Heal Heartburn and Acid Reflux.* New York: John Wiley & Sons, 2001.

Nahin, Richard L., et al. "Costs of Complementary and Alternative Medicine (CAM) and Frequency of Visits to CAM Practitioners: United States, 2007." *National Health Statistics Report* 18 (July 30, 2009): 1–15.

Onken, J. E., et al. "Bromelain Treatment Decreases Secretion of Pro-Inflammatory Cytokines and Chemokines by Colon Biopsies in Vitro." *Clinical Immunology* 126 (2008): 345–352.

Spence, David S., Elizabeth A. Thompson, and S. J. Barron. "Homeopathic Treatment for Chronic Disease: A 6-Year, University-Hospital Outpatient Observational Study." *Journal of Alternative and Complementary Medicine* 11, no. 5 (2005): 793–798.

Von Arnim, et al. "STW 5, a Phytopharmacon for Patients with Functional Dyspepsia: Results of a Multicenter, Placebo-controlled Double-blind Study." *American Journal of Gastroenterology* 102, no. 6 (2007): 1,268–1,275.

amebiasis   An infection of the intestine or liver that is caused by a parasite that can be found in the human intestinal tract or human feces: *Entamoeba histolytica*. About 40 to 50 million people worldwide experience amebiasis each year, and the disease accounts for an estimated 40,000 deaths per year.

Amebiasis is most commonly transmitted through contaminated food or water or contamination that results when people have failed to wash their hands after having a bowel movement and then prepare contaminated food to be consumed by others. The parasite in its cyst form is then transmitted in the food, which is swallowed by the new host. The person's digestive juices break down the cyst, and the parasite is then able to invade the body and grow, unless or until it is diagnosed and treated. The parasite can also be spread during anal intercourse. Usually, only the large intestines of the affected person are involved; however, the liver, lungs, heart, and even brain may also become infected.

Symptoms and Diagnostic Path

The majority of patients remain asymptomatic. Children, pregnant women, elderly individuals, and patients with cancer, alcoholism, human immunodeficiency virus (HIV), and immunodeficiency are more likely to have symptoms.

The infected person who experiences symptoms may not do so for one to three weeks or longer. When they occur, symptoms include ABDOMINAL PAIN, JAUNDICE, DIARRHEA, DYSENTERY, ANOREXIA, fatigue, and weight loss. If untreated, the PARASITIC INFECTION can cause ulcers in the colon and intestinal blockages, and it can also cause death if the parasite invades organs such as the liver or the brain.

Physicians may suspect an amebiasis infection because of a patient's symptoms, but cannot be sure until a stool specimen is analyzed and yields a positive result. Blood tests for amebiasis are also used.

The physician may order a lower gastrointestinal study, such as a sigmoidoscopy or a colonoscopy. A liver abscess may be identified by ultrasound or by a computed tomography (CT) scan.

Treatment Options and Outlook

Medications such as metronidazole (Flagyl) are prescribed to destroy the parasite. Chlorine alone is not adequate to kill the amebic cysts when they are found in contaminated water; the water must be boiled. Disinfection with iodine is also effective. It is best to avoid sexual practices that lead to feco-oral contact.

Risk Factors and Preventive Measures

The infection is more common in poor countries, although outbreaks can occur in developed countries, such as when water is contaminated.

See also CONTAMINATED FOOD OR WATER.

amylase An enzyme that is produced by the body to break down the carbohydrates in food. Saliva includes amylase in the first phase of digestion when food is first eaten. Most of the amylase that is seen in the blood is secreted by the PANCREAS so that the final digestion of carbohydrates can be completed in the intestine. Blood levels of amylase are elevated among patients with PANCREATITIS. Lipase is another pancreatic enzyme that is elevated in pancreatitis.

An acute rise of serum amylase may be seen in bile duct obstruction by a stone, which is then followed by a rapid decline as the stone passes. Amylase is also secreted by the salivary glands and salivary amylase has a limited role in digestion of food. Amylase is derived from the Greek word *amylone*, which means "starch." Smaller amounts of amylase can be found in tissues besides the pancreas and salivary glands. Amylase occurs in several forms (isoforms). The normal values of serum amylase vary depending upon the assay used. Serum amylase levels may be increased in renal failure since kidneys are involved in its excretion. Serum amylase may be bound to other molecules in blood giving rise to macroamylasemia. Macroamylasemia may occur in CELIAC DISEASE, HIV infection, LYMPHOMA, ULCERATIVE COLITIS,

and rheumatoid arthritis. Serum levels may not be increased in all patients with pancreatitis, whereas it may be elevated in gastroenteritis. Many drugs may cause an increase in amylase levels, including aspirin, cimetidine, estrogens, and thiazide diuretics.

amyloidosis A rare disease that is characterized by deposits of amyloid in the organs and tissues. Amyloid is composed of fibrils made up of small subunits of a variety of proteins, many of which may be seen circulating in the blood. The protein fragments may be deposited in the gastrointestinal system, the heart, the kidneys, the brain, the nerves, and the hand. When found in the gastrointestinal system, amyloidosis may cause slow gut motility, and cause GASTROPARESIS and MALABSORPTION syndrome. An estimated one in 100,000 people in the United States carries the genetic mutations for this disease.

There are two forms of amyloidosis: primary amyloidosis and secondary amyloidosis. Primary amyloidosis usually affects the tongue, the gastrointestinal tract, the thyroid gland, the liver, and the spleen. It may also affect the heart and can cause congestive heart failure. Secondary amyloidosis is usually found in conjunction with another disease that is present, such as rheumatoid arthritis or frequent infections. It is more likely to affect the kidneys, liver, and spleen and may also cause skin inflammation. Secondary amyloidosis may cause kidney failure.

Symptoms and Diagnostic Path

Amyloidosis can cause as well as result from disease of other organs. Symptoms of the disease depend upon the organ where the amyloid is deposited and/or on the underlying condition that led to the amyloidosis. In the digestive system, amyloidosis may cause bleeding due to colitis. It may also produce lazy stomach (GASTROPARESIS) and slow intestinal movements, causing constipation, an overgrowth of bacteria in the small intestine, and intestinal pseudoobstruction. Problems in other systems of the body that can be caused by amyloidosis include heart and kidney failure, irregular heart rhythms, heart attack, weight loss, lightheadedness, shortness of breath, and weakness. The disease eventually kills the patient.

The diagnosis of amyloidosis can only be made by a biopsy, the removal and examination of tissue. In primary amyloidosis, the organ that is affected is treated. Gastrointestinal amyloidosis usually does not cause death, and the treatment is directed at the problem. For example, patients who have gastroparesis may be helped by taking PROKINETIC medications, and those patients who have a bacterial overgrowth benefit from taking antibiotics. In cases of hepatic amyloidosis, a liver transplantation is needed. In secondary amyloidosis, the treatment involves treating the underlying cause that has led to amyloidosis.

Risk Factors and Preventive Measures

The risk factors for amyloidosis are unknown, although genetic factors are known to be involved in many cases.

Falk, Rodney H., M.D., Raymond L. Comenzo, M.D., and Martha Skinner, M.D. "The Systemic Amyloidoses." *New England Journal of Medicine* 337, no. 13 (September 25, 1997): 898–909.

Wynbrandt, James, and Mark D. Ludman. "Amyloidosis (genetics)." *The Encyclopedia of Genetic Disorders and Birth Defects.* 2d ed. New York: Facts On File, 2000.

anal cancer   A tumor that occurs in the anus, which is the outlet of the bowel. According to the National Cancer Institute, there were an estimated 5,070 new cases of anal cancer in the United States in 2008, and 680 people died of anal cancer in 2008.

Of all large bowel cancers, anal cancer represents only 1 to 2 percent of the cases. About 65 to 80 percent of patients with anal cancer survive five years or more. Unlike most other forms of digestive cancer, which are adenocarcinomas, most anal cancer (about 70 percent) is of the squamous cell carcinoma type. Anal cancer is often also identified as a sexually transmitted disease because it is associated with the human papillomavirus (HPV), which may be transmitted by anal sex. As a result, one cause of anal cancer is unprotected anal sex. However, not all patients with anal cancer have participated in anal sex.

Symptoms and Diagnostic Path

The primary symptoms of anal cancer are pain as well as bleeding, itching, discharge, and a lump around the anus; however, sometimes there are minimal or no symptoms. The physician performs an inspection of the anal region and does a digital rectal examination (DRE). If anal cancer appears present, the physician performs an anoscopy and a biopsy to remove tissue from the area to check for cancer cells. If anal cancer is diagnosed, the physician usually also orders a pelvic computed tomography (CT) scan and may also order an ultrasound of the anal area. The cancer is staged as to how advanced it is and whether it has spread beyond the anal area.

Many of the symptoms of anal cancer can be seen with other illnesses, and consequently, a person who has these symptoms should not assume that he or she has anal cancer. Only a physician can make that determination.

Treatment Options and Outlook

The treatment of anal cancer depends on the type of the tumor and its location, as well as whether it arises from the anal margin or the anal canal and whether it is an adenocarcinoma or squamous cell carcinoma. The treatment modalities for anal cancer include resection, radiation, or chemotherapy plus radiation therapy. After treatment has been completed, patients should be seen at regular intervals as determined by their doctors.

Anal cancer usually does not spread to distant sites (less than 20 percent spread). When it does spread, the liver is the most frequent site of the distant spread. Such patients are treated with chemotherapy.

Risk Factors and Preventive Measures

Most patients with anal cancer (about 80 percent) are ages 50 to 60 years old. Smoking is associated with an increase in anal cancer rate. Kidney transplantation patients have approximately 100 times greater risk of development of anal cancer. There are no known racial or genetic risks associated with development of anal cancer.

There is a slight preponderance of females over males, except for anal cancer that is associated with human immunodeficiency virus (HIV) infection. While the risk of anal cancer is higher in the HIV population, it is unclear if HIV/AIDS is an independent risk factor for anal cancer.

Studies of females and heterosexual males have indicated that people who have had 10 or more sexual partners, as well as those who have had genital or anal warts, have the highest risk of development of anal cancer. In addition, women with sexual partners who have been diagnosed with sexually transmitted diseases also have an increased risk of anal cancer. Studies also indicate that women with anal cancer are more likely to be diagnosed with vaginal or cervical cancer as well.

The presence of hemorrhoids, fissures, and fistulae does not increase the risk of development of anal cancer.

One preventive measure against anal cancer is to avoid having 10 or more sexual partners.

See also COLORECTAL CANCER; CONDYLOMA ACUMINATUM.

anal warts   See CONDYLOMA ACUMINATUM.

anemia   An illness that is characterized by an insufficiency of red blood cells. For practical purposes, anemia is a reduction in one of the red blood cell measurements, such as hemoglobin, hematocrit, or the red blood cell count.

Symptoms and Diagnostic Path

The key symptoms of anemia are as follows:

- chronic fatigue
- weakness
- headache
- shortness of breath
- sore tongue
- worsening of other illnesses, such as heart disease or cognitive impairment
- DIZZINESS/lightheadedness
- frequent infections
- PICA (a perverted desire to eat nonfoods, such as dirt or clay, or to constantly eat ice [pagophagia], which sometimes results from iron deficiency anemia)

Anemia is identified with a complete blood count (CBC), a test that determines the number of red blood cells, white blood cells, and platelets. In general, anemia is diagnosed if the patient's hematocrit levels on a blood test are less than 41 percent in adult males and less than 36 percent in adult females; however, normal values may vary between laboratories. Anemia is a manifestation of an underlying medical problem; therefore, further testing is needed to determine the specific type of anemia, unless the problem is clearly due to bleeding.

The size of the red blood cells provides clues. Small red blood cell size (microcytic anemia) is seen in iron deficiency, as well as the anemia of chronic disease, and, rarely, with copper deficiency. It is also seen with lead poisoning, sideroblastic anemia, thalassemia, and other hemoglobin disorders.

An increase in red blood cell size (macrocytic anemia) occurs with folic acid and vitamin B_{12} deficiency. It is also seen after cancer chemotherapy and with acute leukemia, alcoholism, liver disease, and hypothyroidism (low thyroid level).

The red blood cell size may also be normal in anemia, especially in mild cases or in anemia that is caused by chronic diseases.

Treatment Options and Outlook

The treatment of anemia depends on the cause of the illness; for example, if the physician believes that it is a temporary problem, such as with a short-term case of iron deficiency anemia, then the use of iron supplements may resolve the anemia. In addition, patients with this condition are advised to eat foods that are rich in iron and following these instructions will usually improve their blood levels. At the same time, the cause of the iron deficiency anemia must be investigated and treated.

Patients who are unable to absorb iron from the intestines need to receive intravenous iron therapy. Patients with folate or B_{12} deficiency need appropriate supplementation of B_{12}. If the anemia is a long-term, chronic problem, then the continued use of supplements may be needed, and treatment is targeted at the cause. In some extreme cases of anemia, bone marrow transplantation is the only way to resolve the anemia completely and to prevent further and more severe consequences.

Patients with sickle cell anemia may require painkilling medications for pain control and may also need transfusions. Bone marrow transplantation (BMT) offers hope for the cure of sickle cell anemia; however it has its own risks. If BMT is undertaken, it should occur before there is irreversible organ damage. BMT requires the identification of patients at high risk for end organ damage as early as possible. Another option is gene therapy, which is experimental, in its infancy, and has the potential to cure SCD.

If the anemia is caused by cancer, chronic kidney disease, or congestive heart failure, then the prognosis is not as good. The patient may be treated with blood transfusions for severe anemia. Patients are frequently treated with high doses of erythropoiesis-stimulating agents (ESAs), which are genetically engineered drugs that were specifically created to treat anemia by simulating the function of erythropoietin, a substance that is naturally made by the kidney and which creates red blood cells. However, in 2007, the Food and Drug Administration (FDA) issued a strong "black box" warning that studies had indicated ESAs were linked to an increased risk for heart attack, stroke, blood clots, and death in some patients with chronic kidney disease. The warning also stated that patients with some forms of cancer (head or neck cancer or breast cancer that had spread) had a higher death risk with these drugs. Even dosages at the recommended levels caused problems in some patients.

Treatment modalities for thalassemia, an inherited form of anemia, include chronic transfusion therapy, chelation to reduce iron load, and splenectomy, which is the removal of the spleen. It is estimated that there are more than 100 different genetic mutations of thalassemia beta; bone marrow transplantation is being increasingly used for the treatment of severe cases. Phlebotomy to reduce iron levels in the body is not an option in transfusion-dependent patients. Iron chelators are used.

Use of chelation therapy early in childhood improves survival of patients with beta thalassemia major. One example of such chelators is deferoxamine. In the circulation and tissues, it binds iron and this bound form of iron is then excreted in the urine, and bile thus removing iron from the body.

Risk Factors and Preventive Measures

The risk for the development of anemia increases with age and it is usually due to the presence of associated severe chronic diseases, such as kidney or heart disease, rather than aging itself. However, women who have heavy menstrual periods are also at risk for the development of anemia.

Race and heredity are other risk factors for anemia: Hereditary forms of anemia include sickle-cell anemia, found in some African Americans, and Fanconi's anemia, found in some Jews of Ashkenazi descent.

Sometimes an individual's own chosen diet can cause iron deficiency anemia, as when a person chooses to eat no meat, poultry, or fish. Vegetarians or others who completely avoid eating meats, poultry, or fish may develop iron deficiency anemia because plants have a lower concentration of iron than is needed by the body. If individuals with this type of induced anemia improve their diet by eating meat, then in most cases, the deficiency is resolved, although iron supplements may also be required for a brief period. Cooking foods in iron utensils can also help to augment their iron content.

Patients with kidney failure who are being treated with dialysis may also have low levels of iron and may also have deficiencies of folic acid. Other factors leading to anemia for dialysis patients include gastrointestinal blood loss, blood loss that results from having multiple laboratory tests, blood retention in the dialysis machine system, and a shortened red blood cell survival time.

In considering patients with iron deficiency anemia, it is important to note that iron supplements should *not* be taken unless they are specifically recommended by a physician, because an iron overload can become a problem when supplements are taken unnecessarily. When a doctor recommends iron supplements, the patient should avoid enteric-coated iron supplements because they may be excreted intact in the stool or they may release iron too far down the intestinal tract to be maximally absorbed.

The ingestion of iron along with cereals, dietary fiber, tea, coffee, eggs, or milk can also reduce its absorption.

Patients should not take iron at the same that they take some other medications, such as antacids because iron absorption is reduced. In addition, iron should be taken with water or juice on an empty stomach for maximal absorption and effectiveness. People with iron absorption problems should also avoid drinking tea with their meals, since it can impair iron absorption.

Some people are unable to absorb sufficient iron in the food that they eat, and only intravenous iron that is given on a regular basis can resolve their anemia. Some good sources of iron are liver, egg yolks, dried fruits, and red meats.

Types of Anemia and Causes

The most common form of anemia is *iron deficiency anemia*, which is a medical problem in which the patient has been bleeding or lacks sufficient iron in the body. Iron deficiency anemia may stem from a gastrointestinal blood loss that is caused by peptic ULCERS, tumors, or the heavy use of NONSTEROIDAL ANTI-INFLAMMATORY DRUGS (NSAIDs). These are medications that are often prescribed to treat many different ailments, such as arthritis, back pain, and other chronic pain disorders. Women and teenage girls who have heavy menstrual periods are also prone to the development of iron deficiency anemia, as are pregnant women.

Anemia of chronic disease is another common form of anemia, and according to Weiss and Goodnough in their article in the *New England Journal of Medicine* in 2005, it is the second-most common form of anemia after iron deficiency anemia. The anemia of chronic disease is caused by such conditions as acute and chronic bacterial and viral infections, parasitic or fungal infections, rheumatoid arthritis, systemic lupus erythematosus, sarcoidosis, INFLAMMATORY BOWEL DISEASE, chronic kidney disease, and the rejection of solid organ transplants. Individuals who have the HUMAN IMMUNODEFICIENCY VIRUS (HIV) are also at high risk for the development of anemia, since they have little or no resistance to infections.

The other main forms of anemia include sickle cell anemia (which is primarily diagnosed among African Americans) and thalassemia (which is primarily diagnosed among people whose family originated in the Mediterranean area and in tropical areas, as in Africa, Indonesia, and southern China). People who have sickle cell anemia are prone to

experiencing a high rate of infections, gallstones, and bone damage.

The most prominent forms of thalassemia are thalassemia alpha and thalassemia beta. Alpha thalassemia is more commonly seen among people from Southeast Asia; beta thalassemia is found among people from the Mediterranean area of the globe. Of the two, thalassemia beta is more severe. It results in an iron overload and skull and facial deformities. Thalassemia beta can also retard growth, can cause heart disease and osteoporosis, and may also lead to other health problems.

Aplastic anemia is another cause of anemia. This is a rare condition in which the bone marrow cannot produce red blood cells. It may be induced by exposure to some drugs, chemicals, or heavy metals. Treatment options include bone marrow transplantation and immunosuppressive therapy.

Fanconi's anemia (FA), named after the 20th-century Swiss pediatrician Guido Fanconi, is another inherited disorder of anemia. It causes a form of aplastic anemia. Children who have Fanconi's anemia have low birth weight, poor growth, microcephaly (a small head), and short stature. Children with Fanconi's anemia may also have heart defects and deafness. Several different mutations of this form of anemia have been identified in the Netherlands as well as among individuals of Ashkenazi Jewish descent. Patients with FA have a high cancer risk, especially for the development of myelodysplastic syndrome, leukemia, and head and neck cancer. Treatment options include androgen therapy and bone marrow transplantation.

PERNICIOUS ANEMIA is an autoimmune disorder that is characterized by the body creating antibodies to intrinsic factor, which is vital for the absorption of vitamin B_{12}. This medical problem leads to a deficiency of vitamin B_{12}.

Sometimes anemia is caused by medications or treatments, such as in the case of chemotherapy that is given to patients in order to treat many forms of cancer. People with chronic alcoholism often have anemia caused by the alcohol suppressing the bone marrow, and producing liver dysfunction, as well as poor nutrition.

Rarely, if a mild anemia is found in a person who is also a regular runner, the problem may be "runner's anemia," which may be caused by the regular and frequent destruction of blood cells during running when the feet hit the hard ground for a long time and/or when blood is lost from the gut.

See also HEMOCHROMATOSIS; IRON; VITAMIN DEFICIENCIES/EXCESSES.

Mitka, Mike, "FDA Sounds Alarm on Anemia Drugs." *Journal of the American Medical Association* 297, no. 17 (May 2, 2007): 1,868–1,869.

Olivieri, Nancy F., M.D. "The g-Thalassemias." *New England Journal of Medicine* 341, no. 2 (July 8, 1999): 99–109.

Weiss, Guenter, M.D., and Lawrence T. Goodnough, M.D., "Anemia of Chronic Disease." *New England Journal of Medicine* 352, no. 10 (March 10, 2005): 1,011–1,023.

anorexia nervosa A very serious EATING DISORDER that is characterized by self-starvation, behavior that, when present, is usually evinced by people (mostly female) who have a distorted body image and who mistakenly believe that they are obese (although the reverse is true and the individual may instead appear starving). They may also fear that they will become obese should they forgo rigidly controlling their eating. The term *anorexia* by itself indicates a lack of appetite; for example, in some cases, elderly individuals are anorexic because they are too ill to eat much and/or are incapable of preparing their own food or feeding themselves; however, these individuals do not have anorexia nervosa.

Symptoms and Diagnostic Path

People who have anorexia nervosa may appear extremely thin or may be slender and intent on losing more weight. The absence of menstruation (amenorrhea) for three or more months is one possible sign of anorexia nervosa. A significant weight loss is a possible indicator, particularly if the individual is less than about 85 percent of the normal body weight for his or her height. Patients with anorexia nervosa exhibit a fear of gaining weight. Female athletes, ballet dancers, and models are at elevated risk of development of anorexia nervosa, since very thin body types are admired by their peers. Females (or males) who have type 1 diabetes may appear thin, and diabetes should be ruled out

as the cause of a recent weight loss. People who have anorexia nervosa sometimes abuse laxatives in order to keep their weight down.

Anorexia nervosa may be diagnosed by an internist or a family practitioner, although sometimes it is diagnosed by a psychiatrist and treated in part as an emotional disorder. The differential diagnosis includes screening for new onset DIABETES MELLITUS, adrenal insufficiency, depression (although the presence of depression does not exclude anorexia nervosa), CROHN'S DISEASE, CELIAC DISEASE, or eosinophilic gastroenteritis and brain tumors. A beta-hCG test should be done to exclude pregnancy in women of childbearing ages.

Treatment Options and Outlook

When medications are prescribed, anorexia nervosa may be treated with antidepressants, such as fluoxetine (Prozac). Therapy is often needed to help the individual adjust the mental image of a distorted body perception to the person's actual appearance. In extreme cases, individuals with anorexia nervosa may need to be hospitalized, either in a standard hospital or in a rehabilitation facility that specializes in treating people with anorexia nervosa. Inpatient treatment is especially indicated if the patient has the following conditions:

- hypotension
- a low pulse rate of less than 50 beats per minute or a fast pulse rate greater than 100 beats per minute
- an extremely severe weight loss resulting in body weight that is 25 to 30 percent below normal body weight
- heart arrhythmias

When a patient's weight increases to within a normal range (about 90 percent of normal body weight), menstruation may resume within about six months.

Risk Factors and Preventive Measures

Anorexia nervosa is commonly considered a problem of teenage girls, but women and males of all ages may exhibit its signs. In rare cases, anorexia nervosa may be confused with Addison's disease, which can produce similar symptoms of extreme weight loss, nausea and vomiting, and weakness and fatigue.

Sometimes in the early stages of Addison's disease, an endocrine disorder of the adrenal glands, patients have weight loss and lack of appetite and may be misdiagnosed with anorexia nervosa. Patients with anorexia nervosa are more likely to have *high* levels of cortisol in contrast with the hypocortisolism seen in Addison's disease. Anorexia nervosa patients are more likely to be hyperglycemic (with high blood sugar); patients with Addison's disease are more likely to be hypoglycemic (with abnormally low blood sugar). Last, anorexia nervosa patients often have low potassium blood levels, whereas Addison's disease patients are hyperkalemic (have excessively high levels of potassium in the blood).

There are no known preventive measures for anorexia nervosa. If the disorder occurs, it should be treated.

See also BULIMIA NERVOSA; LAXATIVES AND LAXATIVE ABUSE.

antacids Over-the-counter medications that significantly neutralize the level of gastric acid in individuals. Antacids are usually used by patients who suffer from acute or chronic indigestion. When antacids are taken infrequently or rarely, they are usually used to treat indigestion or heartburn caused by overeating. However, some individuals take antacids very often and even daily, and such people need medical attention. They may have a peptic ulcer, GASTROESOPHAGEAL REFLUX DISEASE, or a variety of other illnesses that physicians can diagnose and treat. Common antacids contain calcium (Tums), aluminum, and magnesium. Some antacids contain a combination of these elements. Calcium and aluminum cause constipation, whereas magnesium may cause diarrhea.

When treated in the early stages, chronic illnesses that patients sometimes self-treat with antacids may be relatively easy to resolve. Chronic antacid treatment can be expensive and have serious side effects. In addition, if patients treat themselves for years with over-the-counter antacids

before telling a physician about the problem, the condition may have become very serious over that period. At times, the first-time patient may be seen in the hospital emergency room with a possible bleeding ulcer or a food blockage located in the esophagus (such as a piece of meat) in the case of stricture (narrowing) of the esophagus due to gastroesophageal reflux disease (GERD).

See also ACID REFLUX; HISTAMINE-2 BLOCKERS; PROTON PUMP INHIBITORS.

antibiotics Antibacterial medications that are derived from live organisms and that are given to fight diagnosed or suspected bacterial infections. There are many different types of antibiotics, and many of them may have side effects on the digestive system, causing gastrointestinal upset, CONSTIPATION, or DIARRHEA. *Pseudomembranous colitis* may occur as a result of most antibiotics and can cause diarrhea and bleeding. Physicians may advise taking the antibiotic with food or with milk, although some antibiotics may be more effective when taken on an empty stomach.

Patients who know that a particular antibiotic upsets their stomach should advise their physician, who may be able to prescribe a different antibiotic when one is needed. Patients should advise their pharmacist of the problem as well, because pharmacists are aware of medications that are in the same group and can warn patients and doctors away from some medications, particularly newer drugs.

See also *HELICOBACTER PYLORI; LACTOBACILLUS;* THRUSH.

antidepressants Medications that are given to counteract the effects of clinical depression, a state of extreme and clinical sadness characterized by an inability to find joy in former activities and by constant thoughts of death. However, low doses of antidepressants are also often prescribed for individuals to combat other illnesses, such as IRRITABLE BOWEL SYNDROME (IBS), noncardiac chest pain, and other chronic pain conditions. These doses are too low to combat clinical depression but may be efficacious in other disorders.

antidiarrheals Prescribed or over-the-counter (OTC) drugs that are taken to counteract DIARRHEA. Such drugs may be given in the form of oral medication or liquid suspension. If the drug is an OTC medication, such as loperamide (Imodium), the patient is usually instructed to take it after a bowel movement and then again after any subsequent loose stools that occur. If the medication is a prescribed drug, such as diphenoxylate hydrochloride and atropine sulfate (Lomotil), then similar instructions may be given.

It is important to follow the instructions carefully, because taking too many antidiarrheal drugs can lead to CONSTIPATION, whereas taking too few can be ineffectual. Some patients may also need prescribed ANTIBIOTICS depending upon the cause of diarrhea. Patients who have diarrhea that is accompanied by bleeding and weight loss must always consult their physician and not rely on treating themselves with OTC antidiarrheal medications.

See also IRRITABLE BOWEL SYNDROME; LAXATIVES AND LAXATIVE ABUSE.

antiemetics Prescribed or over-the-counter drugs that are taken to prevent nausea and vomiting. Commonly used examples are promethazine (Phenergan) and prochlorperazine (Compazine). Newer and more potent antiemetics include ondansetron (Zofran) and granisetron (Kytril). Among alternative medicines, ginger is a popular remedy for the nausea and vomiting of pregnancy.

See also NAUSEA AND VOMITING.

antioxidants Substances that dispose of the toxic-free radicals that are generated in chemical reactions in the body, thus reducing or preventing damage to body tissues. Antioxidants include vitamins A, C, and E. Many other chemicals, such as selenium, are antioxidants. In addition, vegetables and fruits have ingredients that have antioxidant-like properties. Antioxidants have been identified as possibly effective in preventing cancer and are often added to food or taken as supplements. Some foods, such as tomatoes, are high in various vitamins as well as in antioxidants. Researchers performing a variety of clinical studies are seeking to determine the full extent of the effects of antioxidants.

It should be noted, however, that a systematic review of studies by Bjelakovic and colleagues of synthetic antioxidants (which did not include taking fruits and vegetables) indicated that some substances, particularly beta carotene, vitamin A, and vitamin E, may *increase* the risk for death. The researchers looked at 67 clinical studies with 232,550 participants.

They concluded, "We did not find convincing evidence that antioxidant supplements have beneficial effects on mortality. Even more, beta carotene, vitamin A, and vitamin E seem to increase the risk of death. Further randomized trials are needed to establish the effects of vitamin C and selenium."

See also IRON; SELENIUM; VITAMIN DEFICIENCIES/EXCESSES; ZINC.

Bjelakovic, Goran, D. Nikolova, L. L. Gluud, R. G. Simonetti, and C. Gluud. "Antioxidant supplements for prevention of mortality in healthy participants and patients with various diseases." *Cochrane Database Systematic Review* 2 (April 16, 2008): CD007176.

Bjelakovic, Goran, M.D., et al. "Mortality in Randomized Trials of Antioxidant Supplements for Primary and Secondary Prevention: Systematic Review and Meta-analysis." *Journal of the American Medical Association* 297, no. 8 (February 28, 2007): 842–857.

appendicitis An inflammation of the appendix, an abdominal organ in the lower right side whose purpose is unknown and which appears to be vestigial. The appendix is a small pouch or appendage connected to the cecum, which is the beginning of the colon. The appendix can rupture (burst), endangering other organs and even the person's life. Appendicitis is usually but not always very painful and requires an appendectomy, which is the removal of the entire appendix. (See EMERGENCY ISSUES IN DIGESTIVE DISORDERS.)

The cause of appendicitis is usually a blockage of the appendicial lumen. In young individuals, the blockage occurs as a result of a viral or bacterial infection, causing an increase of the lymph tissue of the appendix and leading to obstruction. In older subjects, the blockage may be due to a hard stool that is impacting the appendix. Appendicitis may also occur among older subjects as a result of cancer, PARASITIC INFECTIONS, or the scarring of the appendix. Rarely, it may occur as a result of COLONOSCOPY. Untreated appendicitis can lead to gangrene and PERITONITIS, which are both life-threatening conditions.

About 250,000 patients per year are hospitalized for the diagnosis of appendicitis in the United States. Many medical problems can mimic the symptoms of appendicitis, such as bladder infections, severe CONSTIPATION, and acute PANCREATITIS. Appendicitis is the most common surgical reason for hospitalizing children, and children younger than age 18 have a rate of about four appendectomies per 1,000.

In one study of 524 patients by Anil Minocha, M.D., and colleagues, those who had had a prior appendectomy were compared to a control group of 469 individuals who had no history of appendectomy. The patients with prior appendectomy (the study group) were more likely to have undergone an ENDOSCOPY (33 percent) than the nonappendectomy patients (21 percent). It is unclear what the clinical significance of this finding is, and further study is indicated. In addition several studies, including one study by Dr. Minocha, have shown that a prior appendectomy may be protective against ULCERATIVE COLITIS.

Symptoms and Diagnostic Path

The general symptoms of appendicitis are as follows; all symptoms do not occur in all individuals.

- acute abdominal pain that starts in the midline near the navel and then localizes on the right side of the lower abdomen, usually for less than 72 hours, and is increasingly severe
- NAUSEA and sometimes VOMITING
- chills and shaking
- constipation or diarrhea
- low fever (about 100°F or 37.7°C)
- lack of APPETITE
- severe pain with gentle pressure on the abdomen, especially in the right lower part

There are no specific blood tests for appendicitis. There is an elevation of the white blood cell count, which is nonspecific, since it may occur due to a variety of causes, including an infection in the body. An ultrasound and computed tomography (CT) scan can identify the illness with a high degree of accuracy. Appendicitis is diagnosed on the basis of presenting symptoms, and the physician may also order tests such as a complete blood count to check for infection and urinalysis to rule out a bladder infection. The doctor may also order either an ultrasound or a computerized tomography (CT) scan to determine whether the appendix appears inflamed. Rarely, a laparoscopy is also performed, and if the laparoscopy confirms appendicitis, then the appendix is removed. In general, surgery is performed when patients are suspected to have acute appendicitis. In many cases an appendectomy can be performed via laparoscopic surgery rather than open surgery.

A 10 to 15 percent error rate (false positive, i.e., no appendicitis is found during surgery) is considered acceptable by experts. This false positive rate is declining as a result of advanced imaging studies that are available now.

Medical history is important Taking a careful medical history is essential to the diagnosis of appendicitis. The pain of appendicitis usually starts in the navel area and then localizes in the right lower abdomen. If abdominal pains have lasted longer than three to five days, the problem is less likely to be appendicitis, especially in a young patient. On the other hand, diagnosis is often delayed in atypical cases and among elderly subjects; in those cases a high rate of complications and even death results.

The doctor also observes the patient. If the patient is an active child with abdominal pains who is running around while also complaining about abdominal pains, the diagnosis is unlikely to be appendicitis, because patients with appendicitis are typically inactive and clearly in severe pain.

Using CT scans for diagnosis According to physicians Rao and colleagues in their article on using a CT scan of the appendix in a 1998 issue of the *New England Journal of Medicine*, CT scan is 93 to 98 percent accurate in diagnosing appendicitis. This is important because sometimes doctors misdiagnose appendicitis or diagnosis is delayed, and a delayed diagnosis increases the risk that the appendix may rupture and that postoperative complications may develop.

The researchers performed an appendiceal CT scan on 100 emergency room patients who were hospitalized for suspected appendicitis or who had been diagnosed with appendicitis and were scheduled for surgery. The researchers found that 53 of the 100 patients actually had appendicitis. The CT scan was 98 percent accurate, and the CT results led to treatment changes for more than half (59) of the patients. The researchers concluded that using a CT scan to check for appendicitis resulted in net savings of $447 per patient.

On rare occasions, appendicitis is diagnosed inadvertently during a colonoscopy examination; however, a colonoscopy should not be used for the diagnosis of appendicitis. In some cases, the colonoscopy has been known to induce appendicitis.

Treatment Options and Outlook

Doctors may not prescribe pain medications when they suspect appendicitis because they do not want the pain to mask any symptoms that can help establish a diagnosis. In cases of appendicitis when the diagnosis is delayed beyond five days or the appendix has ruptured to form an abscess, the illness is initially treated with antibiotics and intravenous fluids, later by surgery.

If the appendix is inflamed and is not removed in a timely manner, it can burst and damage the peritoneum, the sac that covers and protects the abdominal organs. This damage leads to inflammation of the peritoneum, known as peritonitis, and that can be life-threatening.

Some patients may have chronic appendicitis, presenting with chronic pain and fever, and with evidence of a mass or an abscess that is located in the right lower abdomen. Some of these patients may actually have recurrent acute appendicitis that had improved before the perforation occurred. Other causes of pain must be excluded before the diagnosis of chronic appendicitis is made. Surgery may be considered if no other nonsurgical causes of these symptoms are found.

The appendectomy The surgical removal of the appendix (appendectomy) is generally a safe procedure and deaths are rare in the United States (less than 1 percent). On rare occasions, when a patient is too sick to undergo surgery, a colonoscopy has been used to remove pus from the appendix and thus avoid surgery.

Risk Factors and Preventive Measures

Appendicitis is slightly more common among males. Most people diagnosed with appendicitis are below age 40, although individuals older than age 40 may experience it. The incidence of appendicitis peaks from the late teens to the early 20s. Younger children may also have appendicitis, but they are usually at least age two when the problem presents itself.

See also GALLSTONES; LIVER ABSCESS; PAIN.

Minocha, Anil, M.D. "An Endoscopic View of Appendicitis." *New England Journal of Medicine* 339, no. 20 (November 12, 1998): 1,481.

Minocha, Anil, M.D., et al. "Prevalence of Previous Appendectomy among Patients Needing Gastrointestinal Endoscopy." *Southern Medical Journal* 92, no. 1 (1994): 41–43.

Petro M, and A. Minocha: Asymptomatic early acute appendicitis initiated and diagnosed during colonoscopy: A case report. *World Journal of Gastroenterology.* (September 14, 2005), 11, no. 34: 5,398–5,400.

Qdick, Cive R. G., et al. "Appendicitis." In *Essential Surgery: Problems, Diagonsis and Management.* 3d ed. Edinburgh, Scotland: Churchill Livingstone, 2001.

Rao, Patrick M., M.D., et al. "Effect of Computer Tomography of the Appendix on Treatment of Patients and Use of Hospital Resources." *New England Journal of Medicine* 338, no. 3 (January 15, 1998):141–146.

appetite Normal physical desire and need for food. A normal, healthy appetite enables people to know when they are hungry and when they should eat. Sometimes appetite is impaired by temporary or chronic diseases. A chronic lack of appetite may also stem from an emotional disorder, such as depression, or from a physical disorder, such as cancer. Some people are obese because they ignore their natural appetite and eat to excess beyond the point when they feel satiated. In 2002, the substance GHRELIN, which appears to be a sort of appetite thermostat, was discovered. In some individuals, it malfunctions.

Some individuals lose their appetite because of disorders with the sense of taste or smell. If these problems resolve themselves, the normal appetite usually returns.

See also ANOREXIA NERVOSA; BARIATRIC SURGERY; BULIMIA; DIET DRUGS; OBESITY.

ascites   An accumulation of excess fluid in the abdomen that frequently causes visible swelling of the abdomen. Most cases of ascites are caused by liver CIRRHOSIS; it may also be caused by cancer, heart or kidney failure, severe malnutrition, or other medical problems such as blockages in the blood and lymphatic vessels.

Symptoms and Diagnostic Path

Symptoms of ascites include a feeling of pressure and abdominal swelling. The individual may have trouble walking or even breathing. If the physician is unsure of the cause of ascites, he or she may order blood tests, an ultrasound, a computed tomography (CT) scan, or an electrocardiogram.

Treatment Options and Outlook

It is essential that the person with ascites receive medical attention, and hospitalization is also required in many cases.

A physician who knows that an individual has an illness that causes ascites may begin treatment. At least once, all patients with ascites undergo a procedure that is called diagnostic PARACENTESIS, in which the fluid is removed for diagnostic purposes as well as for an evaluation for any complications that the patient is experiencing, such as an infection.

In large-volume paracentesis, several liters of the fluid are removed to help the patient breathe and feel better. Paracentesis is used when ascites is seen for the first time in a patient, usually at the time of every hospitalization (25 percent of those admitted to the hospital have an infection in the ascitic fluid), and then the procedure is performed on an as-needed basis afterward. If the physician is unsure of the cause of the ascites, he or she may order blood tests, an ultrasound, or computed tomography (CT) scan and an echocardiogram.

Treatment for ascites is directed to reducing the excessive fluid and treating the underlying condition and exacerbating factors. Diuretics such as Lasix or Aldactone may help rid the body of fluid. Individuals with ascites are also advised to adopt a salt-restricted diet. In some cases, shunts are implanted to help to move the fluid into the bloodstream via a special catheter or stent. Shunts may be placed surgically or in many cases less invasively by radiologists. Shunts placed by radiologists are called transjugular intrahepatic portosystemic shunts (TIPs).

Antibiotics are required in the case of an infection of ascitic fluid (spontaneous bacterial peritonitis) that occurs in patients who have ascites.

Risk Factors and Preventive Measures

Individuals with liver cirrhosis have an elevated risk for developing ascites. Patients with some forms of cancer have an increased risk for this condition, such as those with cancer of the gallbladder or cancer of the liver. Malnutrition also increases the risk for ascites.

There are no preventive measures against ascites. Diuretics are used to prevent re-accumulation of fluid.

See also BUDD-CHIARI SYNDROME; CIRRHOSIS; EOSINOPHILIC GASTROENTERITIS; GALLBLADDER CANCER; HEMOCHROMATOSIS; LIVER CANCER; MALNUTRITION/STARVATION.

Altman, Roberta, and Michael J. Sarg. *The Cancer Dictionary.* Rev. ed. New York: Facts On File, 2001.
Minocha, A. "A Fatal Case of Paracentesis." *American Journal of Gastroenterology* 94 (1999): 856.

atresia   Usually the absence of a normal opening or a lumen. When present, atresia may be seen as a blockage of any hollow part, for example, a blockage of any part of the small intestine such as the duodenum, jejunum, or ileum. Biliary atresia, as the name suggests, involves the bile ducts. In rare cases, atresia is found in more than one location. Atresia may also occur in newborns at the site of the esophagus or anus, bile ducts, and other locations, requiring surgery. Atresia is most commonly found in newborn infants, although it may also occur in older children and adults.

Atresia is considered the result of a congenital defect. It occurs in about one in 1,500 newborns. Duodenal atresia is associated with Down syndrome, tracheoesophageal fistula and anorectal malformations.

The symptoms of atresia depend on the site involved; for example, infants with intestinal atresia have abdominal swelling, constipation, and vomiting. Surgery is usually required in such cases. Similarly, esophageal atresia can be surgically corrected, allowing the child subsequently to ingest food.

back pain   Pain in the back that may emanate from numerous causes especially from the spine and its related soft tissues. However, back pain may result from even the digestive organs, such as the pancreas (as with PANCREATITIS and cancer of the pancreas) or metastatic colon cancer. Patients with functional bowel disorders like IRRITABLE BOWEL SYNDROME tend to have a higher prevalence of back pain and back surgery. Back pain may also be caused by an infection, such as a urinary tract infection or an infection of the prostate gland in a man.

Back pain is a very common problem for many people, particularly as they become middle-aged or older. Individuals of all races and both genders suffer from back pain. Diagnosing the cause of the back pain can be challenging for physicians, since there are many different reasons for back pain.

Symptoms and Diagnostic Path

Back pain may be mild, moderate, or severe. In diagnosing the cause of back pain, in general, the physician takes a careful medical history from the patient and also orders laboratory blood tests to screen for diseases and infections. Urine tests may be ordered to screen for a bladder infection, which is another frequent cause of back pain. A man is also given a rectal examination, including a manual check of the prostate gland for prostatitis (inflammation of the prostate gland). Frequently, the doctor may order plain X-rays or a computed tomography (CT) and ultrasound, or a magnetic resonance imaging (MRI) scan. A renal ultrasound may be done if kidney problems are suspected.

Treatment Options and Outlook

If the physician does not find any serious illness on the basis of the examination and the results of the laboratory or imaging tests that were performed then he or she may treat the patient for pain by prescribing painkillers or muscle relaxants. Complementary therapies such as massage therapy and acupuncture have also been shown to be of benefit to patients with back pain.

Risk Factors and Preventive Measures

Most Americans are at risk for back pain at some point in their lives.

See also PAIN.

bacteremia   The presence of bacteria in the blood, indicating an active systemic infection. Bacteremia is identified by blood cultures. Bacteremia is a severe condition treated aggressively with ANTIBIOTICS. Initially, broad-spectrum antibiotics such as piperacillin/taxobactam (Zosyn), ampicillin/sulbactam (Unasyn), or imipenem/cilastatin (Primaxin) are started, pending the results of the cultures and antibiotic susceptibility testing. Once the antibiotics that are the most likely to be effective have been identified by the laboratory testing, the initial choice of the broad-spectrum antibiotic may be switched to an antibiotic that is specifically targeted at the particular organism.

Sometimes the source of the origin of the bacteremia, for example, cholangitis or abdominal abscesses, can be identified. In such cases, further treatments, such as therapeutic endoscopy or surgery, may be needed in addition to the antibiotics in order to correct the underlying problem.

balloon distention test   A test that is usually used in the investigation of the esophagus or rectum. Patients who have IRRITABLE BOWEL SYNDROME, in whom the balloon is inserted rectally, sense the balloon at an earlier stage of inflation than do other patients, probably because of problems with HYPER-ALGESIA (a higher sensitivity of the colon/rectum to the stimulus and a low tolerance to pain). Similarly, the inflation of a balloon in the esophagus in patients with noncardiac chest pain results in pain at much lower volumes of inflation than in healthy subjects. The rectal balloon distention test is also sometimes used as part of the testing and investigation of a patient's problems with CONSTIPATION and fecal incontinence.

Sometimes patients with constipation are asked to expel the intrarectally inflated balloon in order for the physician to study the defecatory function. This test is known as the balloon expulsion test.

bariatric surgery Elective surgery that limits the amount of food that the body can digest and absorb by surgically reducing the capacity of the stomach (as with restrictive surgery) or by causing a decreased absorption of nutrients. Some forms of surgery may have both effects. When only the volume of the stomach is restricted, it is known as a gastric restriction procedure. Another form of bariatric surgery is the gastric bypass. Bariatric surgery is also known as weight reduction surgery, and it is used in morbidly obese individuals whose BODY MASS INDEX is 40 or greater. In some cases, physicians perform the procedure on patients whose BMI is 35 and greater if these individuals also have other medical problems that would likely be improved by a significant weight loss, such as diabetes, hypertension, and other problems.

According to the American Society for Metabolic and Bariatric Surgery, an estimated 205,000 people with morbid obesity had bariatric surgery in the United States in 2007.

Gastric banding and vertical banded gastroplasty are restrictive forms of surgery, while malabsorptive forms of bariatric surgery include the long-limb gastric bypass, the biliopancreatic diversion, and the biliopancreatic diversion with duodenal switch. The Roux-en-Y gastric bypass is considered both a restrictive and a malabsorptive bariatric procedure.

It may sometimes be very difficult for patients to obtain medical insurance coverage for bariatric surgery. It may be specifically excluded in some insurance policies because the procedure may be considered cosmetic and not medically necessary by some parties, despite the patient's physician's opinion. However, sometimes medical insurance does provide such coverage, and obese patients should not assume that coverage is never available for bariatric surgery and should investigate the issue with the help of their physician. It should also be noted that Medicare does provide coverage for bariatric surgery if the procedure is preapproved.

Types of Surgery

Bariatric surgery may be performed with an abdominal "open" incision or, in some cases, laparoscopically, through small incisions in the belly. The three most common surgeries used currently are biliary-pancreatic diversion with duodenal Switch, Roux-en-Y gastric bypass surgery (RYGB), and laparoscopic adjustable band (Lap-Band) surgery, and these can all be performed laparoscopically. (The duodenal switch surgery is generally performed only on those with a BMI greater than 50.)

Malabsorptive procedures limit intestinal absorption by restricting the stomach size and also by bypassing the first 75 centimeters of the small intestine. This is done by making a direct connection of the small pouch of the stomach to a loop of the small intestine, and thus reducing the area available for absorption.

Restrictive procedures allow normal digestion to occur, but they decrease the amount of solid foods that patients can eat at one time by limiting the stomach size. After this surgery, the patient can usually only eat one cup of solid food at a time (at most) without experiencing nausea or stomach upset. However, the patient can still drink a lot of high-calorie liquids such as milkshakes if he or she chooses to do so and beat the intent of the surgery. Thus, the potential for weight loss due to restrictive procedures alone is limited, and they may not be effective over the long term in many cases.

According to Brolin in his 2002 *Journal of the American Medical Association* article, the Roux-en-Y operation (which is a combination of a malabsorptive procedure, and a restrictive procedure) is the most effective form of bariatric surgery, giving patients high rates of weight loss compared to the other techniques. In addition, some studies have shown that after having the Roux-en-Y surgery, a majority of patients who had been diagnosed with diabetes or impaired glucose tolerance before their surgery experienced an improvement of their blood glucose level subsequent to the surgery.

In contrast, many patients who have had gastric restrictive surgical procedures have experienced relapses. There are reports of a failure rate as high as 80 percent with vertical banded gastroplasty, and it is falling out of favor. Adjustable gastric banding procedure (Lap-Band) is approved and has largely replaced vertical gastroplasty.

Physicians may limit their patients who have bariatric surgery to those who are older than age 20 and younger than age 60, although some physicians operate on extremely obese adolescents or ELDERLY individuals. Most bariatric surgery patients are female; some males also choose the surgery.

Many physicians require patients who wish to have bariatric surgery to have psychological evaluations to verify that the surgery would be psychologically appropriate and that the patients are not suffering from clinical depression or other emotional disorders. Many physicians require letters of approval for the surgery (preoperative clearance) from the patient's primary care doctor.

All bariatric surgery patients should have a thorough physical examination before the surgery to rule out any undiagnosed medical problems. Some surgeons require a presurgical ENDOSCOPY as well.

Advantages of Bariatric Surgery

The most obvious advantages of weight reduction surgery are the decreased weight and enhanced self-esteem and health experienced by many patients who had previous failures with many different types of diets and prescriptions and over-the-counter diet pills and other weight loss remedies. Patients with diabetes, prediabetes, and hypertension usually improve after bariatric surgery. In addition, patients with sleep apnea may enjoy a remission from this problem, which frequently disappears completely after surgery.

There are other advantages of bariatric surgery for obese patients, according to Brolin:

In women, weight loss resulting from bariatric surgery has a salutary effect on sex hormone balance, menstrual regularity, fertility, and urinary stress incontinence. Women who had previously been infertile have become pregnant and delivered healthy infants following bariatric operations; nutritional status can be maintained for both mother and developing fetus.

However, bariatric surgeons recommend that patients not become pregnant for at least one year after surgery.

Disadvantages of Surgery

All forms of bariatric surgery carry risks for infection and vitamin deficiencies, such as deficiencies of iron, folate, calcium, and vitamin B_{12}, as well as other postoperative medical problems. If the banded gastroplasty is used, the band may break or slip and the surgery has to be redone. There is a risk of death with bariatric surgery, as with all surgeries, although the mortality rate is less than 1 percent, depending on the type of surgery used.

Some patients who have had bariatric surgery may experience dumping syndrome after surgery, developing abdominal cramps, NAUSEA, and DIARRHEA, as well as sweating, dizziness, and even hypotension, particularly after eating carbohydrates. The incidence of dumping syndrome appears to be low after the Roux-en-Y procedure.

A rapid weight loss predisposes patients to gallstone formation, and thus, patients who have had bariatric surgery also have an increased risk for development of gallstones after surgery. Many surgeons check for gallstones before performing bariatric surgery, and if gallstones are found, they may offer patients elective simultaneous cholecystectomy at the time of bariatric surgery. Some physicians give patients medications preventive against the formation of gallstones.

Some patients may require further surgery after their weight reduction surgery, for example, to correct a complication, such as an abdominal hernia.

The Postoperative Period

After the surgery, if the patient eats more than the now-smaller stomach can hold, she or he usually feels nauseated and sick. Most patients benefit by joining a support group of others who have had the surgery, so that they can gain practical tips as well as moral support from people who can identify with and fully understand what they are going through.

Interestingly, some physicians have found that the blood levels of GHRELIN are significantly lower after patients have had Roux-en-Y surgery. Ghrelin is a hormone that is released by the stomach and that apparently affects hunger and satiety, or the feeling of fullness that a person experiences during and after eating. The researchers David E. Cummings, M.D., and his colleagues reported on their findings in 2002 in the *New England Journal of Medicine.*

They compared obese subjects who lost weight through dieting as well as subjects who lost weight through gastric surgery. The subjects who had gastric surgery had significantly lower levels of ghrelin. In contrast, the rates of ghrelin rose in the patients who lost weight through dieting. As a result, the dieters were much hungrier than were the patients who had the gastric bypass.

Said the researchers:

> In summary, 24-hour plasma ghrelin levels increase in response to diet-induced weight loss, suggesting that ghrelin may play a part in the adaptive response that limits the amount of weight that may be lost by dieting. We also found that ghrelin levels are abnormally low after gastric bypass, raising the possibility that this operation reduces weight in part by suppressing ghrelin production. These data, suggest that ghrelin antagonists [blocking medications] may someday be considered in the treatment of obesity.

Criticisms of Weight Reduction Surgery

Bariatric surgery is considered controversial by many experts, and most physicians prefer that patients lose weight through limiting their caloric intake and increasing their levels of exercise; however, such methods may not work well for the morbidly obese person. Another criticism of bariatric surgery is that it causes digestive problems that may not have been present before the surgery, such as GASTROESOPHAGEAL REFLUX DISEASE (GERD), GALLSTONES, GASTROPARESIS, DUMPING SYNDROME,

nausea, and malabsorption of micronutrients such as iron. Death is a rare complication.

Some forms of the surgery may be less likely to cause GERD than others, although every type of bariatric surgery has some effects on the digestive system, since most bariatric surgery involves severely limiting the capacity of the stomach and hence the amount of calories that can be consumed.

See also DIET DRUGS; OBESITY; ROUX-EN-Y STASIS SYNDROME.

Abell T. L. and A. Minocha. "Gastrointestinal complications of bariatric surgery: diagnosis and therapy." *American Journal of Medical Sciences* 331, no. 4 (April 2006): 214–218.

Brolin, Robert E., M.D. "Bariatric Surgery and Long-Term Control of Morbid Obesity." *Journal of the American Medical Association* 288, no. 22 (December 11, 2002): 2,793–2,796.

Cassell, Dana K., and David H. Gleaves, Ph.D. *Obesity and Eating Disorders.* 2d ed. New York: Facts On File, 2000.

Cummings, David E., M.D., et al., "Plasma Ghrelin Levels after Diet-Induced Weight Loss or Gastric Bypass Surgery." *New England Journal of Medicine* 346, no. 21 (May 23, 2002): 1,623–1,630.

DeMaria, Eric J., M.D. "Bariatric Surgery for Morbid Obesity." *New England Journal of Medicine* 356, no. 21 (May 24, 2007): 2,176–2,183.

Dixon, John B., Paul E. O'Brien, Julie Playfair, et al. "Adjustable Gastric Banding and Conventional Therapy for Type 2 Diabetes: A Randomized Controlled Trial." *Journal of the American Medical Association* 299, no. 3 (2008): 316–323.

National Institute of Diabetes and Digestive and Kidney Diseases. "Bariatric Surgery for Severe Obesity." March 2009. Available online: URL: http://win.niddk.nih.gov/publications/gastric.htm. Accessed March 27, 2010.

barium studies   Tests that involve the ingestion or the rectal instillation of barium, a contrast dye, to allow the patient's gastrointestinal tract to show up well under a dark background under a fluoroscope so that the doctor can identify medical problems. Barium may be given orally in a drink, as with an upper gastrointestinal (GI) test and a small bowel series, or may be introduced rectally, as with a barium enema. Barium studies are done when a gastrointestinal illness is suspected. A barium study is one of the options to screen for colorectal cancer; however, a COLONOSCOPY is usually recommended by gastroenterologists for that specific purpose. Biopsy samples cannot be taken and polyps cannot be removed during the barium study. If an abnormality is seen during the test, it is frequently followed up with an endoscopy, at which time a biopsy specimen can be taken.

See also COLORECTAL CANCER.

Barrett's esophagus A precancerous condition that is generally caused by long-standing ACID REFLUX due to GASTROESOPHAGEAL REFLUX DISEASE (GERD). In this case, GERD causes the esophageal lining to become changed to an intestinal type; this abnormality is called an *intestinal metaplasia*.

Symptoms and Diagnostic Path

Barrett's esophagus itself does not cause any symptoms and must be looked for by ENDOSCOPY. A physician may suspect the condition if the patient has long-term GERD.

With Barrett's esophagus, the normally pale lining of the esophagus is altered to a salmon color. The physician takes biopsy samples to examine them under the microscope. If the doctor who is examining the biopsy specimen locates cells that are known as goblet cells, which are not normally found in the esophagus or the stomach but *are* found in the small intestine, then this finding is definitive proof of the presence of Barrett's esophagus. Some experts argue that the presence of goblet cells on biopsy is not a prerequisite.

Treatment Options and Outlook

When Barrett's esophagus is identified, treatment usually takes the form of medications, such as PROTON PUMP INHIBITOR drugs, which are medications that control the acidity of the refluxed food, theoretically to prevent further damage. Indirect evidence suggests that these medications may be helpful; however there is a lack of supporting direct clinical data. Unfortunately, medication does not cure or reverse the disease. There may be some regression of Barrett's esophagus, but the clinical significance of this regression remains to be estab-

lished. The goal of treatment is damage control so that the situation does not further worsen to ESOPHAGEAL CANCER.

Some physicians may recommend surgery as a treatment for GERD, such as laparoscopic fundoplication, which is performed on the stomach and esophagus to prevent the food from moving back up the esophagus from the stomach. However, as with medical treatment, surgery has not been shown to reverse Barrett's esophagus or to reduce the progression to cancer.

Patients with Barrett's esophagus need periodic surveillance by endoscopy, although it is controversial because of the lack of direct evidence based on randomized controlled trials to support its effectiveness. The interval between endoscopies depends on the presence or the absence of dysplasia (abnormal cells). The presence of any dysplasia should be confirmed by an additional pathologist.

Management of Barrett's esophagus is also controversial in the case that high-grade dysplasia is found. Many physicians used to recommend an esophagectomy (removal of the esophagus), since the presence of high-grade dysplasia suggests the high likelihood of progression to cancer in the near future; in fact, cancer cells may already be present in some cases. However, recent data suggest that the risk may be overestimated. Recent guidelines suggest that patients with high-grade dysplasia should not automatically be referred to surgery, but rather that the management should be individualized.

Endoscopic mucosal resection and/or an aggressive surveillance program of endoscopy performed every three months or the use of ablative therapies are alternate options for patients with high-grade dysplasia. Endoscopic ablative therapies include Nd: YAG laser, argon plasma coagulation, photodynamic therapy, or radiofrequency ablation (Halosystem) to ablate the abnormal epithelium in Barrett's esophagus.

The strategy should generally based on the patient's age and coexisting medical problems as well as taking into consideration the local medical expertise that is available. In cases of low-grade dysplasia, physicians may order an endoscopy every six months for a year, and if the condition is stable, once every year thereafter. In patients with Barrett's esophagus without any evidence of dysplasia, the endoscopy is done at one year and thereafter every three years.

A screening esophagogastroduodenoscopy (EGD) for Barrett's esophagus is recommended in patients with chronic, longstanding GERD unless they have had a previous normal EGD. The EGD is an examination of the esophagus, stomach, and upper duodenum with an endoscope (tube fitted with a small camera) passed down the patient's throat into the food pipe. However, as mentioned, screening for Barrett's esophagus is controversial because lack of evidence that it affects outcome. The best candidates for screening are Caucasian males with longstanding GERD. If the EGD does not show any Barrett's esophagus, no further screening endoscopy is needed.

The role of biomarkers associated with carcinogenesis in Barrett's esophagus is evolving. These markers may be an alternative to biopsy samples in order to identify dysplasia in Barrett's esophagus. Potentially useful markers include abnormalities in p53 expression, and abnormal cellular DNA content as seen by flow cytometry.

Risk Factors and Preventive Measures

White males appear to have the greatest risk of development of this condition. Other people at risk are smokers and those who have had acid reflux symptoms for many years.

One important preventive action is to end a smoking habit.

See also ESOPHAGEAL CANCER; ESOPHAGITIS; ESOPHAGUS.

Spechler, Stuart Jon, M.D. "Barrett's Esophagus." *New England Journal of Medicine* 346, no. 11 (March 14, 2002): 836–842.

Behçet's syndrome A rare multisystemic inflammatory disorder that causes lesions and ulcers in the mouth and the genitals. The tissues of the eyes may also be affected. The joints, the digestive tract, the central nervous system, the heart, the kidneys, the skin, the brain, and the blood vessels of patients may be affected as well. The cause of Behçet's syndrome is unknown.

Diagnosis and Treatment

Behçet's syndrome is treated on the basis of the organ that is involved. Medications used to treat Behçet's syndrome include immune suppressant drugs such as prednisone, azathioprine, methotrexate, cyclophosphamide, and cyclosporine; however, a side effect of such treatment is that patients are more prone to infections. Colchicine may be used by patients who have arthritis. Other modalities that have been used include interferon alfa, thalidomide, infliximab, etanercept, intravenous immunoglobulin, and so on.

For further information, contact the following:

American Behçet's Disease Association
P.O. Box 19952
Amarillo, TX 79114
(800) 723-4238 (toll-free)
http://www.behcets.com

Sakane, Tsuyoshi, M.D., et al. "Behçet's Disease." *New England Journal of Medicine* 341, no. 17 (October 21, 1999): 1,284–1,291.

belching The oral release of gas from the stomach, also known as burping. The gas has usually been inadvertently swallowed into the digestive tract. Burping may be further enhanced during times of anxiety and stress. In some cases, the swallowed air may not even reach the stomach before it is expelled by belching. Belching may be seen in patients with GASTROESOPHAGEAL REFLUX DISEASE.

An endoscopy or an upper gastrointestinal X ray is frequently done for patients with chronic belching in order to exclude any serious underlying illness, such as gastric outlet obstruction. In most cases, no cause can be identified. In such cases, the treatment of chronic belching is frequently unsatisfactory.

beriberi A severe deficiency of thiamine (vitamin B_1), a condition that is usually found among children in poor countries. Dry beriberi is a disorder of the peripheral nerves that leads to such symptoms as numbness, tingling, and a burning sensation in the hands and feet, as well as leg cramps. Wet beriberi predominantly involves the heart, leading to heart failure. Cerebral beriberi occurs as a result of an acute illness that is superimposed on a chronic deficiency of thiamine. Cerebral beriberi leads to mental changes and brain damage, and sometimes even to death.

See also MALNUTRITION; VITAMIN DEFICIENCIES/EXCESSES.

beta blockers Medications that are used to treat patients who have heart disease and hypertension. Beta blockers are also useful for the prevention of the bleeding caused by esophageal varices seen in liver CIRRHOSIS. Varices are enlarged dilated veins that usually occur in the esophagus and stomach. The most common cause of varices is liver cirrhosis, and they occur in about one-third to half of patients who have cirrhosis. Bleeding is more likely to occur if the varices are large.

Beta blocker medications may also contribute to the development of GASTROESOPHAGEAL REFLUX DISEASE in some patients. Beta blockers also slow the heart, and some people take a dose of a beta blocker to calm themselves before an anticipated stressful situation, such as before going up to a podium to give a speech to a large crowd.

See also ACID REFLUX.

bile A substance that is produced by the liver and that comprises bile acids, electrolytes, bilirubin, cholesterol, and phospholipids plus water. Bile aids in the digestion of food by assisting in breaking down fats as well as by absorption of nutrients. About half of the bile is stored in the gallbladder between meals. The gallbladder is stimulated by individuals' eating food; eating results in the release of bile into the small intestine, where the bile acts on the food to aid digestion and absorption of nutrients.

See also JAUNDICE; LIVER; LIVER FAILURE.

bilirubin A substance that is formed by the breakdown of heme, a substance present in hemoglobin as well as in some other proteins. Most bilirubin that is produced (250 to 400 mg per day in adults) is derived from hemoglobin; the remaining

20 percent is contributed by other hemoproteins. Increased levels of bilirubin production are found in disorders that are associated with an increased red blood cell turnover, such as hemolytic ANEMIA; liver disorders such as HEPATITIS and CIRRHOSIS; or disorders that cause an obstruction to the flow of bile as in intra- and extra-hepatic obstruction.

Bilirubin is potentially toxic, and it is detoxified by the body and then excreted in both the stool and the urine. Increased levels of bilirubin cause JAUNDICE, which shows up as a yellowing of the skin and eyes. The presence of jaundice may indicate hepatitis, liver cirrhosis, PANCREATIC CANCER, or other diseases.

Infants and Bilirubin

Nonpathologic jaundice may be seen in newborn infants as a result of changes in bilirubin metabolism including increased bilirubin production and decreased bilirubin excretion. In addition, there is an increased enterohepatic circulation leading to an increased bilirubin load in the infant. This results in the mild unconjugated hyperbilirubinemia jaundice seen in most newborns, and it resolves within one to three weeks after birth.

In some newborns, especially preterm babies, the above physiological changes may become exaggerated, resulting in neonatal jaundice. Neonatal jaundice may be caused by other pathological conditions as well and the treatment depends upon the cause.

Babies at birth are screened to assess risk for hyperbilirubinemia and those at high risk undergo phototherapy to prevent hyperbilirubinemia.

Treatment options of severe hyperbilirubinemia include phototherapy and exchange transfusion. Phototherapy involves exposing the infant's skin to light of a specific wavelength. Several light sources are available for use for phototherapy and they use different wavelengths. These options include fluorescent blue light, halogen white light, and fiber-optic blankets or pads. Phototherapy may be administered at home in some cases.

bleeding, gastrointestinal Loss of blood, usually from the stomach or colon, although other parts of the gastrointestinal system may also bleed. Gastrointestinal bleeding may be due to a simple case of hemorrhoids or may indicate a severe disease, such as a peptic ulcer or diverticulosis. It may also indicate colorectal cancer or another cancer. Bleeding from esophageal or gastric varices due to liver cirrhosis is usually massive.

Varices are enlarged dilated veins that usually occur in the esophagus and stomach and are most commonly caused by liver cirrhosis. Other causes of varices include hepatic and splenic vein thrombosis. Varices may also occur elsewhere in the gastrointestinal tract, including the duodenum, colon, and rectum.

Bleeding due to varices is more likely to occur if the varices are large. In such cases, BETA BLOCKER medications may be given to prevent bleeding. Once bleeding has occurred, medications such as octreotide are given and an endoscopic band ligation or sclerotherapy of the varices is performed to control the bleeding. This ligation is followed by banding at regular intervals, along with continued administration of beta blocker medications.

Similarly, diverticulosis also causes massive and painless bleeding. Abnormal blood vessels (arteriovenous malformations) in the gastrointestinal tract may ooze slowly or may cause massive bleeding. One of the screening tests that are done for colon cancer is checking of the stool for occult blood. Colon polyps usually do not bleed unless they are either large or cancerous.

See also COLORECTAL XANCER; OCCULT GASTROINTESTINAL BLEEDING.

blue rubber bleb nevus syndrome   A rare inherited disorder of the skin and the digestive tract. It is characterized by abnormal blood vessels in the gastrointestinal tract and by compressible nodules on the skin, with fewer nodules on other parts of the body. These nodules can cause gastrointestinal BLEEDING, ANEMIA, and even fatal bleeding.

The condition was first noted in 1860, when Dr. Gascoyen described an association between cavernous hemangiomas of the skin and similar lesions in the gastrointestinal tract. It was later named *blue rubber bleb nevus syndrome* in 1958 by Dr. W. Bean. (Some individuals also refer to this medical problem as Bean's syndrome, although that is not its common or official name.) The cause of this condition is unknown.

Symptoms and Diagnostic Path

As mentioned, the color and texture of the blood vessels are the key symptoms of this disorder. The signs of blue rubber bleb nevus syndrome are seen in individuals as young as age two and continue throughout the patient's life. The malformed blood vessels can be found in any part of the body including the central nervous system, thyroid, eyes, mouth, lungs, kidney, liver, spleen, bones, joints, and bladder.

Once a diagnosis is made, there should be a heightened sensitivity by physicians for lesions in the other parts of the patient's body. A search for these lesions, using various imaging and endoscopic modalities, should be considered depending upon the clinical situation. Patients having symptoms from lesions in a particular part of the body should be referred to the appropriate specialist for appropriate treatment; for example, if the lesions are in the thyroid, an endocrinologist should be consulted, or if the lesions are in the kidneys, a nephrologist should be consulted.

Treatment Options and Outlook

If the lesions cause anemia through slow bleeding, then treatment with iron can usually resolve the problem. Smaller lesions may be corrected with minor surgery, but large lesions may require very severe treatments, such as extensive, and even at times disfiguring, surgery. Gastrointestinal areas that are affected can be treated with a laser or with photocoagulation.

The condition is considered very difficult to treat. The illness cannot be cured at the present, and at best the symptoms are managed.

Risk Factors and Preventive Measures

Risk factors for this condition are unknown, and there are no known preventive measures.

body mass index (BMI)   A unisex measurement that takes into account both height and weight, using various equations to provide tables that help physicians, patients, and others to determine whether particular individuals are underweight, normal weight, overweight, or obese. If patients are 100 pounds or more overweight, they are said to be severely or "morbidly" obese, as indicated in BMI tables. Because OBESITY is associated with many serious digestive problems and other medical problems, such as CANCER, GASTROESOPHAGEAL REFLUX DISEASE, and NONALCOHOLIC FATTY LIVER DISEASE (NAFLD), BMI is an important concept.

Using BMI criteria, according to the National Center for Health Statistics, the majority of American adults are either overweight or obese; 35.0 percent of all adults in the United States were overweight, and 25.8 percent were obese in 2006. Among adult females, 28.0 percent were overweight and 25.6 percent were obese in 2006. Among adult males, 41.9 percent were overweight and 25.3 percent were obese. (See Table 1.)

When considering age alone, as can be seen from the table, individuals who were ages 45 to 64 years old had the highest percentage of obesity, or 30.8 percent. Among individuals of different races,

TABLE 1: BODY MASS INDEX AMONG PERSONS AGES 18 YEARS AND OLDER, BY SELECTED CHARACTERISTICS, UNITED STATES, 2006

| Selected Characteristic | Body Mass Index among Persons Ages 18 and Older | | | | |
	Total	Underweight	Healthy weight	Overweight	Obese
Total	100.0	1.7	37.5	35.0	25.8
Gender					
Male	100.0	1.0	31.9	41.9	25.3
Female	100.0	2.5	43.8	28.0	25.6
Age					
18–44 years	100.0	1.9	41.8	33.0	23.2
45–64 years	100.0	1.1	31.4	36.6	30.8
65–74 years	100.0	1.5	31.5	39.4	27.5
75 years and older	100.0	3.3	43.4	35.2	18.1
Race					
White	100.0	1.7	38.2	35.1	25.1
Black or African American	100.0	1.5	29.5	34.4	34.7
American Indian or Alaskan Native	100.0	Unknown	30.0	38.1	30.9
Asian	100.0	4.8	59.3	27.6	8.3
Native Hawaiian or Other Pacific Islander	100.0	Unknown	29.2	37.6	30.8
2 or more races					
Black or African American, and white	100.0	Unknown	28.3	50.9	18.8
American Indian or Alaska Native and white	100.0	Unknown	29.3	39.1	30.5
Hispanic or Latino origin and race					
Mexican or Mexican American	100.0	1.0	30.6	38.7	29.8
Not Hispanic or Latino					
White, single race	100.0	1.8	39.1	34.5	24.7
Black or African American, single race	100.0	1.5	29.6	33.7	35.3
Education					
Less than a high school diploma	100.0	1.6	30.5	38.2	29.7
High school diploma or GED	100.0	1.2	32.6	35.4	30.7
Some college	100.0	1.4	33.0	36.1	29.5
Bachelor's degree or higher	100.0	2.0	43.3	35.9	18.8

blacks had the highest percentage of obesity (34.7 percent), and Asians had the lowest percentage of obesity (8.3 percent).

Individuals who were poor had the highest rate of obesity (29.8 percent) in comparison to those who were near poor (28.5 percent) and those who were not poor (24.9 percent).

In considering marital status, those who were widowed had the highest percentage of obesity (35.4 percent), and those who were never married had the lowest percentage (24.2 percent).

Table 2 illustrates the fattest state and the leanest in terms of BMI; for example, according to the CDC, in 2008, the highest percentage of obese individuals lived in Mississippi (32.8 percent), followed by Alabama (31.4 percent). States that had the lowest percentage of obese people were Colorado (18.5 percent) and Connecticut (21.0 percent).

Some Problems with BMI

One problem with the concept of BMI is that it does not take into account that some people are

	Body Mass Index among Persons Ages 18 and Older				
Selected Characteristic	Total	Underweight	Healthy weight	Overweight	Obese
Family income					
Less than $20,000	100.0	2.4	38.1	31.3	28.2
$20,000 or more	100.0	1.6	37.8	35.7	25.0
$20,000–$34,999	100.0	1.4	37.1	34.4	27.0
$35,000–$54,999	100.0	1.2	34.2	35.7	28.9
$55,000–$74,999	100.0	1.6	36.3	36.1	26.1
$75,000 or more	100.0	2.1	40.9	35.1	21.9
Poverty status					
Poor	100.0	2.2	36.4	31.6	29.8
Near poor	100.0	1.6	36.8	33.1	28.5
Not poor	100.0	1.7	37.9	35.5	24.9
Health insurance coverage, under age 65 years					
Private	100.0	1.5	38.8	34.8	24.8
Medicaid	100.0	1.6	36.8	33.1	28.5
Other	100.0	2.6	32.7	32.8	31.9
Uninsured	100.0	1.3	38.4	34.5	25.7
Marital status					
Married	100.0	1.5	35.3	36.9	26.3
Widowed	100.0	0.9	32.5	31.2	35.4
Divorced or separated	100.0	1.6	35.8	34.4	28.2
Never married	100.0	2.4	42.2	31.2	24.2
Living with a partner	100.0	3.1	37.5	34.0	25.4
Region					
Northeast	100.0	1.6	40.0	34.8	23.6
Midwest	100.0	1.5	37.2	33.5	27.9
South	100.0	1.9	36.5	34.9	26.7
West	100.0	1.9	39.6	36.4	22.1

Source: Adapted from Pleis, J. R., and M. Lethbridge-Çejku. *Summary Health Statistics for U.S. Adults: National Health Interview Survey 2006.* Washington, D.C.: National Center for Health Statistics. 2007, 80–81

TABLE 2: 2008 STATE OBESITY RATES: PERCENT OF OBESE INDIVIDUALS IN EACH STATE

State	%	State	%	State	%	State	%
Alabama	31.4	Illinois	26.4	Montana	23.9	Rhode Island	21.5
Alaska	26.1	Indiana	26.3	Nebraska	26.6	South Carolina	30.1
Arizona	24.8	Iowa	26.0	Nevada	25.0	South Dakota	27.5
Arkansas	28.7	Kansas	27.4	New Hampshire	24.0	Tennessee	30.6
California	23.7	Kentucky	29.8	New Jersey	22.9	Texas	28.3
Colorado	18.5	Louisiana	28.3	New Mexico	25.2	Utah	22.5
Connecticut	21.0	Maine	25.2	New York	24.4	Vermont	22.7
Delaware	27.0	Maryland	26.0	North Carolina	29.0	Virginia	25.0
Washington, DC	21.8	Massachusetts	20.9	North Dakota	27.1	Washington	25.4
Florida	24.4	Michigan	28.9	Ohio	28.7	West Virginia	31.2
Georgia	27.3	Minnesota	24.3	Oklahoma	30.3	Wisconsin	25.4
Hawaii	22.6	Mississippi	32.8	Oregon	24.2	Wyoming	24.6
Idaho	24.5	Missouri	28.5	Pennsylvania	27.7		

Source: Centers for Disease Control and Prevention. *Obesity and Overweight for Professionals: Data and Statistics: U.S. Obesity.* Available online at http://www.cdc.gov/obesity/data/trends.html. Accessed December 8, 2009.

heavily muscled, such as athletes or weightlifters In addition, the BMI does not factor in ethnic or racial differences; for example, some Asian populations generally have smaller body frames and Asian individuals often weigh significantly less than non-Asian people in the United States and other countries. As a result, if physicians rely upon BMI charts alone, some Asians who are categorized as "normal" on the BMI charts may actually be overweight, and they also may be at an increased risk for the development of diabetes and other serious medical problems. On the other hand, some very muscular athletes, such as Shaquille O'Neal, may be considered obese on the basis of BMI tables alone.

However, despite these drawbacks, the body mass index concept is considered by most experts to be a useful one in helping to determine whether most individuals are at a healthy weight.

Children and BMI

The prevalence of obesity among American children has more than doubled over the last 20 years. Because children are rapidly growing, the BMI concept is more complicated and requires consideration of the child's age and sex as well as his or her height and weight. BMI tables for children have also been developed, and they are helpful to parents and physicians. (See Appendix VI for BMI tables for children.)

Children whose BMI for their age is considered to indicate a risk of overweight have a BMI between the 85th and the 94th percentiles. If their BMI is in the 95th percentile or higher for their age and sex, then they are considered to be overweight.

It is also important to keep in mind that a BMI that is normal or overweight at one age would not be normal or overweight for an older child. For example, according to the Centers for Disease Control and Prevention (CDC), a male child with a BMI of 19.3 at age two years would be in the 95th percentile: that is, 95 percent of children have a lower BMI. The child's BMI could actually drop to 17.8 by the time he is four years old, but he would still be in the 95th percentile. The percentiles continue to change; for example, a boy nine years in age who has a BMI of 21 would be in the 95th percentile. When the boy reached the age of 13 years, if his BMI were 25.1, he would still be in the 95th percentile for BMI.

See also ANOREXIA NERVOSA; BARIATRIC SURGERY; BULIMIA; DIET DRUGS.

Pleis, J. R., and M. Lethbridge-Çejku. *Summary Health Statistics for U.S. Adults: National Health Interview Survey 2006.* Washington, D.C.: National Center for Health Statistics, 2007.

botulism   Infection with the botulinum toxin, often through contaminated food or through an open wound. Physicians can usually identify the disease on the basis of the patient's symptoms and the results of laboratory tests done on the patient's stool, vomit, or blood. The outcome of treatment is best when the disease is identified and treated immediately. Physicians administer botulism antitoxins to treat botulism poisoning. In addition, if the doctor thinks that some of the contaminated food may still be present in the digestive system, he or she may administer laxatives or enemas to get rid of it. Human-derived botulinum immunoglobulin (called BIG-IV or BabyBIG) is used to treat cases of botulism in infants as early as possible in the illness. Antibiotics are used in wound botulism in addition to wound debridement.

Patients affected by botulinum toxin generally require hospitalization for several weeks to months (generally one to three months). The overall death rate is 5 to 8 percent.

bowel movement   Expulsion of stool from the rectum and out through the anus. Some people have difficulties with constipation, which is the passage of difficult, infrequent or hard stools. If constipation becomes severe, the individual may suffer from fecal impaction. Other individuals may have chronic loose stools. People who have irritable bowel syndrome (IBS) may have intermittent constipation and/or diarrhea.

Most people have a bowel movement daily or about every other day; however, it is not essential to good health to have a bowel movement every single day, as some people believe. The normal frequency of bowel movements varies over a wide range of three per day to three per week. Irregular bowel movements (constipation or diarrhea, or constipation alternating with diarrhea) in addition to abdominal pain improved by defecation is seen in patients with irritable bowel syndrome.

See also CONSTIPATION; DIARRHEA; FECAL IMPACTION; IRRITABLE BOWEL SYNDROME; LAXATIVES AND LAXATIVE ABUSE.

breath tests   Generally tests that utilize the breath to test for the patient's digestive function and the presence of diseases.

A breath test may be given to determine whether a person is infected with *Helicobacter pylori*, bacteria that are generally harbored within the gastrointestinal system, usually the stomach, when present in the body. After ingesting a specific meal labeled with a small amount of radioactivity, the patient breathes into a device, which measures the level of radioactivity released with radio labeled carbon dioxide that is present in the breath. If the test result is positive for *H. pylori*, treatment is initiated.

Breath tests may also test for gastric emptying time, lactose intolerance, and small bowel bacterial overgrowth.

Breath tests are also administered by police officials to individuals who are suspected of driving while under the influence of alcohol. The breath test reveals whether the driver has a level of alcohol that is above the allowable level in his or her state.

See also HELICOBACTER PYLORI.

Budd-Chiari syndrome   A rare disease that causes the clotting of the veins of the LIVER (hepatic vein) and may consequently cause liver damage.

Symptoms and Diagnostic Path
People who have Budd-Chiari syndrome may have an excessive buildup of fluid in the abdomen (ASCITES), ABDOMINAL PAIN, JAUNDICE, tenderness in the upper right abdomen, and an abnormally enlarged liver and spleen. The diagnosis is based on the patient's medical history and physical examination results plus a Doppler ultrasound of the hepatic veins. A computerized tomography (CT) scan or a magnetic resonance imaging (MRI scan) angiography is used for diagnosis. Venography can be used to confirm the diagnosis, especially if noninvasive studies are negative or nondiagnostic and to plan therapeutic interventions. A liver biopsy may occasionally be performed.

Treatment Options and Outlook
The treatment of Budd-Chiari syndrome depends upon the cause. For example, among patients experiencing clotting of the vein of recent onset, blood thinners such as heparin and clot busters such as tissue plasminogen activator (TPA) are used. Surgery may be needed for decompression.

The prognosis is not good for Budd-Chiari syndrome patients. Most patients die in less than four years. More than 60 percent of patients survive longer than five years after liver transplantation.

Risk Factors and Preventive Measures

Budd-Chiari syndrome is associated with abdominal trauma, lupus, PANCREATIC CANCER, LIVER CANCER, and kidney cancer. It is also associated with PREGNANCY as well as the use of oral contraceptives. In many cases, the cause of this medical problem is unknown. There are no known preventive measures.

See also LIVER FAILURE.

bulimia nervosa An eating disorder in which the individual binges (eats excessively) and then purges (forces herself or himself to vomit) at least twice a week for three or more months. The cause of bulimia nervosa is unknown, but a combination of psychological, biological, family, genetic, environmental, and social factors appear to play roles. Bulimia nervosa affects about 1 to 1.5 percent of adult females and about 1 million to 2 million women in the United States.

Symptoms and Diagnostic Path

Patients with bulimia report feeling that they have no control over their overeating. Bulimic individuals may also abuse laxatives in their efforts to stay slim and may suffer from abdominal cramping or diarrhea as a consequence. They may also abuse diuretics (water pills). Patients with bulimia may also exercise compulsively and feel very distressed if their daily exercise routine cannot be fulfilled; for example, if they cannot run because of extremely bad weather.

Bulimia patients may have abnormal blood electrolyte levels—for example, low levels of potassium. Bulimic patients may have esophagitis caused by constant self-induced vomiting.

Treatment Options and Outlook

Bulimic patients need psychological treatment and may also need to be hospitalized if their weight drops to a very low level and/or if severe fluid and electrolyte abnormalities develop.

Risk Factors and Preventive Measures

Most people with bulimia nervosa are females obsessed about their weight (although, ironically, almost none is obese), although males may also occasionally exhibit these symptoms. About half of the patients who have anorexia nervosa first will subsequently develop bulimia. There are no known preventive measures.

cachexia An abnormal metabolic state causing a wasting away of the body's muscle mass as well as body weight. The term *cachexia* is derived from the Greek words *kakos*, meaning "bad things," and *hexus*, meaning "state of being," It is due to an inadequate intake of nutrition to meet the individual's metabolic needs or the severe stress of illness, which then results in increased metabolic demands that the body is unable to meet.

Symptoms and Diagnostic Path

The following are the primary symptoms of cachexia:

- a lack of APPETITE
- extreme fatigue
- a weight loss of 10 percent or more of body weight
- weakness

Some patients also experience an early satiety (feeling full after eating only a small amount of food), as well as an impaired sense of taste, NAUSEA, and CONSTIPATION.

Treatment Options and Outlook

Patients in a state of cachexia are treated with small, frequent high-fat meals and with nutritional supplements and drugs to stimulate the appetite, such as megestrol acetate, dronabinol (synthetic marijuana), or cyproheptadine. Patients with cachexia may also be given recombinant growth hormone.

Some patients are given drugs in the cytokine modulator class, such as thalidomide. (Thalidomide was a drug that caused pregnant woman to have deformed children in the mid-20th century, but researchers are now finding some use for the drug in treating severely ill patients who are not pregnant.)

Eicosapentaenoic acid (EPA) also known as alpha-3 omega fatty acid may be helpful in some cases. Anabolic steroids are frequently used. Melatonin and amino acid supplements (arginine, glutamine) may help. Patients with a functioning gut who are unable to eat because of their poor appetite or nausea may receive nutrition through feeding tubes. In some cases, nutrition may be administered intravenously as a last resort. However, the risk/cost versus reward value of intravenous nutrition support remains controversial in many instances.

Exercise may also help to increase appetite and inhibit cachexia.

Risk Factors and Preventive Measures

Cachexia is found among severely ill patients with such diseases as acquired immunodeficiency syndrome (AIDS), chronic infections, chronic obstructive pulmonary disease, advanced stages of cancer, congestive heart failure, chronic kidney failure, and other extremely serious illnesses and medical conditions.

See also CANCERS OF THE DIGESTIVE SYSTEM; FEEDING TUBE.

Kotler, Donald P., M.D. "Cachexia." *Annals of Internal Medicine* 133, no. 8 (2000): 622–634.

Campylobacter A common and infectious form of bacteria that is responsible for many foodborne illnesses. However, it was first identified as a cause of abortion in cattle and sheep in the early 20th century. These days it is a common cause of acute DIARRHEA in the United States. The disease caused by *Campylobacter* bacteria is called *campylobacteriosis*. Few people in the United States die of this infection.

There are several varieties of *Campylobacter* bacteria that can cause people to become sick, including *Campylobacter jejuni*, and *C. coli*. *Campylobacter jejuni* (*C. jejuni*) is the most common form of these bacteria. The Centers for Disease Control (CDC) reports that *C. jejuni* is the primary cause of bacterial diarrhea in the United States, infecting an estimated more than 2.4 million people per year, most of whom are either younger than age five or are young adults, aged 15 to 29 years. *C. jejuni* is also responsible for 5 to 14 percent of all the diarrhea that occurs on the globe.

Campylobacter is carried by many birds and animals; thus, they can contaminate the food chain. Chicken is the most common culprit. The organisms may also be transmitted from raw or undercooked poultry products, as well as from contaminated water. These bacteria may also be transmitted by handling of waste from infected humans, animals, or birds. Pets may be carriers of *Campylobacter* bacteria, and pet owners should take special care when removing their pets' fecal material. Pet owners should always wash their hands after changing cat litter, scooping up dog waste, or cleaning a bird's or other pet's cage. Person-to-person transmission is uncommon.

Symptoms and Diagnostic Path

Some people have no symptoms of *Campylobacter* infection. The key symptoms of campylobacteriosis are as follows:

- diarrhea (frequently bloody)
- ABDOMINAL PAIN and cramping
- NAUSEA AND VOMITING
- fever
- tiredness and overall weakness

Less common presentations may include:

- the development of Reiter's syndrome, which causes arthritis and painful urination, as a result of the infection

- rarely, development of Guillain-Barré syndrome (GBS), a paralytic condition that usually occurs two to four weeks after the time of infection and requires hospitalization
- myocarditis and pericarditis
- colitis

The physician observes the symptoms of the patient and may order a stool specimen to identify the bacterium.

Treatment Options and Outlook

No medications are required in most cases, and simple hydration is all that is necessary. The physician may in some cases prescribe ciprofloxacin (Cipro) or erythromycin, especially for those patients who have an impaired immune system due to AIDS, age, or those with severe symptoms such as bleeding.

In general, infected people are ill for two to five days, and most illness resolves on its own. However, some individuals may be in a weakened condition for longer periods.

Risk Factors and Preventive Measures

Most who are infected are younger than age five or are young adults, aged 15 to 29 years. In general, experts recommend the following actions to prevent this food-borne illness:

- washing hands before food preparation
- washing hands after handling raw meat or poultry
- cooking meat thoroughly
- drinking pasteurized milk and clean water
- washing hands after cleaning animal feces or visiting a petting zoo

See also CONTAMINATED FOOD OR WATER.

cancers of the digestive system A disease that is exemplified by the uncontrolled growth of abnormal cells, which are also known as malignant cells. Unless treated, these cells form one or more tumors that continue to grow, eventually causing pain, disability, and death. Cancer can develop in nearly any part of the body, although it is more commonly found in specific particular areas, such as within the lungs, the female breast, the male prostate gland, or the colon. The key types of cancer that may occur within the digestive system include but are not limited to: COLORECTAL CANCER, ESOPHAGEAL CANCER, GALLBLADDER CANCER, LIVER CANCER, ORAL CANCER, PANCREATIC CANCER, SMALL INTESTINE CANCER, and STOMACH CANCER.

Cancer is the number two killer of all individuals in the United States (responsible for 23.1 percent of all adult deaths in the United States in 2006), close behind heart disease (26.0 percent). Among children, cancer is the second-leading cause of death after accidents. However, the most common childhood cancers are not digestive cancers, but rather they are leukemia, brain, and nervous system cancers and other forms of cancer.

According to the American Cancer Society, an estimated 292,540 men and 269,800 women died of all forms of cancer in 2009. Most (30 percent of males and 26 percent of females) died of cancer of the lung and bronchus, followed by breast cancer (15 percent) for women and prostate cancer (9 percent) for men. For men and women, an estimated 9 percent each died of colorectal cancer in 2009, and 6 percent each died of pancreatic cancer. Four percent of males and 2 percent of females died of cancer of the liver and intrahepatic bile duct. Among males, 4 percent died of esophageal cancer. (Esophageal cancer was not listed in the top 10 of causes of cancer deaths among women.)

The cancer death rate has dropped considerably since 1991, when 215.1 per 100,000 deaths were from cancer to a much improved rate in 2006, when the rate was 180.7 per 100,000 deaths.

There are often (but not always) some signs and symptoms to watch out for with any form of cancer, such as a wound that does not heal or unintentional weight loss. In addition, regular medical checkups can screen for many different types of cancer with the use of laboratory tests or specific medical procedures, such as the COLONOSCOPY, which screens for precancerous polyps (which are removed, if found) so that the individual can protect against the development of colorectal cancer.

Another procedure, the SIGMOIDOSCOPY, checks for precancerous polyps, but it does not encompass the entire colon, as with the colonoscopy and thus, some polyps can be missed with this procedure. The fecal occult blood test is a laboratory test that screens for blood in the feces, which, if present, indicates further investigation.

Some digestive cancers, such as colorectal cancer and oral cancer, often can be detected in the early stages of the diseases, when they are readily treated. In contrast, other digestive cancers, such as esophageal cancer, pancreatic cancer, stomach cancer, and liver cancer, often are not detected until they have reached an advanced stage. In the case of liver cancer, the cancer may be preceded by HEPATITIS and CIRRHOSIS, and thus, individuals who have any form of hepatitis/cirrhosis should be sure that their physician orders regular liver function blood tests to check for any changes in the test results, which may be a marker for liver cancer.

Individuals with other diseases in addition to hepatitis have an increased risk for developing a digestive cancer, particularly those with CROHN'S DISEASE, CELIAC DISEASE, or familial adenoma polyposis (FAP).

There are significant racial disparities that have been found between the early diagnosis and the survival rate of whites and blacks. Whites are more likely to be diagnosed at an earlier stage of nearly all forms of cancer, when the cancer is more readily treatable, and whites are also more likely to survive for longer periods than blacks. This issue was addressed by Beth A. Virnig et al. in their 2009 article in *Health Affairs*.

The treatment of cancer depends on the type of cancer that is present as well as its stage (whether it is an early or later stage). In addition, the treatment also depends on whether it is a localized cancer or it has metastasized (spread) to other organs and other factors. Treatment often involves the surgical removal of the tumor and the surrounding tissue. Radiation therapy may also serve as the primary treatment or as an adjunctive treatment. It is also sometimes used as a means to alleviate the pain of cancer that has spread to the bones. When the cancerous tumor cannot be removed or it has spread, chemotherapy may be the chosen treatment. Chemotherapy may also be used to shrink a tumor prior to surgery or radiation treatment. Biological and innovative therapies may also be available as treatments, and in addition, the individual may have an opportunity to gain access to new anticancer drugs by joining a clinical study.

Some people with cancer use complementary and ALTERNATIVE MEDICINE (CAM) as part of their treatment for cancer; however, it should be noted that it is extremely important for individuals to *not* limit their treatment solely to the use of alternative medicine alone *unless* such treatment is specifically recommended by physicians who are oncologists (cancer experts). The risk is that if a patient concentrates on using only CAM, often it will not prevent the cancer from growing and/or from becoming more aggressive. As a result, medical treatment would no longer be effective should the patient later decide in favor of medical treatment. Some types of alternative medicine that may be used in conjunction with medical treatments for cancer are acupuncture and massage therapy, and also herbal remedies such as ginger to control the nausea and vomiting of chemotherapy.

The causes of many forms of cancer are unknown, although it is known that some cancers have a genetic link. However, there are many indications that some forms of digestive cancers are preventable; for example, in their article in *Pharmaceutical Research* in 2008, authors Preetha Anand et al. contend that up to 90 to 95 percent of all cases of cancer are rooted in specific lifestyle choices. (This estimate may be high; hereditary factors also play a role in the development of many forms of cancer.)

Some key lifestyle choices that Anand and colleagues recommend include dietary changes (such as changing from a diet made up of a heavy consumption of fried foods and red meat to a diet that is high in vegetables and fruits); avoiding the excessive use of alcohol and smoking; changing from a sedentary lifestyle and a lack of exercise; and resolving obesity, if present.

Some research has found that people with allergies may have a *lower* risk for the development of cancer than those without allergies, according to Paul Sherman, Erica Holland, and Janet Shellman Sherman, which they reported in a 2008 issue of the *Quarterly Review of Biology*, based on an analysis of hundreds of studies. This inverse relationship (meaning that those with allergies were less likely to develop cancer) was the strongest for some specific types of digestive cancers such as oral cancer, colorectal cancer, and pancreatic cancer. (However, the research also revealed that individuals with asthma had an *increased* risk for the development of lung cancer.)

According to the authors, "The IgE system [part of the immune system] and its associated allergy symptoms may serve a common protective function: the rapid expulsion of pathogens, dangerous natural toxins, and other carcinogenic antigens before they can trigger malignant neoplasia in exposed tissues."

General Signs of Cancer

There are general indicators that a person may have cancer, although the signs and symptoms may indicate many other possible disorders. Anyone with these signs should report them to his or her physician. Each type of cancer also has its own particular signs and symptoms as well. The seven general signs of a possible cancer are:

1. an unintentional or unexplained weight loss
2. an obvious change in the color or the appearance of a mole or a wart
3. a change in bowel habits
4. a lump in the breast or elsewhere
5. a cut or sore that does not heal
6. a discharge that is unusual or unusual bleeding
7. difficulty with swallowing or hoarseness

The National Cancer Institute (NCI) also says that several other signs and symptoms that should be checked for the possible presence of cancer include:

- a new mole or a change in an existing mole
- persistent fatigue with no apparent cause
- a cough that does not go away
- discomfort after eating

Types of Cancer

In considering all forms of cancer (cancers of the digestive system as well as every other form of cancer), the National Cancer Institute estimated that 745,180 men and 692,000 women (for a total of 1,437,180 adults) were diagnosed with cancer in the United States in 2008. The median age at diagnosis for all cancer sites was 67 years. (The median is a statistical measure that means, in this case, that half of the people who were diagnosed with cancer in 2008 were younger than 67 years and half were older—it is a middle point and *not* an average/mean.)

Digestive Cancers

Colorectal cancer is the most common digestive cancer. Some digestive cancers, such as pancreatic cancer or anal cancer, are relatively rare, although they may not be detected until a late stage.

Colorectal Cancer According to the National Cancer Institute, there were an estimated 106,100 new cases of colorectal cancer diagnosed in 2009, and there were 49,920 deaths from colorectal cancer in 2009.

The symptoms of colorectal cancer may include blood in the feces as well as a change in the individual's normal bowel habits. Yet many people have no symptoms in the early stages of colorectal cancer, which is why regular checkups are important. (A physician knows which groups are most at risk for colorectal cancer, by age, gender, race, and so forth and will order the appropriate tests to screen his or her patients.) Colorectal cancer represented 8 percent of all adult male cancer deaths

in 2008 and 9 percent of all adult female cancer deaths, according to the American Cancer Society.

According to data from the Surveillance Epidemiology and End Results (SEER), based on a compilation of data for the period 2001–05, it was estimated that 77,250 men and 71,560 women were diagnosed with colorectal cancer in 2008 in the United States, and that 49,960 adults died of colorectal cancer in 2008. (See Table 1.) The median age at death from colorectal cancer was 75 years. The overall five-year survival rate for 1996–2004 was 64.4 percent. The five-year survival rate by gender and race among those with colorectal cancer was 65.4 percent for white adult males, 65.2 percent for white adult females, 55.5 percent for black females, and 54.7 percent for black males.

Oral Cancer The signs and symptoms of oral cancer may include difficulty with both swallowing and chewing; numbness in the tongue or other parts of the mouth; a sore or irritation in the mouth, and lip or throat; and difficulty moving the jaw or tongue. Often dentists are the first to identify oral cancer in the course of a dental examination. According to the National Institute of Dental and Craniofacial Research, 75 percent of oral cancers are related to the use of tobacco and/or alcohol. This form of cancer is most prevalent among those older than 40 years and is twice as common among men as women.

According to the American Cancer Society, the lifetime risk for men developing oral cancer is 1 in 71. (Data was not provided for women because oral cancer was not in the top 10 lifetime risks for cancer for women.)

TABLE 1: INCIDENCE RATES OF COLORECTAL CANCER BY RACE AND GENDER, 2001–2005, UNITED STATES

Race/Ethnicity	Male	Female
All races	59.2 per 100,000 men	43.8 per 100,000 women
White	58.9 per 100,000 men	43.2 per 100,000 women
Black	71.2 per 100,000 men	54.5 per 100,000 women
Asian/Pacific Islander	48.0 per 100,000 men	35.4 per 100,000 women
American Indian/Alaska Native	46.0 per 100,000 men	41.2 per 100,000 women
Hispanic	47.3 per 100,000 men	32.8 per 100,000 women

Source: Adapted from Ries, L.A.G., et al. eds. "Surveillance Epidemiology and End Results, Cancer of the Liver and Intrahepatic Duct." *SEER Cancer Statistics Review, 1975–2005*. Bethesda, Md.: National Cancer Institute. Available online at http://seer.cancer.gov/csr/1975_2005/. Based on November 2007 SEER submission, posted to the SEER Web site, 2008. Downloaded February 1, 2009.

TABLE 2: OVERALL 5-YEAR SURVIVAL RATES, BY TYPE OF CANCER, RACE (BLACK AND WHITE) AND GENDER

	Colon	Anal	Esophagus	Oral	Pancreas	Liver	Stomach	Small intestine
Black males	54.7	54.9	54.7	36.1	3.6	7.9	21.6	48.2
Black females	55.5	64.5	55.5	52.1	5.4	7.7	27.2	53.7
White males	65.4	61.2	65.4	61.0	5.1	11.0	21.2	59.2
White females	65.2	71.6	65.2	62.9	4.9	12.3	25.5	48.2

Source: Ries, L.A.G., et al. eds. *SEER Cancer Statistics Review, 1975–2005*. Bethesda, Md.: National Cancer Institute. Available online at http://seer. cancer.gov/csr/1975_2005/. Based on November 2007 SEER submission, posted to the SEER Web site, 2008. Downloaded February 1, 2009.

Cancer of the oral cavity and pharynx was diagnosed in 35,310 adults in 2008, according to the National Cancer Institute. The incidence of oral cancer was the highest among blacks, followed by whites. Looking at all the individuals who were diagnosed with oral cancer for the period 1996–2004, more than half survived for five or more years: the overall five-year survival rate was 59.7 percent. Black men had the lowest five-year survival rate or 36.1 percent, followed by 52.1 percent for black women. Among whites, nearly two-thirds survived for five or more years; the five-year survival rate was 61.0 percent for white males and 62.9 percent for white females. (See Table 2.)

Stomach Cancer According to the American Cancer Society, the lifetime risk for men developing stomach cancer is 1 in 88. Data were not provided for women because stomach cancer is not among the top 10 forms of cancer for women. According to the SEER data from the National Cancer Institute, 13,190 men and 8,310 women (for a total of 21,500 adults) in the United States were diagnosed with stomach cancer in 2008. An estimated 10,880 adults died of stomach cancer in 2008. The incidence of stomach cancer was highest among male and female Asians and Pacific Islanders or 18.6 per 100,000 men and 10.5 per 100,000 women. This rate was much higher than the rate for all races of 11.3 per 100,000 men and 5.5 per 100,000 women.

According to Jemal et al., Asian Americans and Pacific Islanders have a much greater exposure to *HELICOBACTER PYLORI* and hepatitis B, which accounts for their higher rate of stomach cancer and liver cancer.

The overall five-year survival rate from stomach cancer, using data for the period 1996–2004, was 24.7 percent.

Signs and symptoms of stomach cancer may include mild nausea, a loss of appetite, heartburn, and a bloated feeling after eating. If the stomach cancer is more advanced, the symptoms may include an unintentional weight loss, stomach pain, jaundice, a buildup of fluid in the abdomen (ASCITES), blood in the stool, and difficulty swallowing.

Esophageal Cancer Esophageal cancer may present with such signs and symptoms as difficulty with swallowing, unintentional weight loss, a persistent cough, and hoarseness.

According to the SEER data, an estimated 148,810 people (77,250 men and 71,560 women) were diagnosed with esophageal cancer in 2008. Males, particularly black males, have the highest risk of developing this form of cancer. The average age at the point of diagnosis was 71 years over the period 2001–05. The median age of death was 75 years. The five-year survival rate, using data from 1996–2004, was 64.4 percent, including 65.4 percent for white males, 65.2 percent for white females, 54.7 percent for black males, and 55.5 percent for black females.

According to the American Cancer Society, cancer of the esophagus represented 4 percent of all adult male cancer deaths. (Statistics were not provided for female cancer deaths—esophageal cancer was included under "all other sites," and 25 percent of all female cancer deaths fell in into this category.)

Gallbladder Cancer Gallbladder cancer is a rare form of cancer; however, according to Mary Denshaw-Burke, et al. in their article online on eMedicine in 2008, it is the fifth-most common form of digestive cancer. Denshaw-Burke and colleagues say that gallbladder cancer stems from inflammation, and in greater than 75 percent of the cases, this inflammation is caused by choles- terol GALLSTONES. The presence of these gallstones increases the risk for gallbladder cancer by four to five times. (Note that most patients with gall- stones do not develop gallbladder cancer, since it is relatively rare.) Other factors associated with inflammation that may lead to gallbladder cancer are ULCERATIVE COLITIS, PRIMARY SCLEROSING CHOL- ANGITIS, and chronic infection with *SALMONELLA* or *HELICOBACTER*.

According to Jemal et al. in their 2007 article for *CA: A Cancer Journal for Clinicians*, there were an estimated 9,250 new cases of gallbladder cancer and other biliary cancer in 2007, including 4,380 men and 4,870 women. There were an estimated 3,250 deaths from gallbladder cancer in 2007.

Individuals with gallbladder cancer may have symptoms of JAUNDICE, abdominal pain, weight loss, fever, nausea, and an abdominal mass; how- ever, these signs may also indicate liver cancer or pancreatic cancer. Itching is another symptom because itching is associated with jaundice. Often there are no symptoms when the cancer is local- ized, and because symptoms usually do not appear until a late stage, gallbladder cancer is usually not diagnosed in its early stages and thus, it spreads to other organs. SEER data is not available specifically for gallbladder cancer.

According to the authors Alan P. Vernook, M.D., and Sabrina Selim, M.D., if gallbladder cancer *is* diagnosed at an early stage, then the five-year survival rate is about 80 percent. However, if the cancer is diagnosed at a late stage, the two-year survival rate is less than 1 percent. Patients with gallbladder cancer as with any other cancer may need narcotics, but physicians must be careful with most narcotics because the liver metabolizes them and the patient with gallbladder cancer may have a malfunctioning liver. NONSTEROIDAL ANTI-INFLAM- MATORY DRUGS (NSAIDs) may be effective. Patients with no appetite may be prescribed Megace, an appetite-stimulating drug.

Native Americans and Mexicans are at the most risk for developing gallbladder cancer.

Liver Cancer According to the National Cancer Institute, about 15,000 men and 6,000 women are diagnosed each year with liver cancer and most are ages 65 and older. In contrast to other forms of cancer, the highest rates of incidence are found among Asian/Pacific Islanders, American Indians/ Alaskan Natives, and Hispanics. (See Table 3.) In considering cancers of the liver and intrahepatic duct, it was estimated that 22,620 new cases were diagnosed in 2009 and that 18,160 people died of these cancers in 2009.

The average age at diagnosis was 65 years old for the period 2001–05. The median age at death was 70 years. The five-year survival rates were poor, or an average of 11.7 percent. Survival rates were as follows: 12.3 percent for white women, 11.0 percent for white men, 7.9 percent for black men, and 7.7 percent for black women. (The sur- vival rates for Asians and other high-risk groups are unknown.)

Cancer of the liver and intrahepatic ducts repre- sented 4 percent of all adult male cancer deaths in 2008, according to the American Cancer Society. The statistic was not reported for female cancer deaths, and instead was incorporated into "all other sites."

TABLE 3: INCIDENCE OF LIVER CANCER, RATES BY RACE AND GENDER, 2001–2005, UNITED STATES		
Race/Ethnicity	Male	Female
All Races	9.9 per 100,000 men	3.5 per 100,000 women
White	8.2 per 100,000 men	2.9 per 100,000 women
Black	13.2 per 100,000 men	4.0 per 100,000 women
Asian/Pacific Islander	21.7 per 100,000 men	8.3 per 100,000 women
American Indian/Alaskan Native	14.4 per 100,000 men	6.3 per 100,000 women
Hispanic	15.0 per 100,000 men	5.8 per 100,000 women

Source: Adapted from Ries, L.A.G., et al. eds. "Surveillance Epidemiology and End Results, Cancer of the Liver and Intrahepatic Duct." *SEER Cancer Statistics Review, 1975–2005.* Bethesda, Md.: National Cancer Institute. Available online at http://seer.cancer.gov/csr/1975_2005/. Based on November 2007 SEER submission, posted to the SEER Web site, 2008. Downloaded February 1, 2009.

Symptoms of liver cancer may include unintentional weight loss, pain in the right upper abdomen, appetite loss and jaundice. Other symptoms are nausea and vomiting, fever, a bloated swollen abdomen and weakness.

Pancreatic Cancer   Cancer of the pancreas is a rare cancer that is often diagnosed in a late stage, making it difficult to treat. Often the first symptom is jaundice, which also frequently indicates that an advanced cancer is present. According to SEER data, an estimated 37,680 adults, including 18,770 men and 18,910 women, were diagnosed with pancreatic cancer in 2008. The median age at diagnosis was 72 years. According to the American Cancer Society, the lifetime risk for adult females developing pancreatic cancer was 1 in 76 in 2002–04. Data were not provided for adult males because pancreatic cancer was not listed among the top ten forms of cancer for males.

The incidence of pancreatic cancer was highest among black males, followed by black females; the rate for black males for the period 2001–05 was 16.2 per 100,000 men, and the rate for black females was 14.3 per 100,000 women. The lowest rates of pancreatic cancer were found among Asian and Pacific Islander and American Indian/Alaska Native females, which groups each had a rate of 8.2 per 100,000 women.

The overall five-year survival rate from pancreatic cancer was a very low 5.1 percent for all races and genders, based on SEER data for the period 1996–2004. Considering black and white races and genders, the five-year survival rates were: 5.4 percent for black women, 5.1 percent for white men, 4.9 percent for white women, and only 3.6 percent for black men.

Small Intestine Cancer   Cancer of the small intestine is a rare form of cancer. Its symptoms may include abdominal cramps, an unintentional weight loss, blood in the stool, and a lump in the abdomen. Black males and females are most at risk for this form of cancer.

Based on SEER data from the National Cancer Institute, it was estimated that 3,200 men and 2,910 women (a total of 6,110 adults) were diagnosed with cancer of the small intestine in 2008, and 1,110 people died from this form of cancer in 2008. The median age at diagnosis was 67 years of age for the period 2001–05. The five-year survival rate for the period 1996–2004 was 57.8 percent. Five-year survival rates by race and sex were: 60.3 percent for white women, 59.2 percent for white men, 53.7 percent for black women, and 48.2 percent for black men.

The Demographics of Cancer Patients

Demographics refers to gender, race and ethnicity, age, and other factors that are associated with an increased risk for developing cancer. In general, males are more at risk for developing cancer than females are; for example, according to the American Cancer Society, the lifetime probability of adult males developing any form of cancer, based on data in the period 2002–04, was one in two; the risk for adult females was one in three. Among digestive cancers, the greatest risk is with colorectal cancer, and the lifetime risk of developing this form of cancer is one in 18 for men and one in 19 for women.

There are distinctive racial differences that are found with the prevalence of many forms of cancer. Based on data from the National Cancer Institute (NCI), black men have the highest risk for most forms of cancer. In general, Asians and Pacific Islanders have a generally lower rate of cancer than do other races and ethnicities with some exceptions. Many people have speculated on the racial disparities among cancer patients. Some experts believe that a lack of access to health care is the main problem, while others believe failure to obtain screening tests for cancer is an issue. Other factors, such as poor diet, smoking, and obesity may also play a role. Other diseases, such as diabetes and hypertension, also may contribute to poor health and cancer risks.

Genetic Risks   If other family members have had cancer, an individual should be screened for cancer as well, particularly in the case of colorectal cancer, stomach cancer, and pancreatic cancer. These forms of cancer have been linked to specific genes; for example, according to Anand, et al., stomach cancer has been linked to the gene TL4, while colorectal cancer has been linked to many genes. Pancreatic cancer has been linked to the gene DPC4.

Racial Disparities   Many studies have indicated that there are racial differences between when cancer is diagnosed at an early stage and also the percentage of long-term survivors of cancer. In nearly every form of cancer, blacks have a clear disadvantage compared to whites. According to Beth A. Virnig, et al., in their 2009 their article in *Health Affairs* on race and cancer, it is crucial to identify blacks with cancer at an early stage, as with many whites.

They say, "Given equal treatment, there is considerable evidence that African Americans and whites could experience equal stage-specific survival. Addressing treatment disparities will not equalize cancer survival if the stage at which diagnosis occurs differs systematically between African Americans and whites. The prognostic impact of late-stage diagnosis is so strongly related to poorer survival that increasing the percentage of cancers diagnosed at an early stage is a prominent goal of the National Cancer Institute."

Virnig and her colleagues also assert that the differences in the early diagnosis and survival of blacks versus whites cannot be explained by either risk factors or screening behavior. The researchers studied the stage of diagnosis for 34 different types of cancers, based on data from SEER. They found that over the period 1992–2003, 190,579 African Americans and 1,517,068 non-Hispanic white adults were diagnosed with cancer. They looked at several factors; for example, one factor considered was cancers that can be screened for, such as colon cancer, renal cancer, breast cancer, and cancer of the cervix. For all four cancers, they found a significantly higher five-year survival rate for whites; for example, the percentage of whites who survived colon cancer for five years was 65.35 percent, compared to 56.47 for African Americans.

In only two types of cancer, of all cancers, did African Americans have an advantage over whites; with gallbladder cancer and with stomach cancer, African Americans had a slightly higher survival rate which was not statistically significant.

The researchers concluded that the factors responsible for the disparities between blacks and whites for early diagnosis as well as five-year survival rates were most likely due to factors within the patients themselves or to an institutional racism. One factor may be a lack of insurance; some studies have found that people who are uninsured or who are on Medicaid are less likely to be screened for cancer. Other possible factors the researchers considered that may be affecting the worse prognosis for blacks included:

- low income and low education
- medical providers who are less educated about cancer or who have a less well established network of providers
- patients' own delay in seeking care, whether from fear or denial
- difficulty in obtaining an initial appointment

The researchers concluded that, "In spite of the growing array of treatments available for patients diagnosed with metastatic disease, the most effective way to improve cancer survivorship is through early detection. Although efforts to eliminate disparities in cancer treatment are important and necessary, they are not sufficient to eliminate disparities in overall cancer survival if the disparities in the stage at which diagnoses are made remain."

Screening for colorectal cancer is very important for blacks. A study of the prevalence of colon polyps that were detected with the colonoscopy among black and white patients with symptoms, reported in 2008 by David Lieberman in the *Journal of the American Medical Association*, revealed that both black men and black women had a significantly higher rate of having large polyps compared to white men and women. In addition, Dr. Lieberman found that black adults older than age 60 had a higher risk of having larger polyps than older white adults. Said the authors, "The differences were especially striking among women. These findings emphasize the importance of encouraging all black men and women to be screened."

Screening for Cancer

The symptoms of digestive cancers generally depend upon the type and site of the cancer, and as mentioned earlier, often there are no symptoms at all in the early stages of cancer. This is why it is important to have regular medical checkups; physicians screen for some types of cancer with specific procedures, such as the colonoscopy, which is used to screen for colorectal cancer. In addition, if precancerous polyps are found during a colonoscopy, they are removed from the colon. The patient will be rescreened for further polyps at periodic intervals depending upon the findings at the initial colonoscopy, enabling physicians to identify and remove any precancerous growths that are present.

If family history indicates, various forms of endoscopies can be used to screen for esophageal cancer, stomach cancer, or liver cancer, although these tests are not routinely performed in the United States. Interestingly, liver cancer is much more common in incidence in Japan than in the United States, but because it is frequently screened for in Japan, the percentage of deaths is lower in Japan than in the United States.

Cancer Staging

When cancer is diagnosed, it is also *staged*, which means that physicians determine the severity of the cancer based upon a biopsy and imaging studies. Biopsy is tissue that includes the tumor, and the physician ascertains other aspects of the staging analysis. Cancer staging varies according to the type of cancer, but "TNM" mode of staging is most commonly used, which means that the tumor itself is graded in terms of how advanced it is, which is the *T* in the TNM staging. The physician also seeks to determine whether the cancer has spread to any surrounding nodes (the *N* in the TNM staging system) where the tumor is located. Finally, the doctor analyzes whether the cancer has metastasized (spread, the *M* in the TNM cancer staging system) at all beyond the original site of the tumor.

The best survivability generally occurs when the tumor is localized; it has not spread to adjacent nodes, and it has not metastasized to distant parts of the body. However, in many cases, the cancer may still be treatable and survivable as long as it has not spread to the bones or the bloodstream. If the cancer has spread to the bones or bloodstream, it can be contained for some period of time, depending on the type of cancer, but it cannot be cured.

Treatment of Digestive Cancers

Treatment of cancer is highly individualized. For example, if the cancer is in its early stages, often surgery or radiation therapy may be used to eliminate the tumor altogether. If the cancer is more advanced, then chemotherapy may be used, in which medications are used to attempt to arrest the spread of the cancer and/or to shrink the tumor. Radiation therapy may also be used to shrink the tumor as well as to treat the pain of advanced cancer.

Newer cancer treatments such as biologic therapy, immunotherapy, and genetic therapy are under development as of this writing.

Lifestyle Choices: Problem Choices

Lifestyle choices can both increase the risk for developing cancer as well as act as a protective factor against the development of cancer, such as the choice to use alcohol to excess (which increases the risk of developing some forms of cancer) or the decision to abstain or limit consumption (which decreases the risk of developing these same forms of cancer). The choice to smoke, overeat, or to avoid vegetables and fruits increases the risk for the development of some forms of cancer.

It is true that individuals who smoke and/or drink to excess have developed a physical and psychological dependence on nicotine and/or alcohol; however, treatment to break these addictions is available for those who are willing to receive it. Many people eschew such treatment. Arguably, no one wishes to be obese; however, with a change in diet and an increase in exercise, most people can attain a healthy weight. Exercise itself is an important protective factor against cancer, even when an individual is not obese. Note that this does not mean that healthy adults who exercise will never get cancer; some do. The risk for developing cancer, however, is lower than among those who fail to exercise.

Smoking and Digestive Cancers   SMOKING is a risk factor for lung cancer, but it is also a risk factor for digestive cancers as well, such as pancreatic cancer, stomach cancer, anal cancer, and cancer of the oropharynx. If the individual who smokes is also a heavy alcohol consumer, the risk for the development of cancer increases markedly.

Alcohol Dependence   According to Helmut K. Seitz, M.D., and Peter Becker, M.D., in their article for *Alcohol Research & Health* published in 2007, alcoholism (alcohol dependence) is a factor in some forms of cancer. Say the authors, "Acetaldehyde itself is a cancer-causing substance in experimental animals and reacts with DNA to form cancer-promoting compounds. In addition, highly reactive, oxygen-containing molecules that are generated during certain pathways of alcohol metabolism can damage the DNA, thus also inducing tumor development. Together with other factors related to chronic alcohol consumption, these metabolism-related factors may increase tumor risk in chronic heavy drinkers."

According to Seitz and Becker, the greatest cancer risk found with alcohol-associated cancer is with the development of cancer of the upper aerodigestive tract, which includes the area of the oral cavity, voice box, and esophagus. In addition, heavy drinking (more than five or six drinks per day) combined with smoking increases the risk for developing these forms of cancer by an astounding 50 times.

According to Key and colleagues, alcohol is a risk factor for oral cancer, esophageal cancer, and probably colorectal cancer.

Obesity According to Anand, et al., obesity is a factor in about 14 percent of all deaths from cancer in men and 20 percent in women. Excessive weight is defined by a BODY MASS INDEX that is equal to or greater than 30 kilograms per square meter (meters of the person's height squared, or the number multiplied times itself). BMI is usually expressed as a single number, for example, a BMI of 30 or greater means that a person is obese. A BMI of 25 to one that is just under 30 means that a person is overweight. The higher that the BMI is, the greater that the risk for cancer is as well as the risk for many other diseases, such as type 2 diabetes and hypertension, and a wide variety of kidney and cardiovascular ailments.

According to Key and colleagues in their article in *Public Health Nutrition* in 2004, overweight and obesity is a known risk factor for the development of adenocarcinoma of the esophagus.

Nutritional Choices In general, a person who consumes a diet that is high in fats, red meats, carbohydrates, and high calories has a greater risk for the development of cancer than a person who consumes a diet that is high in fruits and vegetables and which is also moderate in the number of calories that are consumed. Antioxidants, which are natural chemical substances that are found in both vitamins and minerals, are more likely to be found in a person who consumes a diet that is rich in fruits and vegetables rather than one who relies upon a diet that is heavily dependent on traditional fried fast foods.

Individuals should limit their consumption of preserved meats such as salami, bacon, sausage, and ham as well as red meats such as beef.

According to Preetha Anand and colleagues, diet is linked to as many as 70 percent of all colorectal cancer deaths. This may be because some carcinogens (cancer-causing substances) are ingested, such as nitrites, pesticides, and other harmful items. For example, Anand and colleagues report that the heavy consumption of red meat is a risk factor for colorectal, stomach, pancreatic, and oral cancers.

Earlier articles that analyzed many studies on diet, nutrition, and the prevention of cancer by Timothy J. Key and colleagues reported that salt-preserved foods and a high salt intake are likely to increase the risk for stomach cancer. The authors also noted that drinking very hot drinks or eating very hot foods likely increase the risk for oral and esophageal cancer.

Infections Some types of infections may play a role in the development of cancer, particularly in the case of stomach cancer. The primary infectious culprit in stomach cancer is *Helicobacter pylori*. Hepatitis B and hepatitis C infections are also factors in the development of hepatocellular carcinoma, which is a form of liver cancer. The human papilloma virus (HPV) is a factor in the development of anogenital cancer.

Environmental Carcinogens Anand, et al., report that environmental factors sometimes play a role in the development of some forms of cancer; for example, the nitrates in drinking water can lead to colorectal cancer, while the exposure to radiation, such as carbon, radium, and uranium, is linked to gastric cancer (stomach cancer).

Exercise or Inactivity Regular exercise is protective against most forms of cancer, at least in part because it reduces the risk of obesity. Individuals should consult with their physicians before undergoing an exercise regimen, but most people can perform at least some exercise. Even brisk walking can consume excess calories. As mentioned, exercise is not absolutely protective but rather reduces the risk of cancer.

According to Anand and colleagues, a sedentary lifestyle is linked to an increased risk for cancer of the breast, colon, prostate, and pancreas.

Lifestyle Choices: Protective Factors

Some lifestyle choices are apparently protective against the development of cancer. For example, Anand, et al., report that the consumption of fruits and vegetables is a protective factor against cancer. Fruits that contain lycopene are particularly beneficial, such as watermelon, grapefruit, tomatoes, apricots, and other fruits. Fruits containing resveratrol are apparently protective against many forms of cancer, such as cancer of the pancreas, stomach, and colon as well as others. Resveratrol is present in such fruits as grapes and berries, as well as peanuts. Cercumin is another potentially protective substance with no known toxicities. It is present in the turmeric root.

Other substances that are apparently protective against the development of cancer include ginger, anethold (present in fennel, a spice), and capsaicin. In addition, whole-grain foods have antioxidant capacities. Some vitamins appear protective against cancer, such as vitamin C (which may reduce the risk for cancer of the esophagus, stomach, mouth, and pancreas) and vitamin D, a general protective vitamin.

Regular exercise is a known protective factor against colorectal cancer as well as esophageal cancer.

See also DIET DRUGS; OBESITY; POLYPS.

Ahmedin, Jemal, et al. "Annual Report to the Nation on the Status of Cancer, 1975–2005, Featuring Trends in Lung Cancer, Tobacco Use, and Tobacco Control." *Journal of the National Cancer Institute* 100, no. 23 (December 3, 2008): 1,672–1,694.

Anand, Preetha, et al. "Cancer is a Preventable Disease that Requires Major Lifestyle Changes." *Pharmaceutical Research* 29, no. 9 (2008): 2,097–2,116.

Centers for Disease Control and Prevention, *U.S. Cancer Statistics: 2004 Incidence and Mortality.* Atlanta, Ga.: Centers for Disease Control and Prevention, 2007.

Denshaw-Burke, M.D., et al. "Gallbladder Cancer." eMedicine. Updated June 12, 2008. Available online. URL: http://emedicine.medscape.com/article/278641-overview. Downloaded February 6, 2009.

Jemal, Ahmedin, et al. "Cancer Statistics, 2007." *CA: A Cancer Journal for Clinicians* 57 (2007): 43–66.

Key, Timothy J., et al. "Diet, Nutrition and the Prevention of Cancer." *Public Health Nutrition* 7, no. 1A (2004): 187–200.

Lieberman, David, M.D., "Prevalence of Colon Polyps Detected by Colonoscopy Screening in Asymptomatic Black and White Patients." *Journal of the American Medical Association* 300, no. 12 (September 24, 2008): 1,417–1,422.

Ries, L.A.G., et al., eds., *SEER Cancer Statistics Review, 1975–2005.* Bethesda, Md.: National Cancer Institute. Available online. URL: http://seer.cancer.gov/csr/1975_2005/. Based on November 2007 SEER submission, posted to the SEER Web site, 2008. Downloaded February 1, 2009.

Seitz, Helmut K., M.D., and Peter Becker, M.D., "Alcohol Metabolism and Cancer Risk," *Alcohol Research & Health* 30, no. 1 (2007): 38–47.

Sherman, Paul.W., Erica Holland, and Janet Shellman Sherman. "Allergies: Their Role in Cancer Prevention." *Quarterly Review of Biology* 83, no. 4 (2008): 339–362.

Venook, Alan P., M.D. and Sabrina Selim, M.D. "Cancer of the Gall Bladder." Updated August 19, 2007. Available online. URL: http://www.cancersupportivecare.com/gallbladder.html. Downloaded February 6, 2009.

Virnig, Beth A., et al. "A Matter of Race: Early-Versus Late-Stage Cancer Diagnosis." *Health Affairs* 28, no. 1 (January–February 2009): 160–168.

cancer, anal   See ANAL CANCER.

cancer, colorectal   See COLORECTAL CANCER.

cancer, esophageal   See ESOPHAGEAL CANCER.

cancer, gallbladder   See GALLBLADDER CANCER.

cancer, liver   See LIVER CANCER.

cancer, oral   See ORAL CANCER.

cancer, pancreatic   See PANCREATIC CANCER.

cancer, stomach   See STOMACH CANCER.

Candida   A common yeast that is found in the body. It is a commensal yeast (living with another organism from which they derive a benefit without causing harm) that is normally seen in the oral cavity, gastrointestinal tract, and vagina. *Candida* are not harmful unless an infection occurs. *Candida* organism can cause infections in the skin, mouth, throat, or internal organs when the normal balance of bacteria is disrupted or the person's immune system is suppressed (such as patients who have received organ transplantation, patients with cancer, and patients with acquired immunodeficiency syndrome [AIDS]). A mouth infection of *Candida* is also called THRUSH. The infection may also spread into the bloodstream, especially in immunosuppressed patients. *Candida* infections of other organs, such as the esophagus, liver, lungs, joints, genitourinary system, and heart, may also develop.

Symptoms and Diagnostic Path

Oral thrush may cause no symptoms or may cause a cottony feeling in the mouth, the loss of taste, and painful eating and swallowing. If *Candida* organisms are found on the skin or in the genital area, they usually cause intense itching and may also cause PAIN. Vaginal candidiasis causes itching and discharge and, in some cases, pain during urination and during sexual intercourse. A cottage cheese-like substance in the vagina is characteristic of *Candida* infection, and the infection also produces a distinctive odor.

The male counterpart of candida vaginitis may be *balanitis*, where white patches are seen on the penis causing severe burning and itching. The infection may spread to adjoining areas like the skin.

Oral thrush may be suspected during physical examination and later confirmed by examining oral scrapings with a potassium hydroxide (KOH) preparation. A vaginal examination reveals redness and swelling in the area when *Candida* infection is present, with a curd-like discharge. The presence

of vaginal *Candida* organisms can be confirmed as with oral thrush. The presence of esophageal candidiasis can be confirmed by endoscopy.

Treatment Options and Outlook

Antiyeast creams or drugs are usually effective in combating a yeast infection, and oral antiyeast medications are also efficacious. Some doctors use both oral and topical (used on the skin) medications or intravaginal preparations. Some people, especially patients who are immunocompromised, experience chronic fungal infections and may need to take a "low-maintenance" dose of antiyeast medication. There are also oral drugs that combat fungal infections. Patients in whom *Candida* infection has spread may require intravenous antifungal medications. Patients usually need treatment for about two weeks or more.

In rare cases, a *Candida* infection can become systemic, causing the individual to feel very sick and lethargic, and this condition can be fatal.

Risk Factors and Preventive Measures

People who have some diseases, such as DIABETES MELLITUS, are more prone to development of *Candida* infections than others. Sometimes taking antibiotics can cause *Candida* infections, particularly causing vaginitis in women. An extended dosage of antibiotics is more likely to cause such an infection than is one short course of drugs that is taken for just three to five days.

Vulvovaginitis (an infection of the vulva, or the female external sex organ) may occur in those on birth control pills, during pregnancy or who are using diaphragm or intrauterine devices.

See also *LACTOBACILLUS*.

canker sores   Painful small mouth sores that usually spontaneously resolve in a few days. Various factors have been implicated in causing canker sores, including stress, hormonal factors, food allergies, an altered immune system, heredity, vitamin deficiencies (of B_1, B_2, B_6, and B_{12}), and deficiencies of iron, folic acid, and zinc.

Larger canker sores may require several weeks to heal. Most patients get these ulcers two to four times per year. Occasionally, some patients have canker sores almost all the time. Canker sores are more common during childhood and adolescence and are seen less frequently in adulthood.

Canker sores may also result from infections (herpes), chemotherapy, and systemic illnesses such as CROHN'S DISEASE.

Caroli's disease A rare congenital disease in which the ducts that transport bile from the liver to the intestine are abnormally widened (also called cystic) in one or more places. Caroli's disease may run in families. This condition may result in inflammation, infection, or GALLSTONES. Typical symptoms of Caroli's disease include abdominal pain, jaundice, and fever. Patients with Caroli's disease may experience periodic flare-ups of CHOLANGITIS, which is the inflammation of the bile duct. They may also experience liver abscesses.

Those who have Caroli's disease have a greater risk than others of development of cancer of the bile ducts (cholangiocarcinoma): an estimated 2 to 15 percent of Caroli's disease patients have this form of cancer.

The treatment of choice for Caroli's disease is surgery, which can reduce, but not eliminate, the risk of cancer. The complication of cholangitis is treated with antibiotics. In refractory cases, liver transplantation offers the only hope for patients who have no evidence of cancer.

celiac disease/celiac sprue A severe food allergy that is caused by an allergic reaction to gluten, a substance that is found in wheat, rye, or barley and that leads to damage to the small intestine. The role of oats is controversial in celiac disease, and as of this writing, it appears that pure oats are not a major problem; however, pure oats are difficult to obtain, and hence oats should be avoided in patients with celiac sprue unless the package documents that it is gluten-free and that it was processed in a gluten-free facility. Different patients can tolerate different amounts of gluten. There is no single threshold applicable to everyone. It appears that a daily gluten intake of less than 10 mg per day is unlikely to cause significant intestinal distress.

This disease is caused by an inappropriate immune cell response to the presence of gluten in some foods. In affected people, the immune system perceives gluten in the same way as a foreign invasion. This excites an inflammatory response that causes damage to the intestinal lining of the small intestine, leading to impaired absorption.

Symptoms and Diagnostic Path

Children with celiac sprue may have an enlarged abdomen, chronic DIARRHEA, and delayed growth. Infants may be very pale. Some children have CONSTIPATION rather than diarrhea. Babies and small children with celiac disease may present with abdominal distention and failure to thrive (failure to grow and develop normally). If the condition is not diagnosed and treated, children may have delayed puberty, short stature, and ANEMIA. Older children with celiac sprue may have chronic abdominal pain, defects in the enamel of the teeth, and even emotional disorders, such as depression or irritability.

Celiac sprue usually develops in early childhood, but many cases are identified during adulthood. It may appear for the first time in pregnancy. Adults with celiac sprue have symptoms of diarrhea, weight loss, and excessive gas (flatulence). They may also experience LACTOSE INTOLERANCE. In addition, they may have osteoporosis, abdominal pain, weight loss, hypocalcemia, and other symptoms. Many patients diagnosed with celiac disease were previously diagnosed with irritable bowel syndrome.

About half of all adult patients with celiac disease have iron deficiency anemia. They may also have other vitamin deficiencies, including deficiencies in vitamins B_{12}, D, and K. Many patients have no symptoms at all and may instead have asymptomatic and unexplained iron deficiency anemia.

Other symptoms that may occur in patients with celiac sprue are as follows:

- pale skin
- muscle pain and cramps
- joint pain
- anemia

- edema (excessive retention of water weight)
- extensive bruising (due to insufficiency of vitamin K)

A skin condition known as dermatitis herpetiformis may also be seen. An itchy and burning rash develops and can become blisters that rupture. A rash may be seen on the elbows, knees, buttocks, back, face, neck, and abdomen. Some patients have a deficiency of immunoglobulin A (IgA) antibodies.

Special blood tests of the immune system can be used to detect celiac sprue when physicians suspect that the condition is present. In the past, the patient's blood was tested for antibodies to gliadin; however, this test is outdated and has largely been abandoned. Testing for IgA antibodies to endomysium and/or tissue transglutaminase are usually used, with or without total IgA levels. The antitissue transglutaminase testing is less expensive than the antiendomysial antibody test, but the tests are equally accurate. An antireticulin test is also available, but it is usually not needed and not performed.

Some patients with celiac sprue have IgA deficiency and as such, the IgA antibody tests may be falsely negative in these cases. IgG antibody for tissue transglutaminase may be used in such cases. Physicians also perform a small bowel biopsy for confirmation, which is considered the definitive test to look for damage to the intestinal lining caused by celiac sprue.

Patients are also tested for iron deficiency anemia since it is a very common medical problem among people with celiac sprue. They may also be tested for deficiencies of calcium and vitamin D, which are also frequently seen among patients who have celiac sprue. As mentioned earlier, a vitamin B_{12} deficiency may also be present, although it is less commonly found than are the other types of deficiencies. Some patients with celiac sprue are also deficient in vitamin K.

Treatment Options and Outlook

Doctors put children or adults with celiac sprue on a very strict gluten-free diet. Patients are instructed to avoid all foods that contain any wheat, barley, rye, or oats. Some dessert items and ice creams, and even some vitamin pills contain wheat fillers, and these items must be completely avoided.

An estimated 70 percent of patients with celiac sprue significantly improve on a gluten-free diet, which is the only treatment for celiac sprue. The remaining 30 percent have a poor response. Patients who do not respond to a gluten-free diet may require corticosteroids and other immunosuppressive medications in order to suppress the inflammatory damage that is caused by sprue. Patients with celiac sprue have an increased risk for gastrointestinal cancers. Patients or the parents of children with celiac sprue must be especially vigilant in reading food labels and asking questions about food preparation when not eating at home.

Risk Factors and Preventive Measures

Women have two to three times the risk of having celiac disease as men, and the reasons for this are unknown. The risk for the disease among women declines after age 65.

As indicated by antibody testing, celiac sprue affects an estimated one in every 150 to 300 people in North America and Europe. About one in 4,700 people in the United States has actually been diagnosed with celiac disease; however, according to the National Institutes of Health, there is clear evidence that the disease is underdiagnosed in the United States, as indicated by blood samples drawn from Americans by the Red Cross and then tested for celiac disease. A 2004 NIH consensus conference concluded that as many as one in 133 Americans may actually have the disease based on blood testing.

Celiac sprue is usually diagnosed in children or young adults, although about 20 percent of the cases are diagnosed among people older than age 60. Celiac sprue may also be diagnosed during or after pregnancy, especially among women who are severely anemic after the delivery of the baby. This medical problem is found among all races and ethnicities, although it is rare among Asians and blacks.

People who have celiac sprue are more likely to have other associated autoimmune illnesses, such as type 1 (insulin-dependent) diabetes or autoimmune thyroiditis. An estimated 3 to 8 percent of type 1 diabetes patients also have celiac sprue.

There are no known preventive measures to celiac disease.

See also FOOD ALLERGIES.

Green, Peter H. R., M.D., and Christopher Cellier, M.D. "Celiac Disease," *New England Journal of Medicine* 357, no. 7 (October 25, 2007): 1,731–1,743.

Chagas' disease   An infectious tropical disease caused by the protozoan parasite *Trypanosoma cruzi,* which is transmitted through an insect bite or a blood transfusion. It is also known as American trypanosomiasis. It is a zoonotic parasite, but humans can be infected and suffer illness. About 18 million people worldwide are affected with *T. cruzi,* with an annual mortality rate of about 50,000 patients.

According to researchers Bern, et al., in their 2007 article in the *Journal of the American Medical Association* on Chagas' disease in the United States, about 100,000 people living in the United States have Chagas' disease, although most people were infected while living in other countries.

In Latin America, Chagas' disease has also been transmitted through donated blood after organ transplantation. In the chronic form of the disease, the affected person's life expectancy may be decreased by about nine years.

Chagas' disease was discovered by Carlos Chagas, a physician in Brazil in the 19th century. Chagas' disease is primarily found in Central America and South America, where it is a common problem, and as many as a million people are infected each year. If not diagnosed and treated, Chagas' disease causes a condition known as MEGACOLON, an abnormal enlargement of the colon, and can produce an enlargement of the esophagus (megaesophagus). It may also affect the heart and cause congestive heart failure.

Symptoms and Diagnostic Path

The acute form of the disease occurs from four to eight weeks after infection. Then there is a chronic phase, and if treatment does not occur, the individual will remain infected for the rest of his or her life. Most (70 to 80 percent) infected individuals never have any symptoms and are asymptomatic carriers of the parasite and considered to have an indeterminate form of the disease. However, when chronic disease occurs, the problems usually do not arise until patients are 40 to 50 years of age.

In the acute form of Chagas' disease, which is usually found more among children than adults, the patient has an enlarged spleen, enlarged lymph nodes, fever, rapid heartbeat, and swelling of the legs and face.

In the chronic phase of the disease, which can occur 10 to 30 years after the infection, patients experience a variety of problems. Some patients (about 27 percent) have incurable heart disease. Others (about 6 percent) have enlargements in the digestive tract (megaesophagus, megacolon, etc), which cause severe CONSTIPATION or swallowing problems (dysphagia). Stomach emptying may be delayed. Other patients (about 3 percent) experience neurological symptoms.

The diagnosis of Chagas' disease is based on the symptoms, the results of laboratory tests and imaging studies, as well as the geographical location of the patient. The parasite can only be detected in the acute stage and not during the chronic phase.

According to Bern, et al., as many as 70 to 80 percent of patients infected with Chagas' disease have the "indeterminate" form, which means that they are infected, but have no symptoms or abnormalities, and they have a normal electrocardiogram and normal-appearing esophagus and colon.

Treatment Options and Outlook

In most cases, benznidazole or nifurtimox is used to treat a recently acquired infection, with benznidazole usually the first choice drug because it is better tolerated by patients. In addition, treatment should be given to all immune-suppressed patients. The drugs are not approved by the Food and Drug Administration (FDA) and must be obtained by patients who enter clinical drug protocols managed by the CDC.

Drugs can eradicate the parasite in about 60 to 85 percent of the cases of acute Chagas' disease, but treatment cannot reverse the complications that are seen in the chronic form of the disease. As such, the role of treatment in the chronic stage when complications have occurred is controversial, although it may be reasonable to treat patients even in the chronic stage in the absence of severe heart disease. (Contact the CDC in Atlanta to obtain information about these drugs.)

If the infection is chronic, treatment is symptomatic, depending upon the problems that are seen. According to Bern, et al., the newly diagnosed patient with Chagas' disease should have an electrocardiogram, and if the findings are normal, then the EKG should be given once a year. However, if there is evidence of Chagas' heart disease, then the patient should have a complete cardiac evaluation. Patients with gastrointestinal symptoms should receive barium contrast studies.

Treatment depends partly on the age of the patient, according to Bern, et al. For example, in patient ages 18 years and younger, antitrypanosomal treatment is given in both acute and congenital (contracted from an infected pregnant mother) Chagas' disease as well as reactived infection. If the patient is ages 19 to 50 years old and does not have advanced heart disease, treatment may slow the development of cardiac disease. Treatment is optional for patients older than age 50 since risk of drug toxicity may outweigh the benefits.

Risk Factors and Preventive Measures

People who live in rural areas in poorly constructed houses or huts have greater risk, particularly those who live in houses made of mud or adobe. The insects living in such houses, reduviid insects or kissing bugs, spread Chagas' disease after biting an animal or human who is infected with the disease. Individuals living in the following countries are most at risk for infection with Chagas' disease: Argentina, Belize, Bolivia, Brazil, Chile, Colombia, Costa Rica, Ecuador, El Salvador, French Guiana, Guatemala, Guyana, Honduras, Mexico, Nicaragua, Panama, Paraguay, Peru, Suriname, Uruguay, and Venezuela. Immigrants from these countries to the United States or other developed nations are also at risk as carriers of this disease.

The best prevention is avoidance of sleeping in poorly made houses in developing countries in Latin America. In addition, insects should be promptly destroyed by people living or visiting such areas. Mosquito nets should be used when the person is asleep. Finally, it is important to remember that there are numerous problems associated with screening the blood supplies for Chagas' disease, and thus, if a blood transfusion is required, the patient may contract Chagas' disease from infected blood.

One approach that is used to prevent this problem is to ask prospective blood donors questions that may identify potentially affected individuals and then to exclude from donation those with high risk for infection from donating their blood to a blood bank facility. Eradication programs initiated in several Latin American countries have resulted in reduction in the disease by as much as 70 percent.

See also PARASITIC INFECTION.

Bern, Caryn, et al. "Evaluation and Treatment of Chagas Disease in the United States: A Systematic Review," *Journal of the American Medical Association* 298, no. 18 (2007): 2,171–2,181.

chest pain, noncardiac   Mild to severe discomfort that occurs anywhere in the rib area and is due to causes other than coronary artery disease. Chest pain may be caused by a heart attack; however, there are at least 200,000 cases of noncardiac chest pain in the United States each year. As many as 30 percent of those patients who undergo cardiac catheterization for acute chest pain are found to have normal angiogram results.

According to Lee and Goldman in their 2002 article on acute chest pain in the *New England Journal of Medicine*, of all patients who enter emergency departments reporting acute chest pain, about 15 percent are found to be experiencing myocardial infarction (heart attack) and 30 to 35 percent have unstable angina (heart disease).

When they are not coronary in nature, chest pains may be caused by an ULCER or by the ACID REFLUX that is generated by GASTROESOPHAGEAL REFLUX DISEASE (GERD). Noncardiac chest pains may also be caused by a musculoskeletal problem, such as FIBROMYALGIA, osteoarthritis, rheumatoid arthritis, vertebral disk disease, or other musculoskeletal problems. Musculoskeletal causes may represent up to 20 percent of all noncardiac chest pain causes.

Some patients with chest pains are suffering from ESOPHAGITIS, an inflammation of the esophagus. They may also have other esophageal problems, such as abnormal esophageal motility.

Patients may also have emotional disorders, such as panic disorder or anxiety disorder, which can cause a racing heart as well as chest pains. As many as one-third of all patients who experience noncardiac chest pains may actually be experiencing panic disorders. In addition, the psychological stress of fearing that the chest pains are caused by a heart attack can further accelerate the patient's emotional dismay and distress, worsening the chest pains.

The term *noncardiac chest pain* is actually a misnomer, since it does not exclude all cardiac causes, but only those that are related to coronary artery disease. Thus, noncardiac chest pains also include pains due to microvascular angina of the heart, sometimes called syndrome X. The role of mitral valve prolapse is controversial, but it appears not to contribute to chest pain in most cases.

Symptoms and Diagnostic Path

The primary symptom is acute chest pain. Anyone having chest pain should see a doctor to determine the cause of the pain and should not assume that the problem is solely digestive in nature. Even experienced physicians have had difficulty determining whether their own chest pain indicated a heart condition or a digestive problem. Guessing wrong could mean the difference between life and death.

In most cases, physicians order an electrocardiogram of the heart as well as blood tests for cardiac muscle protein called troponin. Further testing depends upon the results of these tests as well as the patient's risk factors for coronary artery disease. In addition, a coronary angiogram or a myocardial perfusion imaging study with thallium-201 may be ordered. The physician may also order a stress test.

If the results of all of these cardiac tests are negative, further diagnostic evaluation is then needed, including a gastrointestinal evaluation. The physician may need to order esophageal manometry, 24-hour pH monitoring and/or endoscopy to determine whether the noncardiac chest pains are caused by a digestive disorder.

A therapeutic trial of a double-dose proton pump inhibitor such as omeprazole (Prilosec) taken twice a day for eight to 12 weeks may be undertaken. A subsequent reduction in the severity and frequency of symptoms would suggest that the chest pains were related to GERD. In some cases, a referral to a rheumatologist and/or a psychiatrist may be needed.

Treatment Options and Outlook

If the physician is convinced that the problem is musculoskeletal in nature, he or she may order anti-inflammatory medications or painkillers and may also recommend physical therapy.

When patients appear to have emotional disorders that are causing their noncardiac chest pains, doctors may order benzodiazepine (antianxiety) medications or antidepressants. Sometimes beta blocker drugs can help with panic attacks that cause a racing of the heart. A psychologist can also provide assistance by providing cognitive-behavioral therapy, which is a form of therapy that helps patients identify irrational thought patterns and replace them with logical thoughts.

Expectations should be realistic. In many cases, the treatment is suboptimal and only reduces the severity and frequency of chest pains and does not entirely eliminate them.

Risk Factors and Preventive Measures

Many types of problems can cause noncardiac chest pain, such as GERD, rheumatological disorders, and psychiatric disorders.

If the patient has GERD, medications such as proton pump inhibitors and histamine-2 receptor blockers can help alleviate the problem. Patients will be advised to give up smoking and to lose weight if they are obese. They are also advised to avoid large fatty meals, as well as stay away from alcohol, mint, chocolate, onions, and orange juice. In addition, patients are advised to raise the head of their bed, since lying down can exacerbate the symptoms of GERD. They are also told to eat their evening meal at least three hours before retiring to bed.

Relaxation exercises can help in easing the chest pains and acid reflux among patients with GERD.

Patient Confusion over Noncardiac Chest Pains

Chest pains cause nearly all patients to suffer extreme anxiety because they believe they are having a heart attack. Patients go to the emergency room of the nearest hospital and are shocked to have a normal electrocardiogram with or without additional test results and to be told that their heart is fine. Often the pattern repeats itself, and the patient with severe chest pains returns to the emergency room weeks or months later, again convinced that he or she is having a heart attack.

If patients with chest pain are also told that the cause of their problem is unknown, they may become very confused. They may also be offended, thinking that the doctor is accusing them of hypochondria. They are also often uncertain about what to do if the problem occurs again, as it often does. It is best if doctors can help patients to determine a possible cause for the problem. If the doctor thinks that the problem may be digestive in nature, the patient should be referred to a gastroenterologist. In all cases, a cardiac cause must be first excluded before the physician looks for other causes because a heart attack can kill.

See also PROTON PUMP INHIBITORS.

Lee, Thomas H., M.D., and Lee Goldman, M.D. "Evaluation of the Patient with Acute Chest Pain." *New England Journal of Medicine* 342, no. 16 (April 20, 2000): 1,187–1,195.

Minocha, Anil, M.D. "Noncardiac Chest Pain: Where Does It Start?" *Postgraduate Medicine* 100, no. 6 (December 1996): 107–114.

Minocha, Anil, M.D., and Abraham S. Joseph, M.D. "Pathophysiology and Management of Noncardiac Pain." *KMA Journal* 93 (May 1995): 196–201.

children and digestive diseases Children may have many of the same digestive diseases as adults; however, infants are at particular risk for some diseases, such as necrotizing enterocolitis, and older children are more at risk for other diseases. Children in the United States also have an increasing problem with OBESITY. The body mass index (BMI) (a measure that considers height and weight) is further adjusted by age and gender for children. (See Appendix VI for tables on the BMIs of boys and girls at different ages.)

Sometimes the same disease may result from a different cause in a child and in an adult. For example, "spitting up" or even GASTROESOPHAGEAL REFLUX DISEASE (GERD) is fairly common among babies less than one year old. In general, these problems resolve as the child grows. In some cases, however, treatment and even surgery are needed, for example, if the child is not gaining weight and is severely ill. On the other hand, the adult-onset form of GERD frequently does not resolve on its own.

Although not common, infants are at risk for some genetically transmitted diseases, such as HIRSCHSPRUNG'S DISEASE. Children may also contract infectious diseases including PARASITIC INFECTIONS, particularly since they are less careful about cleanliness and personal hygiene than are most adults.

Emotional Problems and Digestive Symptoms

Sometimes children report frequent digestive problems such as stomachaches, which may merit further investigation. If the stomachaches always or nearly always seem to center around the time of an activity that is undesirable to the child, such as going to school or doing housework or schoolwork, then the child may be consciously or unconsciously trying to avoid activities by reporting medical problems. The child is not necessarily lying about the stomachaches, and in fact, he or she may actually experience stomach pain when thinking about or preparing to perform an activity that is deemed unpleasant. Only a physician can make an appropriate diagnosis of a digestive disease or disorder.

It is also true that the child may have a physical basis for complaint; for example, it is possible for children to suffer from the symptoms of GERD, particularly if they are taking medication for asthma.

Children at Risk for Digestive Disorders

Children with diabetes are at higher risk for development of digestive diseases and disorders than are nondiabetics. Children who have some other disorders, such as asthma, have a greater risk for development of digestive diseases, such as gastroesophageal reflux disease (GERD).

See also INFANTS.

Minocha, Anil, M.D., and Christine Adamec. *How to Stop Heartburn: Simple Ways to Heal Heartburn and Acid Reflux.* New York: John Wiley & Sons, 2001.

cholangitis Inflammation and infection of the bile duct as a result of a blockage due to gallstones or stricture (narrowing) causing an obstruction to the normal flow of bile into the small intestine or to other causes. Patients experience fever, jaundice, and abdominal pain. Patients with cholangitis need to be hospitalized and given antibiotics and may need to undergo procedures such as ENDOSCOPIC RETROGRADE CHOLANGIOPANCREATOGRAPHY (ERCP) to remove an existing blockage. Some patients need surgery.

A parasitic infection with roundworm (ascariasis), liver fluke (Clonorchis sinensis), or tapeworm (*Echinococcus granulosus*) in the bile duct may lead to cholangitis.

See also BILE; GALLSTONES; PARASITIC INFECTION.

cholecystitis Inflammation and infection of the gallbladder, which are usually caused by an impaction of the gallbladder opening (the cystic duct) by GALLSTONES. Cholecystitis may also occur in the absence of any gallstones in patients who are otherwise very sick. This is known as acalculous cholecystitis. Acute cholecystitis usually requires cholecystectomy, which is the surgical removal of the entire gallbladder.

choledochal cyst An abnormal cystic dilation of the bile duct. Choledochal cysts are benign but may become cancerous. The choledochal cyst is a rare condition. A choledochal cyst may prevent or slow the bile from going to the intestine, and it may also cause the bile to back up.

Symptoms and Diagnostic Path

Patients with choledochal cysts may suffer from episodes of abdominal pain, JAUNDICE, and PANCREATITIS, although some patients experience no signs or symptoms. Physicians may suspect choledochal cysts when the patient complains of pain and when some laboratory tests, particularly liver enzyme tests, reveal abnormalities. An abnormal mass may rarely be felt by the physician during an abdominal examination. An ultrasound or computed tomography scan can reveal the presence of an abnormal duct. ENDOSCOPIC RETROGRADE CHOLANGIOPANCREA-TOGRAPHY (ERCP) helps confirm the diagnosis. Magnetic resonance cholangiopancreatography is a noninvasive option that may be used as an alternative to the ERCP.

Treatment Options and Outlook

Treatment of choledochal cysts is surgical, with excision of the cyst.

Risk Factors and Preventive Measures

The choledochal cyst may be a congenital birth defect or be acquired during life. When found, it usually occurs during early childhood; however, it can also be seen in adulthood. There are no preventive measures.

See also CAROLI'S DISEASE; LIVER ENZYMES/FUNCTION TESTS.

cholelithiasis See GALLSTONES.

cholera An infectious and dangerous diarrheal disease of the small intestine. It is caused by the bacterium *Vibrio cholerae,* which is found in contaminated water. The organism has almost 200 serotypes, but only a couple of them are capable of causing disease. Cholera can cause severe digestive illness. The bacteria release a toxin that triggers the increased secretion of water and electrolytes in the intestine. Some cases of cholera are spread by contaminated shellfish, particularly bad oysters. If cholera is not treated, it can lead to dehydration and even death.

Cholera is primarily found in less developed countries that are located in Asia, Africa, the Mediterranean, both South and Central America, and Mexico. Most cases that have been identified in the United States can be traced to travelers who have recently returned from Asia or Africa.

The underlying cause of cholera was first uncovered by Dr. John Snow, a British anesthesiologist in the mid-19th century, whose discovery, based on meticulous observations, was described in *Epidemiology* by Leon Gordis. Dr. Snow observed that in one week of 1854, 600 people who were living in several blocks around one particular water pump had all died of cholera. Snow deduced that contaminated water was the cause of cholera, despite the prevailing theory of the time, which was that cholera was caused by a low-lying cloud.

Dr. Snow went from house to house, gathering data on deaths per household and information on where the family obtained their water. Snow found that in houses that were served by several water companies that obtained their water supply from a polluted part of the Thames River, the death rate was 315 deaths per 10,000 houses. But in homes that were supplied water from another company that obtained its water farther upstream, the death rate was only 38 deaths per 10,000 homes.

Symptoms and Diagnostic Path

Most patients do not get any symptoms or have mild symptoms indistinguishable from routine "stomach flu." Symptoms of cholera occur within several hours to about five days from the time of infection. The key symptoms of cholera are as follows:

- watery DIARRHEA
- stool that has flecks that look like rice (rice water stools)
- manifestations of dehydration (dry skin and dizziness), which may be rapid
- extreme thirst and weakness
- abdominal cramps
- severe muscle cramps
- NAUSEA AND VOMITING

Treatment Options and Outlook

Physicians may suspect cholera on the basis of the patient's symptoms and any recent exposure to known epidemics of cholera. If bacteria are collected in a stool sample or culture, they can be analyzed. The bacteria are often seen by specialized examination under the microscope in the procedure known as dark field or phase contrast microscopy of stool. Cholera organisms look like shooting stars.

A stool culture can confirm the presence of cholera. The patient's blood may also be checked for the presence of antibodies to cholera: however,

the antibodies develop one to two weeks after infection and thus, can only confirm the diagnosis retrospectively.

The primary treatment for cholera is to prevent dehydration or to reverse dehydration that is already present with rehydration, and that rehydration may be lifesaving. Most patients can be treated with oral hydration solutions. If the patient's condition is severe, hospitalization is needed, and intravenous fluids are administered.

Physicians may sometimes but not always prescribe antibiotics, which are given to reduce the duration of the sickness and to help limit the spread. Antibiotics such as tetracycline or doxycline are frequently used. Tetracycline is usually not prescribed for children who do not yet have their permanent teeth, because it can permanently discolor teeth that are in the process of formation. Similarly, tetracycline is not used for pregnant women. With children and pregnant women, erythromycin is prescribed instead. Mortality of untreated cases may reach 50 to 70 percent.

Doctors are particularly concerned about the rehydration of children who have cholera. Intravenous fluids are not necessary in the majority of cases. Most children with the disease can be treated with a formula that replaces the salt and water lost from dehydration, and such therapy can prevent the deaths of from 1 million to 2 million children worldwide per year. The World Health Organization has developed an inexpensive oral rehydration solution of sugar and electrolytes. Some studies have found that a rice-based oral rehydration solution is very effective.

Risk Factors and Preventive Measures

The key risk factors are an association with contaminated water or recent travel to a country where cholera often occurs. The ingested bacteria usually are killed by the stomach acid. However, they may survive protected by food or low stomach acidity (higher pH) especially due to antacid intake or rapid stomach emptying. Thus, the risk for infection is increased in those with low stomach acidity due to disease or medications such as antacids or PROTON PUMP INHIBITORS (PPIs) etc.

In parts of the world where cholera is known to be a problem, residents may receive cholera vaccines. People traveling to areas where cholera is a problem may also receive a vaccine before they travel to that area.

In the United States and Canada, the vaccine is given by injection. However, the vaccine is effective only in about 50 percent of cases, and it is not required for travel to other countries. In addition, the vaccine may cause fever and headache, as well as pain at the injection site. If a patient has trouble with breathing or hives after an injection, he or she should seek immediate emergency medical attention.

Travelers Who Wish to Avoid Cholera

Experts report that there are some basic actions that travelers to countries known to harbor cholera can take to limit their risk of contracting the disease.

- avoiding unboiled water
- avoiding ice
- buying no food items from street vendors
- eating no raw vegetables or salads while in the country
- avoiding raw seafood
- drinking only bottled water or treating water with either chlorine or iodine tablets
- drinking carbonated soft drinks
- drinking only hot tea or coffee that is made from boiled water
- consuming only hot cooked foods

See also CONTAMINATED FOOD OR WATER; TRAVEL.

cholesterol A type of body fat (lipid) that is made in the body and is also found naturally in some types of animal foods, such as fish, meat, poultry, eggs, and dairy products. Cholesterol circulates in the body as lipoproteins, including low-density lipoproteins (LDL) and high-density lipoproteins (HDL). LDL, which leads to clogging of the blood vessels, is considered to be a "bad" cholesterol; HDL is a "good" form of cholesterol because it is associated with a lower risk of atherosclerosis

and its complications, such as heart disease and stroke. Consequently, higher levels of HDL are desirable. If the blood vessels become excessively clogged, then the individual is at an increased risk for stroke or heart attack. Those patients may be at risk for digestive system disorders such as intestinal angina, mesenteric thrombosis, and ischemic colitis.

Cholesterol level can be measured in the blood, and if the levels of LDL or total cholesterol are considered too high by a physician, then the patient can be given a diet to follow. In many cases, patients are also given prescribed medications to help lower their LDL level. In general, the type of medication usually considered to treat patients with high LDL level is a drug such as atorvastatin (Lipitor), pravastatin (Pravachol), simvastatin (Zocor) or resuvastatin (Crestor). These medications can effectively lower LDL cholesterol levels by as much as 15 to 60 percent. Some patients with high cholesterol levels may be treated with niacin, but it is poorly tolerated because of its side effects.

CLASSIFICATION OF LDL, TOTAL CHOLESTEROL, AND HDL CHOLESTEROL (MILLIGRAMS PER DECILITER)

LDL Cholesterol

Less than 100	Optimal
100–129	Near optimal/above optimal
130–159	Borderline high
160–189	High
190 and higher	Very high

If patients have diabetes, then the recommended LDL is less than 100.

Total Cholesterol

Less than 200	Desirable
200–239	Borderline high
240 or higher	High

HDL Cholesterol

Less than 40	Low
60 or higher	High

Source: National Cholesterol Education Program. "Third Report of the National Cholesterol Education Program (NCEP) Expert Panel on Detection, Evaluation, and Treatment of High Blood Cholesterol in Adults (Adult Treatment Panel III)." NIH Publication no. 02-5215, September 2002.

Risk Factors

Some individuals have a greater risk for development of health problems associated with their cholesterol level, including individuals with family members who have high cholesterol levels or who fit one or more of the following categories:

- Have diabetes
- Have hypertension
- Are obese
- Are sedentary
- Are black or Native American
- Consume a very-high-fat diet

Recommended Levels of Cholesterol

In 2002, the National Heart, Lung, and Blood Institute released their new guidelines for cholesterol control, which are listed in the table.

Diagnosis and Treatment

As mentioned, cholesterol problems are diagnosed on the basis of blood levels of HDL and LDL, and patients who are diagnosed with cholesterol disorders are usually prescribed dietary modifications and exercise plans. In addition, in some cases, patients are also prescribed medications to help them to lower their LDL level.

Medications alone, however, should not be used to resolve the cholesterol problem, and patients must also make changes to their diet, such as decreasing their level of dietary fat and increasing their fiber consumption. Patients with diabetes as well as cholesterol disorders are urged to make their glucose level as close to normal as possible and patients with hypertension are advised to lower their blood pressure level to as close to normal as possible.

Regular exercise is also usually recommended for patients. It need not be strenuous or difficult, and a mere daily walk can often help to improve health, although strenuous exercise results in better outcomes than mild exercise. Obese patients should reduce their weight to the optimal range. As of this writing, preliminary data suggest that the Atkins Diet, in addition to lowering weight, reduces total cholesterol level and increases the levels of HDL (good cholesterol).

See also FIBER; GALLSTONES.

chromoendoscopy A procedure in which an endoscopy is performed, and a special dye is sprayed on the gastrointestinal wall to the area of interest, using a spray catheter. The dye allows the highlighting of abnormalities on the gastrointestinal wall that may have been ambiguous or otherwise have escaped detection. This procedure is not routinely performed as of this writing because of the lack of good studies showing whether using these special dyes produces better clinical outcomes than using traditional endoscopy without the dyes.

See also ENDOSCOPY.

Churg-Strauss syndrome A rare disease that involves inflammation of the blood vessels (vasculitis) affecting many organs of the body, primarily the lungs, and causing difficulty with breathing, coughing and wheezing, as well as asthma. However, it also affects the digestive system in that many Churg-Strauss syndrome patients also suffer from abdominal pain, appetite loss, diarrhea, gastrointestinal bleeding, colitis, and unintended weight loss. Other organs that may be affected by Churg-Strauss syndrome include the heart, the peripheral nerves, the kidneys, and the liver.

The cause of this medical problem is unknown, although it is suspected that there may be autoimmune factors at work.

See also VASCULITIS, SMALL VESSEL.

cirrhosis Severe and potentially fatal scarring of the liver. Many cases of cirrhosis are caused by years of chronic ALCOHOL ABUSE, although cirrhosis can also occur in individuals who are not alcoholics but instead have viral or autoimmune HEPATITIS or other diseases. Whereas viral hepatitis C is a common cause of cirrhosis in the United States and other countries in the West, hepatitis B is a major cause of cirrhosis in some Asian and African countries. Hereditary disorders such as HEMOCHROMATOSIS (iron overload) and WILSON'S DISEASE (copper overload) also lead to cirrhosis. In addition, it should also be noted that most alcoholics do not develop cirrhosis.

When chronic alcohol consumption does cause cirrhosis, the individual's heavy alcohol intake on a prolonged basis causes inflammation (alcoholic hepatitis) that can then lead to scarring of the tissue in the liver, which is called cirrhosis. When the scar tissue becomes too pervasive, and the liver is unable to function anymore, the individual requires liver transplantation to stay alive. Cirrhosis develops earlier in those who have both hepatitis C and alcoholism than in those who have only one of the conditions.

Malnutrition or viral hepatitis can also lead to cirrhosis. Sometimes a severe reaction to prescription drugs, for example, a reaction to methotrexate, may cause cirrhosis. Cirrhosis is a very serious disease and it increases the risk for the development of LIVER CANCER.

Based on data published by Yoon and Yi in 2008 on liver cirrhosis deaths, liver cirrhosis was the 12th-leading cause of death in the United States in 2005. Yoon and Yee reported that 28,175 people died of liver cirrhosis in 2005. Nearly half of the liver cirrhosis deaths were alcohol-related, and the researchers found that deaths from alcohol-related cirrhosis increased by 2.3 percent from 2004 to 2005. Among those who died, nearly a third were ages 75 to 84 years old and 20 percent were 85 years or older.

Symptoms and Diagnostic Path

Although patients may have no symptoms or signs when they are in the early stages of cirrhosis, indications do develop as the condition of the liver further deteriorates. The following are some of the key indicators of cirrhosis:

- JAUNDICE (yellowing of the skin, caused by bilirubin)
- ASCITES (fluid buildup in the abdomen)
- massive painless bleeding caused by increased pressure in the veins in the esophagus or stomach (varices) that then burst, which is further exacerbated because the patient may also have decreased clotting factors that do not permit bleeding to stop

- nausea and fatigue (which may be mistaken as "normal" reactions of the body to excessive drinking)
- an increased sensitivity to drugs that are metabolized by the liver, which can no longer manage this metabolizing function well, such as a sensitivity to acetaminophen (Tylenol), which can cause severe liver failure in alcoholics at doses much lower than those that can be tolerated by nonalcoholics
- liver cancer, caused by long-standing liver cirrhosis
- altered mental status (hepatic encephalopathy)
- infection in the ascitic fluid (spontaneous bacterial peritonitis)

In a patient with chronic compensated liver disease (in which the liver is diseased but still functioning well enough to not cause problems to the body), the exact diagnosis of cirrhosis can only be made by examining a liver biopsy sample under a microscope. The body needs only a small part of the liver to function. Complications do not occur until most of the liver is gone. In advanced cases, physicians can make a preliminary diagnosis based on a patient's symptoms and signs, such as the presence of jaundice or ascites and the laboratory test findings. However, in early cases of cirrhosis, the patient may be asymptomatic and may also have no laboratory test abnormalities.

In the later stages of the illness, laboratory tests of liver function suggest diagnosis if cirrhosis is present. Imaging tests may also show an enlargement or scarring of the liver, as well as the presence of any complications such as ascites. At the same time, patients who have acute hepatitis due to alcohol or viruses may have damaged but reversible liver function, and these conditions may mimic cirrhosis.

Treatment Options and Outlook

Patients with cirrhosis who drink are advised that they must immediately stop drinking alcohol. If they are alcoholics, they may need hospitalization to undergo detoxification from alcohol. It is difficult for a long-term alcoholic simply to give up drinking; he or she is addicted to alcohol. In addition, the body often responds to the sudden ending of alcohol consumption with severe reactions (acute alcohol withdrawal and even delirium tremens), and with tremors, rapid heart rate and palpitations, seizures, vomiting, and DIARRHEA.

If individuals who are alcoholics completely avoid alcohol, their liver cells may recover completely when the liver is only inflamed (hepatitis) rather than scarred. On the other hand, cirrhosis may be irreversible, although patients may live for years with cirrhosis that is not advanced. As such, the outcome depends on how severely damaged the liver is at the point when the patient becomes abstinent from alcohol. Patients with cirrhosis should also be vaccinated against hepatitis A and B if they have not been exposed to these infections in the past, in order to prevent contraction of viral hepatitis, which would cause further liver damage.

There is no known medical treatment for cirrhosis, and generally, treatment involves identifying and treating the cause of the illness as well as any complications that may arise. LIVER TRANSPLANTATION is the only known definitive cure for cirrhosis. Some physicians recommend medications such as colchicine to help the cirrhotic liver, although this is an investigational therapy. There are also reports that milk thistle, an herbal remedy, helps some patients with certain forms of liver disease.

Risk Factors and Preventive Measures

Other than chronic heavy alcohol consumption, there are other individual risk factors for the development of cirrhosis; for example, cirrhosis death is about 1.5 times more common among nonwhites than among whites in the United States. Hispanic males are especially at risk according to the report from Yoon and Yi, who said that the aged-adjusted rate for all forms of cirrhosis was 1.8 times higher among white Hispanic males than among white non-Hispanic males or black non-Hispanic males. Hispanic females are also at risk, and the rate for white Hispanic females is 1.4 times greater than the rate for white non-Hispanic females and 1.7 times greater than the rate for black non-Hispanic females.

Men are more likely to have cirrhosis than are women.

The only known preventive measures are to avoid drinking to excess and to avoid contracting diseases that can lead to cirrhosis, such as hepatitis.

Yang, Alice L., et al. "Epidemiology of Alcohol-Related Liver and Pancreatic Disease in the United States." *Archives of Internal Medicine* 168, no. 6 (March 24, 2008): 649–656.

Yoon, Young-Hee and Hsiao-ye Yi. *Surveillance Report #83: Liver Cirrhosis Mortality in the United States, 1970-2005.* National Institute on Alcohol Abuse and Alcoholism. Baltimore, Md.: National Institutes of Health, August 2008.

Clostridium A bacterium that causes food-borne illnesses. An illness caused by *Clostridium perfringens,* one of the *Clostridium* bacteria, is also known as the cafeteria germ because many disease outbreaks have resulted from foods left for long periods on steam tables or elsewhere at room temperature. *Clostridium* organisms are ubiquitous in the environment and are commonly found in dust, dirt, and sewage and in the intestinal tract of infected humans and animals.

An infection with *Clostridium perfringens* causes diarrhea and abdominal gas pains within eight to 24 hours of consuming the infected food. Generally, symptoms subside within a day or so, although some minor symptoms may continue for a week or longer. Most patients recover without treatment.

The *Clostridium botulinum* bacteria are extremely dangerous, primarily because they produce a powerful toxin that causes botulism, a severe form of food contamination that also causes food poisoning. However, fortunately, this form of the bacteria is not common.

Another species of the *Clostridium* bacterium, *Clostridium difficile,* is responsible for many cases of antibiotic-induced diarrhea. It is very common, especially among hospitalized patients. Symptomatic patients can be treated effectively with metronidazole or oral vancomycin. In a few cases, the infection cannot be eradicated and patients may suffer from relapse shortly after treatment is stopped.

See also BOTULIS; CONTAMINATED FOOD OR WATER; DIARRHEA.

colic A term that is usually used to describe inter-mittent attacks of abdominal pain, probably charac-terized by spasms of a hollow organ such as the gut. There is no standard definition of the term *colic*. Fre-quently, the term is used by parents and physicians when infants cry for no apparent reason during the first three months of life, and the parents become concerned and seek medical help for this problem. It is a benign and usually self-limited condition.

Colic is a common condition of many infants. A colicky type of pain may also be due to biliary colic in GALLSTONE disease patients and in renal colic in patients who have kidney stones. However, the term *biliary colic* is a misnomer because the pain is steady and not colicky.

See also INFANTS.

colitis See INFLAMMATORY BOWEL DISEASE; ULCER-ATIVE COLITIS.

colon The large bowel, which is a key part of the digestive system. The colon is the final processing component of digestion. It receives about two liters of unabsorbed food remnants, intestinal secretions, and debris in fluid form. Unabsorbed carbohydrates undergo bacterial fermentation in the colon. The colon also absorbs most of the water and then expels the waste in solid form through the rectum and anus.

See also COLORECTAL CANCER.

colonoscopy See COLORECTAL CANCER; COMPLICA-TIONS OF DIGESTIVE DISORDERS; MAJOR DIAGNOSTIC TESTS FOR DIGESTIVE DISEASES.

colorectal cancer A malignant tumor of the colon and/or rectum. Colon cancer forms in the tissue of the colon, which is about four feet long. Rectal cancer forms in the tissues of the rectum, or the last few inches of the large intestine before the location of the anus. According to the National Cancer Institute, there were 108,070 new cases of colon cancer and 40,740 new cases of rectal cancer in 2008. An estimated 49,960 people died of colon

and rectal cancer combined in 2008. Colorectal cancer is the third-leading cause of cancer deaths among both men and women.

According to the National Center for Chronic Disease Prevention and Health Promotion, a divi-sion of the Centers for Diseases Control and Pre-vention (CDC), at least one-third of all deaths of colorectal cancer in the United States could be prevented if everyone age 50 years and older had regular screening tests for the disease.

Colorectal cancer is apparently caused by muta-tions that occur in the cellular deoxyribonucleic acid (DNA) and that then result in excessive and unregu-lated cell growth. Researchers have identified some of these mutations, but it is unknown what triggers normal cells to mutate. However, there is clearly a genetic factor at work, and the risk of the devel-opment of colorectal cancer is increased if one or more family members have had polyps or colorectal cancer. About 25 percent of patients report a fam-ily history of colorectal cancer. Researchers are also studying the impact of diet and nutrition, OBESITY, and other factors that may cause or contribute to the development of colorectal cancer.

One factor that is known about colorectal cancer is that POLYPS, which are small to large outgrowths of the colon, are significant in the development of colorectal cancer. In fact, 95 percent of colon cancer occurs in preexisting adenoma-type polyps. Clinical studies, particularly the National Polyp Study in the United States, have shown that the presence of ade-noma polyps is actually an interim step to the subse-quent development of most colorectal cancer. When these polyps are detected and then removed by phy-sicians (usually during a colonoscopy), the incidence of colorectal cancer is actually reduced by about 60 to 90 percent of the cases. Clearly the colonoscopy is an important diagnostic and preventive tool.

On the basis of clinical research to date, it appears that in most cases, precancerous polyps take about seven to 10 years to develop into cancerous tumors. For this reason, and because colorectal polyps and cancer are more prominently found among middle-aged and older people, it is recommended that people who are age 50 and older undergo colon cancer screening.

If any polyps are found during the colonos-copy, they can be removed, and thus, they cannot develop into colorectal cancer. Further surveillance by physicians is undertaken on the basis of the type and number of polyps identified and removed. It should also be noted that not all polyps are precancerous or cancerous.

Symptoms and Diagnostic Path

There may be no symptoms with the early stages of colorectal cancer. The presence of symptoms is generally not a good sign, because in about half of the cases, by the time that symptoms arise, the cancer has usually spread. If symptoms occur, they may include the following:

- blood in the stool (bright red or very dark)
- a change in bowel habits, such as stools that are narrower than usual
- frequent abdominal pains or cramps or feeling bloated or full
- unexplained DIARRHEA or CONSTIPATION
- unexplained weight loss
- a new feeling that the bowel is not emptying completely (which may indicate an obstruction)
- sustained and unexplained fatigue

There are several ways that doctors screen for and diagnose colorectal cancer. The simplest technique is the *digital rectal examination,* in which the doctor inserts a lubricated finger into the rectum to feel for any abnormalities in the anorectal region. If an abnormality is detected in this examination, the doctor orders further studies. The primary care physician can perform the rectal examination. However, the digital examination can only examine a very small part of the rectum within the reach of the finger, whereas the colon/rectum is about five feet long. Therefore, the rectal examination can help to detect only a small fraction of colorectal cancers. The fecal occult blood test is another screening tool, as are the barium enema, the colonoscopy, and the SIGMOIDOSCOPY. The fecal occult blood test is noninvasive, whereas the colonoscopy, and the sigmoidoscopy are invasive tests. A newer test, the virtual colonoscopy, is noninvasive.

Fecal Occult Blood Test The most commonly used laboratory diagnostic test for colorectal cancer is the fecal occult blood test (FOBT); however, a lack of occult (hidden) blood does not definitively rule out colorectal cancer. Nor does the presence of blood prove that the person has colorectal cancer. Blood in the stool may be caused by HEMORRHOIDS, infection, or another cause. However, when there is blood in the stool, colorectal polyps and/or cancer should be ruled out. As a result, if the FOBT result is positive for occult blood, the doctor usually orders a colonoscopy.

With the FOBT test, individuals are given special cards on which to collect their own small amounts of stool specimens. The laboratory then checks the specimens on the cards for invisible blood (not visible to the eye).

The Virtual Colonoscopy The virtual colonoscopy is a noninvasive procedure that has been developed in recent years and is now one of the recommended options. This procedure involves radiological imaging of the colon without actually introducing a scope into the rectum. However, the preparatory cleansing of the bowel is required for this procedure. Recent data suggests that the efficacy of the virtual colonoscopy may be similar to that of colonoscopy for large polyps. It is, however, likely to miss smaller polyps that are less than 5 millimeters in size. In addition, just as in the case of barium enema, any abnormality that is seen in the virtual colonoscopy will require a follow-up colonoscopy, which does use the scope; for example, if polyps are identified, a follow-up colonoscopy will be needed to remove the polyps.

Invasive Screening Procedures There are also several invasive procedures that are undertaken to detect the presence of colorectal cancer, including the flexible sigmoidoscopy, and the colonoscopy. A gastroenterologist, a physician expert in diagnosing and treating digestive diseases and disorders, usually performs the flexible sigmoidoscopy or the colonoscopy. The sigmoidoscopy and even the colonoscopy may also be performed by physicians who are not gastroenterologists.

The Double-Contrast Barium Enema This procedure is performed by a radiologist. During the double-contrast barium enema, patients are fully conscious. A barium dye is administered through the rectum to bathe and highlight the colon, making it appear opaque on X-rays. Air is then introduced, to give a double contrast and to make the X-ray view clearer. (In a single-contrast barium enema, only the barium is used and the air is not introduced, but the test result is less accurate.) If an abnormality is found by the barium enema, a colonoscopy is then performed. The barium enema does not visualize the lower colon and the rectum very well, and an additional sigmoidoscopy is required to perform a more complete evaluation.

The Colonoscopy and Sigmoidoscopy   The most extensive procedure to check for colon cancer is the colonoscopy, in which the doctor visually inspects the entire colon. In the United States, patients are usually sedated, although sedation is often not used in other countries. The colonoscopy is the best procedure to detect colorectal cancer because it inspects the entire colon and allows physician to take biopsies and/or remove suspicious lesions such as precancerous polyps. Prior to the colonoscopy, the patient is instructed on taking bowel cleansing medications and/or laxatives so that the bowel will be more easily visualized during the procedure.

A sigmoidoscopy is similar to a colonoscopy; however, with a sigmoidoscopy, the doctor inspects only the lower third of the bowel. This procedure may be chosen because it is less expensive than the colonoscopy. However, most experts believe that having a sigmoidoscopy to detect colorectal cancer or precancerous polyps is comparable to having a mammogram breast cancer on just one breast.

The actions that the surgeon can take as a result of the findings during the procedure are dependent on the type of procedure performed. For example, polyps (precancerous growths) can be detected during a sigmoidoscopy, but they cannot be removed by electrocautery unless the colon is completely cleaned out ahead of time, and normally this is not done. Also, if any precancerous polyps are identified during a sigmoidoscopy, the doctor will order a subsequent colonoscopy so that the entire colon can be checked for polyps, which can then be removed. As a result, the patient must have two major procedures instead of one.

The physician's goal is another factor in determining which test is ordered. For example, if the doctor wants to remove any tissue to check for can-cer (a biopsy), this procedure cannot be performed during a barium enema or virtual colonoscopy. The doctor may, however, perform a biopsy during either a colonoscopy or a sigmoidoscopy.

Staging of Cancer   If colorectal cancer is identified, doctors will determine how advanced the cancer is and how fast it is growing in order to determine what treatment to use. This is called staging. Staging is performed using extracted tissue in a *biopsy* as well as using results of imaging studies and surgery. They will then further categorize the cancer, using the Tumor-Node-Metastasis or TNM system, developed by the American Joint Committee on Cancer, which is used to stage all forms of cancer. Staging is important because it helps physicians to determine the recommended course of treatment and assess the prognosis.

With colorectal cancer, the TNM system provides a method of classification that is based on the determination of how deeply the tumor (which is the T) has penetrated through the walls of the colon, as well as whether it has spread to nearby lymph nodes (the N), and whether it has metastasized (the M for metastasis) to distant tissues.

For example, if the finding is that the tumor is categorized as T is $N0$ $M0$, this means that the cancer is in its earliest stage. (T is not a 0 or a 1; it simply stands alone in this stage.)

The worst stage of colorectal cancer is M, irrespective of the T or N stage, and this indicates the cancer has spread to distant sites, such as the liver or lungs. At that point, doctors cannot cure the cancer, and they can only take palliative measures to ease the pain of the patient until death occurs. As opposed to the past, curative resection may be attempted in patients with liver metastasis. In some carefully selected cases, even lung metastasis may be resected as it appears to prolong survival.

If a biopsy will be taken, the patient may wish to ask the doctor the following questions recommended by the National Cancer Institute prior to having the biopsy:

- How will the biopsy be done?
- Will I have to go to the hospital for the biopsy?
- How long will it take? Will I be awake? Will it hurt?

- Are there any risks? What are the chances of infection or bleeding after the biopsy?
- How long will it take me to recover? When can I assume a normal diet?
- How soon will I know the results?
- If I have cancer, who will talk to me about the next steps? When?

If the biopsy shows cancer, the doctor may wish to order other tests. If a colonoscopy was not previously done, it will be done now. The doctor may also order an *endorectal ultrasound*, which is an ultrasound probe inserted in the rectum. This procedure is usually done for rectal and not colon cancer and can show whether a tumor has spread to nearby lymph nodes or other tissues. A chest X-ray may be taken to determine whether cancer has spread to the lungs. A computerized tomography (CT) scan with injected dye may also show if the cancer has spread to the liver, lungs, and other organs. A magnetic resonance imaging (MRI) scan may show if cancer has spread. A PET scan may be done in select cases.

The doctor usually orders a blood test for carcinoembryonic antigen (CEA) because many people with colorectal cancer have a high level of CEA. CEA levels are also used for monitoring after surgery.

Treatment Options and Outlook

The treatment depends on the stage of the cancer and whether it has spread. In general, treatment includes surgery, radiation treatment, or chemotherapy. Before treatment begins, the National Cancer Institute recommends patients ask their doctors the following questions:

- What is the stage of the disease? Has the cancer spread?
- What are my treatment choices? Which do you suggest for me? Will I have more than one kind of treatment?
- What are the expected benefits of the treatment?
- What are the risks and possible side effects of each treatment? How can the side effects be managed?

- What can I do to prepare for treatment?
- How will treatment affect my normal activities? Am I likely to have urinary problems? What about bowel problems, such as diarrhea or rectal bleeding? Will treatment affect my sex life?
- What will the treatment cost? Is this treatment covered by my insurance plan?

With surgery, doctors remove all or part of the cancerous colon/rectum and also any lymph nodes that are found in the area. If the physician finds a small malignant polyp during a colonoscopy, it will be removed. A tumor in the early stages of colon cancer can also be removed through a laparoscopy, which is surgery which uses three or four tiny cuts in the abdomen into which the laparoscope is inserted. The tumor and part of the colon may be removed, and nearby lymph nodes may also be removed. In some cases, open surgery with a large abdominal incision is needed.

Once the tumorous tissue is removed, the doctor usually can reconnect the healthy parts of the intestine but sometimes this is not possible. In that case, the doctor performs a colostomy or ileostomy depending upon the surgery, creating a new path from the body (the *stoma*) for waste material to leave the body. The waste will go into a bag over the opening in the abdominal wall. Many people need the stoma only temporarily until their body heals and then the physician can reconnect the intestines. However, some people, about one in eight, will need a permanent stoma.

According to the National Cancer Institute, the following questions should be asked before surgery occurs:

- What kind of operation do you recommend for me?
- Do I need any lymph nodes removed? Will other tissues be removed? Why?
- What are the risks of surgery? Will I have any lasting side effects?
- Will I need a colostomy? If so, will the stoma be permanent?
- How will I feel after the operation?
- If I have PAIN, how will it be controlled?

- How long will I be in the hospital?
- When can I get back to my normal activities?

While surgery is the only method to cure localized colorectal cancer, radiation therapy may be used as part of treatment of colorectal cancer in advanced cases, and doctors use either external radiation generated by a machine called a linear accelerator or the radiation is implanted in tubes placed in or near the tumor. The side effects to the abdomen and pelvis may include nausea and vomiting, diarrhea, bloody stools, or urgent bowel movements. The skin that is radiated may be sore and tender. The radiation may also cause extreme tiredness. Patients who are recommended radiation therapy by their doctor should ask their physician the following questions before treatment begins:

- Why do I need this treatment?
- When will the treatments begin? When will they end?
- How will I feel during treatment?
- How will we know if the radiation treatment is working?
- What can I do to take care of myself during treatment?
- Can I continue my normal activities?
- Are there any lasting effects?

In some cases, chemotherapy is needed to treat colorectal cancer, as when the cancer has spread. Chemotherapy drugs are usually introduced through an intravenous line or sometimes with a catheter that is placed into the portal vein connecting to the liver. Some forms of drugs are available in pill form. Chemotherapy may cause the patient to feel nauseated, tired, and dizzy, and anticancer drugs may also cause hair loss. Other patients are treated with immune therapy/biological therapy to stimulate the immune system. Patients who will be receiving either chemotherapy or biological therapy should ask their doctor the following questions:

- What drugs will I have? What will they do?
- When will treatment start? When will it end? How often will I have treatments?

- Where will I go for treatment? Will I be able to drive home afterward?
- What can I do to take care of myself during treatment?
- How will we know the treatment is working?
- Which side effects should I tell you about?
- Will there be long-term effects?

Clinical Trials   Another treatment option is to join a clinical trial in which new medications or other therapies are being tested. Frequently, this choice is made when the cancer is in an advanced stage and all other treatment options are exhausted.

Risk Factors and Preventive Measures

Men have a higher incidence of colorectal cancer than women. African Americans, both men and women, have a significantly higher risk for colorectal cancer than that faced by whites in the United States.

The risk for development of colorectal cancer increases with age; about 90 percent of all patients with colorectal cancer are older than age 50 years. Therefore, screening of people who are age 50 and older is very important. Patients who have INFLAMMATORY BOWEL DISEASE (IBD) have a greater risk of the development of colorectal cancer than those without IBD. The risk of colorectal cancer in IBD patients depends upon the extent and duration of the disease.

Tobacco users have more than double (2.5) the risk of development of colorectal cancer of nonusers. Other risk factors for the development of colorectal cancer include the following:

- a family or personal history of colorectal cancer or a history of ovarian cancer, uterine cancer or breast cancer in a woman
- obesity
- a past history of the adenoma type of polyps in the colon
- a high-fat and low-fiber diet
- the presence of ULCERATIVE COLITIS or CROHN'S DISEASE
- alcohol abuse or alcoholism

- physical inactivity/sedentary lifestyle
- a smoking habit
- cholecystectomy
- coronary artery disease
- ureterocolic anastomoses after bladder surgery
- radiation therapy to pelvic area

Genetic changes can also increase the risk for the development of colorectal cancer; for example, hereditary nonpolyposis colon cancer (HNPCC) is the most common form of inherited colorectal cancer, and it represents about 2 percent of all colorectal cancers. This form of cancer is triggered by changes in the HNPCC gene. The average age of diagnosis among individuals with this form of cancer is age 44.

Another form of inherited colorectal cancer is caused by familial adenomatous polyposis (FAP). This condition causes hundreds of polyps to develop in the colon and the rectum. It is caused by a gene known as the APC gene. If this disease is untreated, it generally causes colorectal cancer by the age of 40 years. FAP represents less than 1 percent of all cases of colorectal cancer.

Because the risks for development of colorectal cancer increase with age, people older than age 50 should have the FOBT every year. This is, however, not undertaken if patient has had a colonoscopy. Unfortunately, many people who are 50 years and older do not have a sigmoidoscopy every five years, nor do they have a colonoscopy once every 10 years, and in some of them, colorectal cancer that could have been prevented with such tests develops. More frequent examinations are required for patients who have a higher than average risk of development of colorectal cancer. African Americans have a higher risk of developing CRC, and thus, an earlier screening starting at 45 years instead of 50 has been recommended in this population.

Individuals who drink alcohol or smoke cigarettes should give up these habits to significantly decrease their risk of developing colorectal cancer. Protective factors against colorectal cancer include calcium, magnesium, vitamin B$_6$, physical exercise, aspirin, and other NSAIDs. The majority but not all data suggests that high fiber is protective.

Aspirin: A New Preventive Measure for Those with Past Nonmetastatic Colorectal Cancer A study published in 2009 by Andrew T. Chan, M.D., and colleagues based on a follow-up study of 1,279 men and women diagnosed with colorectal cancer revealed that regular aspirin use after diagnosis of non-metastatic colorectal cancer (cancer that has not spread) is associated with a significantly reduced risk for death from a recurrence of this form of cancer. The researchers found that this relationship was independent of the use of aspirin prior to diagnosis. All individuals who have had colorectal cancer should consult with their physicians about whether aspirin use would be appropriate for them as well as what dosage would be best.

See also ANAL CANCER; COLOSTOMY; FIBER; OCCULT GASTROINTESTINAL BLEEDING.

Chan, Andrew T., M.D, Ogino, Shuji, and Fuchs, Charles, S., M.D. "Aspirin Use and Survival After Diagnosis of Colorectal Cancer." *Journal of the American Medical Association* 302, no. 6 (2009): 649–659.

Minocha, Anil, M.D. *The Gastroenterology Resident Pocket Survival Guide.* McLean, Va.: International Medical Publishing, 1999.

National Cancer Institute. *Cancer Trends Progress Report—2007 Update.* Bethesda, Md.: Department of Health and Human Services, December 2007.

———. *What You Need to Know about Cancer of the Colon and Rectum.* Bethesda, Md.: Department of Health and Human Services, May 2006.

colostomy Surgery that is performed after damage to the colon and/or to the rectum from cancer or other causes, such as diverticulitis. The colostomy creates an opening in the abdominal wall to the colon, through which stools enter either a temporary or a permanent collection bag.

The temporary colostomy allows healing to occur after surgery; later the colostomy is closed and the two disconnected parts of the colon are hooked back together again. In the meantime, patients are trained to empty the bag periodically.

In many cases, the colostomy may be permanent.

See also COLORECTAL CANCER.

complications of digestive disorders Digestive diseases or conditions that are caused or exacerbated to a serious extent and for a variety of different reasons. There are many examples of such conditions; for example, untreated GASTRO-ESOPHAGEAL REFLUX DISEASE (GERD) can lead to the precancerous condition of BARRETT'S ESOPHAGUS, which in turn, rarely, may lead to the development of ESOPHAGEAL CANCER. Liver diseases, such as either viral or alcoholic HEPATITIS, can further lead to the development of CIRRHOSIS (damage and scarring) of the liver, which may worsen to LIVER CANCER. There are also many different complications that are associated with DIABETES MELLITUS, whether the individual is diagnosed with type 1 diabetes (insulin-dependent) or the much more commonly diagnosed type 2 diabetes.

Cirrhosis Complications

Liver cirrhosis refers to the deterioration and scarring of healthy liver tissue. It may be caused by heavy alcohol consumption and/or infection with chronic hepatitis C. It may also be caused by hepatitis B or D. (See HEPATITIS A, B, C, AND D.) In some cases, OBESITY may cause liver cirrhosis, either together with alcoholism or with hepatitis C or by itself. The symptoms of liver cirrhosis include weakness and fatigue, a loss of APPETITE, NAUSEA and VOMITING, weight loss, ABDOMINAL PAIN and bloating, and severe itching.

There are many complications that are associated with cirrhosis, including EDEMA and ASCITES. Edema refers to fluid that collects in the legs, while ascites refers to fluid that collects in the abdomen. Ascites can in turn lead to the development of spontaneous bacterial PERITONITIS (SBP), a serious and sometimes life-threatening infection of the peritoneum. In contrast to secondary peritonitis, there is no overt perforation of the bowel involved in SBP. This is the lining that protects the internal abdominal organs. Individuals with spontaneous bacterial peritonitis may require hospitalization although milder cases have been treated as outpatients on oral medications.

The person suffering from complications of cirrhosis may also bruise or bleed very easily because of low blood clotting factors and/or platelets. Cirrhosis may also lead to JAUNDICE, or a yellowing of the skin tone and of the whites of the eyes as well as a darkening of the urine. Certain forms of cirrhosis are associated with an increased risk for the development of GALLSTONES.

The individual with cirrhosis has an increased sensitivity to medications because the liver is impeded in its ability to metabolize or process medications from the blood. Thus, medications will act longer in the body and they may build up. This factor must be taken into account by the prescribing physician. A common culprit is acetaminophen because of its widespread use among patients.

Hepatic encephalopathy is another complication of cirrhosis, and this condition occurs when the liver fails to remove toxins from the blood, and as a result, they subsequently build up within the body, including the brain. This development can significantly decrease mental functions, and it may also eventually lead to coma. Some signs of hepatic encephalopathy are depressed mental status, personality changes, confusion, memory loss, an increased difficulty with concentration, and a change in the individual's sleep habits.

Liver cancer is another risk for individuals with cirrhosis. Cirrhosis may also lead to *hepatorenal syndrome* (which causes kidney failure) and to *hepatopulmonary syndrome*, which leads to lung failure and these frequently require hospitalization and are potentially lethal.

Cirrhosis may also lead to a malfunction of the immune system, which will increase the risk of developing an infection.

The treatments for the complications of cirrhosis depend on the type of complication, but the goal is to slow down the progression of the development of further scar tissue in the liver, as much as possible. The model for end-stage liver disease (MELD) is a means to evaluate the individual's likelihood of survival for 90 days or more among patients who have advanced cirrhosis. The score is derived from three blood tests, including a test for the international normalized ration (INR) to test the clotting ability of the blood; a test for the amount of BILIRUBIN (bile pigment) in the blood, and a measure of creatinine, which tests for kidney function. Extra points may be added for complications such as hepatocellular cancer. The MELD score is used to triage patients for liver transplantation.

Individuals with cirrhosis should be sure to eat a carefully well-balanced diet, and they may also need to restrict their sodium intake. They should not eat raw shellfish, which may contain a bacterium that could lead to a serious infection. Patients with cirrhosis may sometimes need to consume oral liquid supplements or to be provided their nutrition through a nasogastric tube.

Individuals with cirrhosis should avoid drinking any alcohol or using any illegal drugs, which would further damage the liver. In addition, before taking any medications, including vitamins, minerals or alternative remedies, the patient should check with the doctor first, to ensure that these substances will not be harmful to the liver.

When his or her complications become severe, the individual with cirrhosis may need to receive a liver transplant. Patients with organ transplants of any type must take immunosuppressive drugs for life, so that their body will not reject the organ. Unfortunately, these medications also increase the risk for the development of serious infections as well as cancer.

Complications of Endoscopic Procedures

In addition to the complications that are associated with specific diseases, there are also complications that may occur with the endoscopic procedures used by gastroenterologists for both diagnosis and treatment, although the complication rate is generally very low, according to Giampaolo Angelini and Laura Bernardoni in their chapter on complications associated with lower gastrointestinal tract endoscopy in the book *Intestinal Polyps and Polyposis*, published in 2009.

According to these authors from the Institute of Gastroenterology at the University of Verona in Italy, the death rate for colonoscopies is very close to zero. In addition, the rate of complications is also very low, although complications may occur as late as 30 days of the performance of the procedure.

For example, according to the authors, bleeding rates linked to colonoscopy are less than 1 percent (0.02 percent to 0.03 percent), and the rate of perforations is only slightly higher (0.04 percent to 0.6 percent). The complication rates for therapeutic colonoscopies (colonoscopies in which actions beyond diagnosis are taken such as a dilation or inserting a stent) are somewhat higher, or 0.31 percent to 2.7 percent.

Angelini and Bernardoni also report that cardiopulmonary complications may occur in up to 2 percent of patients who have a colonoscopy. Patients who are at high risk from such complications include those who are:

- pregnant
- obese
- illegal drug users
- alcohol abusers
- ELDERLY
- uncooperative patients

Another issue that is related to potential cardiopulmonary complications is that opiates and benzodiazepine medications are commonly used with the endoscopic procedure, as sedating and painkilling agents. In such cases as when prolonged endoscopic procedures are used, as with the ENDOSCOPIC RETROGRADE CHOLANGIOPANCREATOGRAPHY (ERCP), as well as with procedures that involve children, a short-acting general anesthesia may be needed to cause a greater level of sedation depending on the situation.

If cardiopulmonary complications do occur, the physician may immediately end the procedure and begin to administer medications that will reverse the sedating effects of the medications, such as administering naloxone for an opioid drug that was given or giving flumazenil (Romazicon) to reverse the effects of any benzodiazepine medications that were used to sedate the patient. Drug effects are usually not totally reversible when benzodiazepines have been used. In addition, reversal agents can have their own complications.

With the diagnostic colonoscopy, the most serious risk for the patient is the possible perforation of the colon, and this very low risk increases with the removal of POLYPS by about nine times. The authors provide further information, "Risk factors for perforation are: the presence of inflammatory activity, prior pelvic radiotherapy, the presence of diverticula, and prior abdominal surgery."

Hemorrhage occurs very rarely with the colonoscopy, and the risk is less than 1 percent. However, minor bleeding may occur subsequent to the procedure, which self-heals relatively quickly in most individuals. In some cases, especially those taking NSAIDs, the bleeding may be delayed as long as 28 days.

Other complications with colonoscopy may be the triggering of APPENDICITIS or of acute DIVERTICULITIS. In addition, the patient may, in rare cases, experience *postcolonoscopy syndrome*, with symptoms of abdominal pain and the moderate distention of the abdomen, which may be caused by an excessive introduction of air into the colon.

In their article on complications related to the ERCP, Matthew L. Silviera and colleagues noted that over 500,000 ERCP procedures are performed every year in the United States. They stated that complications included a risk for PANCREATITIS, BLEEDING, and perforation. The authors said that the ERCP was absolutely contraindicated when there was any obstruction in the pharynx or esophagus as well as any problem with active coagulopathy (blood clotting) or a known reaction to contrast dye.

According to the authors, the most common complication of the ERCP is cardiopulmonary depression, which is a slowed heart and breathing with low oxygen, caused by the effect of the sedatives as well as by the scope itself. This complication may represent up to 50 percent of all the possible complications of the ERCP. On the other hand, pancreatitis may occur in as many as 5 to 15 percent of cases of ERCP. However, only 1 percent of the individuals experiencing this complication have a severe reaction. Another risk with the ERCP is a perforation during the course of the ERCP, but the authors say that this risk is less than 1 percent.

They add that more than half of the perforations are associated with underlying anatomic abnormalities, such as ZENKERS'S DIVERTICULUM, benign/malignant esophageal strictures, and other mass lesions. To manage the perforation, fluids are given as well as broad spectrum antibiotics, and drainage is also provided as needed. Surgery may be performed depending upon individual clinical status.

Most complications are short-term (occurring within three days of the procedure) and may include bleeding, infection, or perforation. Long-term complications stem from infections that are linked to inflammatory changes or indwelling stents.

As mentioned above, another complication with ERCP, according to Silviera, et al., is pancreatitis that is caused by the ERCP. Indications of the presence of ERCP-induced pancreatitis are new or worsening abdominal pain, and the need for the patient to be hospitalized for pancreatitis.

Complications of Diabetes Mellitus

Individuals who are diagnosed with type 1 or type 2 diabetes are at risk for digestive complications, such as GASTROPARESIS (a slowed stomach emptying) and chronic CONSTIPATION.

They are also at risk for diabetic ketoacidosis (DKA), a dangerous condition of acute insulin insufficiency that is more often associated with type 1 diabetes than type 2 diabetes, and which can lead to coma and death. According to Ramachandran Cooppan, M.D., and his colleagues in their chapter on acute complications of diabetes in *Joslin's Diabetes Deskbook*, an estimated 100,000 patients are seen in U.S. hospital emergency rooms each year with DKA. The death rate for this condition is less than 5 percent, but it represents a severe health risk. DKA is a combination of hyperglycemia, ketosis, and acidosis, and the blood glucose can be as high as 400 or more, although Coopan and colleagues say it may be between 250 and 300 mg/dl, particularly in patients who have taken some insulin.

The authors state, "The precipitating factors for DKA are mainly infection, concurrent illness, and omission of insulin or inadequate coverage for sick days. Many patients are seen because they have not been taught how to care of their diabetes during a concurrent illness and DKA often precipitates rapidly, so hesitation in self-treatment can be problematic. Even patients who have received education and have had diabetes for many years can make errors in handling sick days. It is not uncommon for patients to state that because of anorexia or poor appetite, they felt it was not necessary to take insulin. This is a major error, especially for a patient with type 1 diabetes who relies completely on exogenous insulin."

Another hyperglycemic crisis in diabetes is called *hyperosmolar hyperglycemic state* (HHS). This condition is found in some individuals with type 2 diabetes who still have some insulin secretion. This leads to a worsening of the hyperglycemia, as with DKA. HHS may be precipitated by severe physiologic stress, such as a mild kidney insufficiency or infections such as pneumonia. Some medications can also precipitate HHS, such as corticosteroids, beta blockers, and diuretics. The key symptom is extreme thirst, urination leading to dehydration that may cause confusion or even coma. The treatment is the aggressive replacement of fluids.

Hypoglycemia is another common problem among diabetics, especially those with type 1 diabetes, and low blood sugar can become a medical emergency. This condition can be severe and may even lead to death if it develops while the person is asleep or while he or she is driving a car. Researchers have found that aggressive glycemic control has a risk of causing hypoglycemia. According to Coopan, et al., the person with diabetes who realizes that he or she has hypoglycemia can take three glucose tablets or four dextrose tablets to reverse the hypoglycemia. They may also drink four ounces of fruit juice, drink about ½ can of regular soda with sugar (not diet soda), eat two tablespoons of raisins or one tablespoon of sugar or jelly.

There are many nondigestive complications that are linked to the diagnosis of diabetes mellitus, such as diabetic nephropathy (chronic kidney disease that is associated with diabetes), diabetic neuropathy (nerve disease that is associated with diabetes), and diabetic retinopathy (an eye disease that can lead to blindness). There are also increased risks for cardiovascular disease, including heart and peripheral vascular disease, and an increased risk for heart attack and the loss of a limb.

GERD Complications

At its simplest and least harmful level, gastroesophageal reflux disease (GERD) is a problem of frequent HEARTBURN. If treated when it is only a minor problem, GERD is generally a very manageable chronic disorder. However, if it is not treated and/or if it is exacerbated by such behavior as SMOKING or drinking alcohol to excess, then the GERD can worsen into becoming a more frequent problem, and the likelihood of the development of Barrett's esophagus is escalated.

According to the National Digestive Diseases Information Clearinghouse, about 1 percent of adults in the United States have Barrett's esophagus, which is usually diagnosed when the individual is about 50 years old; however, the problem may have occurred well before then. It is unusual before the age of five. Men develop Barrett's esophagus at about twice the rate of women, and white men have a greater risk of developing Barrett's esophagus than do men of other races. Barrett's esophagus increases the risk for the development of esophageal cancer. Data is mixed, but overall the risk is low, however, the frequency of Barrett's estimates vary between 1–5 percent. Follow-up of patients with Barrett's reveals that about 0.5 percent per year of those with Barrett's esophagus will develop esophageal cancer. Interestingly, epidemiological data suggests that patients with BE live just as long as those without BE.

Barrett's esophagus is treated similarly to the treatment for GERD; for example, acid-reducing medications are used, including over-the-counter medications as well as prescribed medications such as PROTON PUMP INHIBITORS (PPIs). Examples of some PPIs are esomeprazole (Nexium), lansoprazole (Prevacid), omeprazole (Prilosec, Zegerid), pantoprazole (Protonix), and rabeprazole (Aciphex).

According to the National Digestive Diseases Information Clearinghouse, the following points about Barrett's esophagus should be kept in mind:

- Improvement in GERD symptoms with the use of acid-reducing medications may decrease the risk for developing Barrett's esophagus.

- Barrett's esophagus is diagnosed with an upper gastrointestinal endoscopy and with biopsies.

- Individuals with Barrett's esophagus should have periodical endoscopies and biopsies, on a schedule determined by their gastroenterologist depending upon the presence or absence of dysplasia.

- Endoscopic treatments can be used to destroy Barrett's esophagus, which should then be replaced with normal esophageal tissue. Data on the outcome of such treatments is controversial.

• The removal of most of the esophagus may be recommended if a person with Barrett's esophagus has severe dysplasia (the development of precancerous cells) or cancer and can tolerate surgery. Another viable option is endoscopic ablative treatments and endoscopic mucosal resection with intensive surveillance, e.g. EGD every three months.

• With Barrett's esophagus, the tissue that lines the esophagus is replaced by tissue that is similar to the lining of the intestine.

NSAID-Related Ulcer Complications

NONSTEROIDAL ANTI-INFLAMMATORY DRUGS(NSAIDs) are frequently used to treat individuals with chronic painful conditions, such as arthritis, back pain, and many other PAIN syndromes. However, the regular use of NSAIDs has its risks because it increases the risk for the development of ulcers as well as for complications from ulcers.

In a 2009 article published in the *American Journal of Gastroenterology*, Frank L. Lanza, M.D., and colleagues discussed some guidelines for preventing NSAID-related ulcer complications. They note that as many as 25 percent of regular NSAID users will develop ulcers, and 2 to 4 percent of the ulcers will perforate or bleed. The authors say, "These gastrointestinal events result in more than 100,000 hospital admissions annually in the United States and between 7,000 and 10,000 deaths, especially among those who have been designated as being in a high-risk category."

According to the authors, studies have shown that some individuals have a greater risk for the development of NSAID-related complications than others, such as individuals who are ages 65 years and older, those taking higher than usual dosages of NSAIDs, those taking corticosteroids or anticoagulants in addition to NSAIDs, and those who have been taking NSAIDs for three months or less. In addition, a person with a prior history of a complicated ulcer has an increased risk for developing an ulcer that is caused by NSAIDs if individuals continue taking NSAIDs. NSAIDs can cause gut ulcers and its complications anywhere from the esophagus to the anus.

Other studies have shown that individuals with rheumatoid arthritis who use NSAIDs have an increased risk for complications. The presence of cardiovascular disease also elevates the risk for NSAID complications. Some studies have shown that even the low dosage use of aspirin increases the risk for gastrointestinal bleeding.

An infection with HELICOBACTER PYLORI (H. pylori) as well as the taking of NSAIDs further escalates the risk for ulcer complications.

There are preventive measures that can be taken against the potential development of ulcer complications; for example, the use of proton pump inhibitor medications have been globally effective at reducing NSAID-caused peptic ulcers. Some research has also shown that a double dose of H2RAs are effective at reducing the risk for NSAID-induced ulcers. Medications that are COX-2 inhibitors decrease the risk for ulcers, as well as the risk for complications associated with ulcers; however, most of the medications in the COX-2 inhibitor class have been withdrawn from the market because they were found to increase the risk for serious cardiovascular side effects.

See also MAJOR DIAGNOSTIC TESTS FOR DIGESTIVE DISEASES.

Abell, T. L., and A. Minocha. "Gastrointestinal complications of bariatric surgery: diagnosis and therapy." *American Journal of Medical Science* 331, no. 4 (April 2006): 214–218.

Angelini, Giampaolo, and Laura Bernardoni. "Management and Treatment of Complications in Diagnostic and Therapeutic Lower Gastrointestinal Tract Endoscopy." In *Intestinal Polyps and Polyposis*, edited by Gian Gaetano Delaini, Tomáš Skřička, and Gianluca Colucci, Milan, Italy: Springer Milan, 2009.

Coopan, Ramachandran, M.D., Richard Beaser, M.D., and Greeshma K. Sheety, M.D. "Acute Complications." In *Joslin's Diabetes Deskbook: A Guide for Primary Care Providers*, edited by Richard S. Beaser, M.D. and the staff of Joslin Diabetes Center, 403–427 Boston, 2007.

Lanza, Frank L., M.D., Francis Chan, M.D., and Eamonn M. M. Quigely, M.D. "Complications for Prevention of NSAID-Related Ulcer Complications." *American Journal of Gastroenterology* 104 (2009): 728–738.

Minocha A. "A Fatal Case of Paracentesis." *American Journal of Gastroenterology* 94 (1999): 856.

Minocha, A., and R. Srinivasan. "Ethanol-Acetaminophen Cocktail: The Debate Continues!" *American Journal of Gastroenterology* 93, no. 4 (1998): 661–662.

——— "Conscious Sedation: Pearls & Perils." *Digestive Diseases and Sciences* 43, no. 8 (1998): 1,835–1,844.

Minocha, A., and R. J. Richards. "Pneumothorax Complicating Diagnostic Upper Endoscopy." *American Journal of Gastroenterology* 94, no. 8 (1999): 2,323.

Petro, M., and A. Minocha. "Asymptomatic Early Acute Appendicitis Initiated and Diagnosed during Colonoscopy: A Case Report." *World Journal of Gastroenterology* 11, no. 34 (September 14, 2005): 5,398–5,400.

Siddiqi, A.M., R. D. Hamilton, and A. Minocha. "Malignant Seeding of Percutaneous Endoscopic Gastrostomy (PEG) Tract in Patient with Head and Neck Cancer." *American Journal of Medical Sciences.* 336, no. 3 (2008): 291–292.

Silviera, Matthew L., et al. "Complications Related to Endoscopic Retrograde Cholangiopancreatography: A Comprehensive Clinical Review." *Journal of Gastrointestinal and Liver Disease* 18, no. 1 (2009): 73–82.

condyloma acuminatum (anal warts) The most commonly known venereal disease that is diagnosed in the United States. Most patients who have this disease (about 67 percent) are female. The disease is caused by infection with the human papillomavirus (HPV); more than 70 different types of HPV are currently known.

Some studies have shown that a history of anal warts increases the probability of development of anal cancer, such as a study reported in the *New England Journal of Medicine* in 1997, which was based on telephone interviews with hundreds of men and women who had been diagnosed with anal cancer.

In another interesting study, reported in a 1999 issue of the *Archives of Internal Medicine,* the researchers found that, contrary to popular perception, many lesbians have apparently had unprotected sexual encounters with males. In the sample of nearly 7,000 females who identified themselves as lesbians, 17.2 percent reported having had a sexually transmitted disease (STD). Among the most frequently occurring STDs, experienced by 4.8 percent, were anal or genital warts. Lesbians who said they had had six or more male sexual partners in their life were most likely to have had a sexually transmitted disease (STD). Said the researchers, "Lesbians who had engaged in anal intercourse reported higher rates of STDs and abnormal Pap smears than those who had not engaged in these activities."

Symptoms and Diagnostic Path

Patients may be asymptomatic or may have pain, bleeding, burning, and pruritus in the anal area.

The diagnosis of anal warts can usually be made by a visual inspection by a doctor, although a biopsy may be needed in some cases. Physicians need to exclude condyloma acuminatum from other forms of the disease, such as hemorrhoids, cancer, and condyloma latum, a disease that is linked to infection with syphilis, another venereal disease. Lesions that are present and that look suspicious to the physician can be biopsied to obtain further information and validate (or refute) the presence of condyloma acuminatum.

Treatment Options and Outlook

When condyloma acuminatum has been confirmed, there are various treatment methods. Doctors may choose chemical means to destroy the anal warts, using drugs such as podophyllin, trichloroacetic acid, or 5-fluorouracil/epinephrine gel. Podophyllin should not be used by women who are pregnant or may be pregnant.

Immune-modulating agents such as interferon alfa or iminquimod may be used to treat condyloma acuminatum. Imiquimod is a topical cream; interferon is injected. Patients may also be treated with ablative therapies, such as surgery, cryotherapy (freezing of the anal warts), or laser therapy.

Some physicians also use topical doses of antibacterial drugs such as cidofovir gel or Bacillus Calmette-Guérin (BCG).

Risk Factors and Preventive Measures

In women, condyloma acuminatum is primarily spread through vaginal intercourse, and the greater the number of sexual partners that a woman has, the higher her risk for contracting HPV and subsequent anal warts; for example, women who have five or more sexual partners over the course of five years have about 12 times the risk of infection of women who have had one sexual partner.

Among men, the disease may be spread through either heterosexual or homosexual contact. As with women, the risk of infection increases with the number of sexual partners. In addition, men who are positive for the human immunodeficiency virus (HIV) also have a greater risk for contracting HPV and subsequently having anal warts.

Diamant, Allison L., M.D., et al. "Lesbians' Sexual History with Men: Implications for Taking a Sexual History." *Archives of Internal Medicine* 159 (December 13/27, 1999): 2,730–2,736.

Frisch, Morten, M.D., et. al. "Sexually Transmitted Infection as a Cause of Anal Cancer." *New England Journal of Medicine* 337, no. 19 (November 6, 1997): 1,350–1,358.

constipation   Difficult or infrequent bowel movements. Production of less than three bowel movements per week is often referred to as constipation, but constipation can also include passing very hard stools or frequently having the sensation of incomplete defecation. For example, patients may feel as if they are not "empty" after they do have a bowel movement, and they may feel they need to have another bowel movement.

Symptoms and Diagnostic Path

Constipation may cause back pain and abdominal pain, as well as a generalized feeling of discomfort. Some people struggle with chronic pain associated with constipation that may or may not alternate with diarrhea, a condition that is known as IRRITABLE BOWEL SYNDROME (IBS). Patients can also have IBS without constipation: IBS—diarrhea predominant.

Treatment Options and Outlook

A blockage should be excluded in patients who have constipation. Many cases of general constipation can be resolved by increasing the amount of fiber in the diet and increasing fluid consumption or adding a very mild LAXATIVE. Stool softeners may also help some patients to resolve their constipation. Often, EXERCISE, even as simple as regular walking, can help to resolve problems with constipation.

Doctors may recommend bowel retraining, in which patients are urged to set aside specific times to use the toilet, particularly after meals, when they are more likely to be able to have a bowel movement.

In the most extreme case, which may occur after several days without passing a stool, the feces may become impacted and need to be manually disimpacted by either the individual, a caregiver, or a medical person.

Chronic constipation and straining at bowel movements may lead to the development of hemorrhoids. Patients with constipation that is related to IBS may be treated with a medication called lubiprostone (Amitiza). Biofeedback is also helpful in many cases of constipation, especially those that are characterized by difficult or painful defecation.

Risk Factors and Preventive Measures

Older people have a much greater risk of chronic constipation than younger people, in large part because they generally lead a far more sedentary life. Older people are also more likely to be taking medications that can cause constipation, as well as to have diseases that are linked to problems with constipation, such as DIABETES MELLITUS, Parkinson's disease, or thyroid disease, particularly hypothyroidism (below normal levels of thyroid hormone). Abnormal electrolyte levels, such as low blood levels of potassium, may also cause constipation.

A diet that is poor in FIBER or insufficient in fluids may cause constipation. A sluggish colon can also cause constipation. This particular condition is often seen among patients with diabetes.

See also BOWEL MOVEMENT; FECAL IMPACTION; HEMORRHOIDS; LAXITIVES AND LAXATIVE ABUSE; NARCOTIC BOWEL SYNDROME.

contaminated food or water   Food that is overgrown with bacteria, viruses, or other substances that can cause illness or even death if consumed. Contaminated water is also the cause of the transmission of many diseases. Careful food preparation can prevent many types of food contamination; for example, simply washing the hands after using the toilet gets rid of many contaminants that could otherwise contaminate food.

In addition, cross-contamination should be avoided. Cross-contamination occurs when a contaminated food is placed beside clean food, and the bacteria are able to contaminate it as well. To

COLD STORAGE CHART

Following short but safe time limits helps consumers to prevent refrigerated food from either spoiling or becoming dangerous to eat. In general, according to the United States Department of Agriculture, freezing keeps most food safe indefinitely. As a result, the recommended storage times are provided for quality purposes only.

Product	Refrigerator (40°F)	Freezer (0°F)
Eggs		
Fresh, in shell	3 to 5 weeks	Do not freeze
Raw yolks & whites	2 to 4 days	1 year
Hard cooked	1 week	Does not freeze well
Liquid pasteurized eggs, egg substitutes		
opened	3 days	Does not freeze well
unopened	10 days	1 year
Mayonnaise		
Commercial, refrigerate after opening	2 months	Do not freeze
Frozen Dinners & Entrees		
Keep frozen until ready to heat	—	3 to 4 months
Deli & Vacuum-Packed Products		
Store-prepared (or homemade) egg, chicken, ham, tuna, & macaroni salads	3 to 5 days	Does not freeze well
Hot Dogs & Luncheon Meats		
Hot dogs		
opened package	1 week	1 to 2 months
unopened package	2 weeks	1 to 2 months
Luncheon meats		
opened package	3 to 5 days	1 to 2 months
unopened package	2 weeks	1 to 2 months
Bacon & Sausage		
Bacon	7 days	1 month
Sausage, raw—from chicken, turkey, pork, beef	1 to 2 days	1 to 2 months
Smoked breakfast links, patties	7 days	1 to 2 months
Hard sausage—pepperoni, jerky sticks	2 to 3 weeks	1 to 2 months
Summer sausage—labeled "Keep Refrigerated"		
opened	3 weeks	1 to 2 months
unopened	3 months	1 to 2 months
Ham, Corned Beef		
Corned beef, in pouch with pickling juices	5 to 7 days	Drained, 1 month
Ham, canned—labeled "Keep Refrigerated"		
opened	3 to 5 days	1 to 2 months
unopened	6 to 9 months	Do not freeze
Ham, fully cooked vacuum sealed at plant, undated, unopened	2 weeks	1 to 2 months
Ham, fully cooked vacuum sealed at plant, dated, unopened	"Use-By" date on package	1 to 2 months
Ham, fully cooked		
whole	7 days	1 to 2 months
half	3 to 5 days	1 to 2 months
slices	3 to 4 days	1 to 2 months

(Table continues)

(Table continued)

Product	Refrigerator (40°F)	Freezer (0°F)
Hamburger, Ground & Stew Meat		
Hamburger & stew meat	1 to 2 days	3 to 4 months
Ground turkey, veal, pork, lamb, & mixtures of them	1 to 2 days	3 to 4 months
Fresh Beef, Veal, Lamb, Pork		
Steaks	3 to 5 days	6 to 12 months
Chops	3 to 5 days	4 to 6 months
Roasts	3 to 5 days	4 to 12 months
Variety meats—tongue, liver, heart, kidneys, chitterlings	1 to 2 days	3 to 4 months
Prestuffed, uncooked pork chops, lamb chops, or chicken breasts stuffed with dressing	1 day	Does not freeze well
Soups & Stews		
Vegetable or meat added	3 to 4 days	2 to 3 months
Cooked Meat Leftovers		
Cooked meat & meat casseroles	3 to 4 days	2 to 3 months
Gravy & meat broth	1 to 2 days	2 to 3 months
Fresh Poultry		
Chicken or turkey, whole	1 to 2 days	1 year
Chicken or turkey, pieces	1 to 2 days	9 months
Giblets	1 to 2 days	3 to 4 months
Cooked Poultry Leftovers		
Fried chicken	3 to 4 days	4 months
Cooked poultry casseroles	3 to 4 days	4 to 6 months
Pieces, plain	3 to 4 days	4 months
Pieces covered with broth, gravy	1 to 2 days	6 months
Chicken nuggets, patties	1 to 2 days	1 to 3 months
Pizza, cooked	3 to 4 days	1 to 2 months
Stuffing, cooked	3 to 4 days	1 month

Credit: Food Safety and Inspection Service, "Food Safety Facts: Basics for Handling Food Safely," United States Department of Agriculture, July 2002.

Source: USDA Meat and Poultry Hotline

prevent cross-contamination of foods, items such as chicken, fish, and beef should not be placed near other food. In addition, after cutting up of meat, the cutting board should be thoroughly washed or another cutting board should be used before other items, such as fruits or vegetables, are cut.

It is also very important to discard food by its pass-by date, as well as to throw away food that has been in the refrigerator or freezer for an extended period. The Cold Storage Chart on pages 89–90, which is offered by the Food Safety and Inspection Service of the United States Department of Agriculture, provides helpful guidelines on when various types of foods should be discarded.

In most cases, moldy food should be discarded, because it may be dangerous and because many people are allergic to mold. However, in some cases, such as with some types of meats or cheeses, mold *can* be safely scraped off. The table on pages 91–92 from the Department of Agriculture provides guidelines on the types of food that should be discarded when they have mold and those on

MOLDY FOOD: WHEN TO USE, WHEN TO DISCARD

Note: Anyone who knows he or she is allergic to molds should discard the entire food item containing mold.

Food	Handling	Reason
Luncheon meats, bacon, or hot dogs	Discard	Foods with high moisture content can be contaminated below the surface. Moldy foods may also have bacteria growing along with the mold.
Hard salami and dry-cured country hams	Use. Scrub mold off surface	It is normal for these shelf-stable products to have surface mold.
Cooked leftover meat and poultry	Discard	Foods with high moisture content can be contaminated below the surface. Moldy foods may also have bacteria growing along with the mold.
Cooked casseroles	Discard	Foods with high moisture content can be contaminated below the surface. Moldy foods may also have bacteria growing along with the mold.
Cooked grain and pasta	Discard	Foods with high moisture content can be contaminated below the surface. Moldy foods may also have bacteria growing along with the mold.
Hard cheese (not cheese for which mold is part of the processing)	Use. Cut off at least 1 inch around and below the mold spot (keep the knife out of the mold itself so it will not cross-contaminate other parts of the cheese). After trimming off the mold, re-cover the cheese in fresh wrap.	Mold generally cannot penetrate deep into the product.
Cheese made with mold (such as Roquefort, blue, Gorgonzola, Stilton, Brie, Camembert)	Discard soft cheeses such as Brie and Camembert if they contain molds that are not a part of the manufacturing process. If surface mold is on hard cheeses such as Gorgonzola and Stilton, cut off mold at least 1 inch around and below the mold spot and handle as with hard cheese (above).	Molds that are not a part of the manufacturing process can be dangerous.
Soft cheese (such as cottage, cream cheese, Neufchatel, chevre, Bel Paese) **Crumbled, shredded, and sliced cheeses** (all types)	Discard	Foods with high moisture content can be contaminated below the surface. Shredded, sliced, or crumbled cheese can be contaminated by the cutting instrument. Moldy soft cheese can also have bacteria growing along with the mold.
Yogurt and sour cream	Discard	Foods with high moisture content can be contaminated below the surface. Moldy foods may also have bacteria growing along with the mold.
Jams and jellies	Discard	The mold could be producing a mycotoxin. Microbiologists recommend against scooping out the mold and using the remaining condiment.

(Table continues)

(Table continued)

Food	Handling	Reason
Fruits and vegetables, firm	Use. Cut off at least 1 inch around and below the mold spot (keep the knife out of the mold itself so it will not cross-contaminate other parts of the produce).	Small mold spots can be cut off fruits and vegetables with low moisture content (cabbage, bell peppers, carrots, etc.) It is difficult for mold to penetrate dense foods.
Fruits and vegetables, soft	Discard	Fruits and vegetables with high moisture content (cucumbers, peaches, tomatoes, etc.) can be contaminated below the surface.
Bread and baked goods	Discard	Porous foods can be contaminated below the surface.
Peanut butter, legumes, and nuts	Discard	Foods processed without preservatives are at high risk for mold.

Credit: United States Department of Agriculture's Meat and Poultry Hotline. "Molds on Food: Are They Dangerous?" April 2002

which mold can be scraped off. People who are allergic to mold should avoid all moldy foods.

International Consequences

Sometimes a case of food contamination can affect people in other countries because of the shipping of foods across countries. Reports of contaminated foods affecting Americans and Canadians have been traced back to *Salmonella* infection that was caused by Scandinavian alfalfa sprouts that were grown from imported seeds. In addition, *Shigella* infections in Europeans have been caused by prawns imported from Asia. Serious diseases can sometimes be spread in contaminated food; for example, people in the United States have contracted cholera by drinking fresh coconut milk that was imported from Asia.

Fortunately, the United States, Canada, and many other countries have strict rules regarding the inspection of imported foods, but occasionally problems still occur anyway.

See also BOTULIS; CHOLERA; *ESCHERICHIA COLI; LISTERIA; SALMONELLA*.

CREST syndrome The acronym *CREST* represents a combination of five medical problems: calcinosis (the calcification of tissues), Raynaud's phenomenon (extreme skin color changes that occur in response to temperature changes), esophageal dysfunction, sclerodactyly (the thickening of the skin on the hands and feet), and telangiectasia (the presence of abnormally dilated blood vessels, usually in the face, upper body, or hands). CREST syndrome is also a subset of SCLERODERMA. Some CREST syndrome patients may also have musculoskeletal, cardiac, renal, neurologic, or pulmonary symptoms and signs of disease.

The cause of CREST syndrome is unknown. The diagnosis is based on the presence of the five medical problems that CREST syndrome comprises. Treatments are based on the patient's symptoms; for example, if patients have gastroesophageal reflux disease (GERD) as a component of esophageal dysfunction, they receive recommendations given to other GERD patients, such as raising the heads of their bed and avoiding large fatty meals and other foods that worsen reflux. In addition to using medications, such as acid blockers, patients with Raynaud's phenomenon may be advised to wear gloves and hats, both outdoors and indoors. Vasodilator and immunosuppressive drugs may be beneficial.

See also GASTROESOPHAGEAL REFLUX DISEASE.

Wemple, Mary A., M.D. "CREST Syndrome." eMedicine. Available online. URL: http://www.emedicine.com/derm/topic88.htm. Downloaded January 15, 2003.

Crohn's disease One of two severe chronic idiopathic inflammatory bowel disorders. (The other form of INFLAMMATORY BOWEL DISEASE is ULCERATIVE COLITIS.) Crohn's disease can affect any area of the gastrointestinal tract but most typically affects the ileum (the lower part of the small intestine). Crohn's disease was named after Dr. Burrill B. Crohn, an American physician who first described the disease in 1932. Crohn's disease is uncommon, occurring in about 30 to 100 of every 100,000 people. It is not curable, but it is treatable. Crohn's disease is also known as *regional enteritis.*

Since its clinical features vary widely, some experts believe that Crohn's disease may be more than one disease that has thus far been lumped into one. In addition, according to the National Institute of Diabetes and Digestive and Kidney Diseases (NIDDK), as of 2009, more than 30 genes have been linked to Crohn's disease, and it is believed that more than 100 genes may be associated in some way with susceptibility for Crohn's disease. One gene that is associated with Crohn's disease plays an important part in the Paneth cells, which are specialized intestinal cells. Research has shown that patients with Crohn's disease have intestinal Paneth cells that have diminished or disorganized granules. Similar abnormalities were also noted in mice that were deficient in the autophagy gene (ATG3). Further research may help researchers acquire more genetic data as well as determine how to use this information to help patients with Crohn's disease.

Currently, Crohn's disease may be loosely subdivided by subtypes as

1. inflammatory
2. fistulous
3. obstructive

Symptoms and Diagnostic Path

Individuals with Crohn's disease may have some or all of the following symptoms:

- watery and persistent DIARRHEA (the most common symptom)
- ABDOMINAL PAIN
- weight loss
- deep sores in the anal region
- fever
- irritations of the skin and/or eye
- delayed growth and delayed puberty in children
- MALNUTRITION
- rectal bleeding that may lead to ANEMIA
- arthritis

The patient's medical history and symptoms are considered in diagnosing Crohn's disease. Physicians may also order a stool sample to rule out other diseases (such as parasitic or bacterial infections). Laboratory tests are usually ordered; many Crohn's disease patients have anemia caused by iron deficiencies or from deficiencies of vitamin B_{12}. Individuals with active Crohn's disease may have a high white blood cell count. An upper gastrointestinal and small bowel series may show abnormalities. Physicians usually order a colonoscopy.

During the colonoscopy, the terminal ileum (the most common part of gut involved in Crohn's disease) can usually be entered and examined for evidence of Crohn's disease, both to rule out other diseases, such as IRRITABLE BOWEL SYNDROME (IBS), and to check for colonic inflammation and ulcers and other indications of chronic Crohn's disease. A computed tomography (CT) scan of the abdomen is also a useful investigative tool, especially for the diagnosis of complications. Abdominal ultrasound and radionuclide scans are helpful in select cases.

Crohn's disease is a chronic disease of periodic flare-ups and remissions. Some experts believe that Crohn's disease is an autoimmune disorder, but it is unknown whether this is true. Others believe that in a genetically predisposed individual, the disease may be triggered by infections or a toxin in the fecal stream; however, specific triggers have not been identified to date.

Crohn's disease may cause VITAMIN DEFICIENCIES that must be treated. Other complications may include arthritis, the development of GALLSTONES, kidney stones, inflammation in the eyes or mouth and other diseases, according to the National Institute of Diabetes and Digestive and Kidney Diseases.

Treatment Options and Outlook

Patients who have Crohn's disease may be treated with dietary recommendations of types of foods to avoid (such as fiber and spicy foods), although dietary changes have not been shown to provide much improvement to most patients. The main nutritional problems are that patients may not eat enough, because the disease may induce ANOREXIA (loss of appetite), or patients may be afraid to eat for fear of inducing diarrhea or PAIN in themselves. They also may not drink sufficient fluids, and dehydration may result. In addition, their ability to absorb nutrients may be impaired.

Medications may be given to treat Crohn's disease, including anti-inflammatory drugs such as aminosalicylates like sulfasalazine (Azulfidine) and mesalamine (Asacol and Pentasa).

Corticosteroid drugs are also frequently used for patients who have acute flare-ups, including such medications as prednisone. Steroids may have some distressing long-term side effects, which may end when the patient stops taking the drug, such as weight gain, acne, or difficulty in sleeping. Steroids also cause long-term side effects, especially bone loss or osteoporosis. Both aminosalicylates and steroids may be given by mouth as well as in rectal suspensions by enema.

Antibiotics may also be used to treat the disease, especially metronidazole and ciprofloxacin (Cipro). Immune modulators such as 6-mercaptopurine (6-MP) and azathioprine (Imuran) and methotrexate are also used for long-term treatment. Infliximab (Remicade) is an antibody drug that is effective in treating various types of Crohn's disease, even when conventional therapy has not been effective. Humira and Cimzia are other such antibody drugs that are useful for treatment.

Some patients with Crohn's disease have shown improvement with the administration of growth hormone; a clinical study of 37 adults with Crohn's disease was described in 2000 in the *New England Journal of Medicine*. All of the subjects in the study had a moderate to severe case of Crohn's disease. The patients continued their regular medications during the study. They were all directed to increase their daily protein intake, because some studies have indicated that high-protein diets can improve symptoms.

The subjects who were given growth hormone had significant improvement in their symptoms. The researchers concluded, "Our preliminary study demonstrates that growth hormone may be beneficial in the treatment of patients with chronically active Crohn's disease." As of this writing, the use of this drug for Crohn's disease is still investigational. Growth hormone has also been used with some benefit by patients with Crohn's disease who have growth retardation or short status.

Risk Factors and Preventive Measures

Crohn's disease is most frequently found among people who are between the ages of 15 and 30 years, although people of other ages may also be diagnosed with the disease. There is a genetic risk for the disease, and an estimated 12 to 18 percent of individuals diagnosed with Crohn's disease have other family members who have also been diagnosed with the disease. Those of Jewish ancestry have an increased risk for Crohn's disease.

People who smoke have a higher risk of development of Crohn's disease. This is in contrast to ulcerative colitis, in which smoking is protective against the disease.

Stress does not cause Crohn's disease, but it can worsen the symptoms (as it frequently worsens the symptoms of many chronic diseases).

Most Crohn's disease patients may need surgery at some point in their lifetime to cope with the disease. There are many different types of surgeries that physicians may consider to relieve pain, obstructions, and complications (such as abscess, fistulae, etc.) of the disease.

Ghosh, Subrata, M.D., et al. "Natalizumab for Active Crohn's Disease." *New England Journal of Medicine* 348, no. 1 (January 2, 2003): 24–32.

Minocha, Anil, M. J. Davis, and R. A. Wright. "Small Bowel Endometriosis Masquerading as Regional Enteritis." *Digestive Diseases Sciences* 39, no. 5 (1994): 1,126–1,133.

Minocha, Anil, et al. "Crohn's Disease Complicating Male Genitourinary Tract Without Overlying Cutaneous Involvement." *American Journal of Gastroenterology* 91 (1996): 1,463–1,464,

National Institute of Diabetes & Digestive & Kidney Diseases (NIDDK). *Recent Advances & Emerging Opportunities.* Bethesda, Md.: National Institutes of Health. February 2009.

Slonim, Alfred E., M.D., et al. "A Preliminary Study of Growth Hormone Therapy for Crohn's Disease." *New England Journal of Medicine* 342, no. 22 (June 1, 2000): 1,633–1,637.

Cryptosporidium A protozoon that is found and spread through CONTAMINATED FOOD OR WATER and that causes an illness called cryptosporidiosis. Once inside the body, this microbe infects the lining of the intestinal tract. The most severe outbreak was identified in Milwaukee, Wisconsin, in 1993, when more than 400,000 people became infected with *Cryptosporidium* organisms that were transmitted in a contaminated public water supply.

In 2007, there were more than 10,000 confirmed cases of cryptosporidiosis, according to the Centers for Disease Control and Prevention (CDC), which was double the number of cases that were identified in 2006. Researchers said that more diagnoses may have been made because of the increased use of rapid diagnostic tests or because nitazoxanide, a medication for the infection, was approved for children ages 12 and older and adults in 2005, and hence, doctors had a means of treatment. In addition, more cases may have been diagnosed because there was an actual increase in the number of cases, for unknown reasons.

Testing for this protozoan has indicated that an increased proportion of the cases are caused by *C. hominis* rather than *C. parvum*. *C. hominis* is transmitted by human-to-human contact, while *C. parvum* is transmitted by animal-human contact.

Symptoms and Diagnostic Path

After between five and 28 days from the time of infection, symptoms begin. (Some infected people do not have any symptoms.) They may include the following:

- watery DIARRHEA
- abdominal cramps
- NAUSEA AND VOMITING
- headache
- loss of APPETITE

The disease is difficult to diagnose through symptoms only, since many diseases produce similar symptoms of diarrhea, abdominal cramps, and so forth. A stool sample can detect the disease, but only if the laboratory is specifically alerted to look for *Cryptosporidium* organisms. A routine stool test for ova and parasites may not screen for this protozoan.

Treatment Options and Outlook

Physicians may prescribe nitazoxanide, which was approved to treat the diarrhea of infected children in 2002 and was subsequently approved for children ages 12 and older and adults in 2005. In severe cases, hospitalization is required, and intravenous fluids are needed. Even if hospitalization is not required, it is important for patients to drink plenty of fluids to prevent dehydration.

The best treatment for immunodeficient patients (such as those with AIDS) is an improvement of their immune status, such as giving AIDS patients effective antiretroviral therapy that results in an improved immune system.

Risk Factors and Preventive Measures

People who have a weakened immune system are more prone to become ill, including those with acquired immunodeficiency syndrome (AIDS), cancer, or other diseases that suppress the immune system. Individuals who deal frequently with farm animals are at risk, unless they wash their hands frequently. Even children visiting a petting zoo may contract cryptosporidiosis.

Some simple actions can limit the risks of contracting *Cryptosporidium* infection, including the following:

- filtering drinking water (chlorine does not kill this protozoan)
- washing hands before and after preparing food
- washing hands after changing diapers or working with small children
- washing fruits and vegetables before eating them
- avoiding unpasteurized milk

See also DEHYDRATION; PARASITIC INFECTIONS.

Chen, Xian-Ming, M.D., et al. "Cryptosporidiosis." *New England Journal of Medicine* 346, no. 2 (May 30, 2002): 1,723–1,731.

Hall, Rebecca, and Jonathan Yoder, CDC Division of Parasitic Diseases, *Foodnet News* 2, no. 2 (Spring 2008): 3.

MacKenzie, William R., et al. "A Massive Outbreak in Milwaukee of *Cryptosporidium* Infection Transmitted through the Public Water Supply." New *England Journal of Medicine* 331, no. 3 (July 21, 1994): 161–167.

cultures Scientifically controlled growths of bacteria. Samples are taken from the patients' blood, sputum, feces, or urine, and then they are placed in a culture medium environment that is favorable to growth. The purpose of the culture is threefold: first, to determine whether bacteria are present; next, to identify the particular type of bacteria; finally, to ascertain the specific antibiotics most likely to destroy the bacteria that have been identified. Special culture media are required for certain pathogens.

A culture generally requires at least 24 to 48 hours before the laboratory results may be available to the physician. Some pathogens may take several days to weeks before definite results can be announced. Preliminary results are usually provided to physicians at 24 hours and an update given a day or two later.

If bacterial growth has occurred in the culture, the susceptibility to antibiotics is examined and that information guides the physician to use specifically targeted medications. Growth of some types of bacteria, such as tuberculosis, may take much longer than 48 hours to several days to weeks to occur in a culture. In addition, results of antibiotic sensitivities may also take longer than 48 hours.

See also ANTIBIOTICS.

cyclooxygenase-2 inhibitors A class of medications that are prescribed to treat pain and arthritis inflammation, particularly that caused by chronic illnesses, such as rheumatoid arthritis. These drugs are generally less likely to cause stomach ulcers than are NONSTEROIDAL ANTI-INFLAMMATORY DRUGS, another class of medications used to treat similar illnesses. However, cyclooxygenase-2 (COX-2) inhibitor medications are not risk-free, and some patients experience ulcers and even gastrointestinal bleeding and other side effects as a result of taking these medications.

COX-2 inhibitor medications can also prevent the recurrence of colon polyps in some cases. The role of COX-2 inhibitors in preventing cancer of the colon, stomach and esophagus is being investigated. Celecoxib (Celebrex) is an example of a COX-2 inhibitor. Most have been withdrawn from the market due to increased risks of cardiovascular events.

See also OBESITY; PAIN; ULCERS, PEPTIC.

cystic fibrosis Serious disease that results in a multisystem disease involving the sweat glands and the digestive, respiratory, and reproductive systems. Specifically, there are errors in the cystic fibrosis transmembrane conductance regulator (CFTR) gene. Cystic fibrosis (CF) causes the body to generate copious quantities of thick secretions that clog both the lungs and the pancreas and that also cause a high salt content of the perspiration. It is a disease that interferes with both breathing and digestion. Cystic fibrosis may also cause malabsorption in the intestines, generating an inability of the body to absorb needed nutrients.

Patients with cystic fibrosis have an increased risk of development of gastrointestinal cancers. They may also experience liver disease and even LIVER CANCER. The gene for CF has been identified by researchers as appearing on chromosome 7.

Symptoms and Diagnostic Path

The disease usually appears in infancy, and children with CF have frequent wheezing and coughing and are prone to development of frequent lung infections. However, some patients have few or no symptoms until they reach their teens or early adulthood. If symptoms and signs occur, the key symptoms are problems with respiration and delayed growth.

Other symptoms and signs include the following:

- chronic coughing
- large foul-smelling stools
- sweat that tastes salty as a result of the high level of salt in perspiration
- frequent infections with pneumonia or bronchitis

- failure to thrive in a child
- PANCREATITIS
- GALLSTONES
- infertility
- sinusitis

Treatment Options and Outlook

Cystic fibrosis is not curable, although researchers are seeking a cure through gene therapy. At the present, physicians seek to treat the symptoms and the complications of the disease, whether they are infections, failure to thrive, or other medical problems. Patients may also be advised to eat high-calorie and high-fat diets because of an underweight condition and their difficulty in attaining normal weight. Infections of the lung are treated with antibiotics. Patients should receive an influenza vaccine (flu shot) annually to limit their risk of development of flu. Pancreatic enzyme supplements are given in cases of PANCREATIC INSUFFICIENCY. Patients with cystic fibrosis are also advised to take vitamin and mineral supplements on a regular basis, as well as supplementation during periods of increased sweating, as needed.

Risk Factors and Preventive Measures

Cystic fibrosis occurs predominantly among whites, although some Hispanics also have this disease. An estimated one in 3,300 Caucasians is diagnosed with cystic fibrosis, compared to one in 9,500 Hispanics. The incidence of cystic fibrosis is much lower in other racial and ethnic groups, although blacks in the United States are more likely to have cystic fibrosis than are blacks in other countries. Females with cystic fibrosis usually experience a delayed puberty as well as later problems with fertility. Nearly all (about 95 percent) men with cystic fibrosis are sterile.

The classic symptoms of CF are usually evident to physicians. However, if the symptoms are mild, the patient may sometimes be misdiagnosed with asthma if further testing does not occur.

The sweat chloride test is generally used to diagnose cystic fibrosis. This test determines the presence of elevated chloride levels, an indicator of cystic fibrosis. In addition, results of sinus X-rays and computed tomography (CT) scans are usually abnormal in cystic fibrosis patients. Genetic testing to identify the gene mutations can confirm the presence of cystic fibrosis.

Individuals who inherit the gene for CF are at risk for developing cystic fibrosis. There are no known preventive measures.

Cytomegalovirus (CMV) An extremely common virus that rarely produces problems except among people who are immunocompromised, such as patients infected with the human immunodeficiency virus (HIV), those who have had organ transplantation, patients with advanced cancer, or others who are severely ill.

Symptoms and Diagnostic Path

Common symptoms are fever, fatigue, and swollen lymph glands. CMV may also cause ulcers in the esophagus, leading to painful swallowing. Involvement in the intestines can lead to perforation.

Treatment Options and Outlook

Foscarnet and ganciclovir are two key drugs that have been approved by the Food and Drug Administration (FDA) in the United States to treat patients with CMV. Some individuals who have acquired immunodeficiency syndrome (AIDS) require long-term maintenance therapy on medications for CMV.

Risk Factors and Preventive Measures

Individuals with HIV or with impaired immune systems are at risk. Preventive measures are unknown.

dangerous ingestion of non-food items The hazardous consumption of nonfood solid items, such as toys or other objects. Primarily a problem in INFANTS and toddlers, this issue can also occur in some older children and even adults. For example, in one case of an adult female with trichotillomania, an impulse control disorder in which individuals feel compelled to pull out their hair, the woman not only pulled her hair out but she also swallowed it for years. She nearly died of a giant hairball in her colon, which researchers removed.

Of course the ingestion of non-food items is much more common among toddlers and small children, and it can also be a very risky situation. In several cases described in a 2006 issue of the *Morbidity and Mortality Weekly Report*, several children underwent emergency surgery after they had ingested tiny toy magnets from an older sibling's toy set. In fact, after the magnets were shown to one of the children after he recovered, he responded by saying "Candy!"

In another case, a 20-month-old boy in excellent health complained of stomach pain and vomited several times. The boy's father noticed the child's feet were bluish, and then the child fainted. The child received cardiopulmonary resuscitation (CPR), but he died. An X-ray revealed that the child had swallowed a large object, 30 mm by 6 mm, which was actually nine magnets that had stacked together and compromised the blood supply to the bowel. The magnets had come from an older child's building set.

The Consumer Product Safety Commission has documented at least 19 injuries among children who have consumed magnets. According to the article, caregivers should keep small magnets away from children. If children do consume magnets, their pediatricians should be informed right away.

See also CHILDREN AND DIGESTIVE DISEASES.

Adamec, Christine. *Impulse Control Disorders*. New York: Chelsea House, 2008.
No author. "Gastrointestinal Injuries from Magnet Ingestion in Children—United States, 2003–2006." *Morbidity and Mortality Weekly Report* 55 (2006): 1,296–1,300.

dehydration A condition of an abnormally low level and imbalance of body fluids, usually also associated with electrolyte abnormalities, with the primary symptoms of thirst, dry skin and mucous membranes, and lightheadedness and nausea. The condition can at times be dangerous and even fatal.

The primary causes of dehydration are as follows:

- inadequate fluid intake
- vomiting
- diarrhea
- high fever
- use of diuretic medications or other drugs
- uncontrolled diabetes, causing high glucose levels (hyperglycemia) leading to increased urination
- BLEEDING

Symptoms and Diagnostic Path

Weakness, dizziness, and skin pallor may indicate dehydration. Poor skin turgor is another indicator. (When the skin on the arm is pulled gently, it does not rapidly return to normal and remains pinched longer than usual.) Thirst may be a symptom of dehydration, although severely dehydrated people may occasionally be too ill to feel thirsty, and thus lack of thirst does not necessarily mean that a person is sufficiently hydrated.

The diagnosis of dehydration is based on the medical history, symptoms and physician's observations of the signs of dehydration in the patient and can be verified by blood tests, including a test of electrolytes (sodium, potassium, chloride, and so forth) and blood urea nitrogen (BUN) levels. High BUN levels suggest that dehydration is present. Levels of electrolytes may be low or high. The elevated levels may occur because of a disproportionate loss of water content from the body.

Treatment Options and Outlook

Doctors treat patients with dehydration by seeking the cause of the problem, along with replacing their lost fluids and electrolytes to an adequate level. This is frequently done orally, and if needed, it is performed intravenously. The patient is also urged to consume liquids orally, whenever possible. Severely dehydrated individuals may require hospitalization for a day or longer. After discharge from the hospital, patients should continue to drink sufficient quantities of fluid for at least several days in order to prevent a recurrence of the dehydration. If the physician believes that individuals need antibiotics to fight off infection, they are prescribed. Similarly, treatment of the causes of dehydration, such as diabetes and diarrhea or bleeding also needs to be addressed.

Risk Factors and Preventive Measures

People with DIABETES MELLITUS are at a higher than average risk for experiencing dehydration; however, any person who consumes insufficient fluid or consumes too little fluid to meet increased fluid needs, as occurs with DIARRHEA, can become dehydrated.

Dehydration is a risk for those who are very physically active, and usually the summertime is when risk is greatest for active individuals (as well as inactive people) because of higher levels of perspiration due to the heat.

See also ELECTROLYTES; NAUSEA AND VOMITING.

demographic factors and digestive diseases

Digestive diseases are very common in the United States, and they are also a frequent cause of death; according to the National Commission on Digestive Diseases in 2008, about 236,000 people die each year with the primary cause of their death being a digestive disease. However, most people do not die from digestive diseases; instead, they may suffer unless they receive an appropriate diagnosis and treatment. Many digestive diseases are chronic medical problems and require continuing treatment. There are many differences among people who have digestive diseases, and the prevalence varies by gender, age, and race and ethnicity, as well as education, family income, and other factors, such as the combined factors of gender and ethnicity.

Gender and Digestive Diseases

In considering the serious diagnosis of cancer, men are more likely to be diagnosed with most forms of cancer than women, including COLORECTAL CANCER, ESOPHAGEAL CANCER, LIVER CANCER, SMALL INTESTINE CANCER, and STOMACH CANCER. In the United States, at least in part because they are significantly more likely to exhibit ALCOHOL ABUSE AND ALCOHOLISM, men also have a greater risk for the development of associated diseases, such as CIRRHOSIS of the liver, liver cancer, and stomach cancer, as well as for the diagnoses of alcoholic PANCREATITIS and HEMOCHROMATOSIS than women. (See Table 1 for a breakdown of the estimated male/female incidence of cancer as well as the total incidence in 2008. Note that the *incidence* refers to the number of new cases in the year.)

On the other hand, women in the United States face a higher risk than men for the development of ANAL CANCER, GALLBLADDER CANCER, GALLSTONES, IRRITABLE BOWEL SYNDROME, and PRIMARY BILIARY CIRRHOSIS. They have about the same risk for PANCREATIC CANCER as men. Women also have a greater risk for ever having been diagnosed with liver disease in 2007. (See Table 3.) Females are also slightly more likely to die of gastrointestinal infections than men, according to James Everhart, M.D., in *The Burden of Digestive Diseases in the United States*, published by the National Institute of Diabetes and Digestive and Kidney Diseases in 2008. (See Table 5.)

It should also be noted that men are generally believed to be significantly more likely to suffer from frequent indigestion than are women; how-

TABLE 1: GENDER INCIDENCE OF GASTROINTESTINAL CANCERS IN THE U.S. (2008 ESTIMATED)

Cancer Site	Overall Incidence	Male Incidence	Female Incidence
Anus and anorectum	5,070	2,020	3,050
Colon and rectum	148,810	77,250	71,560
Esophagus	16,470	12,970	3,500
Gallbladder and biliary ducts	9,520	4,500	5,020
Liver and intrahepatic ducts	21,370	15,190	6,180
Pancreas	37,680	18,770	18,910
Small intestine	6,110	3,200	2,910
Stomach	21,500	13,190	8,310
Other digestive organs	4,760	1,470	3,290
Totals	271,290	148,560	122,730

Source: Adapted from U.S. Department of Health and Human Services. "Opportunities and Challenges in Digestive Diseases Research: Recommendations of the National Commission on Digestive Diseases." Washington, D.C.: National Institutes of Health, March 2009. 82.

ever, an increased prevalence of indigestion in men has not been confirmed in some studies, and some research has found the reverse; for example, studies by Anil Minocha, M.D., and colleagues have found dyspeptic symptoms to be more common among women.

Age and Digestive Disease

The federal government maintains statistics on the numbers and percentages of individuals who are diagnosed with many different diseases and disorders. As a result, it is known that in many cases, individuals age 65 and older have an increased risk for most digestive diseases. (See the ELDERLY.) However, some disorders, such as APPENDICITIS are more likely to occur within the first few decades of life, rather than in old age. On the other hand, diverticulitis, ischemic colitis, and digestive cancers occur largely beyond the age of 50 years. (See EMERGENCY ISSUES IN DIGESTIVE DISORDERS.)

In considering the incidence of three common digestive problems, diabetes, ulcers, and liver disease, according to data provided by the National Center for Health Statistics in 2009, 7.6 percent of adults of all ages 18 and older had ever received a diagnosis of diabetes when they were interviewed in 2007, while 6.5 percent had ever received a diagnosis of ulcers. Adults were also asked if they had been diagnosed with a liver disease in the last 12 months in 2007, and 1.2 percent said that they had been.

Of these adults, the largest group of individuals who were ever diagnosed with diabetes were ages 65 to 74 years old (20.3 percent), while the largest percent ever diagnosed with ulcers were 75 years and older (12.6 percent) Among those who had been diagnosed with liver disease in the past year, the largest percent were within the age range of 65 to 74 years (1.9 percent), followed closely by those in the age grouping of 45 to 64 years (1.8 percent). See Table 2 for further data on the percentage of individuals diagnosed with diabetes, ulcers, or liver disease by gender and by age.

In considering numbers alone, in 2007, nearly 17.3 million adults reported having ever been diagnosed with diabetes, while 14.5 million said that they had ever been diagnosed with an ulcer. As for liver disease, about 2.6 million said that they had been diagnosed with a liver disease within the past year.

In an analysis of ambulatory visits (regular doctor visits) and also hospital discharges for all digestive diseases in 2004 (published in 2008), researcher James E. Everhart, M.D., found that elderly people had the highest rates for both ambulatory visits and for hospital discharges. For example, the rate per 100,000 for ambulatory visits for a digestive disease as the first-named diagnosis was 50,483 per 100,000 for those ages 65 and older. The next highest rate that was reported was for those individuals who were ages 45 to 64 years or 30,314 per 100,000. (See Table 3.)

TABLE 2: PERCENTAGES OF INDIVIDUALS AGES 18 AND OLDER WITH DIABETES, ULCERS, AND LIVER DISEASE IN 2007

Selected Characteristic	Diabetes	Ulcers	Liver Disease
Total	7.8	6.5	1.2
Gender			
Male	8.0	6.3	1.1
Female	7.3	6.7	1.6
Age			
18-44 years	2.2	5.2	0.7
45-64 years	10.7	7.4	1.8
65-74 years	20.3	11.0	1.9
75 years and older	17.6	12.6	0.9
Race and ethnicity			
1 race	7.6	6.4	1.1
White	6.8	6.8	1.2
Black or African American	12.3	5.2	0.9
American Indian or Alaska Native	17.2	6.5	Not available
Asian	8.9	3.0	0.9
Native Hawaiian or Other Pacific Islander	20.6	Not available	Not available
2 or more races	10.3	8.0	3.1
Black or African American and white	14.0	Not available	Not available
American Indian or Alaska Native and white	10.5	9.8	5.2
Hispanic or Latino origin and race			
Hispanic or Latino	11.1	4.9	1.6
Mexican or Mexican American	12.5	5.2	1.7
Not Hispanic or Latino	7.3	6.7	1.1
White, single race	6.4	7.2	1.1
Black or African American, single race	12.5	5.1	0.9
Education			
Less than a high school diploma	13.2	9.2	2.1
High school diploma or GED	9.2	6.7	1.3
Some college	7.8	8.0	1.6
Bachelor's degree or higher	6.4	5.3	0.7
Family income			
Less than $35,000	10.4	8.9	1.0
$35,000 or more	6.5	5.7	0.9
$35,000–$49,999	8.2	7.1	1.4
$50,000–$74,999	7.2	5.8	1.1
$75,000–$99,999	5.9	4.6	0.8
$100,000 or more	4.5	5.2	0.6

(Table continues)

(Table continued)

Selected Characteristic	Diabetes	Ulcers	Liver Disease
Poverty status			
Poor	12.2	9.3	2.5
Near Poor	10.6	8.7	1.8
Not poor	6.6	6.1	0.9
Marital status			
Married	7.6	6.0	1.0
Widowed	9.9	7.0	Not available
Divorced or separated	9.2	9.7	2.1
Never married	8.1	5.3	1.3
Living with a partner	6.8	7.6	1.8
Region			
Northeast	6.3	4.9	0.9
Midwest	7.7	7.5	1.2
South	8.3	6.5	1.0
West	7.6	6.4	1.6
Gender and ethnicity			
Hispanic or Latino, male	11.2	4.6	1.1
Hispanic or Latina, female	10.9	5.3	1.9
Not Hispanic or Latino			
White, single race, male	6.8	7.0	1.1
White, single race, female	6.1	7.4	1.2
Black or African American, single race, male	12.2	5.5	1.2
Black or African American, single race, female	12.7	4.9	0.7

Source: Adapted from Pleis, J. R., and J. W. Lucas. "Summary Health Statistics for U.S. Adults: National Health Interview Survey, 2007." Hyattsville, Md.: National Center for Health Statistics, 2009, 31–32.

Note that the actual numbers were lower for older people; for example, they had about 18,342,000 million ambulatory visits compared to 21,430,000 for those ages 45 to 64; however, the rate takes into account the number of people who went to the doctor compared to the entire population (in this case, per 100,000 people), and thus, this measure provides a better perspective of the problem.

In considering people who died from a digestive disease that was the underlying cause of death in 2004, age was clearly a factor, both in sheer numbers as well as in rates; for example, 156,706 people ages 65 and older died of a digestive disease,

compared to the next higher number of 66,806 for those ages 45 to 64 years. The rates of death for those ages 65 and older was 431.3 per 100,000 people, compared to the next highest rate of 94.5 per 100,000 for those ages 45 to 64 years. The lowest death rate (2.2 per 100,000) was among those under age 15 years. See Table 4 for further details.

Older people are also significantly more likely to die from gastrointestinal infections than younger people; according to researcher Everhart, 3,962 people ages 65 and older died of a gastrointestinal infection in 2004, and the rate for this group was 10.0 per 100,000 people. The next closest rate was only 353 deaths for those ages 45 to 65, with

TABLE 3: ALL DIGESTIVE DISEASES, NUMBER AND AGE-ADJUSTED RATES OF AMBULATORY CARE
VISITS AND HOSPITAL DISCHARGES WITH FIRST-LISTED DIAGNOSES BY AGE, RACE,
AND GENDER IN THE UNITED STATES, 2004

Demographic Characteristics		Ambulatory Care Visits		Hospital Discharges	
		Number in thousands	Rate per 100,000	Number in thousands	Rate per thousands
Age (years)	Under 15	10,951	18,010	331	544
	15–44	21,348	16,967	1,112	884
	45–64	21,430	30,314	1,362	1,926
	65+	18,342	50,483	1,779	4,897
Race	White	59,506	24,318	3,526	1,412
	Black	8,733	24,076	531	1,655
Gender	Female	39,531	25,827	2,545	1,592
	Male	32,540	23,017	2,023	1,483
Total		72,071	24,543	4,591	1,563

Adapted from Everhart, James E., M.D. *The Burden of Digestive Diseases in the United States.* Washington, D.C.: National Institute of Diabetes and Digestive and Kidney Diseases, 2008, 4.

a rate of 0.5 per 100,000. See Table 5 for further information.

Race and Ethnicity

In considering racial and ethnic differences and the prevalence of diabetes, ulcers, and liver disease,

TABLE 4: ALL DIGESTIVE DISEASES: NUMBER AND AGE-ADJUSTED RATES OF DEATHS FROM DIGESTIVE DISEASES AS AN UNDERLYING CAUSE, BY AGE, RACE, AND GENDER IN THE UNITED STATES, 2004

Demographic Characteristic		Number of Deaths	Rate per 100,000
Age (years)	Under 15	1,612	2.2
	15-44	11,036	8.8
	45-64	66,806	94.5
	65+	156,706	431.3
Race	White	200,834	77.0
	Black	27,812	99.5
Gender	Female	111,264	63.6
	Male	124,900	97.1
Total		236,164	80.4

Adapted from Everhart, James E., M.D. *The Burden of Digestive Diseases in the United States.* Washington, D.C.: National Institute of Diabetes and Digestive and Kidney Diseases, 2008, 5.

as seen in Table 2, the National Center for Health Statistics data indicates that Native Hawaiians and Pacific Islanders had the highest percentage of diabetes (20.6 percent) in 2007, followed by American Indians or Alaska Natives (17.2 percent).

Individuals of two or more races had the highest rate of reported ulcers, especially those who were American Indian or Alaska Natives combined with white racial ancestry (9.8 percent). With regard to race and the prevalence of liver disease, the highest rates were again among those with two or more races, or 5.2 percent among those of both American Indian or Alaska Native and white racial background.

In considering all visits to physicians for digestive diseases in 2004, as shown in Table 3, whites had many more ambulatory visits than blacks (59,506,000 for whites, compared to 8,733,000 for blacks), but the actual *rates* of visits were very close, or 24,318 visits per 100,000 for whites and 24,076 for blacks. In considering hospital discharges for a digestive disease, the rate was higher for blacks than for whites, or 1,655 per 100,000 for blacks discharged from hospitals compared to 1,412 per 100,000 for whites who were discharged.

As can be seen from Table 4, which depicts the numbers and rates of individuals in the United

TABLE 5: DEATHS FROM GASTROINTESTINAL INFECTIONS: NUMBER AND AGE ADJUSTED RATES OF DEATH BY AGE, RACE, AND GENDER IN THE UNITED STATES, 2004

Demographic Characteristics		Number of Deaths	Rate per 100,000
Age (years)	Under 15	32	0.1
	15-44	49	0.0
	45-64	353	0.5
	65+	3,962	10.9
Race	White	4,104	1.5
	Black	241	1.0
Gender	Female	2,746	1.5
	Male	1,650	1.4
Total		4,396	1.5

Adapted from Everhart, James E., M.D. *The Burden of Digestive Diseases in the United States*. Washington, D.C.: National Institute of Diabetes and Digestive and Kidney Diseases, 2008, 11.

States who died from a digestive disease that was the underlying cause of their death, again, the sheer numbers of deaths for whites were higher than for blacks, but in considering death rates alone, blacks had a higher rate of deaths than whites, or 99.5 per 100,000 for blacks, compared to 77.0 per 100,000 deaths per whites.

Table 5 shows the numbers of deaths and also death rates of individuals who died from gastrointestinal infections, and as can be seen from the table, whites have a significantly higher percentage of death from such an infection, compared to blacks, or 1.5 per 100,000 for whites who died of gastrointestinal infections compared to the rate of 1.0 per 100,000 for blacks. The reasons for this disparity are unknown.

Education

In general, more highly educated people have a lower risk for many diseases, but this risk is never zero for any socioeconomic status, as can be seen in Table 2. For example, among those with diabetes, in considering individuals with less than a high school education, 13.2 percent had ever been diagnosed with diabetes, as seen in Table 1. In comparison, those who were college graduates had a rate of 6.4 percent. With regard to the highest and next highest rates of those who had been diagnosed with liver disease in the past year, the highest rate, or 2.1 percent, was seen among those with less than a high school education. The rates decreased in a linear fashion to the low of less than 1 percent (0.7 percent) for college graduates.

Among those with ulcers, the pattern was not so linear; for example, among those with less than a high school education, the rate was 9.2 percent, dropping to 6.7 percent for high school graduates. However, the rate for the next higher educational level, individuals with some college rose to 8.0 percent. The rate dropped again for those with a bachelor's degree or greater, to 5.3 percent of this group. The reasons for the higher rate among those with some college are not known.

Socioeconomic Status

Socioeconomic status and income are often (but not always) related to a lower risk for digestive diseases and individuals with higher incomes often have a lower risk for issues that lead to health problems, such as OBESITY. Interestingly, however, some researchers have reported that individuals with the highest socioeconomic status are also the most likely to become ill with traveler's DIARRHEA when they travel to high risk countries. (Countries where there are many bacterial diseases that may lead to diarrhea.)

According to Joaquim Gascón in his article on traveler's diarrhea for *Digestion*, "Belonging to a higher socio-economic status seems to carry a significant risk to develop TD [traveler's diarrhea] when people visit a high-risk area."

He notes that travelers who stay at some luxury hotels or who take cruises down the Nile River are at risk for traveler's diarrhea, likely because of the storage conditions of the food over a prolonged period. Adventurous trips to less developed countries may carry a greater risk for traveler's diarrhea among higher income individuals, at least partly because individuals in the United States of lower or middle income socioeconomic status cannot afford the fees involved with expensive trips abroad. It may also be possible that this higher risk occurs because individuals from a higher socioeconomic status may be less likely to have experienced a past exposure to pathogens causing diarrhea than are less wealthy Americans.

Marital Status

In general, married people are healthier than individuals who are widowed, divorced, never married, or living with a partner, although this does not always hold true. For example, in considering those with diabetes, Table 2 shows that the lowest percentage of diabetes occurred among those living with a partner (6.8 percent), followed by those who were married (7.6 percent.) The highest incidence was among those who were widowed (9.9 percent). However, since most people who are widowed are also elderly, this higher rate may be related to age more than marital status.

In considering those with liver disease in the past year, the highest rate was seen among divorced or separated individuals (2.1 percent), and the lowest rate occurred among married people (1.0 percent).

Gender and Ethnicity

Researchers have also looked at the prevalence of diabetes, ulcers, and liver disease in terms of a combination of both gender and ethnicity, as shown in Table 2. For example, the highest rate of diabetes was found among African-American/black females or 12.7 percent, followed by African-American/black males or 12.2 percent. These rates are nearly double those for white males and females.

In considering those with ulcer disease, white single females had the highest percentage, or 7.4 percent, followed by white males at 7.0 percent. The ulcer rate for black males was 5.5 percent followed by 5.3 percent for Hispanic/Latino females.

In considering liver disease, African-American females had the lowest rates or 0.7 percent. The highest rates of liver disease were reportedly among Hispanic or Latin females, or 1.9 percent.

Region of the Country

Some geographic differences have been found with regard to the prevalence of diabetes, ulcer disease, and liver disease. As can be seen from Table 2, the highest prevalence for diabetes was found among those in the South, or 8.3 percent, with the lowest rates seen in the Northeast, or 6.3 percent. With regard to the prevalence of ulcer disease, the highest rates were found among those in the Midwest, or 7.5 percent, with the lowest rates in

the Northeast, or 4.9 percent. Last, with regard to liver disease, the highest rates were found among those in the West, or 1.6 percent and the lowest rates (again) were found in the Northeast, or 0.9 percent. The reasons for these disparities are unknown.

Everhart, James E., M.D. *The Burden of Digestive Diseases in the United States.* Washington, D.C.: National Institute of Diabetes and Digestive and Kidney Diseases, 2008.

Gascón, Joaquim. "Epidemiology, Etiology and Pathophysiology of Traveler's Diarrhea." *Digestion* 73, Supplement 1 (2006): 102–108.

Minocha A., T. L. Abell, W. D. Johnson, and W. C. Wigington. "Racial Differences in Epidemiology of Irritable Bowel Syndrome Alone, Uninvestigated Dyspepsia Alone and the 'Overlap Syndrome' among African Americans as Compared to Caucasians: A Population Based Study." *Digestive Diseases and Sciences* 51 (2006): 218–226.

Minocha, A., W. D. Johnson, and W. C . Wigington. "Prevalence of Abdominal and Pelvic Surgeries in Patients With Irritable Bowel Syndrome: Comparison Between Caucasian and African Americans." *American Journal of Medical Sciences* 335, no. 2 (February 2008): 82–88

National Institute of Diabetes & Digestive & Kidney Diseases (NIDDK). *Recent Advances & Emerging Opportunities.* Bethesda, Md.: National Institutes of Health, February 2009.

Pleis, J. R., and J. W. Lucas. *Summary Health Statistics for U.S. Adults: National Health Interview Survey, 2007.* Hyattsville, Md.: National Center for Health Statistics, 2009.

Wigington, W. C., W. D. Johnson, and A. Minocha. "Epidemiology of Irritable Bowel Syndrome among African Americans as compared to Caucasians: A Population Based Study." *Clinical Gastroenterology and Hepatology* 3 (2005): 647–653.

diabetes mellitus   Diabetes is a serious and common medical problem that is primarily characterized by the failure of the pancreas to create sufficient (or any) insulin, as with type 1 diabetes *or* by the inability of the body to respond to the insulin that is produced by the pancreas (as with type 2 diabetes). These problems with insulin regulation lead to a high glucose level (hyperglycemia) and to multiple digestive problems as well as other serious medical problems. Sometimes people with diabetes also develop hypoglycemia (excessively low blood sugar levels) due to a decreased intake of nutrition while taking antidiabetic medication or for other reasons (such as inadequate nutrition, other illnesses, and an array of other possible causes). When a diabetic patient has hypoglycemia, he or she urgently requires the administration of some form of glucose. Note that diabetes mellitus should *not* be confused with diabetes insipidus, which is another disorder entirely unrelated to type 1 or type 2 diabetes.

About 95 percent of patients with diabetes mellitus have type 2 diabetes, and 5 percent have type 1 diabetes. Type 1 diabetes typically presents in childhood or adolescence, and continued survival is dependent on the administration of insulin. Before the discovery of insulin by the Canadians Frederick Grant Banting and Charles Best in 1921, everyone with type 1 diabetes eventually died at a younger age than the normal life span, usually in childhood, adolescence, or early adulthood. (In addition, at that time, few people were obese, and hence, few people had type 2 diabetes. However, type 2 diabetes was also unknown at that time.)

Now most people with type 1 diabetes can live for many years, assuming that they are diligent about maintaining normal glucose (glycemic) levels. Many individuals with type 2 diabetes live into their elderly years; in fact, type 2 diabetes may not be diagnosed until an individual is age 65 years or older. However, according to the Centers for Disease Control and Prevention (CDC), the death risk from diabetes is about twice that of people without diabetes of the same age. In 2006, diabetes was the seventh-leading cause of death in the U.S. The CDC reported in 2009 that if current trends continued, one in three Americans will develop diabetes at some point in their lives, and individuals with diabetes will lose 10 to 15 years of their lives.

Complications are common in patients with both forms of diabetes; for example, diabetes is the key cause of kidney failure in the United States as well as of blindness and limb amputations that were not caused by accidental injuries. It is also linked to heart disease, stroke, and hypertension as well as nerve damage (diabetic neuropathy). Digestive diseases are common among individuals with both type 1 and type 2 diabetes, although the causes of these diseases are often unknown or in dispute.

According to the CDC, 23.6 million people in the United States had diabetes in 2007 (7.8 percent of the total population), and 5.7 million people of this total had not yet been diagnosed with diabetes. Some racial groups in the United States have a significantly greater risk for diabetes than others; for example, American Indian, Alaska Native, African-American and Hispanic adults have about twice the risk of developing type 2 diabetes compared to whites. Type 2 diabetes is also associated with a family history of the disease.

Obese children are at risk for developing type 2 diabetes, although most people with this disorder are adults ages 40 and older. Elderly individuals also have an increased risk for developing diabetes. Most patients with type 2 diabetes are diagnosed during adulthood, and the broad majority of them have a problem with obesity. If such patients lose weight, their diabetes usually improves or goes away altogether.

Some adults have a condition known as *prediabetes*, which refers to blood glucose levels that are high but not high enough for a diagnosis of diabetes. However, people with prediabetes are at risk for developing type 2 diabetes, as well as heart disease and stroke. About 57 million adults in the United States had prediabetes in 2007.

Individuals with prediabetes are at risk for other disorders; for example, in a study by Gulcan, et al., published in the *American Journal of Medical Sciences* in 2009 on 92 individuals with irritable bowel syndrome (IBS) who were contrasted to healthy control subjects, the researchers found a significantly higher rate of prediabetes in the IBS group. Thus, prediabetes may apparently cause or contribute to the development of IBS.

Some adult females have a disorder known as *gestational diabetes*, which is a form of diabetes that occurs only during pregnancy. It is similar to type 2 diabetes; however, often this disorder is treated with insulin, depending on its severity. Women with gestational diabetes must be closely monitored during pregnancy, both for the health of the fetus as well as the woman's own health. Once the child is delivered, the blood glucose levels usually stabilize on their own within days, although up to 10 percent of women with gestational diabetes are found to have had type 2 diabetes. (They had type

2 diabetes prior to their pregnancy, but it had not been diagnosed.) Women with gestational diabetes also have an elevated risk for the development of type 2 diabetes in later life, and the CDC reports that 40 to 60 percent of women with gestational diabetes will develop diabetes within five to 10 years.

According to Christian A. Koch and colleagues in their 2008 article in the *European Journal of Gastroenterology and Hepatology*, many patients with diabetes suffer from upper and lower gastrointestinal problems and some issues, such as GASTROPARESIS, can worsen glycemic control by altering the actions of some oral diabetes medications. In another article on pain processing in subjects with diabetes mellitus, researchers Jens Brondum Frokjaer and colleagues studied 14 patients with type 1 diabetes and 15 controls without diabetes, reporting on their findings in *Diabetes Care* in 2009. The researchers concluded that diabetes induces changes in the peripheral visceral nerves and the central nervous system, thus increasing the level of gut PAIN.

Some experts believe that up to 75 percent of all patients with diabetes have digestive problems. According to two diabetes specialists, James D. Wolosin, M.D., and Steven Edelman, in their 2000 article in *Clinical Diabetes*:

> The entire GI [gastrointestinal] tract can be affected by diabetes from the oral cavity and esophagus to the large bowel and anorectal region. Thus, the symptom complex that may be experienced can vary widely. Common complaints may include dysphagia, early satiety [fullness after eating], reflux [acid reflux], constipation, abdominal pain, nausea, vomiting, and diarrhea. Many patients go undiagnosed and undertreated because the GI tract has not been traditionally associated with diabetes and its complications.

People with diabetes may sometimes experience acutely severe digestive problems that may become life-threatening. Drs. Sikander Mesiya and Anil Minocha explain further in their 1998–99 *Southern Medical Journal* monograph: "Acute problems include stress gastritis during ketoacidiosis, acute pancreatitis and acute cholecystitis [inflammation and infection of the gallbladder]. Most problems

are, however, chronic, and may manifest with remissions and relapses."

In a study of thousands of subjects, including 423 diabetics (nearly all with type 2 diabetes) reported by Peter Bytzer, M.D., and colleagues in *Archives of Internal Medicine* in 2001, the patients with diabetes had a greater prevalence of both upper and lower gastrointestinal symptoms than did the nondiabetics. For example, 26 percent of the diabetic patients had bowel symptoms, compared to about 19 percent of the nondiabetic subjects. In addition, 15.6 percent of the diabetics had DIARRHEA (more than three bowel movements per day, along with urgency and loose or watery stools) compared to 10 percent of the nondiabetics. The diabetic subjects also reported more problems with dysphagia (difficulty swallowing) (5.4 percent) than the nondiabetic subjects (1.7 percent).

The most common digestive problems that appear to be associated with diabetes are gastroparesis (slow stomach emptying) and GASTROESPHAGEAL REFLUX DISEASE (GERD). Other common problems are CONSTIPATION and fecal incontinence. In addition, diarrhea may sometimes become a chronic problem and one that is also difficult to manage in diabetics.

Constipation

Constipation is another common problem among individuals with diabetes, although often the cause is difficult to ascertain. It may be linked to autonomic neuropathy, or it could be tied to the use of some medications, such as calcium channel blockers. In general, poor glycemic control is a major factor in constipation, according to Malagelada.

Treatment of constipation in patients with diabetes is generally the same as the treatment for those without diabetes (such as stool softeners, the recommendation for an increased ingestion of fiber, and an increased fluid intake, etc.); however, the addition of acarbose (Precose) as well may also improve constipation, according to Malagelada. In some cases, fiber intake may be restricted.

Diarrhea

As many as 20 percent of all diabetics may have chronic problems with diarrhea. Diarrhea may be caused by an abnormal motility or by secretions of the intestines, as well as by diabetic neuropathy or a bacterial overgrowth present in the small intestine. However, Malagelada says that the cause of diarrhea in diabetics is generally not well understood and, as a result, probably has many different triggers. Visceral neuropathy may be one cause, and there may also be dysfunctions in neuroendocrine peptides, which are some natural chemicals that affect the digestion of food. Sometimes medications such as metformin are implicated in chronic diarrhea.

Antidiarrheal medications such as loperamide and codeine are used to treat diabetic diarrhea. Octreotide (Sandostatin) is also used.

Fecal Incontinence

Elderly individuals with diabetes are especially at risk for fecal incontinence (accidental loss of control of the bowels), and according to Malagelada, as many as 20 percent of diabetics suffer from fecal incontinence. In general, this problem is age-related, and is also linked to diabetic neuropathy as well as to the use of multiple medications. FECAL IMPACTION (excessive levels of stools that have not passed) may also cause fecal incontinence. Improved glycemic control can improve fecal incontinence as can the use of biofeedback therapy.

Gastroesophageal Reflux Disease

Some studies have found that subjects with diabetes have a greater risk for GERD than other patients; for example, in their study reported in 2004 in the *Journal of Gastroenterology and Hepatology*, Nishida and colleague found that among 241 patients with diabetes, 25.3 percent had GERD compared to a control group of subjects with hepatitis C, who had a GERD rate of 9.5 percent.

Individuals with GERD are advised to avoid eating before bed or lying down after eating (such as taking a nap after lunch). Medications for HEARTBURN, both over-the-counter (OTC) and prescribed drugs, are also often helpful.

Gastroparesis in Individuals with Diabetes

Gastroparesis can make it very hard for individuals with diabetes to maintain normal glucose levels. Yet it is very important to manage gastroparesis

because this disorder can seriously impede the management of glucose levels in diabetics. If the food stays too long in the stomach, it can harden into masses that are known as *bezoars*, which lead to nausea and vomiting and even stomach obstruction. A further problem is that chronic gastroparesis often leads to the development of gastroesophageal reflux disease. In some cases, the delayed emptying of the stomach is the direct result of nerve damage that was caused by diabetes, a condition that is known as *gastroparesis diabeticorum*.

Gastroparesis in diabetics is associated with diabetic autonomic neuropathy, or damage to the nerves that control automatic functions such as digestion. Common symptoms of gastroparesis are bloating and also nausea and vomiting as well as early satiety (fullness). Other signs may include a lack of appetite, fluctuating blood glucose levels and weight loss, as well as spasms of the wall of the stomach.

Gastroparesis is treated with dietary recommendations, such as eating five or six small meals per day rather than three large meals. A liquid diet may be recommended until the gastroparesis improves. A low-fiber diet may also be recommended as well as a diet of low-fat foods. Some medications such as prochlorperazine and Zofran® can help with the symptoms of nausea and vomiting, and prokinetic medications (metaclopramide, erythromycin, domperidone) can also stimulate muscle stomach contractions, making digestion easier. Domperidone is not approved by the FDA in the United States. Cisapride, an effective promotility agent, was withdrawn from the market in the United States.

According to the dietitians Carol Lee Parrish and Joyce Green Pastors in their article on the nutritional management of gastroparesis in individuals with diabetes in *Diabetes Spectrum* in 2007, diabetics with gastroparesis should avoid chewing gum because it increases the swallowing of air and can exacerbate gastroparesis. They also recommend that specific types of foods, such as peppermint, chocolate, fat, and caffeine all should be avoided by patients with gastroparesis because these foods work to lower the esophageal sphincter pressure, a goal that is undesirable with gastroparesis.

The two dietitians also note that the chronic nausea and vomiting that may be associated with gastroparesis can lead further to dehydration, malnutrition, inadequate medication delivery, hyperglycemia, and electrolyte issues, and it can also severely impede the individual's quality of life. According to the authors, "Clinically, patients with gastroparesis are at risk for fluid, electrolyte, and nutrient deficits and in patients with diabetes, erratic glycemic control. Treatment is targeted at correcting fluid, electrolyte, and nutritional deficiencies, reducing symptoms, and correcting the precipitating cause of [exacerbations of] gastroparesis, if possible."

If these measures fail to resolve the gastroparesis, the patient may be treated with a feeding tube into the small bowel (jejunum) or with even parenteral nutrition (nutrients introduced directly into the bloodstream) although parenteral nutrition is avoided unless it becomes an absolute necessity. Sometimes a gastric neurostimulator is surgically implanted. Injections of botulinum toxin (Botox®) to the pylorus muscle of the stomach may also be tried to temporarily paralyze the stomach muscle so that the food can move through the gastrointestinal system more easily, although this is not a common use of Botox.

In a very small study of eight patients with diabetic gastroparesis treated with Botox injections into the pylorus, reported by Brian E. Lacy, M.D., and colleagues in 2004 in *Diabetes Care*, Botox was injected endoscopically, and the subjects improved significantly, with improvements in nausea and vomiting as well as abdominal pain. However, some of the patients subsequently required higher dosages of their daily insulin. Controlled studies have not confirmed this benefit. Further studies with more subjects are needed to determine whether Botox is a viable option for the treatment of diabetic gastroparesis.

According to Juan-R. Malagelada, M.D., in his chapter on gastrointestinal syndromes caused by diabetes in *Contemporary Diabetes: Diabetic Neuropathy: Clinical Management*, "Diabetic gastroparesis is an electromechanical motility disorder that in many instances involves not only the stomach, but also the upper small bowel."

An overproduction of prostaglandins in the smooth muscles of the stomach may be the chief culprit of gastroparesis, while acute hyperglycemia

also plays a role. Other diseases such as chronic PANCREATITIS and CELIAC DISEASE may also be implicated in gastroparesis. Malagelada says that 30 to 50 percent of diabetes patients experience a delayed emptying of gastric solids, while another 20 percent may have speeded up gastric emptying.

Life-Threatening Digestive Disorders in Diabetes

Some digestive disorders that may occur to individuals with diabetes can be life-threatening, such as acute pancreatitis or CHOLECYSTITIS (gallbladder inflammation and infection). According to a study that was reported by Rebecca A. Noel and colleagues in a 2009 issue of *Diabetes Care*, subjects with type 2 diabetes had a more than double (2.83) increased risk for pancreatitis and a nearly double or 1.91 increased risk for serious biliary (gallbladder) diseases such as cholelithiasis, cholecystectomy (gallbladder removal), or acute cholecystitis when compared to those without diabetes. The researchers had a very large database of subjects: They studied data on 337,067 subjects with type 2 diabetes when compared to another 337,067 subjects without diabetes.

The researchers found a pancreatitis incidence of 422 cases per 100,000 patient-years in those with diabetes compared to 149 cases per 100,000 patient-years in the nondiabetic subjects. They also noted that there was a high rate of pancreatitis among younger subjects with type 2 diabetes, and the researchers suggested that further research was needed to study this issue in greater depth.

Medications Used to Treat Diabetes

Diabetes is managed primarily by medication and by nutritional adaptations. Individuals with type 1 diabetes are treated with a variety of short-, medium-, and long-acting forms of insulin. Individuals with type 2 diabetes are usually treated with oral medications, such as drugs in the sulfonylurea class, including glimepride (Amaryl), chlorpropamide (Diabinese), glyburide (Micronase), and glipizide (Glucotrol, Glucotrol XL). They may also be treated with medications in the category of meglitinides, including such drugs as repaglinide (Prandin) or nateglinide (Starlix). Both sulfonylurea and meglitinide medications stimulate the pancreas to secrete higher levels of insulin.

They are also called hypoglycemic agents because they lower glucose levels.

Biguanides are medications that decrease the glucose production of the liver. Medications in this class are various formulations of metformin (Glucophage, Glucophage XR, and Romet).

Thiazolidinediones (TZDs) are sometimes administered to help the body use glucose more efficiently. Medications in this particular class of drugs include rosiglitazone (Avandia) and pioglitazone (Actos). Sometimes alpha glucosidase inhibitors are prescribed to slow the digestion of carbohydrates, including such medications as acarbose (Precose) or miglitol (Glyset).

A newer drug is the DPP-4 inhibitor, which affects both the alpha and beta cells in the pancreas that regulate glucose levels. This medication is called sitagliptin (Januvia). Sometimes individuals with type 2 diabetes (as well as some patients with type 1 diabetes) use noninsulin injectable drugs to control their diabetes, including exanatide (Byetta) or pramlintide (Symlin, Symlinpen). Some patients receive combinations of injectable insulin plus oral medications.

Recommendations for Individuals with Diabetes

Individuals with all forms of diabetes (type 1, type 2, or gestational diabetes) should perform blood tests on a frequency recommended by their physicians. They should then act on the information that the blood test reveals; for example, if the blood glucose levels are high, then it is important to limit carbohydrates for the rest of the day. If blood glucose levels are low (hypoglycemia), the individual should ingest carbohydrates to bring the levels up to normal.

All individuals with diabetes who smoke should stop SMOKING because smoking accelerates problems with both diabetes and digestive disorders, in addition to worsening diabetes-associated complications, such as serious heart disease, eye disease, and other medical problems. Physicians also urge people diagnosed with diabetes to obtain regular exercise to improve their health.

Individuals with diabetes should also limit their alcohol consumption because alcohol provides only empty calories and can lead to alcohol abuse or alcoholism in some individuals. Alcoholics are notoriously poor at monitoring their own chronic medical conditions, including diabetes.

See also ALCOHOL ABUSE AND ALCOHOLISM.

Brøndum Førkjaer, Jens, et al. "Central Processing of Gut Pain in Diabetes Patients with Gastrointestinal Symptoms." *Diabetes Care* 32, no. 7 (July 2009): 1,274–1,277.

Bytzer, Peter, M.D., et al. "Prevalence of Gastrointestinal Symptoms Associated with Diabetes Mellitus: A Population-Based Survey of 15,000 Adults." *Archives of Internal Medicine* 161 (2001): 989–1,996.

Fennell, Diane. "Gastroparesis." Diabetes Self-Management. Available online. URL: http://www.diabetesselfmanagement.com/articles/diabetes-definitions/gastroparesis/print. Accessed July 1, 2009.

Gulcan, E., et al. "Increased Frequency of Prediabetes in Patients with Irritable Bowel Syndrome." *American Journal of Medical Science* 338, no. 2 (August 2009): 116–119.

Koch, Christian A., and Gabriel I. Uwaifo. "Are Gastrointestinal Symptoms Related to Diabetes Mellitus and Glycemic Control?" *European Journal of Gastroenterology* 20, no. 9 (2008): 822–825.

Lacey, Brian E., M.D., et al. 'The Treatment of Diabetic Gastroparesis with Botulinum Toxin Injections of the Pylorus." *Diabetes Care* 27, no. 10 (2004): 2,341–2,347.

Malagelada, Juan-R., M.D. "Gastrointestinal Syndromes Due to Diabetes Mellitus." In *Contemporary Diabetes: Diabetic Neuropathy: Clinical Management*, edited by N. Veves, A., and R. Malik, 2nd ed. Totowa, N.J.: Human Press, 2007. 433–451.

Mesiya, Sikander, M.D., and Anil Minocha, M.D. "Gastrointestinal Disease in Diabetes Mellitus." *Southern Medical Journal* (1998/1999): 33–38.

Nishida, T., et al. "Gastroesophageal Refulux DIse Related to Diabetes: Analysis of 241 Cases with Type 2 Diabetes Mellitus." *Journal of Gastroenterology and Hepatology* 19, no. 3 (2004): 258–265.

Noel, Rebecca A., et al. "Increased Risk of Acute Pancreatitis and Biliary Disease Observed in Patients with Type 2 Diabetes." *Diabetes Care* 32, no. 4 (2009): 834–838.

Parrish, Carol Lee, and Joyce Green Pastors. "Nutritional Management of Gastroparesis in People with Diabetes." *Diabetes Spectrum* 20, no. 4 (2007): 231–234.

Petit, William Jr., M.D., and Christine Adamec. *The Encyclopedia of Diabetes*. 2nd ed. New York: Facts On File, 2010.

Wolosin, James D., M.D., and Steven V. Edelman. "Diabetes and the Gastrointestinal Tract." *Clinical Diabetes* 18, no. 4 (2000): 148–151.

diarrhea An increase in the frequency and/or fluidity of stools. If diarrhea has lasted for at least four weeks or longer, it is considered a chronic medical problem. Diarrhea is a symptom that is caused by many different infections and by chronic as well as acute illnesses. In the United States, about 8 million people per year see a physician to report diarrhea, and of these individuals, about 250,000 are hospitalized. Some individuals experience a chronic problem of having diarrhea that may alternate with CONSTIPATION, in addition to experiencing abdominal pain that improves with defecation, a condition that is known as IRRITABLE BOWEL SYNDROME (IBS).

Most cases of acute diarrhea resolve spontaneously. However, if the problem continues and the individual is untreated, diarrhea can sometimes become life threatening, particularly to infants or to very elderly individuals. Diarrhea can also be dangerous for others who have a compromised immune system, such as people who have the human immunodeficiency virus (HIV), cancer, or other serious illnesses.

Symptoms and Diagnostic Path

Physicians ask patients with diarrhea how many bowel movements they are having per day and how long the problem has occurred. Most patients do not require laboratory testing; however, laboratory tests, such as the complete blood count (CBC) and stool studies, can indicate whether an infection is present. Electrolyte tests and tests of renal (kidney) function may be ordered to help the doctor determine the harmful effects of diarrhea, such as DEHYDRATION. Physicians may also order a stool sample analysis to test for both infections and other diseases that are causing the problem.

Treatment Options and Outlook

Most cases of acute diarrhea are self-limited and do not require any specific treatment except adequate hydration. Diarrhea is usually treated with over-the-counter (OTC) or prescribed medications. Minor cases of diarrhea may be treated with antidiarrheal medications, rest, and plenty of fluids.

Patients with diarrhea that is associated with bleeding, fever, severe weakness and lethargy, or weight loss should seek medical attention promptly.

In addition, replacement of fluids and electrolytes is important to prevent dehydration. Some individuals may need to be hospitalized so that they can receive an intravenous replacement of fluids.

Risk Factors and Preventive Measures

Diarrhea may be a temporary condition that is caused by a minor or serious illness, indigestion, food-borne illnesses, or contaminated food or water. Diarrhea may be caused by bacteria or viruses or by another agent altogether, such as by a parasitic disease such as AMEBIASIS. Diarrhea may also result as a side effect from taking some medications. In fact, many different medications produce diarrhea as a side effect, including many antibiotics, antiarrhythmic drugs (medications for the heart), antidepressants, antihypertensive drugs, and diuretics.

Infections with bacteria or parasites in the gastrointestinal tract may also cause diarrhea. Many people who travel to other countries experience diarrhea to such an extent that "travelers's diarrhea" is a diagnosis.

Washing hands before preparing food or eating is one preventive measure against contracting infections or viruses. However, sometimes no matter how careful an individual is, he or she may develop diarrhea, and in that case should see the physician if needed.

See also CONSTIPATION; CONTAMINATED FOOD OR WATER; DIVERTICULOSIS; DYSENTERY; PARASITIC INFECTIONS.

diet drugs Prescribed or over-the-counter medications or herbal remedies that are taken to reduce appetite so that an overweight or obese individual may lose weight more easily. An estimated 5 million people in the United States take prescribed drugs for weight loss, and many millions more take over-the-counter diet drugs. People buy over-the-counter diet remedies in pharmacies and supermarkets as well as through the Internet. There are also print and television advertisements that promote over-the-counter diet drugs.

Medications for weight loss are recommended for some patients who have a BODY MASS INDEX (BMI) of greater than 30 or greater than 27, if there are obesity-related problems that diet and exercise have failed to correct. Diet drugs should not be used by the following individuals:

- Children
- The elderly (older than age 65 years)
- Pregnant or breastfeeding women
- Individuals who have pulmonary hypertension
- Patients who have uncontrolled systemic hypertension
- Patients who have unstable heart disease

In the past, amphetamines were used as diet drugs, but today this category of drugs is not recommended for this use in the United States and in other countries. Some researchers are also looking at the efficacy of some antidepressant drugs, such as bupropion (Wellbutrin) in producing weight loss. Most studies have shown that most diet drugs do not produce massive weight losses and that the weight that is lost is usually regained when the person stops taking the drug.

Studies on Newer Medications

Researchers are seeking better drugs to control overweight and obesity. Sometimes drugs that have not worked out well in treating other illnesses have had a side effect of causing weight loss, and thus researchers have subsequently performed separate studies to determine whether those medications would help obese people. An antiepileptic drug, zonisamide (Zonegran), has been tested for its efficacy in weight loss by some researchers.

In a study reported in 2003 in the *Journal of the American Medical Association*, the researchers Gadde and colleagues gave obese subjects zonisamide or a placebo over 16 weeks. All patients were also placed on a hypocaloric (low-calorie) diet, and their compliance was monitored with self-rated food diaries. There were 55 women and five men; of these subjects, 51 completed the protocol. The zonisamide therapy was started at 100 mg orally with a gradual increase to 400 mg. A further increase to 600 mg was made for those patients who had lost less than 5 percent of their body weight after 12 weeks.

The researchers found that zonisamide, combined with a low-calorie diet, was significantly more effective than placebo in producing weight loss. Over the 16-week period, the weight loss in the zonisamide group was an average of 5.9 kg (a 6.0 percent loss), whereas in the placebo group, the average loss was 0.9 kg (a 1.0 percent loss). One reported side effect of zonisamide was fatigue.

In a study reported by Ettinger and colleagues in 2003 in the *Journal of the American Medical Association*, researchers tested the effect of a genetically engineered form of ciliary neurotrophic factor (CNTF) manufactured by Regeneron. This protein had originally been tested as a treatment for amyotrophic lateral sclerosis (ALS) patients, but it had caused significant weight loss in nonobese subjects because it apparently suppresses hunger signals from the hypothalamus.

Researchers decided to test its efficacy on obese patients over 12 weeks. One hundred and twenty-three patients completed the clinical study. Patients taking the protein achieved a significant weight loss when compared to subjects in the placebo group; however, adverse effects were reported, such as nausea as well as pain at the injection site of the medication.

All prescribed diet drugs are offered for short-term use; however, many obesity experts believe that people for whom an antiobesity drug is effective have to continue to use it over the long term, much as patients who have hypertension continue taking hypertension medications once their blood pressure has improved.

Primary Prescribed Diet Drugs

In the United States, the key prescribed diet drugs are sibutramine (Meridia) and orlistat (Xenical). Orlistat also reduces serum cholesterol level. Phentermine was formerly combined with fenfluramine (Pondimin) or dexfenfluramine (Redux): the phen–fen combination. The combined drug was removed from the consumer market in 1997 in the United States because of an associated problem with a heart valve disease. Phentermine and diethylpriopion are approved only for short-term use (12 weeks).

The side effects of sibutramine are a mild increase in blood pressure, dry mouth, constipation, and headache. It should not be used by those who have a history of heart disease or stroke.

Orlistat's side effects are fecal urgency and incontinence, flatulence, increased frequency of defecation, and oily spotting. An estimated 9 percent of patients discontinue taking orlistat specifically because of these troublesome side effects, although the side effects generally decrease over time. Orlistat decreases the absorption of vitamins A and E, and for this reason, some physicians recommend vitamin supplements to patients who are treated with this drug.

Leptin has been shown to cause a reduction in food intake and to be effective for obese animals and humans; however, its effect is modest and it is not approved for use in the United States.

An Analysis of the Users of Prescribed Weight Loss Medications

In one analysis of the use of diet drugs, in a 2001 issue of the *Annals of Internal Medicine*, the authors reported that 2.5 percent of adults in the United States used prescription weight loss medications over the period 1996 to 1998. Women were four times more likely to use prescribed diet drugs than men. Hispanic women, at a usage rate of 3.2 percent, were more likely than whites or blacks (both at 2.4 percent) to use these drugs.

The pills were most heavily used by females between the ages of 25 and 44 years. Disturbingly, as many as one-quarter of the individuals taking prescribed weight loss drugs were *not* overweight in terms of their BMI. Hispanic women were most likely to be using these drugs inappropriately. BMI is a measure derived from height and weight that enables physicians to determine whether individuals are overweight or obese. People who are not overweight or obese should not take any diet drugs, whether they are prescribed or over-the-counter medications.

Use of Over-the-Counter Diet Drugs

In past years, phenylpropanolamine was the primary ingredient in many over-the-counter diet medications; however, because studies showed such drugs increased the risk for heart attack and stroke, these drugs were withdrawn from the market by manufacturers in 2000.

Before 2004, many drugs contained ephedra or ma huang (*Ephedra sinica*), a stimulant combined with caffeine to aid in weight loss. However, ephedra is dangerous for people with hypertension, heart disease, diabetes, and other medical problems. It is also true that some individuals have purportedly died as a result of taking drugs that contain ephedra. Because ephedra is considered an herb under the 1994 Dietary Supplement Health and Education Act, it is not directly under the control of the Food and Drug Administration (FDA) in the United States. However, the Food and Drug Administration after issuing numerous warnings against using ephedra banned the drug in the United States in 2004.

The ingestion of green tea has been shown to produce weight loss. Some use guar gum (derived from the Indian cluster bean) as a weight loss remedy.

In a study reported in a 2001 issue of the *Journal of the American Medical Association,* researchers contacted more than 14,000 individuals in Florida, Iowa, Michigan, West Virginia, and Wisconsin and asked them about their use of over-the-counter diet medications. Ten percent of the consumers reported having used or currently using diet drugs. Most users were obese young women (28 percent), but some users (8 percent) were normal-weight women who apparently wanted to be thinner. There were no ethnic or racial differences among those using over-the-counter diet drugs.

For more information on weight loss, contact the following organization:

Weight-Control Information Network (WIN)
1 WIN Way
Bethesda, MD 20892
(877) 946-4627
Web site: www.niddk.nih.gov/health/nutrit/nutrit.htm

See also BARIATRIC SURGERY; OBESITY.

Blanck, Heidi Michels, Laura Kettel Khan, and Mary K. Serdula, M.D. "Use of Nonprescription Weight Loss Products: Results from a Multistate Survey." *Journal of American Medical Association* 286, no. 8 (August 22/29, 2001): 930–935.

Ettinger, Mark P., M.D., et al. "Recombinant Variant of Ciliary Neurotrophic Factor for Weight Loss in Obese Adults: A Randomized, Dose-Ranging Study." *Journal of the American Medical Association* 289, no. 13 (April 9, 2003): 1,826–1,832.

Gadde, Kishore M., M.D., et al. "Zonisamide for Weight Loss in Obese Adults: A Randomized Controlled Trial." *Journal of the American Medical Association* 289, no. 14 (April 9, 2003): 1,820–1,825.

Khan, Laura Kettel, et al. "Use of Prescription Weight Loss Pills among U.S. Adults in 1996–1998." *Annals of Internal Medicine* 134, no. 4 (2001): 282–286.

Wirth, Alfred, M.D., and Jutta Krause. "Long-Term Weight Loss with Sibutramine: A Randomized Controlled Trial." *Journal of the American Medical Association* 286, no. 11 (September 19, 2001): 1,331–1,339.

Yanovski, Susan Z., M.D., and Jack A. Yanovski, M.D. "Obesity." *New England Journal of Medicine* 346, no. 8 (February 21, 2002): 591–602.

digestion and absorption The process by which foods are broken down and nutrients, vitamins, minerals, and other substances are absorbed and used by the body as building blocks and as a source of energy. The process of digestion and absorption is complex and ongoing and is accomplished over several hours.

Food is processed in the stomach and the small intestines for about three hours in each. Thus, digestion does not start with the intake of food and end when a meal is finished. Instead, the food eaten for breakfast and a midmorning snack is still being digested, absorbed, and assimilated while the individual is eating lunch, and digestion and absorption continue continuously until at some point it slows while the individual sleeps for seven or eight hours.

Digestion and absorption normally work very well every day for most people. However, sometimes the digestive system experiences temporary or long-term problems that require treatment.

Lack of Absorption of Vitamins or Minerals

In some cases, because of disease or medical problems, patients absorb too much or too little of needed nutrients. For example, some people cannot absorb vitamin B_{12} from the food that they eat, so they must take supplemental doses of it. Others suffer from iron deficiency anemia and must take supplemental doses of iron in order for their body to function normally. Others have deficiencies of other substances, such as magnesium or potassium.

Patients with short bowel syndrome have an insufficient length of the small intestines to meet their needs for nutrient absorption and may need to rely upon parenteral nutrition. Patients with hemochromatosis absorb too much iron and suffer from an overload that can lead to liver cirrhosis and heart problems.

Missing or the Wrong Level of Enzymes Can Be the Problem

In other cases, there is a problem with the specific enzymes that are needed for digestion; for example, patients with chronic pancreatitis cannot produce enough digestive enzymes to digest food. Since these enzymes are needed for digestion, those who have this problem must obtain these enzymes through an external source (pills or capsules) to survive.

Other Illnesses, Such as Thyroid Disease

Sometimes other systems in the body may cause problems with digestion. For example, if patients have a thyroid disease, they may have a sped-up metabolism, caused by hyperthyroidism (high levels of circulating thyroid hormone), or, conversely, they may have a very sluggish metabolism, which is caused by hypothyroidism (low levels of thyroid hormone). Both of these conditions can affect the appetite and digestion. Diagnosis and treatment of the underlying thyroid disease usually resolve any digestive problems that the condition has caused.

Malfunctions of Digestive Organs

Sometimes organs within the digestive system malfunction and may prevent normal digestion and absorption. Organs may have blockages or benign or cancerous tumors that can impede or prevent the normal digestive processes. Organs can also become inflamed and irritated, interfering with the normal digestive process. In addition, slow gut may lead to a small-intestine bacterial overgrowth, causing malabsorption.

Behavior Can Cause Digestive Problems

The individual can impair normal nutrition, for example, by failing to eat sufficient amounts of food or by eating large quantities of food that lead to obesity and resulting digestive difficulties. Other behavior, such as alcoholism or drug addiction, can cause damage to the digestive system. Depending on how severe the damage is, the digestive system may recover if the abusive behavior ends, or the damage may be irreversible. Examples of the results of abusive behavior are alcoholic liver cirrhosis and narcotic bowel syndrome.

Infections Impede Digestion

Parasitic or other infectious diseases may make normal digestion difficult or impossible until they are identified and treated. Some infections are spread by contaminated food or water. Many times it is difficult to determine the source of an infection, and the best the doctor can do is to identify the disease and treat it.

Inherited Defects

Some individuals have hereditary medical problems such as a risk for development of diabetes, that make digestion difficult if diabetes develops, unless or until they are treated. For this reason, physicians obtain a complete medical history in addition to performing a physical examination when a patient consults them about a medical problem.

Food Allergies and Food Intolerances

Patients may also have food allergies (in which an immune reaction to a food develops) such as peanut allergy or food intolerances (symptoms that occur in response to eating certain foods, which may be due to the body's lacking a substance that is needed to digest them, such as lactase needed for the digestion of lactose) of which they are unaware. Some allergies are mild, others are very severe. In addition, food intolerance may also range from mild to severe in scope.

The Impact of Aging

As individuals age into middle age and then the elderly years (ages 65 and older), the digestive system may become more sluggish, the patient becomes less active, and the risk for development of digestive diseases and/or worsening of existing diseases becomes great. It is also true that older people are much more likely to be using three or more medications than younger individuals. Because many medications can cause digestive difficulties, such as diarrhea or constipation, it is not surprising that many elderly people have difficulties with digestion and problems such as constipation and fecal impaction.

The Impact of Technology

Diseases and illnesses that physicians could not treat in past years are now treated routinely. Canadian scientists have discovered how to graft cells from the pancreas of deceased individuals into living patients with insulin-dependent diabetes, curing their diabetes. Physicians have found many ways to treat and even cure digestive cancers, through surgery, chemotherapy, and radiation therapy. Nearly every month has new revelations about potential ways physicians can help people of all ages to cope with their digestive problems.

See also CHILDREN; CONSTIPATION; DIABETES MELLITUS; DIARRHEA; DIGESTIVE SYSTEM; ELDERLY; INFANTS.

digestive enzymes   Substances that are secreted by the body to aid in digesting food. AMYLASE is secreted by the salivary glands as well as the pancreas. Other enzymes are trypsin, chymotrypsin, and carboxypeptidases A and B, all of which are enzymes that transform proteins into amino acids. Lipase is an enzyme that breaks down fats into fatty acids and glycerol. Lactase breaks down milk sugar, which is known as lactose. A deficiency of lactase leads to LACTOSE INTOLERANCE.

Other digestive enzymes include maltase, which breaks down maltose, and sucrase, which digests sucrose.

Some people do not secrete sufficient digestive enzymes, as a result of disease, inflammatory processes, PARASITIC INFECTIONS, and other medical problems. They may need supplemental enzymes; for example, pancreatic enzymes may be needed in cases of chronic pancreatitis. Supplemental pancreatic enzymes are also used to decrease the pain caused by chronic pancreatitis.

digestive system   The series of interconnected organs that together work to process food, beginning with the mouth, where the salivary glands start processing food that has been ingested. The food then passes into the esophagus, the "food tube" that joins to the stomach, which is the digestive organ where the solid large pieces of food are processed into smaller-sized particles for delivery to the small intestine, where most of digestion and absorption occurs.

Enzymes in the small intestine break down the food further. The liver, pancreas, and gallbladder are also involved in processing food. The pancreas releases special enzymes to break the food down into its elements of carbohydrates, fats, and proteins. Note: the pancreas is a dual-purpose gland, in that it also secretes the hormone insulin, which helps utilize carbohydrates and maintain a normal blood sugar level. When that function goes awry, diabetes results. However, a person can have diabetes and still have normal pancreatic digestive function, because different parts of the pancreas handle the release of digestive juices and insulin.

The liver produces bile, which is released into the duodenum at meals. Bile juice helps in the processing of the fat. Between meals, the bile that is secreted by the liver is stored and concentrated in the gallbladder, which releases it at mealtime.

The small intestine further breaks down the food and nutrients as fluids and electrolytes that are absorbed into the body. The unused waste products move into the colon, where there is further processing and fluid absorption and conversion of liquid waste matter into solid waste occur. This matter is eliminated in a bowel movement, usually within about a day or two after the food is first consumed.

See also COLON; DIGESTION AND ABSORPTION; ESOPHAGUS; LIVER; PANCREAS.

digital rectal examination (DRE)   The physician's gloved manual examination using a finger. It involves insertion of a finger into and examination of the rectum and (in men) also of the prostate gland, for the purpose of identifying cancer, hemorrhoids, polyps, or other serious medical conditions or problems.

The rectal examination generally takes about 30 seconds. The digit is the lubricated finger of the physician; the examination is usually performed during a routine physical examination. Most physicians recommend that the rectal examination be a standard part of the annual physical examination. This is particularly true for men, because the DRE may sometimes detect abnormalities of the prostate gland, an indicator of prostate disease or prostate cancer.

Most men and women detest having a rectal examination and may consider it the worst part of the physical examination. They may try to deter the physician from performing the rectal examination or even refuse to have one. They may not realize the importance of the examination and the major findings that may result from it, which sometimes may save their life.

See also ANAL CANCER; COLORECTAL CANCER.

diverticulitis   An inflammatory infective condition that is a complication of chronic DIVERTICULOSIS, which is the presence of pouches (diverticula), usually in the colon. Many people have diverticulosis (although most of them do not realize this, and it is undiagnosed), but do not have diverticulitis. If the diverticulitis is acute, however, it is a painful condition that may produce mild to severe pain. Patients with diverticulitis may experience CONSTIPATION and loose stools. In some cases, diverticulitis can become very severe and even life threatening.

The conditions of diverticulosis and diverticulitis are frequently confused by many patients because of their similar-sounding names. To distinguish the two conditions, keep in mind that diverticulosis is the *cause* of the problem and diverticulitis, when it occurs, is the resulting complication of diverticulosis.

Diverticulitis results from a tiny perforation in the diverticular pouches, which causes the pouch and the surrounding area to become infected and inflamed. Diverticulitis usually involves a diverticulum on the left side of the colon, although it can occur anywhere along the colon.

Symptoms and Diagnostic Path
Some symptoms of diverticulitis are fever, abdominal pain that is usually located in the left lower abdomen, CONSTIPATION or DIARRHEA, indigestion, gas, and bloating. Patients also have a belly that

is sore to the touch, especially on the left side. Blood test results may suggest the presence of an infection.

The diagnosis of diverticulitis is based on clinical grounds. An ultrasound and computed tomography (CT) scan are also helpful. When physicians suspect diverticulitis, they do not perform a colonoscopy because this procedure can exacerbate the problem by causing the inflamed pouch to burst and spill its contents.

Treatment Options and Outlook

Patients with diverticulitis are prescribed a liquid diet and a course of antibiotics. Patients with severe cases of diverticulitis may need to be hospitalized and may, rarely, require surgery.

When the condition has resolved, physicians may then order a colonoscopy to rule out the presence of cancer that is masquerading as diverticulitis. Patients with recurrent bouts of diverticulutis require surgery for an excision of the involved segment.

Risk Factors and Preventive Measures

About 5 to 10 percent of people in the United States and Canada older than 45 years may have an attack of acute diverticulitis. Diverticulitis is less of a problem in such places as Asia and Africa, where fewer people have diverticulosis.

Some patients with diverticulitis are younger individuals, and an estimated 10 to 20 percent of patients with diverticulitis are younger than 50 years. It is also possible, although not common, for children and adolescents to experience diverticulitis. There are no preventive measures.

diverticulosis A condition in which small pouches (diverticula) occur, usually in the colon. It usually causes no symptoms. Diverticulosis is common in the United States, Canada, and Western European countries, perhaps because of the low fiber in the diet of most citizens. Diverticulosis is rare in Asian and African populations.

Most people older than the age of 60 years have diverticulosis, but the majority of them have no symptoms or problems with this condition. Many people do not even know that they have diverticu-

losis unless they are informed by their doctor of the presence of the condition, for example, after they undergo a barium enema or COLONOSCOPY. Diverticuli may also occur in the small intestine, often as a result of a disease such as SCLERODERMA.

Diverticulosis may lead to DIVERTICULITIS, which is a condition in which the pouches become inflamed and infected. Diverticulosis and diverticulitis are frequently confused because of the similarity of the names. However, diverticulosis is the cause and diverticulitis, when it occurs, is the result.

Symptoms and Diagnostic Path

Many people with diverticulosis have no symptoms; however, some individuals have vague symptoms, such as abdominal cramping. This is called painful diverticular disease. Patients who also have diverticulitis (inflammation of the diverticuli) experience left lower abdominal pain with fever and a belly that is sore to the touch. Blood test results may also suggest the presence of an infection. Diverticula are a common cause of lower gastrointestinal bleeding, which is usually painless and massive, often requiring a blood transfusion.

The diagnosis of diverticulosis is often made incidentally, when a colonoscopy, sigmoidoscopy, or barium enema is performed. The diagnosis of diverticulitis, on the other hand, is made on clinical grounds with or without noninvasive imaging studies, and a colonoscopy or barium enema is not performed in such circumstances, since the inflamed pouch may actually burst and worsen the patient's condition, even becoming life-threatening.

A colonoscopy would be performed within a few weeks after the diverticulitis was resolved, to make sure there was no other medical problem such as cancer, which could mimic a bout of diverticulitis. Diverticulitis and diverticular bleeding usually do not occur simultaneously. Patients who have lower gastrointestinal bleeding require a colonoscopy to look for the cause of the bleeding, including diverticulosis, and to allow the physician to treat the bleeding lesion as appropriate.

Treatment Options and Outlook

People who have diverticulosis are advised to drink plenty of water and to eat fruits and vegetables each day so that they have sufficient fiber to help move fecal material through the colon. Some physicians routinely advise patients who have diverticulosis to avoid eating popcorn or nuts, which may get trapped into the diverticular pouches and cause diverticulitis. This dietary modification recommendation is considered controversial.

See also MECKEL'S DIVERTICULUM.

dumping syndrome A condition in which after a person eats food it travels very rapidly (within 30 minutes) directly from the stomach into the jejunum of the small intestine.

There are two types of dumping syndrome: early and late. Early dumping syndrome is caused by the rapid and uncontrolled entry of food into the small intestine. Late dumping syndrome involves the release of an increased quantity of insulin, which results in reactive hypoglycemia (low blood sugar level).

Symptoms and Diagnostic Path

The symptoms and signs differ in early dumping syndrome and late dumping syndrome. The key symptoms of early dumping syndrome, which occur shortly after eating, are sweating, heart palpitations, weakness, abdominal pain, and nausea that may be accompanied by vomiting and even by syncope (fainting). In late dumping syndrome, the symptoms occur a few hours after eating, and they may include anxiety, restlessness, tremors, a rapid and pounding heartbeat, and even mental confusion.

Doctors diagnose the illness on the basis of the symptoms and a careful medical history, particularly noting past surgeries. The recommended treatment for dumping syndrome is that the patient eat small and frequent meals that are high in fat and proteins and low in carbohydrates. Solids and liquids are generally separated, and patients are advised to drink their liquids *between* meals, rather than with them, as is the usual custom. Octreotide is used for patients who still have problems despite complying with these recommendations. Sometimes anticholinergic drugs may be taken before meals to decrease the effect of dumping syndrome.

Risk Factors and Preventive Measures

Dumping syndrome may sometimes be a result of surgery, such as elective BARIATRIC SURGERY. Some obese individuals have this surgery to lose large amounts of weight. Other forms of gastric surgery may be responsible (for example, surgery for a peptic ulcer).

dysentery An infectious disease that is often caused by CONTAMINATED FOOD OR WATER, and that causes severe bloody DIARRHEA and stomach upset. People who are living in poor countries, especially children, can die of dysentery. Some forms of dysentery, such as bacillary dysentery, are caused by *SHIGELLA* bacteria. AMEBIASIS also causes dysentery.

dyspepsia Abdominal pain or discomfort in the upper abdomen that is presumed to have originated in the upper gastrointestinal system. Pain is exacerbated by food intake, and there may be accompanying nausea, vomiting, and bloating. Dyspepsia may indicate a minor or a more serious condition. The main causes of dyspepsia are gastroduodenal ulcer, atypical GASTROESOPHAGEAL REFLUX, and GASTROPARESIS; occasionally gastric cancer may cause dyspepsia.

Other Digestive Causes

Dyspepsia may have a variety of other causes. *HELICOBACTER PYLORI* may be the culprit that causes chronic dyspepsia as a result of ulcer disease. However, whether *Helicobacter pylori* alone, without the presence of an ulcer, can cause dyspepsia is a controversial issue among experts. Excessive gastric acid may be seen in as many as 20 percent of all patients with dyspepsia. Other patients may have problems with GASTROPARESIS, very slow emptying of the stomach contents into the intestines. In some cases, dyspepsia may be a symptom of gastrointestinal cancer.

Most of the time, however, despite investigations, no specific cause of the dyspepsia can be found, and consequently, the diagnosis is nonulcer dyspepsia (dyspepsia with no ulcer).

Nondigestive Causes of Dyspepsia

Other causes, some of which may emanate from outside the gut which are also considered in the diagnosis of dyspepsia include the following:

- angina pectoris of the heart (atypical angina)
- abdominal aortic aneurysm
- intestinal angina
- biliary colic
- PANCREATIC CANCER
- PANCREATITIS

Diagnosis of the Cause of Dyspepsia

Physicians determine the cause of the dyspepsia by taking a careful medical history, performing a physical examination of the patient, and ordering appropriate tests. The major causes of dyspepsia can be best evaluated by an upper gastrointestinal endoscopy. An alternate option is for the physician to order upper gastrointestinal X-rays. In the case of young and healthy patients without alarming symptoms such as weight loss or bleeding, the physician may elect simply to test the patient for the presence of *Helicobacter pylori,* and if the finding is positive, treat the patient as if he or she has an ulcer without specifically testing for ulcer.

See also ENDOSCOPY; ULCER, PEPTIC.

Bytzer, Peter, M.D., and Nicholas J. Talley, M.D. "Dyspepsia." *Annals of Internal Medicine* 134, no. 9, part 2 (2001): 815–822.

Fisher, Richard S., M.D., and Henry P. Parkman, M.D. "Management of Nonulcer Dyspepsia." *New England Journal of Medicine* 339, no. 19 (November 5, 1998): 1,376–1,381.

Minocha, A., et al. "Helicobacter Pylori Is Associated with Alterations in Intestinal Gas Profile Among Patients with Non-ulcer Dyspepsia." *Digestive Disease Sciences* 39, no. 8 (1994): 1,613–1,617.

Minocha, Anil, et al. "Alterations in Upper Gastrointestinal Motility in Helicobacter Pylori Positive Non Ulcer Dyspepsia." *American Journal of Gastroenterology* 89, no. 10 (1994): 1,797–1,800.

dysphagia   Difficulty and sometimes choking with swallowing. Dysphagia may be due to an inability to transfer food from the throat to the esophagus, which is called transfer dysphagia. This problem may be seen in patients with stroke, DIABETES MELLITUS, Parkinson's disease, and other medical problems. Another type of dysphagia is esophageal dysphagia, wherein the transfer occurs normally, but the transit through the esophagus is impaired, as is found with chronic GASTROESOPHAGEAL REFLUX DISEASE (GERD). The esophagus (food tube) in GERD can become constricted, often as a result of years of untreated disease.

In severe dysphagia, even tiny pieces of food may be blocked, and then if the condition worsens, even fluids cannot pass through. Such blockages need to be treated before normal feeding can resume. Benign strictures can be dilated by using dilators. In the case of a stricture due to cancer, an esophageal stent can be placed to maintain the patency of the esophageal lumen. Treatment of ACHALASIA involves pneumatic dilation, surgery, and sometimes botulinum toxin (Botox). GERD is not the only cause of dysphagia; patients may have SCLERODERMA, an enlarged heart, CANCER, or other medical problems. Those who experience dysphagia should have a medical evaluation.

See also BARRETT'S ESOPHAGUS.

Lavu, Kalyana, M.D., Thomas Matthew, and Anil Minocha. "Effectiveness of Esophageal Dilation in Relieving Non-Obstructive Esophageal Dysphagia and Improving Quality of Life." *Southern Medical Journal* 97, no. 2 (February 2004): 137–140.

E

eating disorders   Medical and psychological problems that lead to either excessive undereating or extreme overeating. The three most common eating disorders are ANOREXIA NERVOSA, BULIMIA NERVOSA, and a third category of eating disorder is "eating disorders not otherwise specified," which includes disorders such as binge eating disorder. In the case of binge eating disorder, the individual has periods of excessive eating behavior which usually leads to OBESITY.

Physicians use the concept of BODY MASS INDEX to determine whether individuals are underweight, normal weight, overweight, or obese. Whether they are too thin or obese, individuals who have any form of an eating disorder are obsessed with food and consider it paramount to their self-image.

Symptoms and Diagnostic Path

An extreme preoccupation with food is a key indicator of an eating disorder. Both the anorexic and the obese person, despite the disparities in their weight and appearance, constantly think about food. In the case of the obese person, when food is desired, it is usually consumed. Conversely, the anorexic is also obsessed with food, but primarily with thoughts of *avoiding* food, to maintain the current body weight. (Some anorexics also want to lose more weight.) The person with bulimia nervosa induces vomiting to rid herself of excessive food. This eventually affects the enamel of the teeth.

With the individual who has anorexia nervosa, the person is usually obviously emaciated and looks starving. Females with anorexia nervosa often stop menstruating, and they may exercise to excess. The individual with anorexia may weigh her or himself several times per day. Individuals with anorexia nervosa have an increased risk for death from complications such as cardiac arrest, fluid imbalances, and electrolyte imbalances.

Other symptoms of anorexia nervosa may include the following, which occur over time:

- brittle hair and nails
- thinning bones
- dry and yellowish skin
- muscle weakness and muscle loss
- ANEMIA
- severe CONSTIPATION
- low blood pressure
- slowed breathing and pulse
- a lower body temperature, causing the person to feel cold frequently
- lethargy

With the person who has bulimia nervosa, the behavior is characterized by periods of excessive eating followed by a behavior meant to purge the body, such as induced vomiting or the excessive use of laxatives or diuretics, fasting, or extreme exercising. People with bulimia nervosa may have a normal body weight, but they desperately fear gaining weight and are extremely unhappy with their bodies, as are all individuals with eating disorders. However, the bulimic behavior, particularly the induced vomiting, is usually performed in secret and hidden from family members and others.

Individuals with bulimia nervosa may have electrolyte imbalances, oral diseases, and gastrointestinal diseases stemming from their purging behavior. Other symptoms of bulimia nervosa include the following:

- chronic sore throat
- swollen glands in the neck and below the jaw
- sensitive decaying teeth and worn tooth enamel, caused by refluxed stomach acids during induced vomiting episodes
- GASTROESOPHAGEAL REFLUX DISORDER
- intestinal irritation caused by laxative abuse
- kidney disease caused by abuse of diuretics
- severe DEHYDRATION caused by excessive purging of fluids

With binge eating disorder, the individual feels a loss of control over eating, although excessive eating is not followed by purging of food or excessive exercising or fasting. Most people with binge eating disorder are overweight or obese; however, their symptoms are not as obvious as with individuals who have anorexia nervosa or bulimia nervosa. People who are binge eaters also experience shame and guilt over their behavior but may have great difficulty with changing their behavior. Individuals with binge eating disorder may also have problems with anxiety and depression.

Treatment Options and Outlook

If the eating disorder causes severe health problems, as in extreme cases of anorexia nervosa or bulimia nervosa, then the patient may need to be hospitalized for malnutrition and treated. Medications may be used to treat the person with anorexia nervosa, such as drugs that are antidepressants, antipsychotics, or mood stabilizers. Individual psychotherapy is often used, as is group psychotherapy and family counseling.

With bulimia nervosa, the patient may receive both nutritional counseling and psychotherapy. Fluoxetine (Prozac) is the only medication approved by the Food and Drug Administration (FDA) for the treatment of bulimia; however, other antidepressants may be prescribed "off-label" to treat depressive symptoms. Cognitive-behavioral therapy (CBT) is often used for eating disorders. With CBT, the individual is taught to recognize and challenge irrational thoughts. A combination of CBT and antidepressents may offer the best chance for response, especially in difficult to manage cases of eating disorders.

Individuals with binge eating disorder may be treated with antidepressants and are sometimes treated with appetite suppressants as well. Often psychotherapy, particularly CBT, is used to treat this disorder.

Note that the FDA has warnings on some antidepressants, particularly selective serotonin reuptake inhibitors (SSRIs) such as Prozac and other drugs in this class. Some studies indicate that there is an increased risk for suicidal thinking among adolescents and young adults up to age 24 years who take these medications. As a result, individuals should be closely monitored during the first weeks of treatment for any worsening of suicidal thoughts, depression or unusual behavior such as agitation, sleeplessness, or the withdrawal from normal social situations.

Risk Factors and Preventive Measures

Anorexia nervosa and bulimia nervosa are more common among females, while both males and females may exhibit binge eating characteristic of binge eating disorder. According to the National Institute of Mental Health (NIMH), females account for about 85 to 95 percent of all cases of anorexia nervosa and bulimia nervosa and 65 percent of all cases of binge eating disorder.

Individuals with eating disorders often have other serious psychiatric problems such as anxiety disorders or depression. In addition, they may have serious health problems such as kidney and/or heart disease.

See also DIET DRUGS.

Cassell, Dana K., and David H. Gleaves. *Obesity and Eating Disorders*. 2d ed. New York: Facts On File, 2000.
National Institute of Mental Health. *Eating Disorders*. Bethesda, Md.: National Institutes of Health, 2007. Available online. URL: http://www.nimh.nih.gov/health/publications/eating-disorders/summary.shtml. Downloaded May 3, 2008.

E. coli See ESCHERICHIA COLI.

elderly In many cases, the elderly (those who are ages 65 years and older) have an increased risk for suffering from many types of digestive diseases and disorders compared to younger individuals, including having diagnoses of CANCERS OF THE DIGESTIVE SYSTEM as well as such diseases as type 2 DIABETES MELLITUS, DIVERTICULITIS, and peptic ULCERS. In addition, many older people suffer from multiple medical problems, and consequently, they may also have a significantly weakened immune system compared to their younger counterparts. Another issue is that often existing medical problems presage an impending risk for other health problems; for example, many older people suffer from both hypertension and diabetes, and these conditions together are the top two risk factors for the development of kidney failure, eventually ultimately necessitating the receipt of either dialysis or a kidney transplantation in order for the continued survival of the individual.

Many elderly people may suffer from seemingly relatively minor problems, such as TASTE IMPAIRMENTS, which, however, may significantly decrease their appetite and lead to other health problems, such as VITAMIN DEFICIENCIES or even MALNUTRITION. In addition, according to the Food Safety and Inspection Service (FSIS) of the U.S. Agriculture Department, in the case of many adults ages 75 and older, should they contract an illness from CONTAMINATED FOOD, they are more likely to become sicker than others and to require hospitalization, and they are also more likely to die from such an infection. (See Appendix IV for the major pathogens that can cause food-borne illnesses in the United States, including the source of the pathogen, the symptoms that they cause and the potential impact on infected individuals.)

The elderly also have an increased risk for suffering from many chronic digestive disorders, such as GASTROESOPHAGEAL REFLUX DISEASE (GERD), DIVERTICULITIS and DIVERTICULOSIS, DYSPHAGIA, HIATAL HERNIA, and CONSTIPATION. GERD can lead to BARRETT'S ESOPHAGUS and then to ESOPHAGEAL CANCER. Some older individuals also have a problem with ALCOHOL ABUSE (also known as *alcohol dependence*), which in turn increases their risk for the development of CIRRHOSIS of the liver, LIVER CANCER, and LIVER FAILURE, as well as for serious injuries that are caused by falls, traffic accidents, and various other injuries that are directly related to the physical and mental impairments that are caused by a state of intoxication.

Other older individuals may have a problem with LACTOSE INTOLERANCE, while others may experience other difficulties with the digestion of their foods; for example, they may have slowed stomach emptying, also known as GASTROPARESIS. Chronic CONSTIPATION is very common among older people, as are symptomatic HEMORRHOIDS. Older individuals may also have a slowed immune system, causing them to be at greater risk for a wide variety of infectious diseases that can affect the digestive system.

Alcohol Dependence

Many older people who are alcoholics have been addicted to alcohol for years, although some older people begin their drinking in later years because of loneliness and depression, particularly widowed elderly women. Alcohol dependence is a risk factor for many different digestive disorders, including liver cirrhosis and liver cancer, as well as liver failure. The liver is the organ that metabolizes alcohol, and chronic alcoholism has the potential to damage not just the liver but also other organs such as the pancreas and the heart.

Alcohol dependence over the long term often leads to vitamin deficiencies as well as malnutrition and other health problems and can also lead to dementia. In addition, intoxication increases the risk for injuries, particularly falls, which may lead to fractures among older people. Many older people who suffer from fractures, particularly hip fractures, have considerable difficulty with recovery.

It is also important to note that many prescription and over-the-counter medications interact with alcohol, often to a dangerous level, and according to the National Institute on Alcohol Abuse and Alcoholism (NIAAA) in their 2007 report on harmful medication interactions with alcohol, older people are more likely to take one or more medications that interact with alcohol than younger people. In addition, alcohol stays in the system of an elderly person longer because aging slows down the body's ability to break down alcohol. It is also important to note that alcohol affects a woman's body faster than a man's body because women generally have less water in their bodies than do men. Consequently, women are more susceptible to alcohol-related damage, such as harm to the liver.

Many different medications may interact with alcohol, and some interactions are extremely serious. For example, older individuals who are taking commonly prescribed pain medications for arthritis, such as celecoxib (Celebrex), naproxen, (Naprosyn), or diclofenac (Voltaren) and who also consume alcohol are at risk for developing stomach bleeding and ulcers, as well as problems with their liver. In another example, those who take frequently used medications prescribed for type 2 diabetes, such as metformin (Glucophage, Glucophage XL), glyburide (Micronase), or tolbutamine (Orinase) and who also drink alcohol risk the development of abnormally low blood sugar levels as well as rapid heartbeat and sudden changes in their blood pressure.

Individuals who take antibiotics for infections and who also drink alcohol are at risk for stomach problems, vomiting, liver damage, and many other medical issues. Note that the individual does not need to meet the criteria for alcoholism to incur these risks but could simply drink heavily while taking medications, leading to an increased risk for serious interactions. (See the table.) Of course these interactions could occur to individuals of any age; however, elderly people are much more likely

TABLE: COMMONLY USED MEDICINES (BOTH PRESCRIPTION AND OVER-THE-COUNTER) THAT INTERACT WITH ALCOHOL

Symptoms/Disorders	Medication (Brand Name)	Medication (Generic Name)	Some Possible Reactions with Alcohol
Allergies/colds/flu	Alavert Allegra, Allegra-D Benadryl Clarinex Claritin Claritin-D Dimetapp Cold & Allergy Sudafed Sinus & Allergy Triaminic Cold & Allergy Tylenol Allergy Sinus Tylenol Cold & Flu Zyrtec	Loratidine Fexofenadin Diphenhydramine Desloratidine Loratidine Brompheniramine Chlorpheniramine Chlorpheniramine Chlorpheniramine Cetirizine	Drowsiness, dizziness, increased risk for overdose
Angina (chest pain), coronary heart disease	Isordil	Isosorbide Nitroglycerin	Rapid heartbeat sudden changes in blood pressure, dizziness, fainting
Anxiety, epilepsy	Ativan Klonopin Librium Paxil Valium Xanax	Lorazepam Clonazepam Chlordiazepoxide Paroxetine Diazepam Alprazolam	Drowsiness, dizziness, increased risk for overdose, slowed or difficulty breathing, impaired motor control, unusual behavior and memory problems
Arthritis	Celebrex Naprosyn Voltaren	Celecoxib Naproxen Diclofenac	Ulcers, stomach bleeding, liver problems
Blood clots	Coumadin	Warfain	Occasional drinking may lead to internal bleeding; heavier drinking my cause bleeding or may have the opposite effect, resulting in possible blood clots, strokes, or heart attacks
Cough	Delsym Robitussin Cough Robitussin DAC	Dextromethorphan Guaifenesin + codeine	Drowsiness, dizziness; increased risk for overdose

(Table continues)

(Table continued)

Symptoms/Disorders	Medication (Brand Name)	Medication (Generic Name)	Some Possible Reactions with Alcohol
Depression	Anafranil Celexa Desyrel Effexor Elavil Lexapro Luvox Norpramin Paxil Prozac Serzone Wellbutrin Zolfot Herbal preparations such as St. John's Wort	Clomipramine Citalopram Trazodone Venlafaxine Amitriptyline Escitalopram Fluvoxamine Desipraine Paroxetine Fluoxetine Nefazodone Bupropion Sertraline	Drowsiness, dizziness; increased risk for overdose; increased feelings of depression or hopeless in adolescents (suicide)
Diabetes	Glucophage Micronase Orinase	Metformin Glyburide Tolbutamide	Abnormally low blood sugar levels, flushing reaction (nausea, vomiting, headache, rapid heartbeat, sudden changes in blood pressure)
Enlarged prostate gland	Cardura Flomax Hytrin Minipress	Doxazosin Tamsulosin Terazosin Prazosin	Dizziness, light-headedness, fainting
Heartburn, indigestion, sour stomach	Axid Reglan Tagamet Zantac	Nizatidine Metoclopramide Cimetidine Ranitidine	Rapid heartbeat, sudden changes in blood pressure (metoclopramide); increased alcohol effect
High blood pressure	Accupril Caprozide Cardura Catapres Cozaar Hytrin Lopressor HCT Lotensin Minipress Vaseretic	Quinapril Hydrocholorothiazide Doxazosin Clonidine Losartan Terazosin Hydrochlorothiazine Benzapril Prazosin Enalapril	Dizziness, fainting, drowsiness; heart problems such as changes in the heart's regular heartbeat (arrhythmia)
High cholesterol	Advicor Altocor Crestor Lipitor Mevacor Niaspain Pravachol Pravigard Vytorin Zocor	Lovastain + Niacin Lovastatin Rosuvastatin Atorvastatin Lovastatin Niacin Pravastatin Pravastatin + Aspirin Exetimibe + Simvastatin Simvastatin	Liver damage (all medications); increased flushing and itching (niacin), increased stomach bleeding (pravastatin + aspirin)
Infections	Acrodantin Flagyl Grisactin Nizoral Nydrazid Seromycin Tindamax	Nitrofurantoin Metronidazole Griseofulvin Ketokonazole Isoniazid Cycloserine Tinidazole	Fast heartbeat, sudden changes in blood pressure; stomach pain upset stomach, vomiting, headache or flushing or redness of the face; liver damage (isoniazid, ketokonazole)

Symptoms/Disorders	Medication (Brand Name)	Medication (Generic Name)	Some Possible Reactions with Alcohol
Muscle pain	Flexeril Soma	Cyclobenzaprine Carisoprodol	Drowsiness, dizziness; increased risk of seizures; increased risk for overdose; slowed or difficulty breathing; impaired motor control; unusual behavior; memory problems
Nausea, motion sickness	Antivert Atrarax Dramamine Phenergan	Mexlizine Hydroxyzine Dimenhydrinate Promethazine	Drowsiness, dizziness; increased risk for overdose
Pain (such as headache, muscle ache, minor arthritis pain), fever, inflammation	Advil Aleve Excedrin Motrin Tylenol	Iburprofen Naproxen Aspirin, Acetaminophen Ibuprofen Acetaminophen	Stomach upset, bleeding and ulcers; liver damage (acetaminopnen); rapid heartbeat
Seizures	Dilantin Klonopin	Phenytoin Clonazepam, Phenobarbital	Drowsiness, dizziness; increased risk of seizures
Severe pain from injury, postsurgical care, oral surgery or migraines	Darvocet-N Demerol Fiornal with codeine Percocet Vicodin	Propoxyphene Meperidine Butalbital + codeine Oxycodone Hydrocodone	Drowsiness, dizziness; increased risk for overdose; slowed or difficulty breathing; impaired motor control; unusual behavior; memory problems
Sleep problems	Ambien Lunesta Prosom Restoril Sominex Unisom Herbal preparations (chamomile, valerian, lavender)	Zolpidem Eszopiclone Estazolam Temazepam Dephenhydramine Doxylamine	Drowsiness, sleepiness, dizziness, slowed or difficult breathing, impaired motor control, unusual behavior, memory problems. Increased drowsiness

Adapted from: National Institute on Alcohol Abuse and Alcoholism. *Harmful Interactions: Mixing Alcohol with Medicines.* National Institutes of Health. 2007

to be taking at least several medications for arthritis, back pain, and so forth.

Cancer

Older individuals have an increased risk for nearly all forms of cancer compared to younger individuals; however, because cancer treatment often can be painful and difficult to manage, some experts have hypothesized that there may be circumstances when it may not be reasonable to treat certain elderly individuals for their cancer. Refuting this theory (at least as far as COLORECTAL CANCER is concerned), researchers K. M. Devon and colleagues studied patients age 50 to 74 and 75 years and older.

The researchers found that the five-year survival rate among those who had surgery for colorectal cancer was virtually identical between the two age groups: 74.0 percent for the younger group and 74.7 percent for the older group. The researchers wrote, "Long-term colorectal cancer-related outcomes in the older group are similar to outcomes in younger patients, suggesting that the decision to operate should not be based on age alone."

Chronic GERD that is untreated may lead to the development of Barrett's esophagus, a precancerous condition that changes the lining of the esophagus to an intestinal type and which increases the risk for esophageal cancer.

Diabetes Mellitus and the Elderly

Type 2 diabetes is very common among older people; for example, according to the National Center for Health Statistics, 20.3 percent of those ages 65 to 74 have been diagnosed with diabetes, compared to about half that level (10.7 percent) among those ages 45 to 64 years old and an even lower level among those in the age range of 18 to 44 years, or 2.2 percent. In addition, the health problems that are associated with diabetes are an increasing burden for the elderly, such as diabetic retinopathy, a leading cause of blindness, and diabetic nephropathy, the primary cause of kidney failure in the United States.

Good glycemic control, the attention of their physicians and carefully complying with their doctors' recommendations are all means to decrease (although not to eliminate) the health risks and complications of diabetes.

Diverticular Disease

Diverticular disease is common among older people, particularly DIVERTICULOSIS. According to Giuseppe Comparato and colleagues in their article for *Digestive Diseases* in 2007, only about 5 percent of those under age 40 have diverticulosis; however, among those ages 65 and older, the prevalence is about 65 percent. The majority of patients have no symptoms, but about 15 to 20 percent are symptomatic. About 5 percent develop diverticulitis, an inflammation of the diverticula, and a smaller number develop complications, such as hemorrhage, obstruction, and the development of abscesses.

Diverticulitis causes abdominal pain that may be severe and most often occurs in the lower left quadrant, along with fever and elevated white blood cell count. A computerized tomography (CT) scan can help make the diagnosis. Individuals with diverticulitis are treated with medications and strongly advised to increase their fiber intake in their diet. Antibiotics are given to treat diverticulitis. A low threshold should be exercised for admitting elderly patients to hospitals and treating them aggressively since they have a higher risk for complications. Some patients may need surgery.

If the pockets of diverticulosis should undergo a perforation, usually a microperforation, it leads to diverticulitis, and this can be a serious and even a life-threatening situation especially in elderly. (See EMERGENCY ISSUES IN DIGESTIVE DISORDERS.)

Diverticular bleed is a massive painless bleed that usually requires hospitalization and blood transfusions. Management options include colonoscopy, embolisation by interventional radiologists, and surgery.

Some individuals have no symptoms from their diverticulosis, while others experience mild constipation or bloating and mild pain. Diverticulitis, however, can be severely painful for the individual.

Diverticular disease may stem at least in part from a diet that is insufficient in daily FIBER, and as a result, it is generally treated with a high-fiber diet as well as pain medications and/or surgery, as needed.

Gastroesophageal Reflux Disease

Gastroesophageal reflux disease (GERD), often referred to as chronic HEARTBURN, is a common problem among many older people. They may have developed GERD because of the side effects of the medications that they take as well as from medication interactions that may occur. Sometimes older people mistake their GERD-related chest or abdominal pain as a heart attack; however, it is always important to rule out a possible heart attack, even in a person with long-term GERD.

Severe Chronic Constipation

Older people often fail to drink sufficient fluid, leading to DEHYDRATION. Because many elderly people lead very sedentary lives, they are often at an elevated risk for developing constipation, including severe constipation. Contrary to popular belief, it is not necessary to have a bowel movement every day. But if the older person does not have a bowel movement for several days, and when he or she does have one, the stools resemble hard pellets that are difficult to pass, then this generally indicates a constipation problem. According to experts, constipation is a common problem among older people, ranging up to 28 percent of the elderly population. However, the incidence of constipation rises to greater than 80 percent of nursing home residents, according to G. C. Spinzi in his article for *Digestive Diseases* in 2007

In many cases, simply increasing the fiber level of the diet can help considerably. (Increasing fiber will not help if the individual has GASTROPARESIS, a condition of slowed stomach emptying or an overall slow gut.) In general, the diet should be rich in fruits and vegetables as well. In addition, it is advisable to decrease the amount of caffeine that is consumed, because caffeine can be very constipating for many people. Caffeine is found in coffee, tea, chocolate, and many soft drinks. Substituting water for such drinks is a good idea, although it may be best to taper off from caffeine because a sudden withdrawal by a previously heavy user can lead to headaches and irritability.

Note that doctors often diagnose constipation based on the Rome criteria, while patients define it by how they feel. According to Spinzi, according to the Rome criteria, the patient must have two or more of the following symptoms for at least 12 weeks in the past year:

- straining to make a bowel movement at least 25 percent of the time
- hard or lumpy stools in at least 25 percent of all bowel movements
- a feeling of incomplete evacuation in at least 25 percent of the bowel movements
- a feeling of a blockage or anorectal obstruction in more than 25 percent of bowel movements
- manual movements to cause bowel movements to occur, in more than 25 percent of bowel movements
- fewer than three bowel movements in a week

Spinzi also notes that medications cause constipation in about 40 percent of all cases of chronic constipation, including such medications as antihistamines, antidepressants, calcium channel blockers, diuretics, iron pills, narcotics, NONSTEROIDAL ANTI-INFLAMMATORY DRUGS (NSAIDs), and other medications. Sometimes the dosage of medications can be adjusted downward or a non-constipating (or less-constipating) medication can be substituted.

Malnutrition

Some elderly people fail to eat an adequate diet, leading to MALNUTRITION, which is a great threat to their health and self-reliance. They may have decreased ability to taste their food, making food less appetizing and appealing. Older people may

also have delayed gastric emptying due to a variety of reasons, including diabetes, infection, gastro-duodenal surgery, or medications, and this may cause a prolonged feeling of fullness in the stomach in addition to possible nausea, vomiting, and early satiety.

According to Vincenzo Di Franceso and colleagues in their 2007 article in *Digestive Diseases*, the problem of eating a diet that is too low in calories is alluded to as the "anorexia of aging." The authors say, "Dysphagia and poor mastication [chewing of food] interfere with nutritional status either directly or indirectly, by reducing taste sensation. Many drugs, which are widely used in the elderly, may cause anorexia." The authors say that medications that are used to treat gastrointestinal disorders may cause anorexia, such as histamine-2 antagonists, PROTON PUMP INHIBITORS (PPIs), and psyllium. In addition, medications taken for the cardiovascular system, such as digoxsin, amiodarone, furosemide, spironolactone, and theophylline, may lead to loss of appetite.

Malnutrition can lead to a further negative health spiral, according to the authors. They say, "Malnutrition has a dramatic impact on health in the elderly; it impairs the immune system thus increasing the frequency and severity of infectious diseases. In fact malnourished old people have particularly low levels of CD4+ T-helper cells. Malnutrition may cause anemia as well as cognitive decline, osteopenia, altered drug metabolism and sarcopenia. Malnourished elderly run a higher risk of hospitalization, delayed discharge from the hospital and mortality."

Other Digestive Problems

There are a broad array of other digestive diseases and disorders that older people may develop. For example, according to the National Commission on Digestive Diseases in their 2009 report, swallowing disorders are very common among elderly people who are residing in nursing homes, and as many as 30 to 40 percent of nursing home residents have such a problem, compared to about 7 percent of the elderly who are not living in nursing homes.

Dysphagia can lead to an inability to eat an adequate diet, and it also increases the individual's risk for the development of pneumonia. According to the National Commission on Digestive Disease, at least 37 to 45 percent of individuals have post-stroke dysphagia. Most individuals suffering from stroke are elderly individuals.

Medications and the Elderly

Many older people take at least three or more prescribed medications as well as using many over-the-counter (OTC) remedies, while some use ALTERNATIVE MEDICINE as well, including herbs, vitamins, and dietary supplements. There are several common issues that relate to older people and their medications. One is that often the dosage of medication that is needed by an older person may be significantly lower than what is the normally prescribed dosage for younger people. This is in part due to multiple factors, including slowed stomach emptying, changes in body muscle/fat, slowed metabolism of medications, etc.

Another issue is that many medications can interact with one another, increasing or decreasing the effect of other drugs as well as causing unintended and sometimes very serious consequences; as a result, it is very important for the elderly person to advise his or her physician about all medications that are taken, including OTC and alternative remedies such as herbs or dietary supplements. For example, some older people take warfarin (Coumadin), a prescribed blood thinning medication. They should stay away from other drugs that thin the blood, including foods and herbal remedies such as St. John's wort or vitamins such as Vitamin A and E, as well as cranberry, fenugreek, ginkgo biloba, and glucosamine because the increased blood thinning action caused by all of these medications could lead to an incidence of dangerous bleeding, which could be fatal.

Many doctors recommend that elderly individuals obtain all of their medications from one pharmacy, so that the pharmacist can track the drugs and identify any possible or likely interactions before they occur.

A third issue relating to medication use surrounding the elderly is that their failure to comply with the medication regimens that have been ordered by their physicians is a common problem. (It is also a common problem among younger people as well but may be worse among the elderly.) The older

person may forget to take the medications altogether because of dementia or poor memory or may purposely decide to stop taking them, for a wide variety of reasons. Yet medication compliance is important, and failure to follow the doctor's orders could lead to health problems or even death.

See also ADAPTATIONS TO DAILY LIVING AND LIFESTYLE FACTORS; DEMOGRAPHIC FACTORS AND DIGESTIVE DISEASES.

Comparato, Giuseppe, et al. "Diverticular Disease in the Elderly." *Digestive Diseases* 25 (2007): 151–159.

Devon, K. M., et al. "Colorectal Cancer Surgery in Elderly Patients: Presentation, Treatment, and Outcomes." *Diseases of the Colon & Rectum* 52, no. 7 (2009): 1,272–1,277.

Di Franceso, Vincenzo, et al. "The Anorexia of Aging." *Digestive Diseases* 25 (2007): 129–137.

Food Safety and Inspection Service. *Food Safety for Older Adults.* Washington, D.C.: U.S. Department of Agriculture, September 2006.

Gold, Mark, M.D., and Christine Adamec. *The Encyclopedia of Alcoholism and Alcohol Abuse.* New York: Facts On File, 2010.

Kandel, Joseph, M.D., and Christine Adamec. *The A-to-Z Guide to Elder Care.* New York: Checkmark Books, 2009.

National Institute on Alcohol Abuse and Alcoholism. *Harmful Interactions: Mixing Alcohol with Medicines.* Bethesda, Md.: National Institutes of Health, 2007.

Spinzi, G. C. "Bowel Care in the Elderly." *Digestive Diseases* 25 (2007): 160–165.

U.S. Department of Health and Human Services. *Opportunities and Challenges in Digestive Diseases Research: Recommendations of the National Commission on Digestive Diseases.* Bethesda, Md.: National Institutes of Health, March 2009.

electrolytes   Essential chemical substances in the body, both within the cells and in the body fluids, including the blood. Electrolyte levels can become low when an individual has DEHYDRATION, fever, vomiting, and DIARRHEA, as a result of infection or disease. Electrolytes can be replaced with oral hydration solutions or by intravenous feeding in the hospital.

In a matter of hours, illnesses such as cholera can cause massive fluid loss and electrolyte imbalance which can be fatal. Ironically, intravenous potassium is given as part of the three-drug "cocktail" (very high dosages are given) that is used in a lethal injection to execute convicted prisoners.

Mild electrolyte imbalances can be resolved with preparations available at most pharmacies. For example, for children who have mild electrolyte imbalance, the electrolyte Pedialyte may be recommended.

See also CHOLERA.

emergency issues in digestive diseases Some digestive diseases or disorders either are or they may readily become life-threatening conditions, and thus, they require urgent medical attention, as with APPENDICITIS, massive gastrointestinal bleeding, and a severe GALLBLADDER attack that is precipitated by GALLSTONES. In such cases, the individual should not drive him or herself to the doctor's office or hospital. Depending upon the clinical situation, either an ambulance or others in the family or at work should drive the ill person to the hospital emergency room. In these cases, it is best to call 911 so that life-saving medical attention can be provided by emergency medical staff before leaving the site where the ill person is located as well as providing care en route to the hospital.

It should also be noted that some medical problems that may seem like emergencies to the individual often are not actual emergencies, such as the severe pain that can accompany GASTROESOPHAGEAL REFLUX (GERD) and which may seem like a heart attack. However, the reality is that it may actually be a heart attack, even if the person has previously been diagnosed with GERD.

Acute Cholecystitis: A Gallbladder Attack

Cholelithiasis refers to gallbladder stones, and there were 3,114 people of all ages who died of cholelithiasis and other disorders of the gallbladder in 2006, according to the National Center for Health Statistics within the Centers for Disease Control and Prevention (CDC). Of this number, 1,738 were female, and 1,376 were male.

According to Robert A. Casillas, M.D, and colleagues in their 2008 article in *Archives of Surgery*, an early laparoscopic cholecystectomy is the best means of treating acute cholecystitis (gallbladder inflammation and infection). They analyzed the results of 173 patients diagnosed with acute cholecystitis, including 71 treated with an early cholecystectomy and 102 treated with only antibiotic therapy.

Of those who were treated with antibiotics only, the antibiotic therapy was unsuccessful in 45 patients. In addition, of the patients for whom antibiotics did not work, 26 of them had to have a cholecystectomy at a later date, and 19 subjects had a percutaneous cholecystostomy. Cholecystotomy is usually done in cases of poor surgical candidates and involves draining the gallbladder by putting in a drain via an incision in the belly directly into gallbladder. Such a procedure is done by surgeons as well as interventional radiologists.

The researchers concluded that an early laparoscopic cholecystectomy markedly reduced the hospital length of stay for patients and did not incur any major complications in the patients. According to Casillas and colleagues, general surgeons perform about 700,000 laparoscopic cholecystectomies in the United States, and they believe that more of these procedures should be performed.

The researchers said, "In our experience, early LC [laparoscopic cholecystectomy], compared with any other treatment strategy, results in significantly reduced LOS [length of stay in the hospital]. Reduced LOS is likely associated with reduced overall cost for those patients who will ultimately require surgery."

They also added, "Reasons for slow adoption of early LC at our institution and others may include lack of acceptance of current evidence; a persistent, if misguided, belief in the idea of 'cooling off' a 'hot' gallbladder, patient factors such as delayed presentation or comorbidities [other diseases]; surgeon convenience; or resource constraints such as surgeon availability or timely access to operating rooms."

Acute Pancreatitis

An inflammation of the pancreas, acute PANCREATITIS, requires urgent medical attention. ALCOHOL ABUSE and gallstones are the leading causes of acute pancreatitis, but there are many other possible causes, such as an infection, a malignant tumor, CYSTIC FIBROSIS, a scorpion bite, hypercalcemia (excessive levels of calcium in the bloodstream), and the use of some medications. About 2 percent of the cases of acute pancreatitis are fatal, according to the National Commission on Digestive Diseases. This is primarily because of complications that affect other organs, such as the cardiovascular system, the lungs, or the kidneys.

Acute pancreatitis is diagnosed by the individual's symptoms and medical history, the clinical examination, laboratory tests (serum amylase and lipase) as well as with imaging choices, such as computerized tomography (CT) scanning. In fact, experts report that a special CT scan called the spiral CT with contrast dye is best to identify acute pancreatitis. Other tests that may be used to diagnose acute pancreatitis are ultrasound imaging or magnetic resonance imaging (MRI) with gadolinium.

An ENDOSCOPIC RETROGRADE CHOLANGIOPANCREA-TOGRAPHY (ERCP) diagnostic test will identify acute pancreatitis that has persistent stones in the bile duct. On the other hand, the stone may sometimes have passed, and the ERCP findings may be normal. Before the patient with gallstones is discharged from the hospital, he or she frequently will also need surgery to remove the gallbladder (a cholecystectomy). In many cases, however, surgery is postponed for a few weeks.

The patient with severe acute pancreatitis needs to be treated in the intensive care unit (ICU) of the hospital and must be very carefully monitored because of the high risk for death from complications arising due to pancreatitis. Some patients with acute pancreatitis will develop bacterial or fungal infections, which will need to be treated as well. Enteral nutrition, or feeding the patient nutritional fluids with a tube through the nose, preferably into the small bowel and bypassing the stomach, may also be used. However, intragastric feeding has been found to be equally effective in many cases. Patients may also be put on parenteral nutrition depending upon the clinical situation.

Appendicitis

The severe inflammation of the appendix and its rupture is a dangerous situation for anyone experiencing this problem. Many individuals with appendicitis are children or adolescents, but appendicitis can occur in anyone. Fortunately, the death rate with appendicitis is low, and only 424 individuals of all ages died of appendicitis in the United States in 2006, according to the National Center for Health Statistics. According to the National Commission on Digestive Diseases, about 325,000 case of appendicitis are diagnosed each year, usually in the second decade of life (ages 10 to 20).

Sometimes the disorder is managed with high dosages of antibiotics intravenously, as when the patient is in an advanced state of pregnancy or when surgery would be dangerous for another reason. For example, in a 2009 issue of *Obstetrics & Gynecology*, Brett C. Young, M.D., and colleagues discussed a case of a woman at 27 weeks of gestation who was diagnosed with a ruptured appendix and who was treated with antibiotics intravenously. She recovered, but her symptoms recurred again at 32 weeks, and she was again treated with antibiotics. The woman had a cesarean section at 34 weeks when she experienced preterm labor.

An emergency appendectomy can be performed in an open incision in the abdomen, as it has been done for many years, or it may also be performed as a laparoscopic procedure.

In a study by Hong-Bo Wei and colleagues and reported in 2009 in *Surgical Endoscopy*, the researchers analyzed the results of 220 patients, including 108 who underwent open appendectomy (OA) and 112 who had a laparoscopic appendectomy (LA). The researchers found that the LA group was significantly associated with a shorter hospital stay, or an average 4.1 days for the LA group compared to 7.2 days for the OA group.

The LA group also had a shorter time to returning to a general diet or an average of 20.2 days for the LA group versus 36.5 days for the LA group. The LA group was also associated with a shorter time to returning to normal activity (9.1 days for the LA group vs. 13.7 days for the OA group) and to the patient being able to go back to work (21.2 days for the LA group vs. 27.7 days for the OA group).

The researchers said, "Laparoscopic appendectomy is a useful tool in the treatment of acute appendicitis. Its advantages lie in its minimal invasiveness, its better cosmetic outcome, its lower rate of complications based on surgical expertise and state-of-the-art equipment. It can be recommended as an adoptable method for the routine patient with appendicitis."

The time is not far off when the appendectomy will be done using an endoscope and making the cut through the stomach wall to reach the appendix and take it out. This does not involve any external incisions in the abdominal wall and patients could conceivably be discharged shortly after the procedure. The first such patient was treated in India by Dr. N. Reddy. It is an experimental procedure and is being done in select centers in the United States as part of an investigational tool.

Sometimes a laparoscopy is used as a diagnostic tool to determine if a patient actually has appendicitis; however, according to Roland E. Andersson, the use of diagnostic laparoscopy in young women of reproductive age is associated with considerable risk. Andersson says, "Historically, this method of diagnosis has been associated with a high frequency of management errors, especially in women of reproductive age, with high proportions of unproductive surgical explorations of the abdomen and delayed diagnoses that led to increased suffering of the patient and costs to society."

Andersson also noted that a spontaneous improvement of appendicitis commonly occurs, and that not all patients will need to have an appendectomy. He notes that if the diagnosis of appendicitis is unclear, diagnostic imaging can be used to help ascertain the correct diagnosis of the problem.

It should be noted that acute appendicitis may be diagnosed inadvertently during colonoscopy. While a colonoscopy is generally contraindicated during an acute episode of appendicitis, the procedure has been used to drain pus from the appendix in a poor surgical risk patient.

Gastrointestinal Bleeding

Severe gastrointestinal bleeding can be a life-threatening problem for an individual. Such a problem may even be precipitated simply by the use of prescribed blood thinners such as warfarin (Coumadin, Jantoven) that are combined with other substances, such as vitamin E or gingko biloba, which further thin the blood to often dangerously low levels. Even common over-the-counter (OTC) painkillers such as aspirin or naproxen can interact with warfarin to the extent of causing gastrointestinal bleeding.

Individuals who must take warfarin regularly to avoid the risk of blood clots should wear a medical bracelet with this information so that if they are ever injured or unconscious and thus unable to report the medications that they take, the information will be readily available to medical staff, and drug interactions can be thus avoided. The medical bracelet should provide the individual's name, the reason for the use of warfarin, as well as the name and phone numbers of emergency contacts.

Some research has indicated that medications that are used to prevent cardiovascular disease, commonly known as complex antithrombotic therapy (CAT), or the use of two or three antithrombotic medications, can increase the risk of gastrointestinal bleeding. These medications are in the category of anticoagulant-antiplatelet (ACAP) therapy, aspirin-antiplatelet (ASAP) therapy, aspirin-anticoagulant (ASAC) therapy, or TRIP, which is aspirin-anticoagulant-antiplatelet. Patients between ages 60 to 69 years who are prescribed CAT have the highest risk for GI bleeding.

Other Causes of Gastrointestinal Bleeding The use of prescribed or OTC NONSTEROIDAL ANTI-INFLAMMATORY DRUGS (NSAIDs) to treat commonly occurring painful conditions such as arthritis or back pain can lead to gastrointestinal bleeding, as well as leading to the vomiting of blood and the appearance of bright red blood, coffee ground emesis (vomit), or black, tarry stools. These are emergency symptoms that should be immediately reported to the physician.

Individuals who are on kidney dialysis or who have an impaired kidney are at risk for gastrointestinal bleeding because of blood platelet abnormalities.

According to Deborah D. Proctor, M.D., in her article in *Clinics in Chest Medicine* in 2003, upper gastrointestinal (GI) bleeding is about five times more common than is lower GI bleeding. Proctor also noted that 30 percent of those with upper GI bleeding are ages 65 years and older. She also notes that 80 percent of GI bleeds are self-limited—they eventually stop; however, the danger is that bleeding may restart within 48 to 72 hours, and patients whose GI bleed starts again usually have a worse prognosis.

Vomiting Blood If an individual vomits blood, this is a dangerous situation that requires urgent medical treatment. The individual who vomits blood (also known as *hematemesis*) may have CIRRHOSIS of the liver leading to varices. Peptic ulcer disease is also a common cause of an upper GI bleed. It is usually caused by *H. pylori* or NSAID drugs. Another possibility of the cause of acute GI bleeding and the vomiting of blood could be the ingestion of a poison or an excess of a substance such as iron. Vomiting blood may also indicate a severe ulceration of the esophagus. The cause could be frequent vomiting, causing ulcers in the esophagus. HYPEREMESIS GRAVIDARUM is an example of a case of extreme vomiting in a pregnant woman. Sometimes the junction between the esophagus and stomach get torn when a patient is vomiting or even just retching. It is called a Mallory-Weiss tear, and the bleeding usually is self-limiting in most cases.

Identifying and Treating Severe Gastrointestinal Bleeding If the gastroenterologist suspects that a patient has a problem with upper gastrointestinal bleeding, the doctor will often perform an esophagogastroduodenoscopy (EGD), a diagnostic test that allows for visualization as well as treatment. (See MAJOR DIAGNOSTIC TESTS FOR DIGESTIVE DISEASES.) According to Jonathan Cohen, M.D., and colleagues, the EGD is a mainstay therapeutic treatment for upper gastrointestinal bleeding, especially with such problems as a bleeding peptic ulcer, unless it is contraindicated for some reason.

Lower GI bleeding usually originates in the colon (in about 75 percent of the cases). A colonoscopy can help the physician to determine the source of the bleeding. Other tests to help localize the source of the bleeding include an RBC bleeding scan, arteriography, CT, angiography, etc. Arteriography also allows for procedures such as embolization, etc. to help the bleeding stop.

Perforated Ulcer

Ulcers are painful enough for many patients, but a perforated ulcer is an emergency condition. According to the National Center for Health Statistics, 3,323 people of all ages died of a peptic ulcer in the United States in 2006.

According to Bertleff and colleagues in their 2009 article in the *World Journal of Surgery*, a perforated peptic ulcer can be treated with either laparoscopic surgery or open surgery. They studied 101 patients with symptoms of perforated peptic ulcer (PPU). They compared the results of 49 patients receiving a laparotomy (open surgery) versus 52 patients receiving laparoscopic surgery.

The researchers found that the operating time was significantly longer for the patients receiving laparoscopic surgery (75 minutes) than for those in the open group (50 minutes). The researchers said that the laparoscopy group's surgery may have taken longer because the suturing in the laparoscopy is more difficult than with the open surgery.

Complications were about the same between the two groups; however, 4 percent of the laparoscopic group and 8 percent of the open group died. The researchers found no significant difference in the two groups in terms of the length of stay in the hospital or the incidence of complications in the postoperative period.

Studies have found a significantly decreasing rate of perforated peptic ulcers compared to past years; for example, Michael Hermansson and colleagues studied the rates of ulcer complications, and they reported a significant decrease in the incidence of peptic ulcer complications after the introduction of PROTON PUMP INHIBITORS (PPIs) in 1988. The rate of the use of nonsteroidal anti-inflammatory drugs (NSAIDs) for painful conditions such as arthritis, back pain, and so forth was still very high, but PPIs help to reduce toxicity that NSAIDs generate and promote healing.

Bertleff and colleagues also agreed that the need for surgery for peptic ulcer disease (PUD) has dramatically declined, by as much as 50 to 80 percent and for the reason of much more effective acid-reducing medications.

In some cases, clips and even glue (not approved by the FDA) may be applied endoscopically to close the perforation site.

Hospital Emergency Room Visits for Acute Gastrointestinal Illnesses

In an analysis of hospital emergency room visits for acute gastrointestinal illnesses from 1997 to 2006 in the United States, Bechien U. Wu, M.D., and colleagues found that there were approximately 3.9

million visits to the emergency room for patients with an upper gastrointestinal hemorrhage, 2.2 million visits for appendicitis, 1.2 million visits for cholecystitis, and 1.6 million visits for acute pancreatitis. The average waiting time before being seen ranged from an average of 48 minutes for the patients with acute pancreatitis to 61 minutes for those with cholecystitis. There was also a delay in the clinical evaluation in 24 percent of the cases.

One finding that apparently surprised the researchers was that race and ethnicity were significant factors for Hispanic whites, who had to wait longer for to be seen and treated for their digestive disease. For example, the waiting time for non-Hispanic whites being treated for acute pancreatitis was 42.1 minutes, and the wait was 48.0 minutes for non-Hispanic blacks. However, for Hispanic whites with acute pancreatitis, the wait was nearly double, or 81.4 minutes. With regard to appendicitis, the wait for non-Hispanic whites was 43.5 minutes, and it was an even shorter wait of 36.1 minutes for non-Hispanic blacks. But for Hispanic whites with appendicitis, the wait was 91.2 minutes, again, about twice the waiting time. The researchers speculated that the language barrier could be a factor in the delayed waits for Hispanic whites; for example, perhaps extra time was needed to wait for a language interpreter.

The researchers stated:

This finding is consistent with other national trends, but the extent of the disparity for the disease studied was striking. These findings, coupled with recent United States census data that indicate Hispanics to be the fastest-growing segment of the population (accounting for 13.3% of the total US population in 2002), reinforce the need for further efforts to be placed on implementing measures that will help reduce future disparities in ED [emergency department] care. Possible interventions include programs to expand the availability of language interpreters and improve cultural awareness. In addition, efforts to expand ED and urgent care services in Hispanic communities and implementation of language-concordant care in Spanish may help improve overall access as well as reduce the burden on already over-crowded existing EDs.

See also COMPLICATIONS OF DIGESTIVE DISORDERS; DEMOGRAPHIC FACTORS AND DIGESTIVE DISEASES.

Andersson, Roland E. "Laparoscopy for Suspected Appendicitis." *Nature Reviews: Gastroenterology & Hepatology* 6 (2009): 390–391.

Bertleff, Mariëtta J.O.E., et al. "Randomized Clinical Trial of Laparoscopic Versus Open Repair of the Perforated Peptic Ulcer: The LAMA Trial." *World Journal of Surgery* 33 (2009): 1,368–1,373.

Casillas, Robert A., M.D., Sara Yegiyants, M.D., and J. Craig Collins, M.D. "Early Laparoscopic Cholecystectomy Is the Preferred Management of Acute Cholecystitis." *Archives of General Surgery* 143, no 6 (2008): 533–537.

Cohen, Jonathan, M.D., et al. "Quality Indicators for Esophagogastroduodenoscopy." *American Journal of Gastroenterology* 101 (2006): 886–891.

Fiumara, Karen, and Samuel Z. Goldhaber. "A Patient's Guide to Taking Coumadin/Warfarin." *Circulation* 119 (2009): e220–e222.

Heron, Melonie, et al. "Deaths: Final Data for 2006." *National Vital Statistics Report* 57, no. 14 (April 17, 2009). Available online: URL: http://www.cdc.gov/nchs/data/nvsr/nvsr57/nvsr57_pdf. Accessed March 29, 2010.

Minocha, A. "An Endoscopic View of Acute Appendicitis." *New England Journal of Medicine* 339 (1998): 1,481.

Petro M., Minocha A. "Asymptomatic Early Acute Appendicitis Initiated and Diagnosed during Colonoscopy: A Case Report." *World Journal of Gastroenterology* 11, no. 34 (September 14, 2005): 5,398–5,400.

Proctor, Deborah D., M.D. "Critical Issues in Digestive Diseases." *Clinics in Chest Medicine* 24 (2003): 623–632.

U.S. Department of Health and Human Services. *Opportunities and Challenges in Digestive Diseases Research: Recommendations of the National Commission on Digestive Diseases.* Bethesda, Md.: National Institutes of Health, March 2009.

Wei, Hong-Bo, et al. "Laparoscopic versus Open Appendectomy: A Prospective Randomized Comparison. *Surgical Endoscopy* 24, no. 2 (2009): 266–269.

Wu, Bechien U., M.D., Peter A. Banks, M.D., and Darwin L. Conwell, M.D. "Disparities in Emergency Department Wait Times for Gastrointestinal Illnesses: Results from the National Hospital Ambulatory Medical Care Survey, 1997–2006." *American Journal of Gastroenterology* 104 (2009):1,668–1,673.

Young, Brett C., M.D., et al. "Medical Management of Ruptured Appendicitis in Pregnancy." *Obstetrics & Gynecology* 114, no. 2 (2009): 453–456.

encopresis Accidental bowel movement, a problem that usually occurs in small children. Technically, *encopresis* may be defined as a repeated passage of feces in inappropriate places for at least once a month for three months. This frequency and duration criteria are appropriate for patients who are older than four years: younger children may not be fully toilet trained. The possibility of physical abuse should be excluded in small children with encopresis. Some patients with encopresis may have CONSTIPATION with FECAL IMPACTION.

endoscopic retrograde cholangiopancreatography (ERCP) An endoscopic procedure in which the pancreatic and biliary ducts can be examined by the physician, who is usually a gastroenterologist. The ERCP is usually an outpatient procedure, although sometimes a patient may be observed overnight in the hospital after the procedure, depending on the interventions that are undertaken during the procedure. The ERCP is used to diagnose suspected disorders of the bile ducts and the pancreas. Some conditions that may be diagnosed with an ERCP are bile duct stones, strictures (narrowing), and cancerous tumors.

Preoperative antibiotics are administered in cases of suspected bile duct obstruction before ERCP. The patient is given local anesthetic medication to numb the throat before the ERCP, as well as intravenous sedatives to calm him or her during the procedure. Sometimes general anesthesia is used. The physician places the endoscope down the throat. The scope is propelled downward to the duodenum until the doctor reaches the ampulla, where the openings of both the biliary and the pancreatic ducts lie. The doctor then inserts a catheter through the endoscope and penetrates the opening, passing the catheter into the ducts, and then injects radiocontrast dye. Examination under fluoroscopy is performed, and X-rays of the area are taken.

The ERCP not only is a diagnostic procedure but can also be used for therapeutic purposes. For example, a physician who notes a stone in the bile duct can make a cut in the ampulla to widen the opening and can remove the stone with instruments that are inserted through the scope. Similarly, a stricture of the duct can be dilated.

The doctor also may take a biopsy sample to test for cancer.

The aftereffects of ERCP may be a sore throat and feeling of bloating or abdominal pain. In about 5 to 10 percent of patients who have this procedure, pancreatitis may develop. This is an inflammation of the pancreas that may require hospitalization. Death is a rare complication.

See also ENDOSCOPY.

endoscopy A procedure that is performed usually by a physician who is also a gastroenterologist in which a device (the endoscope) is inserted into the gut to visualize the inside of the digestive system. Surgeons and physicians in other specialties may also perform endoscopies. The endoscopy may be an upper endoscopy or a colonoscopy of the colon. Biliary endoscopy is another form of endoscopy. The enteroscopy procedure examines the small intestine.

In an upper endoscopy or esophagogastro-duodenoscopy (EGD), the endoscope is inserted through the throat and into the stomach of the patient for the purpose of detecting the presence of any diseases and disorders of the esophagus, stomach, and duodenum: cancer of the esophagus or stomach, GASTROESOPHAGEAL REFLUX DISEASE, hiatal hernia, peptic ulcer, or a variety of other digestive ailments. The cause of upper gastrointestinal bleeding can be identified and treated as needed.

In biliary endoscopy, or endoscopic retrograde cholangiopancreatography (ERCP), physicians can observe the bile and pancreatic ducts and see any obstructions that may be present such as stones, stricture, or cancer. Occasionally, specialized endoscopes with an ultrasound transducer attached may be used to take sonographic pictures from inside the gut.

In most cases, sedation (also known as conscious sedation or twilight sleep) is administered to the patient; however, some physicians believe that the procedure is actually safer when it is performed without sedation, and it is also less expensive to perform the procedure without sedation. Most endoscopies in the United States are undertaken with sedated patients. In addition, newer and narrower ultrathin endoscopes make sedation less necessary because these endoscopes can be introduced either transnasally (through the nose) or transorally (through the throat) with much less discomfort to the patient.

Reasons Why Gastroenterologists Order Endoscopies

Physicians perform at least 10 million endoscopic procedures each year. In a survey of 276 gastroenterologists nationwide in the United States on the reasons why they performed endoscopies, reported in a 2000 issue of *Gastroenterology* by David A. Lieberman and his colleagues, the researchers found that upper endoscopies (EGD) were most frequently performed to evaluate the cause of abdominal pain or dyspepsia (23.7 percent). Other reasons for performing endoscopies included dysphagia, or difficulty in swallowing (20 percent); acid reflux symptoms (17 percent); suspicion of gastrointestinal bleeding (16.1 percent); and nausea/vomiting (10.9 percent). Other primary reasons for performing endoscopy were checking a patient who had Barrett's esophagus and evaluating chest pain.

Association of Endoscopies with Other Diseases

In an interesting study to determine whether the appendix may play a role in immune-modulation of the gut, Minocha and colleagues studied 524 patients, 55 who had previously had appendectomy and 469 in the control group who had not had this surgery. These findings were reported in a 1999 issue of the *Southern Medical Journal*.

The researchers did find a significant association in individuals who had an appendectomy and needed an endoscopy after the appendectomy (if one was performed). The previous appendectomy group had a rate of 33.46 percent of endoscopies versus the rate of 20.55 of the patients who had not had an appendectomy.

See also COLORECTAL CANCER; SIGMOIDOSCOPY.

Brugge, William R., M.D., and Van Dam, Jacques, M.D. "Pancreatic and Biliary Endoscopy." *New England Journal of Medicine* 341, no. 24 (December 9, 1999): 1,808–1,818.

Lieberman, David A., et al. "Patterns of Endoscopy Use in the United States." *Gastroenterology* 118, no. 3 (2000): 619–624.

Minocha, Anil, M.D., and Radhika Srinivasan, M.D. "Conscious Sedation: Pearls and Perils." *Digestive Diseases and Sciences* 43, no. 8 (August 1998): 1835–1,844.

Minocha, Anil, M.D., et al. "Prevalence of Previous Appendectomy among Patients Needing Gastrointestinal Endoscopy." *Southern Medical Journal* 92, no. 1 (January 1999): 41–43.

Newman, Julliana. "Radiographic and Endoscopic Evaluation of the Upper GI Tract." *Radiologic Technology* 69, no. 3 (January/February 1998): 213–227.

Van Dam, Jacques, M.D., and Brugge, William R., M.D. "Endoscopy of the Upper Gastrointestinal Tract." *New England Journal of Medicine* 341, no. 23 (December 2, 1999): 1,738–1,748.

Wood, Bradford J., and Razavi, Pouneh. "Virtual Endoscopy: A Promising New Technology." *American Family Physician* 66, no. 66 (July 1, 2002): 107–112.

enema   Procedure in which the colon is evacuated (emptied) through the external introduction of water and chemicals into the rectum, thus inducing a bowel movement. Enemas can be self-performed or may be given by other individuals. They are usually used for severe constipation or for emptying of the colon of waste before medical procedures, such as the SIGMOIDOSCOPY or colonoscopy. Enemas may be self-administered through insertable packaged chemicals that can be purchased at pharmacies or supermarkets or may be administered by medical personnel in the home or hospital. Fleet enemas are the most popular brand used; however, different medications are found in different forms of Fleet enemas.

An enema is not the same as a barium enema, which is a procedure performed by a doctor in which barium is inserted into the rectum so that the colon is highlighted and shows up well on X-rays.

enteral nutrition   Food that is provided to a patient through a tube that is placed into the stomach or small intestine and is also called tube feeding. Enteral nutrition may be provided in a long tube that is inserted into the nose and travels to the stomach or the small intestine. Alternatively, it may be provided via a small tube that is inserted directly through the abdominal wall into the stomach or intestine, which can be placed by a physician during an endoscopy or surgery. Radiologists can also place such tubes.

Enteral nutrition is provided to individuals who are unable to eat normally because of illness and/or incapacity but have a functional gut. On the other hand, patients for whom enteral feeding cannot be administered into the gut, such as those who have bowel obstruction, require parenteral nutrition.

See also FEEDING TUBE; PARENTERAL NUTRITION.

enterovirus   A common virus in the picornavirus family that is found worldwide. The virus generally multiplies within the intestinal tract. The coxsackievirus is an example of an enterovirus, as are the poliovirus and echovirus. To identify them better, since 1970, enteroviruses that have been identified have been given numbers, starting with enterovirus 68.

Some enteroviruses can trigger severe diseases, such as encephalitis and meningitis. Older people, small children, and people who have a weakened immune system are usually affected more severely by enteroviruses than other people; for example, enterovirus 71 has been associated with some deaths among children age five and younger.

Transmission of Enteroviruses

Medical researchers believe that enteroviruses are spread by fecal–oral contamination (as occurs after a person does not wash his or her hands after using a toilet and then touches others or touches items that others touch, such as food), and they may be spread through respiration as well (by an infected person's breathing on someone and transmitting the disease).

Symptoms

The symptoms caused by enterovirus vary; they often include nausea, vomiting, and diarrhea, as well as abdominal pain.

Diagnosis and Treatment

Physicians suspect and clinically diagnose an enterovirus illness on the basis of symptoms. Laboratory diagnosis is based on the identification of the virus in the cell culture. Other methods include detection of enterovirus RNA by polymerase chain reaction (PCR) or retrospectively by serologic methods. Cell culture is cumbersome and expensive and is not commonly performed except in cases of mass infections. A blood test for serology may be helpful in select cases.

Patients are treated with antiemetics (to control vomiting) and antidiarrheal drugs (to limit diarrhea). Dehydrated patients may need to be hospitalized, particularly if they are infants, elderly people, or individuals who have a weakened immune system.

See also ANTIDIARRHEALS; ANTIEMETICS; CONTAMINATED FOOD OR WATER; DIARRHEA; NAUSEA AND VOMITING.

Raphael Dolin, M.D. "Enterovirus 71—Emerging Infections and Emerging Questions." *New England Journal of Medicine* 341, no. 13 (September 23, 1999): 984–985.

enzyme   See DIGESTIVE ENZYMES.

eosinophilic gastroenteritis (EG)   A rare disease that is often misdiagnosed as IRRITABLE BOWEL SYNDROME or other disorders. In EG, any part of the gastrointestinal tract, from the ESOPHAGUS to the COLON and including the BILE ducts, can be affected. The disorder affects both adults and children. It is likely caused by an allergic reaction to foods or airborne allergens.

Symptoms and Diagnostic Path

Common symptoms of EG include NAUSEA AND VOMITING, ABDOMINAL PAIN, and DIARRHEA. According to Fouad J. Moawad and colleagues in their 2009 article on EG, the most common symptom is a DYSPHAGIA for solid food. Some patients experience weight loss; others have problems with MALABSORPTION. Patients may also have ANEMIA and fecal blood less as well as weight loss. EG may mimic other conditions such as PANCREATIC CANCER and APPENDICITIS in its symptoms. In addition, PARASITIC INFECTIONS may cause similar symptoms as EG, and thus, the patient's stool needs to be evaluated for parasite.

The gut may become rigid and lead to intestinal obstruction. Patients may also have a fluid-filled abdomen (ASCITES).

Eosinophilic gastroenteritis can be suspected with results from laboratory tests and confirmed by a biopsy of the affected region of the stomach and small intestine or colon, which can be taken during an upper gastrointestinal ENDOSCOPY or colonoscopy as needed. The mucosa of the gut may appear normal in many cases on endoscopy but histopathology of biopsies may suggest otherwise. Therefore, if the disease is suspected, biopsies are done even if the mucosa is normal. In addition, some laboratory tests may provide abnormal results for patients with EG with malabsorption, such as a reduced serum iron concentration and a prolonged prothrombin time. Peripheral eosinophil counts are frequently elevated with EG patients, although they are normal in about 20 percent of patients with EG.

According to Moawad and colleagues, the esophagus of the person with EG has concentric rings, longitudinal furrow, and other characteristic findings that are common in a patient with EG.

Treatment Options and Outlook

Mild cases of EG can be treated symptomatically; for example, antidiarrheal medications are given to patients to treat diarrhea, and iron supplementation is given in cases of an iron deficiency. A targeted elimination diet after appropriate testing may benefit some patients. The treatment also usually includes the administration of a steroid, such as prednisone. The steroid is administered to patients for two weeks; then the dosage is tapered over two more weeks A few patients may require prolonged treatment. Some patients are administered systemic corticosteroids in an inhalant form. Another form of treatment is to dilate the esophagus if there is a stricture (this is done very carefully, since such patients are at high risk for perforation).

EG patients may experience flares of the disease months or years later, requiring short-term dosages of prednisone, which are tapered off. Some patients have also been treated with oral cromolyn, ketotifen, montelukast, etc., with benefit in some patients although data from randomized controlled trials is lacking.

When allergies are suspected, patients undergo skin prick testing, and if allergies are confirmed, those substances are avoided. The most common substances found to be the causal allergens when patients with EG have food allergies are dairy eggs, wheat, soy, peanuts, and seafood. Avoiding these substances bring improvement to an estimated two-thirds of patients with EG.

Risk Factors and Preventive Measures

EG is most likely an allergic disorder. EG may be caused by intestinal parasites; often the cause cannot be determined. Approximately 50 percent of patients who have EG have other allergic disorders, such as asthma, eczema, or rhinitis, while others may just show increased serum IgE levels.

According to Ahsan Baig and colleagues, most cases of EG are found in whites, with some cases found among Asians. Most patients are in their 30s to their 50s, but patients can be of any age. Males are slightly more likely to have EG than females.

See also FOOD ALLERGIES.

Ahsan Baig, Muhammad, M.D., Abdul Qadir, M.D., and Javeria Rasheed, M.D. "A Review of Eosinophilic Gastroenteritis." *Journal of the National Medical Association* 98, no. 10 (2006): 1,616–1,619.

Moawad, Fouad J., Ganesh R. Veerappan, and Roy K. Wong. "Eosinophilic Esophagitis." *Digestive Diseases Science* 54 (2009): 1,818–1,828.

Escherichia coli (E. coli) Common bacteria normally found in the colon of humans and animals, some strains acquire certain genetic material and they can become pathogenic to cause infection. *E. coli* may also be found in contaminated foods, such as meat or other foods that are prepared under unsanitary conditions.

Sometimes swimmers contract *E. coli* from swimming in water or swimming pools that are contaminated with feces and are inadequately chlorinated.

Types of E. coli

There are several forms of harmful *E. coli,* such as enterohemorrhagic *E. coli* (EHEC). This bacterium causes bloody diarrhea, and it may also lead to kidney failure in adults and children who have weakened immune systems. The most common harmful form of EHEC that is found in the United States as of this writing is O157:H7, which can severely harm the intestinal lining as well as cause hemolytic uremic syndrome (HUS), which can be fatal. Antibiotics are not useful against *E. coli* O157:H7, and treatment is symptomatic. Other harmful types of *E. coli* are also found in the United States.

Foods in Which E. coli is Most Commonly Found

Although any food can theoretically be contaminated by *E. coli*, this bacterium has been found most frequently in the following types of foods:

- raw or undercooked hamburger
- lettuce
- salami
- unpasteurized milk, apple cider, and apple juice
- contaminated well water

Symptoms of E. coli O157:H7 Infection

Common symptoms of the most frequently found strain of *E. coli* (O157:H7) are as follows:

- watery or bloody diarrhea
- nausea
- painful abdominal cramps

Some patients also have low-grade fever and may experience vomiting. If the disease is caused by contaminated food, the patient's symptoms usually start within two to five days of the time the food is ingested. Symptoms may last up to eight days.

Other Types of E. coli Infection

Enterotoxigenic *E. coli* (ETEC) is usually the cause of "traveler's diarrhea," an infection that develops when tourists consume contaminated food or water.

Another form of *E. coli* is enteropathogenic *E. coli* (EPEC). This form causes diarrhea that lasts two weeks or longer. It is transmitted through contaminated water or infected animals.

Diagnosis and Treatment

The physician diagnoses patients with *E. coli* infections on the basis of symptoms as well as results from laboratory stool sample tests. Generally, patients are advised to rest and to drink plenty of water to prevent dehydration. Antibiotics are not effective for diarrheal illness in most cases, and they are usually not prescribed. However, antibiotics may be helpful in selected cases of traveler's diarrhea.

Preventing E. coli Infections

To prevent the food-borne transmission of *E. coli*, experts recommend that individuals take the following actions:

- Avoiding raw and undercooked beef products
- Drinking no unpasteurized milk or juices
- Washing fresh fruits and vegetables, whether they are to be eaten raw or cooked

See also CONTAMINATED FOOD OR WATER; DIARRHEA; TRAVEL.

esophageal cancer A malignant tumor of the ESOPHAGUS, the food tube that lies between the throat and the stomach. The esophagus is sited behind the trachea (the windpipe) and travels downward; the average length of the adult esophagus is 10 inches.

There are two basic types of esophageal cancer: squamous cell carcinoma and adenocarcinoma. Squamous cell carcinoma usually occurs in the upper esophagus, while adenocarcinoma occurs in the lower esophagus, especially near the gastroesophageal junction. According to research published in 2009 by Ahmedin Jemal and colleagues in *CA: A Cancer Journal for Clinicians*, there were 16,470 new cases of esophageal cancer in 2009, including 12,940 in men and 3,530 in women. There were also an estimated 14,530 deaths from esophageal cancer, including 11,490 men and 3,040 women who died. The incidence of squamaous cell carcinoma has been decreasing in recent decades. Most cases of esophageal adenocarcinoma are preceded by BARRETT'S ESOPHAGUS, a precancerous condition that occurs after years of untreated GASTROESOPHAGEAL REFLUX DISEASE (GERD).

Symptoms and Diagnostic Path

Many patients have no symptoms in the early stages of esophageal cancer. When symptoms occur, they may include some or all of the follow-ing indicators:

- difficulty in swallowing (DYSPHAGIA)
- weight loss
- pain in the throat or between the shoulder blades of the back
- chronic cough
- chronic hoarseness
- vomiting

Physicians diagnose esophageal cancer on the basis of the patient's symptoms, the findings of the physical examination, and the results of testing. The most frequently appearing symptom is dys-phagia, which is difficulty with swallowing foods or even liquids that may be accompanied by PAIN when eating or drinking is attempted. Initially, the dysphagia occurs with solids only. Progres-sively, it gets worse, and difficulty in swallowing liquids indicates a more severe dysphagia than is found when patients have difficulty with eating solid foods only. The patient may also be hoarse and constantly clear the throat. Another indicator is weight loss when a patient has not tried to lose weight. In this case, weight loss is usually caused by the patient's difficulties with eating as well as the effect of meeting the increased metabolic demands due to cancer.

The presence of esophageal cancer may be suggested by an abnormal result found with the barium swallow test of the esophagus, in which barium is swallowed by the patient and the phy-sician observes its passage down the esophagus by using a fluoroscope. In the case of abnormal barium swallow results, and in many cases without a barium swallow, the doctor usually recommends an ENDOSCOPY, in which a slender tube with a camera lens is inserted down the patient's throat. The endoscopy enables the physician to view the interior of the esophagus on the monitor, and he or she can also take biopsy specimens (small tissue samples) to check for cancer.

Other tests may include a computed tomog-raphy (CT) scan, endoscopic ultrasound, and a bone scan to determine whether cancer has spread beyond the esophagus.

If the test results and the subsequent biopsy findings reveal that the patient has esophageal cancer, the disease is staged: The physician deter-mines how advanced the cancer is and how fast it is growing. The doctor also seeks to determine whether the cancer has spread (metastasized) to other organs; if it has, the disease is usually not curable, although patients may try treatments in attempts to delay any further spread of cancer, as well as to provide symptomatic relief.

Physicians also check for any spread to nodes in the surrounding area; if there is spreading, the prognosis is not good. Lymph nodes are tiny immune organs that work to remove toxins from the body. Progression to the lymph nodes in cases of esophageal cancer tends to occur early. Once cancer involves the lymph nodes, this indicates a poorer prognosis.

Treatment Options and Outlook

Assuming that the cancer has not reached a stage in which treatment would be futile, the most common form of treatment is surgical resection, which is removal of the part of the esophagus that is cancerous. The stomach may be pulled up and hooked to the remaining healthy esophagus, or the removed part may be replaced with a part of the patient's colon.

After surgery, the patient may need to receive nutrition intravenously, at least for a while, because swallowing is difficult or painful. Alternatively, during the surgical resection, the FEEDING TUBE may be inserted into the small intestine, directly through the abdominal wall, and liquid nutrition can be provided until patients can eat without it again.

In addition to surgery, physicians may use radiation therapy and/or chemotherapy, which is the use of drugs given to destroy cancer cells. In patients in whom cancer has spread beyond the limits of a curative resection, a stent (tubing that is made of synthetic material) may be placed into the esophagus to keep it open so that the patient may swallow. Laser and photodynamic therapy may also be used.

The patient may also be offered an opportunity to join a clinical trial, a formal study of drugs or treatments that are being tested for their effectiveness in combating esophageal cancer (or other cancers or diseases). When a patient with an advanced form of cancer joins a clinical trial, he or she may have access to an experimental medication or treatment that is not otherwise available.

Risk Factors and Preventive Measures

In the United States, men are about twice as likely to have esophageal cancer as women. Age is another factor in the development of esophageal cancer, and the risk is greatest for individuals between the ages of 50 and 70 years. According to James E. Everhart, M.D., in *The Burden of Digestive Diseases in the United States*, published in 2008, about two-thirds of all new cases of esophagus squamous cell cancer in 2004 occurred to those ages 65 and older. The same was true for esophageal adenocarcinoma.

Everhart also reports that blacks had the highest incidence of esophageal squamous cell cancer, or 3.2 per 100,000 people, followed by whites and Asian/Pacific Islanders, who each had a rate of 1.7 per 100,000 people. The rates were lowest for Hispanics, or 0.7 per 100,000 individuals.

With regard to the incidence of esophageal adenocarcinoma in 2004, Everhart reported that the rate was higher among males (3.8 per 100,000) than females (0.6 per 100,000). In considering race and ethnicity, the highest rates were among whites, or 3.4 per 100,000, followed by Hispanics at 0.7 per 100,000 people. The highest rates worldwide are found in China, Iran, France, and South Africa.

Other factors that are associated with esophageal cancer are a low intake of fresh fruits and vegetables, ACHALASIA, the presence of the human papillomavirus, and lye-induced strictures of the esophagus. Environmental exposure to radiation or asbestos may also play a role in the development of esophageal cancer.

The differences in risk factors for squamous cell and adenocarcinoma include the following:

1. Alcohol is an increased risk for squamous cell cancer but not adenocarcinoma.
2. Adenocarcinoma is more common among whites; squamous cell cancer is found more often among blacks.
3. Barrett's esophagus is not a risk factor for squamous cell cancer.

Everhart, James E., M.D., ed. *The Burden of Digestive Diseases in the United States*. Washington, D.C.: National Institute of Diabetes and Digestive and Kidney Diseases, 2008.

Jemal, Ahmedin, et al. "Cancer Statistics, 2009." *CA: A Cancer Journal for Clinicians* 59 (2009): 225–249. Available online. URL: http://caonline.amcancersoc.org/cgi/reprint/59/4/225?ijkey=b939af835bcd5e 227911f9c2e179a4502a3fe4f7. Accessed August 18, 2009.

esophagitis An inflammation of the ESOPHAGUS (the upper food tube). The esophagus may also be ulcerated, in the condition called ulcerative esophagitis. Esophagitis may be caused by a disease, such as GASTROESOPHAGEAL REFLUX DISEASE, or other factors, such as use of medications (such as tetracycline). It may also be caused by infections.

Symptoms and Diagnostic Path

Individuals who have esophagitis may have chest pain and experience painful swallowing of foods or even liquids. Other symptoms of esophagitis include nausea and vomiting. Fever may be seen in some cases of infectious esophagitis. Physicians take a complete medical history and examine the throat. An ENDOSCOPY is frequently indicated in many cases of esophagitis, especially of suspected infectious esophagitis.

Treatment Options and Outlook

If the physician finds that the patient is infected with CANDIDA organisms or a viral infection, then appropriate medications can be prescribed. If the doctor believes that other illnesses, such as diabetes, are predisposing the patient to esophagitis, in addition to fighting the infection, he or she urges the patient to work hard to reach a blood glucose level that is as close to normal as possible.

If the patient's esophagitis is caused by medications, doctors should consider another medication as well as advise the patient to take the drug while in an upright position with at least a glass of water. Sometimes changing from a capsule to a tablet form of the medication can help resolve much of the problem.

Risk Factors and Preventive Measures

Esophagitis may also be induced by infections, such as *Candida* infection (particularly by *Candida albicans*), CYTOMEGALOVIRUS, and herpes. Patients who have a weakened immune system, such as those who have HUMAN IMMUNODEFICIENCY VIRUS (HIV) or cancer, are more prone to development of such infection.

People in the following categories are more likely to have infectious esophagitis than others:

- patients with diabetes
- patients who are alcoholics
- patients who are on chemotherapy drugs
- patients who have had organ transplantation and are taking immunosuppressive drugs

Some patients have had ulcers in the esophagus as a consequence of an infection with viruses.

Pill Esophagitis Sometimes esophagitis is caused by medications; the disorder is called pill esophagitis. The key drugs that induce this form of esophagitis include tetracycline antibiotics, iron, ascorbic acid, and potassium chloride. Tetracycline used for acne in adolescents, and alendronate (Fosamax) used to treat osteoporosis in the elderly are both common culprits in causing pill esophagitis. The form of the drug is also significant; for example, according to Drs. Minocha and Greenbaum, gelatin capsules are more adhesive in nature and thus, more likely to stick to the tissue in the esophagus. An additional problem occurs if patients take medicine at bedtime while lying down. The authors write: "Sometimes even large quantities of water may fail to dislodge the tablet stuck in the esophagus. Similarly, swallowing in a supine position [lying down] delays esophageal transit. Esophageal clearance of pills taken at bedtime is also delayed by marked decreases in salivation and swallowing that occur during sleep."

See also BARRETT'S ESOPHAGUS; ESOPHAGEAL CANCER; DYSPHAGIA.

Minocha, Anil, M.D., and David S. Greenbaum, M.D. "Pill-Esophagitis Caused by Nonsteroidal Antiinflammatory Drugs." *American Journal of Gastroenterology* 86, no. 8 (1991): 1,086–1,089.

esophagus The food tube that connects the throat to the stomach. The esophagus is a part of the digestive system. If problems arise, the esophagus may become inflamed (ESOPHAGITIS). If an individ-

ual has chronic GASTROESOPHAGEAL REFLUX DISEASE, in which some food that has already been acidified by the stomach travels backward up the esophagus, this condition can cause esophagitis. Chronic acid reflux may also cause BARRETT'S ESOPHAGUS, a precancerous condition. Infections caused by viruses or fungi may occur in the esophagus of patients who have a compromised immune system, such as patients who have acquired immunodeficiency syndrome (AIDS). The incidence of cancer of the esophagus is rising in the United States.

See also ACID REFLUX; ESOPHAGEAL CANCER.

exercise Physical activity that achieves the goals of improving digestion, maintaining a healthy weight, and improving an individual's overall physical and emotional health. Physicians believe that at least some form of exercise is advisable for most people. Exercise reduces the risk of medical problems such as constipation. It can also decrease the risk of some diseases; for example, a study reported in 1999 in the *New England Journal of Medicine* found that physical activity (or inactivity) is an independent risk factor for decreasing (or increasing) the risk of a cholecystectomy among women.

Many experts believe that walking, one of the simplest exercises that can be performed, is recommended for most ambulatory people. Even elderly individuals who are wheelchair bound may be able to perform some simple exercises. Exercise reduces not only the risk of heart disease, but also the risk for development of many cancers, including cancers of the digestive system.

Tailoring Exercise

Exercise should be tailored to the individual's health and abilities, and any medical problems that are present should also be considered. For example, individuals who have GASTROESOPHAGEAL REFLUX DISEASE should avoid exercises that cause abdominal strain, such as weightlifting.

National Problems with Physical Inactivity in the United States

A lack of physical activity and exercise can lead to problems such as overweight and obesity. Many people in the United States are physically inactive,

EXAMPLES OF MODERATE AMOUNTS OF PHYSICAL ACTIVITY*

Common Chores	Sporting Activities
Washing and waxing a car for 45–60 minutes	Playing volleyball for 45–60 minutes
Washing windows or floors for 45–60 minutes	Playing touch football for 45 minutes
Gardening for 30–45 minutes	Walking 1¾ miles in 35 minutes (20 min/mile)
Wheeling self in wheelchair for 30–40 minutes	Basketball (shooting baskets) for 30 minutes
Pushing a stroller 1½ miles in 30 minutes	Bicycling 5 miles in 30 minutes
Raking leaves for 30 minutes	Dancing fast (social) for 30 minutes
Walking 2 miles in 30 minutes (15 min/mile)	Water aerobics for 30 minutes
Shoveling snow for 15 minutes	Swimming laps for 20 minutes
Stairwalking for 15 minutes	Basketball (playing a game) for 15–20 minutes
	Jumping rope for 15 minutes
	Running 1½ miles in 15 minutes (15 min/mile)

*A moderate amount of physical activity is roughly equivalent to physical activity that uses approximately 150 calories of energy per day, or 1,000 calories per week. Some activities can be performed at various intensities; the suggested durations correspond to expected intensity of effort.

and that is one reason for the high rate of obesity. According to the National Center for Health Statistics in their 2002 Advance Data report, 35.4 percent of men and 40.9 percent of women ages 18 and older were physically inactive in 1997–98. The percentages of people who are physically inactive increase with age: nearly half (47.9 percent) of people 65 to 74 years are physically inactive.

In looking at exercise and race and ethnicity, whites (34.5 percent) and Asians (38.2 percent) have the lowest rates of physical inactivity; more than half of blacks (50.2 percent) and Hispanics (53.2 percent) are physically inactive.

Physical activity is clearly correlated with education. Among people with less than a high school education, 60.1 percent are physically inactive. Of people who have a high school diploma in the United States, 43.3 percent are inactive. The least inactive group (which, turning it around, means the most physically active group) were people who have a master's degree or higher level of education: only 21.8 percent were physically inactive.

In considering the geographic region of the country, the most inactive people are found in the South (44.2 percent) and the least inactive people in the West (32.2 percent).

See also ANOREXIA NERVOSA; BULIMIA NERVOSA; EATING DISORDERS; OBESITY.

failure to thrive (FTT) Condition in which an INFANT or a small child up to the age of two years old does not eat adequately and shows markedly abnormal growth (or no growth) as well as development that is much slower than is normally expected for a child in this age group. Rather than growing and increasing proportionately in weight, as is normal for healthy children, some children who have failure to thrive (FTT) are actually losing weight, causing concern or alarm.

For about 1 to 5 percent of children younger than age two who are admitted to the hospital, failure to thrive is diagnosed. Children in orphanages may experience failure to thrive, particularly when they receive minimal care and caregivers vary from day to day.

Studies of children who have FTT have shown that about half are below the 5th percentile in terms of growth and weight—that means that 95 percent of all other children are taller and weigh more. Some people also use the term *failure to thrive* to describe ELDERLY patients who are losing weight and declining in health, but not as a result of any apparent medical problem. However, most experts use the term exclusively to describe severely undernourished and late-developing infants and children.

The failure to thrive is a cause for concern for both parents and pediatricians, because the condition can lead to (or can indicate already-existing) developmental delays and/or emotional problems. Some experts believe that FTT may indicate a neuroendocrine disturbance resulting from emotional deprivation; however, one should not assume that children with FTT have uncaring parents unless there is clear evidence of child abuse or neglect.

There are two classifications of failure to thrive: organic and nonorganic. Organic failure to thrive may be caused by a chronic severe medical problem; it may also be an indicator of a genetic disorder with an early onset. Organic causes of FTT include the following medical problems:

- gastroesophageal reflux disease (GERD)
- postnatal infections
- CYSTIC FIBROSIS
- Milk protein intolerance
- HUMAN IMMUNODEFICIENCY VIRUS (HIV) infection
- intestinal parasites
- congenital heart disease

In contrast, nonorganic failure to thrive may result from social disruption, an emotional disorder, starvation, maternal drug addiction, or other causes. Severe abuse and neglect are also causes of nonorganic failure to thrive among some children.

Risk Factors

Mothers in poor neighborhoods and who are drug abusers are more likely to have children who are diagnosed with FTT. Malnourished mothers are also more likely to have infants who fail to thrive. There appears to be an increased incidence of FTT among some children who are receiving Medicaid, as well as among those who are homeless or living in rural areas.

Symptoms of Failure to Thrive

Infants with failure to thrive usually appear listless, apathetic, and weak. They may appear malnourished and exhibit poor muscular development. Some babies with FTT exhibit behavior that is characteristic of this condition; for example, according to *The Encyclopedia of Child Abuse*, "Infants suffering from the sensory deprivation associated with FTT often maintain a posture in which the arms are held out, flexed at the elbow with the hands up and legs drawn in. This position of apparent surrender is held for long periods of time."

Diagnosis and Treatment

Laboratory tests cannot diagnose the presence of failure to thrive, but they are a useful adjunct. Thus, tests, including a complete blood count (CBC) and a complete metabolic profile, should be done judiciously. Laboratory tests to search for a cause should be ordered on the basis of clues obtained from the medical history and the physical examination.

Tests can only screen out other medical problems, such as infections, low thyroid level, vitamin deficiencies, or other medical illnesses. Physicians base a diagnosis of failure to thrive on a comparison of the child's past height and weight to his or her current height and weight as well as to those of children who are of the same age. If the child is not growing or is actually losing weight, then the physician actively seeks to identify the problem and resolve it.

The physician is in close contact with the family, assisting them with ways to help the child improve. If the doctor thinks that the family is in some way causing the child's failure to thrive, he or she must report the family to the authorities who oversee and investigate child abuse and neglect accusations. Some physicians may worry that placing the child in foster care could cause further harm; however, if the underlying problem is abuse or neglect, then remaining with the family could cause further deterioration of the child's health or even the death of the child.

See also MALNUTRITION.

Clark, Robin E., Judith Freeman Clark, with Christine Adamec. *The Encyclopedia of Child Abuse.* 2d ed. New York: Facts On File, 2000.

familial juvenile polyposis (FJP) A hereditary condition with an onset in childhood in which a patient has at least 10 POLYPS (abnormal growths of tissue) of the juvenile type. This condition occurs in one in 100,000 live births. These polyps can lead to the development of COLORECTAL CANCER. Children with a family history of this condition should be screened for familial juvenile polyposis. Familial juvenile polyposis is different from familial adenomatous polyposis (FAP): up to 20 percent of patients with FJP develop cancer, whereas in FAP, the long-term risk of cancer is 100 percent.

In late childhood or early adolescence, patients with this condition have rectal bleeding. In most cases, the polyps are located in the colon, but sometimes they may also be seen throughout the digestive tract. Rarely, they may be found only in the stomach. The polyps usually range in size from five millimeters to five centimeters.

Symptoms and Diagnostic Path

Although many patients with this condition have no symptoms, especially in the early stages, if symptoms do occur, they may include the following:

- visible blood in the stool
- DIARRHEA or CONSTIPATION
- ABDOMINAL PAIN
- rectal prolapse of the polyp
- intestinal obstruction
- fatigue due to ANEMIA

Familial juvenile polyposis patients are also at increased risk for development of cancer of the colon, which may occur at an average age of 37 years.

Polyposis can be diagnosed with a colonoscopy, barium enema, or sigmoidoscopy; colonoscopy gives the most comprehensive results. If polyps are present and they are few in number, they are removed by the physician, usually during a colonoscopy. A biopsy can help distinguish juvenile polyps from other kinds of polyps.

Treatment Options and Outlook

Colonoscopic polypectomy with regular periodic surveillance colonoscopy is probably adequate therapy when only a small number of polyps are present. Prophylactic surgery may be used for patients who have a large number of polyps, as well as those who have large polyps that cannot be removed by an endoscopy or patients with a strong family history of colon cancer. An upper endoscopy or an upper gastrointestinal X-ray with a small bowel X-ray is also recommended as part of the surveillance of patients with familial juvenile polyposis, starting at the age of 25 years.

Risk Factors and Preventive Measures

Children with a family medical history of familial juvenile polyposis should be screened for this disorder. There are no known preventive measures against the initial development of this disease.

See also ENDOSCOPY; MULTIPLE LYMPHOMATOUS POLYPOSIS.

fasting Purposely avoiding consuming food and sometimes fluids as well for a given period. Fasting may be done for a religious purpose or because of a belief that fasting somehow "cleans out" the body. Fasting may be perceived as therapeutic, but it can become dangerous if it extends beyond the duration that an individual's body can handle. Individuals who are also avoiding fluids may experience severe DEHYDRATION.

Fasting may be undertaken on physician orders, for example, before ENDOSCOPY or an ultrasound test for the gallbladder. Prolonged fasting may also be appropriate in situations in which food intake may worsen a condition, as in acute PANCREATITIS. However, if fasting is continued for more than several days, PARENTERAL NUTRITION is administered.

See also ANOREXIA NERVOSA; DIET DRUGS.

fecal impaction A condition of severe constipation in which the person's stools become stuck and cannot be moved normally through a bowel movement, often because they are very hard and solid, and bowel movements are too sluggish.

Symptoms and Diagnostic Path

In most cases, the person has not had a bowel movement for at least two or three days, and possibly for a much longer period. On occasion, the person who has fecal impaction may have loose stools, which are liquefied stools that are trying to pass around the blockage that is being caused by the impacted stool.

Treatment Options and Outlook

If the person who has fecal impaction cannot cause the removal of the feces with the use of laxatives or enemas, he or she must be disimpacted manually by medical personnel or others to resolve the blockage created by the stool and allow bowel movements to occur. Over the long term, individuals who have been diagnosed with fecal impaction are often advised to take stool softeners and/or laxatives on a regular basis, along with drinking plenty of fluid, to prevent a recurrence of the problem. The treatment for fecal impaction is individualized by the physician, on the basis of the patient's clinical situation and on the cause that precipitated the impaction.

Risk Factors and Preventive Measures

The problem of fecal impaction is most commonly found among elderly individuals in nursing homes, as well as among those who have severe physical and/or mental and/or developmental disabilities. Sometimes use of medications that strongly slow action of the gut can lead to fecal impaction, particularly prolonged use of narcotic painkillers, which can lead to narcotic bowel syndrome.

See also CONSTIPATION; NARCOTIC BOWEL SYNDROME.

feeding tube A flexible cylindrical tube into which nutrition formula is placed when a person is unable to eat and swallow food normally, such as after a severe accident or serious medical procedure, or during a severe chronic illness. In addition, some very weak older people or younger individuals who are permanently disabled may need to receive nutrition through a feeding tube on a regular basis. The feeding tube may be inserted through the nose down through the throat and threaded directly into the stomach. A patient's nutritional and fluid needs are calculated on the basis of his or her height and weight and then delivered through the tube.

Patients requiring long-term feeding may have a feeding tube placed directly into the stomach (gastrostomy) or the small intestine (jejunostomy) through the abdominal wall, bypassing both the nose and the throat. These tubes can be placed by gastroenterologists, surgeons, and radiologists, using different techniques.

See also ENTERAL NUTRITION; PARENTERAL NUTRITION.

fiber Vegetable matter from plant cell walls, which is often included in the diet as an aid to bowel function and helps to protect against the development of cancer. Fiber is found in such items as wheat bran and some fruits and vegetables, as well as in oats, beans, peas, and other vegetables. A high-fiber diet may also help to lower high CHOLESTEROL levels. It can also often prevent problems with constipation. Commercial forms of fiber that are available in the United States include Metamucil, Citrucil, and Fibercon, as well as many other brands.

Some experts believe that the risk of development of colorectal cancer can be reduced by increasing the amount of dietary fiber. In a study reported in a 2003 issue of the *Lancet,* the researchers described their study of dietary fiber intake and the subsequent development of colorectal cancer in more than a half-million individuals ages 25 to 70 years old in 10 European countries who participated in the European Prospective Investigation into Cancer and Nutrition (EPIC). According to the researchers, fiber reduced the risk of colorectal cancer development in some individuals: "In populations with low average intake of dietary fibre, an approximate doubling of total fibre intake from foods could reduce the risk of colorectal cancer by 40 percent."

A high-fiber diet is not always advisable; for example, it is not recommended when a person has severe GASTROPARESIS or megacolon, because it can worsen both conditions. Often people who have DIABETES MELLITUS have gastroparesis.

See also COLORECTAL CANCER; CONSTIPATION.

Bingham, Sheila A., et al. "Dietary Fibre in Food and Protection against Colorectal Cancer in the European Prospective Investigation into Cancer and Nutrition (EPIC): An Observational Study." *Lancet* 361, no. 9368 (May 3, 2003): 1,496–1,501.

fibromyalgia syndrome (FMS) A chronic and widespread muscle pain disorder that is also often associated with the ACID REFLUX that occurs in people who are diagnosed with GASTROESOPHAGEAL REFLUX DISEASE. In addition, many people who are diagnosed with fibromyalgia also have arthritis and IRRITABLE BOWEL SYNDROME as well as several other chronic pain disorders, such as migraines and irritable bladder. An estimated six million people in the United States have fibromyalgia. It is unknown how many people have this medical problem worldwide.

Researchers such as Roland Staud, M.D., at the University of Florida in Gainesville, have found in clinical studies that people who have fibromyalgia are more pain-sensitive than others and that their pain lasts longer. Despite this research finding, there are still many medical doctors and other experts who persist in believing that fibromyalgia is not a "real" medical problem, and that people exhibiting such symptoms should be referred to psychiatrists for treatment, rather than to rheumatologists or pain management centers.

Symptoms and Diagnostic Path
Rheumatologists have identified 18 specific "tender points" throughout the body that people with fibromyalgia may have, and if an individual experiences pain when at least 11 of these points are gently pressed, then the physician may diagnose fibromyalgia. These tender points may be very painful to the touch, although the physician cannot feel any bumps or other differences from other areas. (Tender points are not the same as trigger points, which are painful areas that the physician can actually feel when touching them.)

Other symptoms of fibromyalgia include overall muscle stiffness (particularly stiffness that is experienced in the morning, when the patient first wakes up) and extreme fatigue. Some patients also experience a mild form of mental confusion that some experts have labeled "fibro fog," in which they forget appointments and lose items, symptoms that are also common to adults who have attention deficit disorder. Most people with fibromyalgia also have chronic sleep problems, including difficulty in falling asleep and/or frequent wakening. These sleep problems may be part of the reason for the confusion.

In addition to palpating the tender points that are commonly associated with fibromyalgia, physicians usually order laboratory tests (such as blood and urine tests) to rule out other medical problems. There are no specific medical tests that detect fibromyalgia. It is also possible—and indeed it is common—for patients to have both fibromyalgia and other illnesses. Generally, physicians diagnose fibromyalgia on the basis of physical examination, medical history, and results of laboratory tests.

Treatment Options and Outlook

Fibromyalgia is treated by some experts with recommended lifestyle changes, such as the avoidance of foods and drinks that contain caffeine, including soft drinks and chocolate. Some individuals who have fibromyalgia improve by avoiding citrus fruits and foods that contain monosodium glutamate (MSG), a flavor enhancer that is added to many canned and frozen foods. Weight loss among individuals with FMS who are obese may also help to improve the condition, and exercise is also recommended; however, exercise should not be overly vigorous, since some fibromyalgia patients may tire rapidly and may be injured more readily than others.

Individuals with fibromyalgia may need medications such as nonsteroidal anti-inflammatory medications or painkilling drugs. Some doctors believe that guaifenesin, a cough medicine, may be helpful in treating fibromyalgia. Guaifenesin is a mild analgesic and a mild muscle relaxant, and it may make some individuals feel better, although it is not a cure for fibromyalgia. Mild doses of antidepressants may help some patients, even when they are not depressed. Such drugs can also help improve problems with sleep.

Massage therapy and/or meditation may be helpful. Patients should avoid vigorous and painful massages, which can exacerbate overall pain. Some patients improve with hypnotherapy.

Some physicians also treat the pain of fibromyalgia with botulinum toxin (Botox) injections into several painful areas. (Botox is also used by cosmetic surgeons to rid the face of facial wrinkles temporarily.) Botox treatment for fibromyalgia is controversial, and it is also very expensive. Beyond some anecdotal reports from some physicians of success with their patients, it is still unknown as of this writing whether Botox injections are a good treatment for fibromyalgia.

Risk Factors and Preventive Measures

Fibromyalgia is a condition that is more commonly diagnosed among women than men (although men can have fibromyalgia, too, as can children), and it is also diagnosed most frequently among females of childbearing age, although it is not known whether this group most often has a diagnosis of FMS because physicians assume that older or younger individuals (or men) never have fibromyalgia.

See also PAIN.

Staud, Roland, M.D., and Christine Adamec. *Fibromyalgia for Dummies,* 2nd ed. New York: John Wiley & Sons, 2007.

fish oil Generally capsules that contain oil extracted from fish. Fish oil has anti-inflammatory qualities, but it can cause digestive problems such as abdominal discomfort, heartburn, or diarrhea. However, when it is enteric-coated, fish oil can be tolerated by most people.

In one small study of 78 patients with Crohn's disease who were in remission, reported in a 1996 issue of the *New England Journal of Medicine,* the researchers found that the group who took fish oil had significantly fewer relapses of Crohn's disease symptoms (28 percent in the fish oil group versus 69 percent in the placebo group). Fish oil may be helpful for patients with ULCERATIVE COLITIS. It can also lower triglyceride levels in the body.

See also ALTERNATIVE MEDICINE; CROHN'S DISEASE.

fissure A small crack or tear in the anal opening. It may be caused by straining to have a bowel movement or passing a very hard stool. Fissures may also be caused by TUBERCULOSIS, herpes infection, acquired immunodeficiency syndrome, cancer, INFLAMMATORY BOWEL DISEASE, and other disorders that should be considered.

The patient who has a fissure experiences severe pain that worsens during defecation as well as during a routine digital rectal examination by a physician. There may also be some bleeding associated with a fissure. Physicians treat most patients with fissures with sitz baths, rectal suppositories, or creams containing corticosteroids and local anesthetics. Patients are also advised to eat a high-fiber diet to keep their stools soft so that the fissure has an opportunity to heal. Some patients are given nitroglycerin ointments. Botulinum toxin injection is also useful. Chronic fissures may require surgery.

Pfenninger, John L. "Common Anorectal Conditions. Part III. Lesions." *American Family Physician,* July 1, 2001.

fistula An artificially created passage between two hollow organs or between an organ and an external part of the body. Fistulas usually develop as a result of damaged tissues' contacting with each other and uniting during healing. If the fistula causes harm, it requires medical treatment or surgery. Examples of different types of fistulas are gastrocolic (the stomach and the colon), rectovaginal (the rectum and the vagina), colovesical (the colon and the urinary bladder), and enterocutaneous (the intestines and the skin).

Conditions that can cause fistula formation include CROHN'S DISEASE, DIVERTICULITIS, and cancer. A fistula can also occur as a complication of abdominal surgery.

fluid and electrolyte balance Levels of fluids and electrolytes in the body. To retain normal health, the body needs to maintain a healthy level of fluids and electrolytes. Sometimes, the fluid and electrolyte levels can become unbalanced as a result of disease, such as gastroenteritis, excessive vomiting, sweating, or severe infections.

Some medications can also cause fluid losses. In such cases, patients need fluid and electrolyte replacement. In acute cases of imbalances, some patients may even require hospitalization so that they can receive intravenous fluid and electrolyte replacements. When a patient's condition is stabilized, he or she can usually drink sufficient fluids to maintain a normal level of fluids and electrolytes.

Most individuals who have diarrhea can replenish their fluid and electrolyte levels by drinking fluids. People who exercise heavily often drink the commercial product Gatorade, which was developed by researchers at the University of Florida. Patients who have low potassium levels caused by some diuretic drugs such as furosemide (Lasix) often routinely take potassium supplements.

See also DEHYDRATION; DIARRHEA; ELECTROLYTES.

food allergies An immune response of the body to certain foods that causes the body to release protective chemicals that may lead to reactions that may sometimes be severe and even life-threatening. Some food allergies are extreme and may be fatal, such as a severe allergic reaction to eating peanuts. Some individuals are extremely allergic to common substances such as wheat. In other cases, the allergy may be a mild one.

Infants may be allergic to either cow's milk or soy milk. Children may be allergic to shellfish, cow's milk, peanuts, soy, wheat, eggs, tree nuts (walnuts, hazelnuts, and so forth), and fish. Adults with food allergies are most likely to be allergic to peanuts, tree nuts, fish, and shellfish.

Sometimes people may believe that they have become ill from a food allergy when, in fact, the food that they ate may have been contaminated with bacteria or other pathogens. Before assuming that a food allergy is present and fastidiously avoiding a food, patients should first consult their physician.

Digestive diseases may also be misdiagnosed as food allergies by patients. Persistent nausea and vomiting or chronic HEARTBURN may be an indicator of another serious disease rather than a reaction to a particular food, and patients should consult physicians for diagnosis and treatment. Untreated diseases such as GASTROESOPHAGEAL REFLUX DISEASE or duodenal or gastric ulcers can become worse over time, when untreated.

Food Allergies versus Food Intolerances

A food allergy is *not* the same as a food intolerance. A food intolerance may cause an adverse reaction, but it is not a reaction that is immunological in nature; for example, a lactase deficiency in a person may cause LACTOSE INTOLERANCE. The person is not allergic to milk or milk products; instead, he or she is unable to digest them because of an innate lactase deficiency. Such individuals can either avoid milk products or take an over-the-counter remedy that helps digest these products. Another type of food intolerance is a reaction to food colorings or to some chemical additives, such as monosodium glutamate (MSG). The individual does not respond with an allergic reaction but instead may feel ill after consuming foods to which he or she is intolerant.

Symptoms and Diagnostic Path

There are a variety of symptoms and signs of food allergies, ranging from a skin reaction to asthma and all the way to the most severe reaction, which is anaphylaxis, a medical emergency in which the allergic reaction usually occurs within a few minutes and can be rapidly fatal. The patient experiences nausea and vomiting, and the patient's tongue swells up. In addition, the patient's throat and the air passages start to close, and the patient experiences low blood pressure and then shock. If a person has a true anaphylactic reaction to a certain food, then the individual usually responds rapidly to the administration of epinephrine (adrenaline). Additionally, steroids and antihistamines may be used, depending on the severity of the allergic reaction.

If a patient has been treated and any crisis has passed, the physician attempts to work with the individual to analyze what foods were eaten in relation to when the reaction occurred. For example, a food eaten a week before a reaction is unlikely to have caused the reaction, since it would have been digested and excreted days before.

Treatment Options and Outlook

Doctors may recommend an elimination diet, in which specific foods, such as eggs or nuts or other suspected foods, are avoided. The patient observes whether he or she feels better when not consuming these foods. In some cases, physicians use scratch tests, in which a small amount of the suspected food extract is scratched on the skin, to determine whether there is any allergic reaction. Physicians may also use blood tests to check for food allergies, such as the radioallergosorbent test (RAST) and the enzyme-linked immunosorbent assay (ELISA). These tests determine whether there is a food-specific reaction in the blood.

Once the physician determines that there is a food allergy, and the food or foods to which the patient is allergic, the patient is then instructed to avoid these foods. Sometimes this can be difficult. For example, peanuts and peanut oil are added to many foods; consequently, patients must carefully read the labels on food products. In addition, when eating out, it is important to advise the waiter that the patient is highly allergic to whatever the food is and that the waiter should check with the chef to make sure the problem food is not included in the meal. When dining with friends or others, it is very important to share the information about the food allergy.

Risk Factors and Preventive Measures

Patients who have shown allergic reactions to food in the past are at risk for other food allergies. Some gastrointestinal disorders and symptoms may be caused by food allergies, such as EOSINOPHILIC GASTROENTERITIS. Food allergies also appear to run in families, and if a parent or sibling is highly allergic to a food, other family members may need to be tested for the allergy as well.

People who are allergic to one food are often allergic to other similar foods. This phenomenon is called cross-allergy. For example, if a person is allergic to shrimp, he or she may also need to avoid all shellfish, including lobster, crab, and crayfish.

Children and adults who have known severe food allergies should wear medical bracelets that state their allergies, their doctors' names, and other emergency information. They should also carry a syringe of epinephrine (adrenaline) to self-inject in the event of an emergency. Parents of minor children should be certain to alert school authorities and make sure that epinephrine is readily available for emergency use. Many schools have a no-drug policy, so children may be prevented from carrying their own syringe, even with a prescription. For this reason, it is imperative that other individuals are trained and alerted to treat the child, if necessary.

Food Allergies in Children

Food allergies in children can be particularly difficult for parents who cannot be with their children constantly to watch them, particularly as the children get older; in addition, children may be resistant to refusing foods to which they are allergic, simply because they want to avoid embarrassment. Parents must make it clear to children that it will be far more embarrassing to have a severe allergic reaction requiring hospitalization than to tell people about their food allergy and/or to refuse a food or fluid to which they are allergic.

Anaphylaxis: It Can Be Fatal

As mentioned, the most severe allergic reaction to food is anaphylaxis. If untreated, the patient dies. The patient becomes rapidly sick and sicker and requires emergency medical attention. Patients who know that they are allergic to foods should self-inject with epinephrine if it is available. In the United States, the 911 emergency phone number should also be called immediately for an ambulance to treat patients with a reaction to a life-threatening food allergy.

The foods most commonly found to cause anaphylaxis in children are nuts, peanuts, and seafood.

See also CELIAC SPRUE.

functional bowel disorders   Disorders of the functioning of nerves and muscles of the gastrointestinal system that cause diarrhea, constipation, and pain, such as in IRRITABLE BOWEL SYNDROME. There is no grossly apparent (visible to the naked eye) structural damage to the organ involved in a functional bowel disorder; thus, irritable bowel syndrome causes no visible damage to the colon. Thus, the diagnosis is primarily or solely made by taking the patient's medical history and performing a physical examination, as well as by excluding other mimicking diseases by ordering tests such as blood tests, X-rays, and ENDOSCOPY.

In addition to irritable bowel syndrome, other functional bowel disorders include functional dys-

pepsia, noncardiac chest pain, and functional heartburn, for which the causes are unknown. Visceral hypersensitivity or a lowered pain threshold is seen in these patients. Treatments include use of antidepressants to increase the patient's pain threshold.

See also CONSTIPATION; DIARRHEA.

fundoplication   A surgical treatment for GASTROESOPHAGEAL REFLUX DISEASE, which is also called Nissen's fundoplication. The procedure may be performed laparoscopically, or it may be accomplished through a large open incision in the abdomen. A part of the stomach is wrapped around the junction of the esophagus and the stomach in order to tighten the junction and to prevent the reflux of gastric contents back into the esophagus. In a modification of the Nissen's fundoplication procedure the surgeon creates a partial wrap (270 degrees) rather than a 360-degree wrap around the esophagus; this modified procedure is used for patients with impaired esophageal motility.

See also ACID REFLUX.

fungi   Yeast or mold that cause infection, such as *Candidiasis* species or THRUSH. In addition to infection in other organs, fungal infection occurs in the digestive organs among patients whose immune function is suppressed or suboptimal, such as patients who have acquired immunodeficiency syndrome (AIDS). Sometimes diabetes patients experience a fungal infection in the esophagus, leading to pain during swallowing of food. Oral medications can be administered to treat fungi. If the fungus is external, antifungal creams are recommended by physicians. Sometimes intravenous medications are needed to eradicate the fungus, especially if it has spread to the bloodstream.

See also *CANDIDA; LACTOBACILLUS*.

gag reflex   The natural tendency of the throat to prevent swallowing that may occur if a noxious substance, fluids, or foods touches the back of the tongue and the throat (the back of the pharynx, or soft palate). This reflex does not have any relation to the swallowing process and lack of this reflex does not imply impairment of swallowing mechanisms.

Testing the Gag Reflex

The gag reflex can be checked by touching or stroking the posterior pharynx on one side with a cotton swab and then comparing this response to the response elicited by touching the other side. About 15 to 30 percent of normal individuals do not have a gag reflex response to this test. The test result is most informative when the responses are asymmetric (differing from one side to the other).

Gag Reflex and Endoscopy

Many people worry that because of the gag reflex they cannot endure endoscopy, a procedure in which a tube is inserted down the throat so that the physician can inspect both the esophagus and the stomach. However, most people have little or no problem with this procedure, and the gag reflex does not prevent the doctor from performing the endoscopy.

Abnormal Gag Reflexes

An abnormal gag reflex may be elicited in patients who have swallowing problems after a stroke or who are in a coma. However, the absence of the gag reflex does not mean that this absence is the cause of dysphagia.

The gag reflex is abnormal and asymmetric in diseases involving cranial nerves IX and X.

An abnormal gag reflex is not protective and its absence does not affect the swallowing function.

gallbladder   The digestive organ that stores bile that is manufactured by the liver. When the gallbladder malfunctions, stones and infection may develop. GALLSTONES usually do not cause symptoms, but they can block the flow of bile to the duodenum, causing CHOLECYSTITIS, CHOLANGITIS, or PANCREATITIS, which can be extremely painful and sometimes even life-threatening. If the gallbladder must be surgically removed, patients can continue to digest their food and function without it. Most cases of cholecystectomy (removal of the gallbladder) are currently undertaken laparoscopically.

See also GALLBLADDER CANCER.

gallbladder cancer   Malignant tumor of the gallbladder or the bile duct. About 5,000 people are diagnosed with gallbladder cancer each year in the United States. Many cases of gallbladder cancer are detected by chance during surgery for other gallbladder problems, such as GALLSTONES.

Symptoms and Diagnostic Path

Patients with gallbladder cancer are usually asymptomatic or have nonspecific symptoms until the disease is advanced. The symptoms and signs, when present, include the following:

- pain in the upper right abdomen
- NAUSEA AND VOMITING
- lack of APPETITE

- JAUNDICE
- pruritus (very itchy skin)
- hepatomegaly (enlarged liver)
- ASCITES (fluid buildup in the abdomen)
- weight loss
- dark urine (the color of cola)
- intolerance of fatty foods

The patient who has symptoms indicative of gallbladder disease is usually evaluated with an ultrasound, which can rule out gallstones. If gallbladder cancer is present, the ultrasound may show localized thickening and irregularity of the wall of the gallbladder. An endoscopic ULTRASOUND (an ultrasound done through the endoscope rather than through the skin and the abdominal wall) is superior but is not widely available as of this writing. A computed tomography (CT) scan may also be done for diagnosis as well as identification of spread of the cancer to other adjacent organs.

Treatment Options and Outlook

If the cancer has not advanced beyond the gallbladder, surgery is usually considered to be the best treatment for most patients. For T1 tumors (the earliest stage of gallbladder tumors), the five-year survival rate is about 80 to 90 percent. Survival rates drop with an advance in the level of the tumor.

Risk Factors and Preventive Measures

Gallbladder cancer is two to three times more commonly found among women than among men. (There are no gender differences found among people with cancer of the bile duct.) There are also racial and ethnic differences in risks, and Native Americans have the highest risk for gallbladder cancer, followed by natives of Israel, Mexico, Chile, and northern Japan.

A study of more than 42,000 Danish patients with gallstone disease over the period 1977 to 1989, which was reported in a 1999 issue of the *British Journal of Cancer,* found a linkage between gallstones and the later development of digestive cancer. Patients with gallstone disease who did not have a cholecystectomy (the removal of the entire gallbladder) had an increased risk for gallbladder

cancer, LIVER CANCER, and cancers of the extrahepatic duct and the pancreas. Patients who did have cholecystectomy had an increased risk for cancers in the ampulla of Vater, which is also known as the hepatopancreatic ampulla. This is an enlargement of the major duodenal papillae that receive the common bile duct and pancreatic duct.

Patients who have had PANCREATIC CANCER may also be at an increased risk for development of gallbladder cancer.

In general, patients who have previously had the following diseases, disorders, or exposures have the greatest risk of development of gallbladder cancer:

- those with existing gallstones
- those who have a calcified wall of the gallbladder
- people who are carriers of typhoid bacteria
- people who have POLYPS in the gallbladder
- obese individuals

There are no known preventive measures. See also CANCERS OF THE DIGESTIVE SYSTEM.

gallstones   Yellow, black, or brown stonelike material that can cause severe PAIN when they become lodged in the ducts carrying bile from the liver or the GALLBLADDER to the small intestine. Individuals may have one gallstone or many of them.

The presence of stones in the gallbladder, called cholelithiasis, may lead to a chronic inflammation of the gallbladder known as chronic CHOLECYSTITIS. If gallstones are lodged in the bile ducts, this condition is known as choledocholithiasis. About 15 to 20 percent of gallstone patients have choledocholithiasis, which can lead to inflammation of the bile ducts as well as to PANCREATITIS. When impacted in the cystic duct, gallstones cause acute cholecystitis.

Most gallstones (about 90 percent) comprise cholesterol; others may comprise many different materials. Cholesterol gallstones are yellow. Noncholesterol gallstones are either black or brown. People who have some blood diseases (such as thalassemia and sickle cell anemia) are more likely to have noncholesterol gallstones. Individuals who have liver CIRRHOSIS may also have black or brown gallstones. Brown stones are often related to parasitic or bacterial infections. Coffee, aspirin, and vitamin C appear to protect against gallstones.

Gallstones can be as small as one grain of sand or as large as a golf ball.

Symptoms and Diagnostic Path

In general, the following symptoms and signs may indicate the presence of gallstones, although only a physician can confirm the diagnosis. It is important to keep in mind that in most patients gallstones produce no symptoms, and health problems related to them never develop. When patients are symptomatic, the symptoms that indicate gallstones may actually be indicators of other serious problems, such as a heart attack, APPENDICITIS, ULCERS, or pancreatitis.

Pain characteristics of biliary colic gallstones may include the following:

- Pain in the upper and right abdomen that has lasted for at least 30 minutes to several hours.
- Pain lasting longer than six hours suggests acute cholecystitis (inflammation of the gallbladder). The term biliary *colic* is a misnomer, since the pain is not colicky but constant.
- Pain may be preceded by a heavy meal.
- Pain may radiate to the center, between the patient's shoulder blades.
- Pain may radiate to the tip of the right shoulder.
- Pain may be accompanied by NAUSEA AND VOMITING.
- Pain may be accompanied by restlessness.

Symptoms such as bloating, vague abdominal discomfort, and gas occur with the same frequency as in other conditions such as ulcers.

Unless the patient has emergency symptoms, in many cases, doctors identify gallstones during routine tests for other medical problems, with tests such as ULTRASOUND. Ultrasound is considered the best test for identifying gallstones; however, it is possible that gallstones will not be identified by an ultrasound examination, especially when the stones are in the bile duct.

Other tests that doctors may order include blood tests to identify infection, JAUNDICE, or pancreatitis as well as magnetic resonance imaging (MRI) tests to check for blocked bile ducts or computed tomography (CT) tests to check for gallstones in the ducts as well as for inflammation of the gallbladder and the pancreas. Blood test results that show elevated levels of liver enzymes and bilirubin may indicate biliary duct stones (choledocholithias). Elevated blood levels of amylase and lipase may indicate the presence of bile duct stones and/or pancreatitis.

One older diagnostic test is oral cholecystography, in which patients took one dose of a contrast dye, and the gallbladder was imaged in plain X-rays. This test is not usually chosen today because it is cumbersome and takes several hours. In addition, this test is no more accurate than the ultrasound test.

Treatment Options and Outlook

If gallstones are identified, and the physician believes that the patient's problems are related to the gallstones, usually the physician recommends surgery to remove the entire gallbladder. This surgery not only removes existing gallstones but ensures that additional gallstones will not develop. Rarely, stones may develop in the bile duct after the removal of the gallbladder.

Surgery to remove the gallbladder is called cholecystectomy; an estimated 500,000 patients in the United States have cholecystectomy every year. In most cases, the surgery is performed laparoscopically: It is done through multiple small incisions in the abdomen. A cholecystectomy is not performed if gallstones are not causing symptoms except in cases when a condition carries a high risk for disease or cancer, such as calcified gallbladder or a large gallbladder POLYP.

If surgery is not considered advisable for some reason, because the patient is a poor surgical risk or the patient declines surgery, then doctors may prescribe nonsurgical therapy. A functioning gallbladder as assessed by oral cholecystography is an essential prerequisite to nonsurgical therapy. Ursodiol (Actigall) is a medication that help to dissolve the gallstone. The drug works only on cholesterol gallstones, but since this form of gallstone is the more common, most patients have the potential to benefit from this therapy. This drug is not very effective for large, multiple, or calcified stones. The drug may take months or longer to dissolve existing stones and may cause some DIARRHEA as a side effect. In addition, this therapy may be ineffective in many cases depending on the type and size of stones.

Contact dissolution is a method whereby a needle is inserted into the gallbladder and a solvent such as methyl tert-butyl ether (MTBE) is injected to dissolve the stone. The factors affecting effectiveness are the same as bile acid therapy. Complete stone dissolution may be achieved in 65 percent of the cases, and selected patients are subsequently recommended oral dissolution therapy to prevent recurrence of stones. However, this method of treatment has a significant risk for complications. This method is also not widely available as of this writing.

Another treatment for gallstones is extracorporeal shockwave lithotripsy (ESWL). In this treatment, the gallstones are broken up by shock waves that are administered; however, patients may have severe pain after their treatment. The best candidates for this treatment are patients who have only one gallstone with a diameter of less than two centimeters that is radiolucent. Some physicians use the procedure when there are multiple stones with an aggregate size of three centimeters.

Lithotripsy is followed by administration of ursodiol, as described earlier. ESWL is not a very popular method because of its poor efficacy relative to laporoscopic surgery, and it is used only for patients at poor surgical risk.

Risk Factors and Preventive Measures

An estimated 15 to 20 percent of the population in the United States has gallstones at some point in their life. Native Americans in the United States have the highest risk of development of gallstones. Worldwide, people in Scandinavian countries are at high risk for gallstones, and as many as half the population in these countries has gallstones by the age of 50.

Although almost anyone can have gallstones, there are some key risk factors among patients that doctors look for:

- OBESITY is a major risk factor, especially among women.

- High levels of estrogen caused by PREGNANCY, birth control pills, or hormone replacement estrogen that is given to menopausal women increase risk.

- Race and ethnicity: Native Americans, particularly the Pima of Arizona, have the highest risk of development of gallstones. An estimated 70 to 80 percent of all Pima women have gallstones by the age of 30. Native Americans are followed by Mexican Americans in high risk of development of gallstones.

- Gender: Women between the ages of 20 and 60 have double to triple the risk of the development of gallstones as men.

- Age: People age 60 and older have a higher risk than younger individuals.

- Medications: People taking cholesterol-lowering drugs like clofibrate or antibiotics like ceftriax have a high risk.

- Patients who have had bariatric surgery as a treatment for severe obesity have a risk of development of gallstones after surgery of about 30 percent.

- Presence of diabetes raises risk.

- Presence of CROHN'S DISEASE increases risk.

- Very rapid weight loss raises risk.

Agrawal, Sangeeta, M.D., and Sreenivasa Jonnalagadda, M.D. "Gallstones, from Gallbladder to Gut." *Postgraduate Medicine* 108, no. 3 (September 1, 2000): 143–153.

Minocha A, Greenbaum D. S. "Effect of Nonsteroidal Anti-Inflammatory Drugs on Formation of Gallbladder Stones. *Veterinary and Human Toxicology* 36, no. 6 (1994): 514–516.

gas Air that is produced as a normal part of the digestive process. When gas is expressed through the mouth, the process is called burping, and when it is expressed through the rectum, it is called farting or flatulence. The gas that is belched is usually the air that is swallowed and does not stem from the colon. On the other hand, the gas of flatus is produced in the colon as a result of bacterial fermentations of the unabsorbed carbohydrates.

Gas production in the colon is normal; there is always some gas in the gut. There is a wide range in the number of flatulent expulsions that people may have. Elderly subjects expel small amounts but more frequently than younger individuals.

A variety of measures are used by patients who have "excessive gas," such as avoiding gas-producing foods and taking over-the-counter medications such as alpha-D-galactosidase enzyme (Beano), simethicone, and activated charcoal. However frequently, treatment is unsatisfactory.

If the gas problem is a severe one, individuals should see their physician to determine whether there is another underlying problem.

See also BELCHING.

gastroesophageal reflux disease (GERD) A chronic digestive disease whose primary characteristic is a chronic backflow (reflux) of food and digestive juices from the stomach into the esophagus and sometimes as far as high up into the mouth as well. Millions of people in the United States and Canada suffer from GERD. Many people with GERD are untreated (other than by taking over-the-counter antacids) because they do not realize that they have the illness or they do not know about the seriousness of this chronic illness over time.

Chronic GERD can lead to damage of the upper food tube called the ESOPHAGUS (the condition of ESOPHAGITIS), and it may also cause a narrowing (stricture) of the esophageal passage so that the individual has difficulty in swallowing (DYSPHAGIA). GERD that has been untreated for many years may also lead to BARRETT'S ESOPHAGUS, a precancerous condition of the esophagus that can ultimately lead to cancer.

The cause of GERD is usually not excessive acid level, but rather it is acid that is in the wrong place. There are a variety of different potential factors contributing to GERD, and the physician may have difficulty determining a specific cause; for example, GERD may be related to a genetic factor; it may also be caused or exacerbated by OBESITY. However, most of the time there is no clear cause, and most reflux occurs during transient lower esophageal relaxations.

Symptoms and Diagnostic Path
The key symptoms of chronic GERD are frequent HEARTBURN and entry of a sour (acid)-tasting fluid into the mouth. Many other atypical symptoms may occur; they may include:

- asthma
- chronic throat clearing
- hoarseness and cough
- possible difficulty in swallowing
- frequent episodes of bronchitis and recurrent pneumonia
- frequent ear, nose, and throat infections

Some people who have GERD may also experience severe chest pains that even physicians may confuse with heart attack; a heart attack should always be ruled out by a physician before GERD is considered as a possibility. It is also possible to have both heart disease and GERD.

GERD is often diagnosed on the basis of the presence of a clinical history of chronic heartburn alone. In general, the physician takes a full medical history and performs a complete physical examination of the patient.

In some cases, the patient may have an upper ENDOSCOPY, in which a special instrument is inserted down the throat and into the esophagus and then into the stomach. Besides detecting damage to the esophagus due to GERD, this test can detect other medical problems, such as hiatal hernias, ulcers, or STOMACH CANCER. The endoscopy results are normal in about half of the cases of patients with GERD; in those cases, it is known as nonerosive reflux disease (NERD).

Treatment Options and Outlook
People diagnosed with GERD may be treated with medications, lifestyle recommendations, and even surgery, although surgery is not the usual treatment. However, some surgeons believe that almost every patient who has GERD requires surgery. Many patients can improve their medical status by taking simple actions such as giving up SMOKING or avoiding certain types of foods.

Recommended medications Many patients are treated with a drug in the PROTON PUMP INHIBITOR (PPI) class, such as omeprazole (Prilosec), pantoprazole (Protonix), rabeprazole (Aciphex), lansoprazole (Prevacid), or esomeprazole (Nexium).

Generic versions of omeprazole are available. Some patients are treated with a medication in the histamine-2 inhibitor class (also known as H-2 blockers) such as cimetidine (Tagamet) or ranitidine (Zantac), which are effective in about half of the cases. PPIs are superior to histamine-2 blockers and are effective in about 90 percent of patients. There are other possible medications that may have potential for relieving GERD such as baclofen, and new ones are continually in development by pharmaceutical companies.

Drugs to be avoided Some medications should be avoided whenever possible by people who have GERD, because they may further aggravate the condition. Examples of drugs that patients should try to avoid are:

- progesterone
- calcium channel blockers
- bisphosphonate type medications for osteoporosis (Fosamax®)
- NONSTEROIDAL ANTI-INFLAMMATORY DRUGS
- tricyclic antidepressents

Some experts also believe that herbal remedies such as goldenseal and peppermint may worsen the condition, although good studies to address this issue are lacking. Anecdotally, many patients feel that these herbs help them with their heartburn and indigestion.

Risk Factors and Preventive Measures

Certain categories of people are more prone to development of GERD than others, such as people who:

- have diabetes
- have hypothyroidism (low level of thyroid hormone)
- have a HIATAL HERNIA
- have chronic CONSTIPATION and straining to move the bowels
- smoke
- have asthma
- are pregnant

- have decreased production of saliva (caused by medications and/or aging)
- are overweight
- have gastroparesis

GASTROPARESIS (slow stomach emptying) and gastroduodenal surgery each predispose patients to the development of GERD.

Another common risk factor for GERD and esophagitis is the regular use of nonsteroidal anti-inflammatory drugs (NSAIDs), which are medications that are usually prescribed for arthritis and related illnesses. Medications such as calcium channel blocker medications that are taken to treat hypertension or heart disease can also cause or contribute to the development of GERD. A variety of other medications may cause GERD, including estrogen or progesterone preparations taken by menopausal women and sumatriptan (Imitrex) taken for migraine headaches, as well as antidepressants such as amitriptyline (Elavil), doxepin (Sinequan), and nortriptyline (Pamelor).

Lifestyle changes Most doctors strongly advise GERD patients to make changes in their lifestyle as preventive measures to a GERD attack, such as raising the head of their bed, so they are less likely to experience acid reflux at night. Patients with GERD should not go to bed for at least two to three hours after eating a meal. Avoid bedtime snacks.

Patients who are overweight are urged to lose weight because obesity may worsen the symptoms of GERD. Patients are also urged to exercise but should avoid weightlifting and other strenuous exercises, instead concentrating on walking and riding a stationary bicycle or participating in other forms of low-impact aerobic activity.

Dietary changes may improve symptoms; for example, patients should forgo consuming large fatty meals, alcohol, chocolate, onions, orange juice, and carbonated beverages.

Patients who smoke should stop smoking immediately. SMOKING aggravates many medical conditions, including GERD.

See also ACID REFLUX; CHEST PAIN, NONCARDIAC; HISTAMINE-2 BLOCKERS.

Madan A., and A. Minocha. "Despite high satisfaction, majority of gastro-oesophageal reflux disease patients continue to use proton pump inhibitors after antire-flux surgery." *Alimentary Pharmacology & Therapeutics* 23, no. 5 (2006): 601–605.

Minocha, Anil, M.D., and Christine Adamec. *How to Stop Heartburn: Simple Ways to Heal Heartburn and Acid Reflux.* New York: John Wiley & Sons, 2001.

gastrointestinal bleeding   See BLEEDING, GASTRO-INTESTINAL; OCCULT GASTROINTESTINAL BLEEDING.

gastroparesis   A delayed emptying of the stomach. In the early stages of gastroparesis, the patient's main problem is the stomach's delaying of the emptying of solids. If the condition worsens further, there is also a delay in the emptying of liquids from the stomach to the small intestine. This condition makes a normal three-meal-a-day schedule difficult because the food from breakfast may still be in the stomach when food from lunch is eaten.

Symptoms and Diagnostic Path

Some people have no symptoms of gastroparesis, others have symptoms or signs, which include:

- NAUSEA AND VOMITING
- ANOREXIA (lack of appetite)
- early satiety (feeling of fullness that occurs soon after eating)
- bloating
- ABDOMINAL PAIN and distention
- ACID REFLUX

Physicians generally suspect that their patients have gastroparesis on the basis of their symptoms, and they confirm the diagnosis with a gastric emptying test, after first excluding the presence of a gastric obstruction with either the upper gastrointestinal X-ray or an ENDOSCOPY.

Treatment Options and Outlook

A low-fiber diet is usually recommended for people who are diagnosed with gastroparesis (because fiber may exacerbate the condition), as is eating five or six small meals per day rather than three large meals. Some patients are placed on a liquid diet. A person who has diabetes and gastroparesis should try to maintain a blood sugar level that is as close to normal as possible in order to improve gastric emptying.

There are several medications used for treating gastroparesis, and in the United States, meto-clopramide (Reglan) is frequently prescribed. However, metoclopramide can cause tremors and parkinsonian effects. Another drug, domperidone, works as metoclopramide does but without causing the same parkinsonian side effects; however, it has to be made in pharmacies on a special order. Some patients obtain the medication from foreign countries over the Internet. Some physicians have also used erythromycin to treat gastroparesis, but it is effective only for short periods.

Some conditions improve with a special device that is implanted to treat gastroparesis. The Food and Drug Administration (FDA) has approved the implantation of a gastric electrical stimulator or stomach pacemaker (Enterra Therapy), which is similar to the pacemaker of the heart on a limited basis. However, this treatment is used only in severe cases for humanitarian use only in patients with diabetic or idiopathic gastroparesis. Injection of botulinum toxin (Botox) into the pylorus may help improve gastric emptying of people who have diabetic gastroparesis, although the literature is controversial on this issue.

In patients who are unable to eat, an endoscopic insertion of a percutaneous endoscopic jejunostomy (PEJ) or a surgical jejunostomy may be done. In this procedure, a tube is placed through an incision in the abdominal wall into the small bowel, bypassing the stomach. As a result, food is directly fed into the intestine rather than into the stomach through the mouth. Some patients need to be fed via long-term intravenous nutritional methods.

Risk Factors and Preventive Measures

Gastroparesis may be caused by or linked to diseases such as DIABETES MELLITUS, neurological disorders, thyroid disease, or peptic ulcer. Older people (ages 65 and older) are more likely to experience gastroparesis.

Gastroparesis may also be caused by medications, which can have the side effect of slowing the process of digestion. Examples of types of drugs that can have that effect are antidepressants, tranquilizers, and calcium blocker medications. In many cases, no cause of the gastroparesis can be found, and it is often believed to be triggered by a viral illness.

SMOKING is also known to exacerbate gastroparesis, and smokers are urged to stop smoking immediately to prevent the problem from worsening. (Even if the smoker does not yet have a problem with gastroparesis, it is advisable to quit smoking before the condition develops.)

See also FIBER.

ghrelin　A hormone that was discovered in 1999. Ghrelin is released by the stomach and appears to affect appetite and satiety (a feeling of fullness after eating) directly. Preliminary studies indicate that suppression of ghrelin may become a treatment for OBESITY. Comparisons of patients that have lost weight by dieting or by gastric bypass surgery have demonstrated that the gastric bypass patients experienced significant drops in their blood level of ghrelin after the surgery.

Because obesity is a major problem in the United States, Canada, and many other developed countries, the finding that blood levels of ghrelin apparently can increase or decrease an individual's appetite appears to be a major breakthrough. Some researchers anticipate that ghrelin antagonist medications will be developed to create a new diet drug that will help many patients who are overweight or obese.

See also BARIATRIC SURGERY; DIET DRUGS.

Giardia/giardiasis　*Giardia* is the protozoon that causes the infection giardiasis. In the United States, most infections are caused by *Giardia lamblia*, which harbors in the human intestinal tract and is also found in human feces. Giardiasis is generally a nonfatal and common infection of the small intestine. Giardiasis is transmitted usually through contaminated water. Cooking of food kills *Giardia* cysts, hence the food-borne spread is uncommon and only occurs when cysts contaminate food that is uncooked or after it has been cooked.

Symptoms and Diagnostic Path

Most people with giardiasis (as many as two-thirds) have no symptoms. When symptoms do occur, they generally appear within one to three weeks or longer after infection and may include the following:

- DIARRHEA
- bad-smelling and oily feces
- ABDOMINAL PAINS
- loss of APPETITE
- GAS
- NAUSEA AND VOMITING

Doctors may particularly suspect giardiasis if other individuals in the same environment (such as a day care center) have already been diagnosed with giardiasis; however, the only certain way to confirm giardiasis is with an analysis of a stool sample or duodenal aspirate. Generally, three samples are required because *Giardia* organisms may be missed otherwise. Testing for *Giardia* stool antigen is also very sensitive.

Treatment Options and Outlook

Medications help most patients and prevent further transmission. However, asymptomatic patients may not need treatment unless they are food handlers or children in order to prevent spread of infection. The medication that is most commonly used to treat giardiasis is metronidazole. Other medications that may be used include quinacrine, furazolidone, and paromomycin.

Risk Factors and Preventive Measures

Periodic outbreaks of giardiasis occur in institutions via person-to-person contact, especially those that cater to small children, and at functions such as large picnics. Person-to-person transmission also occurs among male homosexuals. People at high risk include infants, children, and those immunocompromised, such as those with acquired immunodeficiency syndrome (AIDS).

Food handlers are at risk as are children because of their failure to wash their hands. There is no vaccine to protect against *Giardia* organisms; however, simple precautions can and should be taken by people to limit the incidence of infection, including the following actions:

- Wash hands after using the toilet.
- Avoid unwashed fruits or vegetables unless the surface of the food can be peeled away.
- Keep children who attend a day care center who have severe diarrhea at home, to prevent infecting other children.
- Boil drinking water if *Giardia* organisms may be present. Iodine treated water is better than chlorine treated water.

Note that with babies, breast milk may offer some protection for infants since it contains some IgA antibodies.

See also CONTAMINATED FOOD OR WATER; PARASITIC INFECTIONS.

glucose   Blood sugar. Normal levels of glucose are essential to good health. High levels constitute hyperglycemia and are characteristic of DIABETES MELLITUS, in which low insulin levels occur. In diabetic patients, insulin may have to be taken every day in injections in order to maintain the blood glucose level. Patients who have type 2 diabetes may be treated with oral medications and not need insulin.

Low levels of blood glucose are known as hypoglycemia. Sometimes people who have diabetes may take insulin but eat inadequate amounts of food; they may then experience unusually low glucose levels. Low glucose levels can lead to mild symptoms, or, in extreme cases, even to coma. Because of this problem, diabetes patients frequently carry candy, fruit, or another form of sugar for use in an emergency.

Certain tissues in the body, such as the brain, red blood cells, bone marrow, parts of the eyes, and kidneys, can utilize only glucose as an energy source.

guaiac   A substance that is used in fecal occult blood testing to screen patients for colorectal cancer. Guaiac is a gumlike or resinous substance that is obtained from two tree species: *Guaiacum officinale* and *Guaiacum sanctum*. The test was discovered by Van Deen in 1864, who found that guaiac changes color when it is applied to stool that contains blood.

Various tests that are based on guaiac are used. Guaiac tests do produce some false positive results, such as those caused by the patient's eating red meat, turnip, or horseradish before having the test or ingesting stomach-irritant drugs that cause gastritis, such as aspirin. On the other hand, the ingestion of vitamin C before testing can cause a false negative test result.

heartburn Occasional or chronic acidic feeling behind the chest that is usually caused by acid reflux. Chronic heartburn is also known as GASTRO-ESOPHAGEAL REFLUX DISEASE; however, sometimes even a heart attack may produce a burning pain in the chest, and distinguishing between acid reflux and heart attack can be difficult. Chronic heartburn can occur in the absence of any espheageal/cardiac disease and is called functional heartburn.

See also ACID REFLUX.

Helicobacter pylori (*H. pylori* or **HP**) Common bacteria that are found in the stomach of many people in the United States and other countries and that are the primary cause of peptic ulcers. In addition, sometimes an infection with *Helicobacter pylori* (HP) precedes certain forms of stomach cancer. In the past, HP was also associated with other medical problems, such as heart disease and short stature, but these links have been scientifically refuted.

One association based on scientific data was found by researchers who looked at studies of people infected with HP in Japan; their findings were reported in the *New England Journal of Medicine* in 2001. The research showed that infected people had a higher risk of development of gastric cancer when they were compared to those patients who were not infected with HP. In one study 1,526 Japanese patients who had duodenal or gastric ulcer or other serious gastric problems were evaluated for an infection with HP. Of these patients, 280 individuals were infected. The patients were then followed up for about eight years. The researchers found that about 3 percent of the patients who had been diagnosed with HP developed gastric cancer, whereas cancer developed in none of the uninfected patients.

Some Historical Background

Until the late 20th century, most physicians worldwide believed that ulcers were caused by stress, diet, or acid; however, in 1982, the Australian physicians Marshall and Warren theorized that ulcers are actually caused by bacteria. In fact, Dr. Marshall consumed some HP bacteria and caused the development of an infection. He contracted gastritis, had antibiotic treatment, and was cured of both gastritis and HP.

Despite this research, for a while, most physicians worldwide refused to believe that bacteria could cause gastritis or ulcers, believing instead that the primary causes were diet and/or stress, and consequently they ridiculed Marshall and Warren. It was not until 1994, when the National Institutes of Health (NIH) in the United States confirmed the association between HP and ulcers and the NIH then recommended that antibiotics be used to prevent recurrence of HP-induced ulcers, that most physicians began to accept that *Helicobacter pylori* is the true culprit in the majority of ulcers. This was a dramatic paradigm shift for physicians worldwide.

Risk Factors for Contracting HP

Although HP is more commonly found in poor countries, the bacteria are ubiquitously present in every society. Researchers report that the incidence of infection in developed countries is 20 to 50 percent, whereas it is greater than 80 percent in poor countries. Generally, the bacteria are contracted by children and harbored in the stomach unless or until they are eradicated by antibiotics.

Risk of Development of an Ulcer Caused by HP

People infected with HP have a much higher risk of development of ulcers, although not everyone who has had HP infection has an ulcer. Researchers report that the risk of development of a peptic ulcer among people who are infected with HP is about 15 percent.

Interestingly, Dr. Minocha and his colleagues have found that patients who have a prior history of having a tonsillectomy have a significantly reduced risk of being infected with HP, possibly because patients with bad tonsils are more likely to have used antibiotics in the past, thus eradicating the HP infection in the stomach. The same patients are also likely to undergo subsequent tonsillectomy. Thus, the possible linkage between HP and tonsillectomy may be merely an association and not a cause-and-effect relationship.

Another possibility is that the tonsils serve as a kind of collecting place for bacteria, although researchers are not sure whether this is true. Minocha's findings were reported in 1997 in the *Journal of Clinical Gastroenterology.*

Symptoms and Diagnosic Path

Most individuals who are infected with HP have no symptoms. Most have chronic gastritis and a few patients develop ulcers. Symptoms of indigestion in the presence of HP but without an overt ulcer are usually not relieved by eradicating the HP.

Diagnosis of HP

If physicians suspect that HP is the underlying cause of the patient's problem, they can confirm the diagnosis with the urea breath test, or with blood tests or stool antigen tests. In addition, if an endoscopy is performed, the physician can take a biopsy of extracted tissue to determine whether it is infected with HP. Physicians usually do not test patients who have endoscopy for HP unless they also suspect that they may have a problem related to HP *and* they intend to treat the HP. If the patient has no symptoms, then it is not considered necessary to confirm or refute the presence of HP. Therefore, patients who are receiving long-term treatment for GASTROESOPHAGEAL REFLUX DISEASE (GERD) are usually not tested for HP. Interestingly, HP may be protective against GERD.

In the breath test, the patient ingests a urea-laden meal that is laced with minute amounts of radioactivity. The patient then merely breathes into a device that measures the presence of radioactivity, and a high level of radioactivity or radio labeled carbon dioxide indicates infection with HP. This test is highly reliable for adults and children older than age six but may not be available at some clinics. Blood testing for HP is considered relatively inexpensive and thus is used by many physicians; however, it is only a screening test, as it tests for antibodies. The blood test cannot be used for testing whether bacteria have been eradicated after treatment because antibodies may persist for years even after HP has been eradicated.

The stool test for HP is also highly reliable and can be used to confirm after treatment that HP has been eradicated.

Treatment Options and Outlook

HP is a very resistant bacterium. Single-drug regimens are ineffective. Once HP has been diagnosed, physicians usually treat patients with combination therapy, with at least two and usually three or more antibiotics for about two weeks. Some doctors confirm that HP is truly eradicated from their patients after the treatment is complete by examining for HP with a stool antigen test or a breath test. A 2002 article in the *Annals of Internal Medicine* revealed that the stool antigen test successfully identifies patients who continue to be infected.

See also ANTIBIOTICS; BREATH TESTS; DYSPEPSIA; STOMACH CANCER; ULCERS, PEPTIC.

Minocha, Anil, M.D., et al. "Alterations in Upper Gastrointestinal Motility in *Helicobacter pylori*-Positive Nonulcer Dyspepsia." *American Journal of Gastro-enterology* 89, no. 10 (1994): 1,797–1,800.

Minocha, Anil, M.D., et al. "*Helicobacter pylori* Is Associated with Alternations in Intestinal Gas Profile among Patients with Nonulcer Dyspepsia." *Digestive Diseases and Sciences* 39, no. 8 (August 1994): 1,613–1,617.

Minocha, Anil, M.D., C. A. Racakowski, M.D., and Robert J. Richards, M.D. "Is a History of Tonsillectomy Associated with a Decreased Risk of *Helicobacter pylori* Infection?" *Journal of Clinical Gastroenterology* 25, no. 4 (1997): 580–582.

Uemura, Naomi, M.D., et al. "*Helicobacter Pylori* Infection and the Development of Gastric Cancer." *New England Journal of Medicine* 345, no. 11 (September 13, 2001): 784–789.

Vaira, Dino, M.D., et al. "The Stool Antigen Test for Detection of Helicobacter pylori after Eradication Therapy." *Annals of Internal Medicine* 136, no. 4 (February 19, 2002): 280–287.

hemochromatosis   A disease that is caused by the excessive absorption of iron from food that is consumed, resulting in excessive and potentially very harmful deposits of iron into the liver, pancreas, heart, and other organs. Most people absorb about 10 percent of the iron from the food they eat, but individuals with hemochromatosis absorb up to 30 percent of the iron that they consume, and over time (if the disease is undiagnosed and untreated), they have from five to 20 times more iron than the body needs. Because the body has no easy way to rid itself of the iron, it is stored in the organs. If untreated, this disease causes damage to the organs and it can be fatal. Hemochromatosis increases the risk for the development of CIRRHOSIS (liver inflammation) and liver cancer. (See LIVER CANCER.)

Less than 1 percent of people in the United States are at risk for hemochromatosis. In most cases, hemochromatosis is a hereditary disease that is caused by a defect in the *HFE* gene. In a few cases, however, the disease does not appear to have a genetic link, and the cause is sometimes unknown.

Symptoms and Diagnostic Path

The diagnosis of hemochromatosis is usually delayed since symptoms do not develop until the late stages of the disease. When physicians observe that a patient has a constellation of abnormal blood tests or diseases that are commonly caused by hemochromatosis, they screen for the disease by blood testing.

Common early symptoms of hemochromatosis include the following:

- fatigue
- joint pain
- weakness
- weight loss
- ABDOMINAL PAIN

When hemochromatosis continues untreated, the following diseases may develop:

- liver disease (CIRRHOSIS, liver cancer, and LIVER FAILURE)
- pancreatic damage (which may cause diabetes)

- low thyroid level
- adrenal gland damage
- cardiac problems, such as congestive heart failure or heart arrhythmias

Physicians generally order the following tests to screen their patient for hemochromatosis: serum iron, serum transferrin, and serum ferritin. If the tests show an abnormally high level of iron, doctors may then order a blood test that checks for the *HFE* genetic mutation. A positive test result confirms the presence of hemochromatosis, whereas a negative test result does not exclude hemochromatosis but does make it less likely. In addition, doctors may also order a liver biopsy to test for iron in the liver, to determine whether the liver is damaged, and, if it is damaged to evaluate the extent of the damage.

It should also be noted that very high serum ferritin levels even greater than 1,000 ng/mL may occur in association with bilateral congenital cataracts that are associated with hemochromatosis, but without tissue iron overload. This is known as hereditary hyperferritinemia-cataract syndrome.

Treatment Options and Outlook

It is very important to treat hemochromatosis because if it is not treated, patients may develop the following conditions:

- liver cancer
- heart disease
- male impotence
- female infertility or premature menopause
- diabetes
- thyroid deficiency
- arthritis
- cirrhosis of the liver

The treatment for hemochromatosis sounds to many people like a throwback to medieval times when patients were "bled" to be treated. Hemochromatosis is one of the few diseases in which patients actually benefit from bloodletting. For most patients with hemochromatosis, the removal of the excessive levels of iron are required through a phlebotomy, which is the same procedure that is used when blood is donated. Each 500 ml of blood removed gets rid of about 200–250 mg of iron from the body. About a pint of blood is removed at a time, and the process takes about an hour. How many phlebotomies are needed depends on how high the iron level is in the blood. In general, most people with hemochromatosis need to have the procedure once or twice a week for about a year. After the iron level has dropped to a safe level, the procedure is usually needed only a few times a year.

If the disease is treated in time, and before the development of liver cirrhosis, patients have a normal life expectancy. Patients start to feel better and have an increased energy level shortly after phlebotomy; however, patients with already damaged joints and hypogonadism do not revert to the predamaged condition.

Risk Factors and Preventive Measures

Individuals diagnosed with hemochromatosis should urge their blood relatives to be tested for the disease so that they can be treated. All close biological family members should be tested, including parents, grandparents, siblings, and children.

Most people with hereditary hemochromatosis are whites of northern European descent. An estimated one in 200 whites carries the hemochromatosis gene and is at risk for development of the disease. Symptoms usually begin in middle age.

Men have a five times greater risk of developing hemochromatosis than women. In general, the disease develops in men between ages 30 and 50, while in women, the average age of onset is 50. In many cases, people who are diagnosed with the disease have no symptoms at the time of diagnosis.

People with hemochromatosis should avoid eating raw fish (sushi) or shellfish. Some harmful bacteria thrive in the presence of high iron in the body, and cooking destroys germs that are harmful to such individuals with hemochromatosis. Alcohol intake results in increased iron absorption and can worsen liver disease. As such, alcohol should either be avoided or limited, and women should drink no more than one drink a day and men should drink no more than two drinks per day; however, if the patient has any liver damage, alcohol should be completely avoided.

Individuals with hemochromatosis should avoid taking any iron supplements or any vitamin pills or other drugs that include iron. It is all right to eat food that includes iron. Individuals with hemochromatosis should also avoid taking vitamin C supplements.

Secondary Iron Overload A secondary iron overload may be caused by an increased absorption of iron that is related to the inability of the body to produce sufficient red blood cells, also known as ANEMIA due to ineffective erythropoiesis. It may also be related to chronic liver disease and sometimes to the excessive use of iron supplements. In some cases, an increased iron level may be caused by repeated and multiple blood transfusions or the administration of intravenous iron. In cases of hereditary hemochromatosis, the symptoms do not appear until adulthood; nonhereditary hemochromatosis may appear in infancy or childhood.

Juvenile Hemochromatosis A rare form of hemochromatosis occurs in childhood, and it is termed juvenile hemochromatosis or type II hemochromatosis (JH) I. The affected gene is called HJV. In this case, the disease has been mostly reported from Italy. Patients with juvenile hemochromatosis may have more severe heart problems, diabetes, and hypogonadism than the severe liver disease experienced by patients with the more common form of hemochromatosis.

Neonatal Hemochromatosis Neonatal hemochromatosis (NH), also called neonatal iron storage disease, was first noted in 1957, but only about 100 cases have been identified since then. This medical problem is believed to be related to an intrauterine infection that causes babies to be born with excessive levels of iron in their liver. Babies who have NH are usually small for gestational age or premature. The PREGNANCY of their mothers was often complicated by intrauterine growth retardation, placental edema, or other serious problems. The baby's distress is usually noted shortly after birth.

INFANTS with NH have liver failure, and hypoalbuminemia, hypoglycemia (low blood sugar level).

Usually ASCITES (fluid in the abdomen) and hyper-bilirubinemia (excessive levels of bilirubin in the blood) develop. The prognosis of the babies is poor, and they usually die without LIVER TRANSPLANTATION. NH should be suspected in very sick newborns with evidence of liver disease and in cases of late intrauterine fetal demise.

African Iron Overload   Another form of hemochromatosis is called African iron overload, or bantu hemosiderosis, which was once believed to be caused by an increased level of iron that was absorbed through the alcohol in iron drums. It is now believed instead that this form of hemochromatosis is a genetic disorder, but it is different from the disease related to the *HFE* gene.

See also DIGESTION AND ABSORPTION; IRON; VITAMIN DEFICIENCIES/EXCESSES.

Allen, Katrina J., M.D., et al. "Iron-Overload-Related Disease in *HFE* Hereditary Hemochromatosis," *New England Journal of Medicine* 358, no. 2 (January 17, 2008): 221–230.

Murray, Karen, M.D., and Kris V. Kowdley, M.D., "Neonatal Hemochromatosis." *Pediatrics* 108, no. 4 (October 2001): 960–964.

National Institute of Diabetes and Digestive and Kidney Diseases. *Hemochromatosis*. Bethesda, Md.: National Institutes of Health, April 2007.

hemorrhoids/hemorrhoidal disease   Hemorrhoids are normal in the human body and present at birth. Hemorrhoids are a cushion of widened blood vessels called the hemorrhoidal plexus. However, when the term *hemorrhoids* is used, physicians and others are referring to hemorrhoidal disease, as when hemorrhoids are causing problems, such as bleeding, by becoming enlarged or irritated, or when a blood clot forms within them.

Hemorrhoids are said to be internal when they are located inside the lower rectum, whereas hemorrhoids that are located around the anus are called external hemorrhoids. Both internal and external hemorrhoidal problems may coexist in the same patient. The true incidence of hemorrhoidal problems is not known; it is believed that at least 4 percent of the adults in the United States experience such problems.

Symptoms and Diagnostic Path

Hemorrhoids cause few or no problems in most individuals. In some cases, however, they cause minor or severe painless bleeding, as well as pain and itching. Other features may include the protrusion of an internal hemorrhoid through the anus and pain resulting from the blood clots that lie within the hemorrhoids. Fecal soiling may also occur.

Hemorrhoidal disease is often diagnosed by a physician by taking a complete history of the patient and performing a physical examination, including a routine rectal examination. Anoscopy (examination of the anal canal) can be performed in the office.

Rectal bleeding, either overt or invisible, should not be automatically attributed to hemorrhoids, unless other causes such as cancer have been excluded, since the two can coexist. Hemorrhoids can also be diagnosed during a routine sigmoidoscopy or colonoscopy, and such a procedure is usually performed not just to diagnose hemorrhoids but also to exclude the presence of any other disease that might cause hemorrhoidal symptoms.

Treatment Options and Outlook

Patients who are experiencing pain and itching from hemorrhoids may gain benefit from taking sitz baths (shallow soaking baths). Small tubs that fit over the toilet can be used for this purpose, or the patient may soak in the bathtub. Cold packs over the anal area may help, if they are recommended by the patient's doctor. Medications or over-the-counter (nonprescribed) suppositories can be purchased at pharmacies, and some suppositories are prescribed. Because of the risk of side effects, creams and suppositories, especially those containing hydrocortisone, should not be used by patients longer than one week, unless recommended by a physician.

Minimally invasive procedures for hemorrhoids include rubber band ligation, laser therapy, sclerotherapy (injection of chemicals into hemorrhoids to obliterate them), and cryosurgery. Sometimes surgical removal of hemorrhoids is needed, especially if the patient is experiencing severe and protruding hemorrhoids with frequent bleeding and pain and medical treatments are not relieving the symptoms. However, complications can follow surgery, and the physician weighs the risks versus the benefits of surgery before embarking on the surgical course.

Patients are also advised to avoid sitting on the toilet for a long period. In addition, constipation should be prevented whenever possible, and regular exercise, such as walking, can often help with this problem.

Risk Factors and Preventive Measures

Hemorrhoids occur in both sexes and are seen most commonly in people who are between 45 and 65 years old. The exact cause of hemorrhoidal disease remains to be established. Some key risk factors include straining during defecation, chronic constipation or diarrhea, prolonged sitting, advancing age, pregnancy, and abdominal or pelvic tumors. Medication may indirectly caused hemorrhoids by drying out the stool and making passing it difficult.

In many cases, patients can manage and improve their own hemorrhoid symptoms by taking specific actions, such as increasing the level of FIBER in their diet and the quantity of water they drink so that having bowel movements becomes easier. Some patients may also take laxatives or stool softener medications if they are advised to do so by their physicians.

See also CONSTIPATION; FECAL IMPACTION.

hepatitis A Inflammation of the liver that is caused by an infectious virus. Other viruses can also cause hepatitis; however, the five primary forms of viral hepatitis are hepatitis A, B, C, D, and E. (There are also causes of liver inflammation other than viruses, such as ALCOHOL ABUSE AND ALCOHOLISM and use of some drugs.) Chronic hepatitis B and C can lead to cirrhosis (inflammation of the liver), which, in turn, can cause liver cancer of the hepatocellular carcinoma type.

Hepatitis A is a common form of hepatitis. It is contracted through consuming food or water contaminated with the virus. Some outbreaks are attributed to the consumption of raw or half-cooked shellfish that are contaminated. Transmission of hepatitis A through blood and blood products is rare. The incidence of hepatitis A in the United States is 1.5 per 100,000.

Symptoms and Diagnostic Path

There are a range of symptoms that may be experienced by a person with hepatitis A. These symptoms are common to other illnesses, and only a physician can properly diagnose the presence of hepatitis, with appropriate laboratory tests. The common symptoms of hepatitis A include the following symptoms (not everyone has these symptoms, and most people with hepatitis A have no symptoms at all):

- fatigue
- nausea
- lack of APPETITE
- ABDOMINAL PAIN
- DIARRHEA

Hepatitis A can be diagnosed with a blood test to check for antibodies to hepatitis A. Presence of serum IgM anti-HAV indicates acute hepatitis A. Levels of liver enzymes such as serum alanine aminotransferase (ALT) are typically elevated in individuals who have any form of viral hepatitis.

Treatment Options and Outlook

Treatment for acute hepatitis is supportive, and most patients do not require hospitalization unless the hepatitis is severe. Patients with hepatitis must avoid all alcohol, which would cause further liver damage. The liver metabolizes alcohol and alcohol injures the liver by causing alcoholic hepatitis. As a result, since people with viral hepatitis have a liver that is already in a weakened condition, alcohol can further exacerbate the problem and must be avoided. Hepatitis A does not progress to chronic hepatitis. Severe cases may require LIVER TRANSPLANTATION.

Risk Factors and Preventive Measures

People who are at most risk for contracting hepatitis are those who fit one or more of the following categories:

- reside with someone who has the disease
- are children who attend day care
- are adults who work in a day care center

Maternal-fetal transmission of hepatitis A has not been reported. Injection needles and transfusion products are a minor source of disease. Hepatitis may occasionally affect more than the liver, causing arthritis, optic neuritis, spinal cord problems, thrombocytopenia (low platelets), and aplastic anemia. Hepatitis A is more likely to produce symptoms in adults than in children.

Children and adults can be vaccinated against hepatitis, and the Centers for Disease Control and Prevention (CDC) recommends universal vaccination for hepatitis A for all children aged 12 to 23 months. Adults generally have a vaccination for hepatitis only if they are in a high-risk category: travelers going to an endemic area where hepatitis is known to be prevalent, children and adults living in endemic areas, and chronic liver disease patients.

A passive immunity can be quickly achieved by giving patients pooled immunoglobulin after an acute exposure to hepatitis A. Pooled immunoglobulin already includes the antibodies; it is used *after* the person has had a potential exposure, in order to provide immunity quickly against the virus that has already entered the system. It is also given in cases when there is potential to be exposed soon (travel to endemic area) Both immune serum globulin and HAV vaccine may be given simultaneously if the exposed person belongs to a high-risk group for repeated exposure.

Basic good hygiene can protect against contracting hepatitis A, such as washing the hands before eating or before preparing food or after using the toilet. If a person travels to another country, it is best to drink only bottled water or soft drinks while there and to avoid using ice. Any fruits or vegetables should be thoroughly washed before they are eaten. It is best to eat fruits or vegetables that can be peeled, such as oranges or carrots.

See also CIRRHOSIS; LIVER; LIVER FAILURE.

hepatitis B   Another common form of hepatitis is hepatitis B, which is caused by the hepatitis B virus. Unlike hepatitis A, hepatitis B is caused by contact with body fluids of an infected person, such as the blood or the semen. Worldwide, there are an estimated 300 million persons infected with hepatitis B, or about 5 percent of the global population.

Symptoms and Diagnostic Path
The symptoms of hepatitis B are virtually identical to those of any other form of hepatitis, such as hepatitis A. Most patients with hepatitis B have no symptoms when they acquire the infection. Acute hepatitis B can progress to chronic hepatitis and even CANCER.

A doctor who suspects hepatitis B may order blood tests to confirm the diagnosis. These tests check the blood for hepatitis B virus and/or antibodies against the virus. In some cases, the doctor also orders a liver biopsy, which is the removal of a small amount of tissue from the liver. The biopsy can show whether the virus is affecting the liver and, if so, how severely.

Treatment Options and Outlook
Hepatitis B patients are treated with injections of interferon or with oral medications such as lamivudine, adefovir, entecavir, or telbivudine. Some patients experience total liver failure and must have LIVER TRANSPLANTATION in order to stay alive. Hepatitis B also increases the risk for the development of liver cancer.

Risk Factors and Preventive Measures
Individuals who are at risk for contracting hepatitis B are those who:

- have sex with an infected person without a condom
- are men who have sex with other men
- share a needle used by an infected person
- have body piercing or a tattoo performed by a facility that reuses needles or tools used on an infected person
- are born to a mother who has hepatitis B
- get a needle stick with infected blood (a problem for some health-care workers)
- are medical personnel
- share a toothbrush with an infected person
- have an organ transplantation

Vaccines for hepatitis B can protect individuals from the disease. These vaccines are given to newborn infants, as well as to older children and adults. Universal vaccination of all newborns is the rule. Catch-up vaccination implies vaccination of children who were born before universal neonatal vaccination was implemented amd most of these children are school-age. The vaccine is given in three injections spread over about six months. All three shots must be received for protection against hepatitis B.

Behavioral ways to protect against contracting hepatitis B include the following:

- using a condom when having sex
- avoiding using needles that have been used by others to self-inject drugs
- avoiding using the personal items of another person, such as a toothbrush, razor, or any item that could have any blood on its surface
- not having body piercing or tattooing, or, if they are done, making sure that the person doing the piercing or tattooing uses clean tools by observing that they are removed from sterile packaging

See also CIRRHOSIS; LIVER; LIVER FAILURE.

hepatitis C   A very common viral infection of the liver, hepatitis C is caused by the hepatitis C virus. It is transmitted through body fluids, such as blood. The sexual transmission of hepatitis C is uncommon.

Chronic hepatitis develops in about 60 to 85 percent of the cases of hepatitis C. In about 10 to 20 percent of hepatitis C patients, CIRRHOSIS of the liver develops over time (about 20 years). This risk is accelerated if patients are diagnosed when they are older than age 50, and the risk is further exacerbated if they consume alcohol or have concurrent hepatitis or the human immunodeficiency virus (HIV) infection.

Symptoms and Diagnostic Path

Most people who have hepatitis C have no symptoms or signs until the advanced stages of liver disease. Those who do have symptoms experience the same nonspecific flulike symptoms experienced by hepatitis A or B patients: fatigue, abdominal pain, fever, lack of appetite, and DIARRHEA

Physicians usually detect hepatitis C through a blood test. Initially, an HCV antibody test is done. HCV levels also are measured and are useful in guiding treatment. If hepatitis C is found, the physician may order a liver biopsy to determine how severe the hepatitis is and whether the liver has sustained damage.

Treatment Options and Outlook

There are several different forms of hepatitis C. Genotype 1 is the predominant form found in the United States. It causes more severe disease and is more refractory to medical treatment. Genotypes 2 and 3 cause less severe disease among infected individuals, and these forms of hepatitis C also respond to treatment better even with shorter course of treatment.

Hepatitis C is usually treated with two medications, interferon and ribavarin, unless the case is very mild. In that instance, physicians may postpone treatment while they continue to monitor the patient. The pegylated form of interferon is usually used. If the liver is very damaged, the patient may need LIVER TRANSPLANTATION.

Risk Factors and Preventive Measures

Individuals who are at risk for contracting hepatitis C include the following groups:

- those who have injected drugs with needles that were used by others
- people who have experienced a prick from a needle that has infected blood (a problem faced by some health-care workers)
- INFANTS born to a woman who has hepatitis C
- those who have had body piercings performed by people using equipment infected with hepatitis C (new needles and sterilized equipment should be used for each person)
- individuals who had blood transfusions or organ transplantation before 1990 in the United States or Canada or in the present in poor countries
- people who use intranasal cocaine

- people who have kidney dialysis
- rarely, those who have had sexual contact, especially if one or both partners have other sexually transmitted diseases (however, the risk is minimal to nonexistent if a couple have been in a monogamous relationship for more than five years and the infected person has not yet transmitted the hepatitis to the partner)

There is no vaccine that is available against hepatitis C as of this writing. Actions that an individual can take to limit the risks of contracting hepatitis C are as follows:

- Never share drug needles.
- Wear surgical gloves if the blood of another person must be touched.
- Avoid using another person's toothbrush or other item that may have blood on it.
- Avoid body piercing or tattooing or make sure that the equipment used is sterile.
- If having sex with multiple partners, make sure that males use condoms.

See also CIRRHOSIS; LIVER; LIVER FAILURE.

hepatitis D   Hepatitis D is a rare form that is mostly found in southern Italy, some areas of the former Soviet Union, and Romania. Hepatitis D is primarily spread through the sharing of contaminated needles for drug use. It is also known as the delta virus. It is a defective virus and does not occur independently, but only as a coinfection in patients who also have hepatitis B. Hepatitis D may infect the subject at the same time that he or she is infected with hepatitis B, or chronic hepatitis B patients may be infected later with hepatitis D. Worldwide, 5 percent of hepatitis B carriers also have hepatitis D.

Symptoms and Diagnostic Path

The symptoms of acute hepatitis D are the same as those of all other forms of hepatitis. Diagnosis can be made with blood tests for the virus. Blood is tested for hepatitis B since its presence is essential for hepatitis D. Tests for presence of the HD antigen are not yet widely available. Total (IgM and IgG) anti-HDV antibody testing confirm the diagnosis.

Treatment Options and Outlook

Interferon is used for treatment of patients who are candidates for this therapy, such as patients with chronic hepatitis D and active liver disease as evidenced by abnormal liver enzymes and/or chronic hepatitis on liver biopsy. This is because chronic hepatitis D can be a severe liver disease, and interferon treatment is more likely to be effective in patients with a short duration of infection. Asymptomatic hepatitis D carriers with normal liver enzyme levels do not require therapy, but should be observed to see if more active liver disease develops. The role of foscarnet (Foscavir) in treatment appears promising.

Risk Factors and Preventive Measures

Prevention of hepatitis D involves the same measures used to prevent hepatitis B.

See also CIRRHOSIS; LIVER; LIVER FAILURE; LIVER TRANSPLANTATION.

hepatitis E   Hepatitis E is a form of hepatitis that is rare in the United States and Canada. It is transmitted through contaminated water or food.

Symptoms and Diagnostic Path

The symptoms of hepatitis E infection are the same as those of hepatitis A, B, and C. Often there are no symptoms. Fulminant LIVER FAILURE may occur, especially among pregnant females in the third trimester. It does not cause long-term infection.

Treatment Options and Outlook

Doctors can diagnose the presence of hepatitis E with blood tests. There is no specific treatment for the illness, and generally supportive care is provided. Most patients improve within days to weeks. No chronic hepatitis is caused by hepatitis E.

Risk Factors and Preventive Measures

Person-to-person transmission of hepatitis E is uncommon and less than that for hepatitis A. International travelers and people living in areas where there is an outbreak of hepatitis E are at risk for contracting hepatitis E. The highest attack rate occurs among persons between 15 and 40 years.

There is no vaccine for hepatitis E. International travelers should avoid drinking tap water while in other countries and should wash their hands before eating or preparing food and after using the toilet.

See also CIRRHOSIS; LIVER; LIVER TRANSPLANTATION.

Farci, Patrizia, et al. "Treatment of Chronic Hepatitis D with Interferon Alfa-2a." *New England Journal of Medicine* 330, no. 2 (January 13, 1994): 88–94.

Herrine, Steven K., M.D. "Approach to the Patient with Chronic Hepatitis C Virus Infection," *Annals of Internal Medicine* 136, no. 10 (May 21, 2002): 747–757.

Lieber, Charles S. M.D. "Alcohol and Hepatitis C." *Alcohol Research & Health* 25, no. 4 (2001): 245–254.

Zamani, Saeed, and Steven K. Herrine. "Viral Hepatitis." In *20 Common Problems in Gastroenterology*. New York: McGraw-Hill Medical Publishing Division, 2002.

hereditary pancreatitis   An inherited condition that causes inflammation of the pancreas. Cases of hereditary pancreatitis constitute only a small fraction of all cases of pancreatitis. The condition usually appears before the 20th birthday (usually around age 10) and in some cases may appear before the age of five years. The condition may be mild at first, with increasingly severe occurrences of attacks.

Computed tomography (CT) and ultrasound scans help doctors to diagnose pancreatitis, but these imaging tests do not indicate that the illness is hereditary. An ENDOSCOPIC RETROGRADE CHOLANGIOPANCREATOGRAPHY (ERCP) may be needed in some cases, especially to determine whether surgery is indicated. Genetic testing for hereditary pancreatitis may be undertaken after obtaining full informed consent from a child's parents or guardian. However, not all genetic mutations have been described. Diagnosis is made by the clinical picture, imaging studies, genetic markers, and recognition of the genetic pattern.

See also PANCREAS; PANCREATITIS.

heredity and environment   Both inherited factors as well as the general environment and lifestyle choices of an individual combine together to affect the development of digestive diseases as well as the severity of any diseases that do present in an individual. For example, a person may have an inherited predisposition toward the development of ESOPHAGEAL CANCER. According to the National Commission on Digestive Diseases, chromosomes 9p, 17p, 5q, and 18q are associated with an elevated risk for the development of esophageal adenocarcinoma.

Similarly, chronic idiopathic INFLAMMATORY BOWEL DISEASE also has strong familial risks, and it is most commonly found among individuals of Ashkenazi Jewish ancestry, although individuals of any race or ethnicity may develop inflammatory bowel disorders. (Chronic idiopathic inflammatory bowel disorders include CROHN'S DISEASE and ULCERATIVE COLITIS although about 10 percent of patients may be classified as indeterminate.) Researchers have speculated that as many as 100 different genes may be implicated in the development of Crohn's disease.

Personal choices made by an individual also affect the likelihood of developing a digestive disease; for example, individuals with a hereditary risk for a digestive disease may aggravate their own risk factors by their behavior. For example, an individual who is at an inherited risk for ESOPHAGEAL CANCER may choose to smoke and drink alcohol, further increasing the risk for the development of esophageal cancer. Conversely, they could also mitigate their risk factors somewhat by *not* SMOKING and *not* drinking.

Note that it should not be assumed, if the person at genetic risk continues to drink and smoke, that it is entirely the person's fault should he or she develop this form of cancer; however, individuals with known genetic histories toward a digestive disease, particularly in the cases of their biological parents or siblings, are well advised to take any actions that could decrease or at least not increase the risk for the development of the disease.

Looking at Inherited Risks and Digestive Diseases

As research on genetic issues continues, scientists are finding increasing genetic links to many different digestive diseases, such as cancer, CELIAC

DISEASE, Crohn's disease, and a broad array of other diseases. In many cases, scientists either already have or are working on mapping the exact genetic location linked to the disease.

Autoimmune Disorders and Digestive Diseases According to Andrea Cassinotti, M.D., and colleagues in their article on the human leukocyte antigen (HLA) in the *American Journal of Gastroenterology* in 2009, a review of existing studies indicate that HLA is apparently linked to the development of such autoimmune digestive diseases as celiac disease, inflammatory bowel disease, PRIMARY SCLEROSING CHOLANGITIS and PRIMARY BILIARY CIRRHOSIS. The HLA system involves genes that are located on chromosome 6.

According to the authors, the inheritance of certain HLA alleles affect not only the incidence of the disease but also its severity. For example, HLA-DQB1*0201 is linked to the development of severe intestinal disease. Other HLA alleles are associated with an increased risk for an earlier than normal onset of celiac disease. Immunological blood tests can be used to test for antibodies among those individuals with symptoms suggesting that they may have celiac disease.

Celiac Disease Andrea Cassinotti and colleagues noted that studies have shown that there is a 10 percent risk that a person with celiac disease will also have a sibling with the disease. In addition, the risk of the as-yet unaffected sibling could be further ascertained ahead of time by the genetic testing of HLA genes. The authors also noted that individuals with type 1 diabetes have an increased risk for celiac disease, and that there are some HLA alleles that are common to both diseases.

The authors said, "Autoantibody screening for celiac disease in type-1 diabetes has been recently suggested to prevent long-term celiac disease-related complications and to improve diabetes control. The role of HLA typing in such a screening program is currently under debate."

According to the National Commission on Digestive Diseases, about 3 million people in the United States have celiac disease and one in 22 individuals with celiac disease also have a relative with the disease. Celiac disease is an immune-mediated disorder that affects the gastrointestinal tract of those individuals with this disease. According to the National Commission on Digestive Diseases, celiac disease is largely attributed to specific genetic markers, such as HLA-DQ2 and HLA-DQ8. If it is undiagnosed and untreated, celiac disease can lead to serious vitamin and mineral deficiencies as well as to the development of osteoporosis and other key health problems.

Cystic Fibrosis According to the Online Mendelian Inheritance on Man (OMIM), which reports on information regarding the genetic location for many diseases, the genetic locations of the gene causing CYSTIC FIBROSIS are located at both 7q31.2 and 19q13.1. This disorder is caused by mutations in the cystic fibrosis conductance regulator on chromosome 7.

Colorectal Cancer COLORECTAL CANCER has been linked to many different genets, according to OMIM. Some of the genes map loci identified so far include: 17q24, 17p11.2, 17p13.1, 15q15, 14q32.3, 14q24.3, 11q13, 11p11.2, 1p13.2, 9q32-q33, 8p22-p21.3, 5q21-q22,4q32, 3q26.3, 1p35, 2p25, 22q13, and 20q13.2-q13.3. According to the National Commission on Digestive Diseases, about one-third of all patients with colorectal cancer have a first or second degree relative with colorectal cancer. This is one reason why screening for colorectal cancer on a schedule determined by a gastroenterologist is so important. Any precancerous POLYPS found during the colonoscopy can be easily removed by the physician. If cancer has already developed, treatment can begin immediately.

Diabetes Type 2 diabetes has been linked to many different genetic loci, according to OMIM. It is also a consequence of HEMOCHROMATOSIS. Type 1 diabetes has been mapped to the following locations: 12q24.2, 1p13, 7p21, 6p21.3, tpter-p21, and Xp11.23-q13.3. Among identical twins, when one twin has type 1 diabetes, the other twin also has type 2 diabetes in 30 to 50 percent of the cases, indicating that there is also an environmental factor that is present and which may trigger the onset of the disease—although that factor is unknown as of this writing.

Esophageal Cancer Researchers have known for many years that there is a familial risk for the development of esophageal cancer. Esophageal squamous cell carcinoma has been linked to several different genetic loci, according to the OMIM, including 16q23.2-q24.1, 13q12.11, 9q32, 8p22, 2p22-p21.3, and 3p22.

Gallbladder Disease According to the OMIM, one form of cholelithiasis (GALLBLADDER disease) is linked to the ABCB4 gene on chromosome 7q21. In addition, there are genetic susceptibilities to gallbladder disease that include the development of GALLSTONES and that have been identified among Mexican Americans at risk. Some genetic research has also shown that a key factor in the formation of cholesterol gallstones is the hypersecretion of cholesterol into the bile.

Hemochromatosis An iron overload disease first identified in 1865, hemochromatosis has a strong hereditary component, which was first described in 1935. According to the OMIM, hemochromatosis is linked to gene map locus 6p21.3 and 20p12, but it is usually caused by a mutation on chromosome 6p21.3. Hemochromatosis can lead to liver CIRRHOSIS, LIVER CANCER, diabetes, and heart failure. If treatment is initiated before the disease has advanced, then these complications can usually be avoided.

Inflammatory Bowel Disease According to Grishma J. Joy and colleagues in their article in *Practical Gastroenterology* in 2009, there is an association between NOD2/CARD 15 gene mutations on chromosome 16 and an earlier age of onset, ileal involvement and the need for both initial and repeated bowel resections among those with inflammatory bowel disease (IBD). Research has also shown that African Americans are more likely to have ileocolonic or colon disease than Caucasians (whites).

Studies have shown that the first-degree relatives of individuals diagnosed with IBD have a 5-20 times greater risk for IBD than those from unaffected families. Up to half of identical twins may have IBD, compared to 5 to 10 percent of nonidentical twins.

The National Institute of Diabetes & Digestive & Kidney Diseases (NIDDK) has reported that as of 2009 more than 30 different genes have been linked to Crohn's disease and as many as 100 genes may be linked to Crohn's disease. This genetic risk for Crohn's disease has been known for years although the actual genes have not been identified until recent years.

Ulcerative Colitis Mark S. Silverberg and colleagues reported in *Nature Genetics* in 2009 that the genetic location for ulcerative colitis has been identified on chromosomes 1p36 and 12q15. According to the researchers, DNA samples were taken from 1,052 people diagnosed with ulcerative colitis, and in addition, pre-existing data from 2,571 European controls was also used. The most likely candidate genes that were linked to ulcerative colitis were identified as PLA2G-E, IFNG, IL26, and IL22.

Pancreatic Cancer First degree relatives of those who have had pancreatic cancer are the most at risk for inheriting a genetic predisposition toward the development of pancreatic cancer. President Jimmy Carter's brother died of pancreatic cancer, as did his father and sister, and pancreatic cancer as well as bone and breast cancer killed his mother. In studies of families in which two or more first-degree relatives had pancreatic cancer, the average age of diagnosis was 62.8 years.

Primary Sclerosing Cholangitis A rare liver disease, primary sclerosing cholangitis (PSC) has a genetic link to HLA according to Cassinotti and colleagues, who say that there is a 100 times increased risk of the disease occurring to a sibling when another sibling has this disease. The authors also state that there are many links between PSC and HLA, although no specific shared susceptibility has been identified to date and the genetic locus has not been mapped as of this writing.

Stomach Cancer STOMACH CANCER, also known as gastric cancer, has been linked to many different genes. The genetic susceptibility may be triggered by infection with *HELICOBACTER PYLORI*. Stomach cancer is also associated with Type A blood as well as with the development of PERNICIOUS ANEMIA.

Environmental Risks

Sometimes the environment itself presents risks to the individual, as when the person is exposed to toxic materials on the job or elsewhere, in the case of lead poisoning or poisoning with other toxic substances. Fortunately, such instances are relatively rare in the United States, as far as is known. However, there are many common bacteria that are easily transmissible in society, and that often cause disease. *Helicobacter pylori* (*H. pylori*) lives in the stomach of millions of individuals in the United States, although most people who harbor this bacterium do not develop the ULCERS caused by *H. pylori*.

Some common bacteria cause transient discomfort such as bacteria that cause DIARRHEA. Poor food preparation can lead to food contamination and a resulting overgrowth of bacteria, which leads to food poisoning, which is characterized by nausea and vomiting as well as diarrhea.

Personal Lifestyle Choices

Individuals make lifestyle choices that directly affect their lives and their digestive systems. For example, the smoking habit is very damaging to the body and increases the risk for the development of cancer as well as other harm to the body. The choice to drink alcohol to excess also affects the body, increasing the risk for digestive cancers and other disorders. It should be noted that people who are addicted to tobacco and alcohol may believe that it is a personal choice to smoke or drink; however, there are medications and treatments to end these addictions and decrease the risk of harm to the body.

Overeating and failing to exercise are lifestyle choices that lead to OBESITY, a major problem for at least one-third of the adult population of the United States, according to the Centers for Disease Control and Prevention (CDC). These are also choices that increase the risk for the development of type 2 DIABETES MELLITUS, as well as many forms of cancer, including colorectal cancer.

Smoking   Smoking worsens the course of many diseases, such as Crohn's disease and GASTROPARESIS (slowed stomach emptying). It is also a risk factor for the development of ANAL CANCER, esophageal, and oral cancer. Smoking is also a known risk factor for pancreatic cancer. Smoking does not cause diabetes, but doctors report that it makes its management much more difficult. Individuals who have digestive ulcers have a worsening of their condition if they smoke.

In a study of 97 patients with PRIMARY BILIARY CIRRHOSIS, reported by Claudia O. Zein and colleagues in *Hepatology* in 2006, the researchers found that advanced disease was directly related to cigarette smoking, and among those who smoked, the consumption of tobacco was higher in those with more advanced symptoms.

Paradoxically, smoking has opposing effects in two types of inflammatory bowel disease; it has a protective role in ulcerative colitis, but it is harmful in Crohn's disease. However, the many health problems that smoking causes need to be taken into account for those who have ulcerative colitis.

Drinking Alcohol   Drinking alcohol, and particularly drinking alcohol to excess, clearly increases the risk for some digestive diseases, such as alcoholic hepatitis and cirrhosis, and it also worsens the prognosis for existing diseases, such as GASTROESOPHAGEAL REFLUX DISEASE (GERD). Excessive drinking leads to liver cirrhosis and finally, to the development of liver cancer.

Some long-term drinkers develop diabetes because of harm that has occurred to the pancreas. They may also develop PANCREATITIS and increase their risk for the development of pancreatic cancer. An estimated 80 percent of all cases of pancreatitis are caused by either gallstones or alcoholism. Chronic alcoholism can lead to an increased risk for ANEMIA. Alcoholism also increases the risk for the development of colorectal cancer. Heavy drinkers are also at risk for oral cancer.

People who abuse alcohol for an extended period are at risk for MALNUTRITION as well as for mineral and VITAMIN DEFICIENCIES, particularly a deficiency of folic acid, vitamin B_{12} and vitamin A. In addition, long-term heavy drinkers are at a considerable risk for a severe thiamine (vitamin B_1) deficiency, which can lead to WERNICKE'S ENCEPHALOPATHY. Alcoholics are also often deficient in other important minerals such as ZINC.

About half the patients suffering from MALLORY-WEISS SYNDROME are alcoholics. Mallory-Weiss tear is caused by internal gastrointestinal bleeding in the area where the esophagus joins the stomach. It may be caused by vomiting or retching, a common behavior among people who are alcoholics.

Obesity   Excessive weight increases the risk for the development of some cancers as well as the onset of type 2 diabetes. In addition, OBESITY is linked to many other digestive disorders, such as gastroesophageal reflux disease, colorectal cancer, and even asthma. About one-third of all Americans are obese, and two-thirds are either obese or overweight. A sedentary lifestyle combined with abundant high-calorie food is largely responsible for the prominence of obesity in the United States today, and individuals must actively seek to gain a more healthy body through exercising and saying no to calorie-laden choices if they wish to attain better health and also live a longer life. Obesity and central adiposity (fat belly) is also linked to the development of BARRETT'S ESOPHAGUS, according to the National Commission on Digestive Diseases in their 2009 report.

Combined Personal Lifestyle Choices Some lifestyle choices worsen the outcome of diseases even more than each factor alone. For example, smoking and drinking work together to increase the risks for the development or the worse prognosis of gastroesophageal reflux disease. Smoking and drinking also increase the risk for the development of esophageal cancer. In addition, the risk of developing head and neck cancer is 200 times greater for heavy smokers and drinkers than for others.

The common combination of obesity and lack of exercise increases the risk for most diseases, as does the combination of excessive weight and smoking. The greater the number of poor choices made by an individual, the higher the likelihood that he or she will suffer from one or more serious digestive diseases. When combined with a genetic risk for a disease, the risk is raised even higher.

See also ALCOHOL ABUSE AND ALCOHOLISM; DEMOGRAPHIC FACTORS; EMERGENCY ISSUES IN DIGESTIVE DISORDERS; ELDERLY.

Cassinotti, Andrea, M.D., et al. "HLA and Autoimmune Digestive Disease: A Clinically Oriented Review for Gastroenterologists." *American Journal of Gasteroenterology* 104 (2009): 195–217.

Joy, Grishma J., Raymond K. Cross, and Mark H Flasar. "Race and Inflammatory Bowel Disease." *Practical Gastroenterology* Series #48 (2009): 23–33.

Silverberg, Mark S. "Ulcerative Colitis Loci in Chromosomes 1p36 and 12q15 Identified by Genome-Wide Association Study." *Nature Genetics* 2,009, no. 4 (2009): 216–220.

U.S. Department of Health and Human Services. *Opportunities and Challenges in Digestive Diseases Research: Recommendations of the National Commission on Digestive Diseases*. Bethesda, Md.: National Institutes of Health, March 2009.

Zein, Claudia O., et al. "Smoking and Increased Severity of Hepatic Fibrosis in Primary Biliary Cirrhosis: A Cross Validated Retrospective Assessment." *Hepatology* 44, no. 6 (2006): 1,564–1,571.

hernia, hiatal A medical condition that is caused by the sliding of a section of the upper part of the stomach into the chest through an opening in the diaphragm (esophageal hiatus). It may be a very dangerous condition, but in most cases, hiatal hernias are not symptomatic, and they remain undiagnosed and are not a problem for most people who have them.

The hiatal hernia may be a sliding hernia or a paraesophageal hiatal hernia. In sliding hiatal hernia, part of the stomach along with the junction of the stomach and the ESOPHAGUS slide up into the chest. In the case of paraesophageal hiatal hernia, the junction stays at the level of the diaphragm, whereas part of the stomach moves into the chest cavity. The combination of the two may be seen in some cases.

Symptoms and Diagnostic Path

As mentioned, in most cases, there are no symptoms or signs of a hiatal hernia. A few patients may have ulcers in the hernia and may experience gastrointestinal bleeding as well as ANEMIA. The paraesophageal hernia can become twisted in a life-threatening fashion, and the patient may enter an emergency room with severe upper abdominal pain. If hiatal hernias cause severe symptoms, they can be surgically repaired.

Treatment Options and Outlook

In many cases, the surgery can be performed laparoscopically, through small incisions that are made in the abdomen. In many cases, however, the treatment for the hiatal hernia is the same as for GERD; for example, physicians recommend lifestyle changes, such as advising obese patients to lose weight, which may result in the reduction of the hiatal hernia, along with recommending acid blocking drugs.

Risk Factors and Preventive Measures

People who are obese have a greater risk of the development of hiatal hernia than others. The presence of GASTROESOPHAGEAL REFLUX DISEASE (GERD) worsens a hiatal hernia.

Minocha, Anil, M.D., and Christine Adamec. *How to Stop Heartburn: Simple Ways to Heal Heartburn and Acid Reflux.* New York: John Wiley & Sons, 2001.

Hirschsprung's disease (HD) A severe disease of the colon that causes a loss of nerve cells in part of the COLON/rectum and is usually diagnosed for the first time in INFANTS or small children and occasionally in adults. The disease was named after Harald Hirschsprung, a Danish pediatrician who wrote about the condition in 1888. In the case of infants and children who have the disease, a pediatric gastroenterologist should be consulted for treatment. Adults should be treated by a gastroenterologist.

The disease causes severe CONSTIPATION, and sometimes the child who has Hirschsprung's disease (HD) is unable to have BOWEL MOVEMENTS; blockage and backup result. This condition may lead to abdominal distention and even perforation of the colon, which may be fatal to the child. The cause of the disease remains to be established; the potential causes for problems include lack of migration of appropriate nerve cells during pregnancy or the damaged or destroyed nerve cells in the rectum/colon. The affected part does not relax to accommodate the passage of stool, causing functional obstruction. Only a small segment of the rectum and the sigmoid colon is involved in about 75 percent of cases; however, in about 10 percent of cases of Hirschsprung's disease, the entire colon is affected.

Hirschsprung's disease occurs in about one in every 5,000 births. About 20 percent of infants born with HD die in infancy,

Symptoms and Diagnostic Path

The majority of cases of Hirschsprung's disease present within the first few weeks of birth. Among newborns, infants with Hirschsprung's disease may vomit green bile after eating and may also have a swollen abdomen. There may be a delay in the passage of the first stool. These infants may have problems with DEHYDRATION and FAILURE TO THRIVE. These babies are usually very fussy because they are extremely uncomfortable as a result of both GAS and constipation.

Small children and school-age children who have Hirschsprung's disease also have major problems with constipation, although some may have DIARRHEA at some times. In addition, children with this disease usually have slower growth and development rates than other children their own age.

Infants and children who have Hirschsprung's disease may contract a severe, life-threatening infection called enterocolitis. If a child who has the disease shows any of the following indicators, the physician should be called immediately:

- bleeding from the rectum
- swollen abdomen
- vomiting
- diarrhea
- fever

Adults and adolescents who have Hirschsprung's disease may be severely constipated. Adults also may have a dilated colon and rectum caused by the disease. Doctors may suspect Hirschsprung's disease because of a patient's symptoms and/or a family medical history of HD, although other medical problems, such as IRRITABLE BOWEL SYNDROME (IBS) in adults, may be diagnosed instead unless tests are ordered.

The barium X-ray is one test used to diagnose Hirschsprung's disease; in this test, barium is inserted into the anus and the colon so that the physician can take X-rays in which the barium highlights the colon. The barium enema reveals the narrow affected area of the colon/rectum and the proximal dilated colon. If a patient has a chronic problem with severe constipation, particularly a newborn baby who is suffering from chronic severe constipation, the physician may use diatrizoate meglumine (Gastrografin) rather than barium. Gastrografin is a water-soluble contrast dye that has the effect of a stool softener as well as a highlighter of the intestine on X-rays.

Anorectal manometry to test for pressure—relaxation responses in the anorectal region—is a test that is done on adults. A biopsy is considered to be the best diagnostic tool for HD. The biopsy result shows whether nerve cells are missing from the colon/rectum and definitively proves the presence of HD when it is present.

Treatment Options and Outlook

Surgery is usually the treatment of choice for HD. There are different methods of performing the procedure; all involve removing the damaged part of the intestine and then connecting the healthy intestine as close as possible to the anus to preserve the anal sphincter.

Surgery results in normal or near-normal anorectal function in most cases. An estimated 70 to 90 percent of children are able to have five or fewer stools daily after the operation. Some children have diarrhea for a while, and others may subsequently have problems with constipation. These problems can usually be treated by stool softeners or other medications ordered for the patient. There is a minimal operative mortality rate, and long-term problems, such as fecal soiling, occur in about 10 percent of patients.

Risk Factors and Preventive Measures

Familial forms of Hirschsprung's disease stem from a genetic mutation that leads to lack of function in part of the colon; usually all children in a family do not have the disease. Several different genetic mutations have been identified in patients with HD. The disease may also occur sporadically, with no known familial relationship. Researchers say that it is not caused by anything that a pregnant woman does or does not do during her pregnancy.

Males are about four times more likely to be diagnosed with this medical problem than females. Hirschsprung's disease is associated with some cases of Down syndrome, and it occurs in about 6 percent of individuals diagnosed with Down syndrome.

There are no known preventive measures.

Eng, Charis, M.D., "The *RET* Proto-Oncogene in Multiple Endocrine Neoplasia Type 2 and Hirschsprung's Disease." *New England Journal of Medicine* 335, no. 13 (September 20, 1996): 943–951.

histamine-2 blockers Medications that block the acid secretion caused by body chemicals known as histamines. Histamine-2 blockers (H-2 blockers) are used to treat such patients as those who have chronic acid reflux problems, gastroesophageal reflux disease (GERD), or peptic ulcer. Treatment may be short term or long term, depending on the clinical situation. Patients who do not respond well to H-2 blockers are treated with more potent acid blockers called proton pump inhibitors.

The commonly known H-2 blockers include cimetidine (Tagamet), ranitidine (Zantac), famotidine (Pepcid), and nizatidine (Axid). H-2 blockers cut back on the production of acid in the stomach, allowing the ulcerated stomach to heal and helping the patient with GERD to feel better.

H-2 blockers are also available over-the-counter although the doses are lower than prescribed drugs. Studies have shown that prescribed H-2 blockers are effective in about half of cases of GERD. Sometimes over-the-counter H-2 blockers, including Tagamet HB, Zantac 75, and Pepcid AC, may be used for occasional indigestion.

See also ACID BLOCKING AGENTS; ACID REFLUX; GASTROESOPHAGEAL REFLUX DISEASE; PROTON PUMP INHIBITORS; ULCERS.

hormones Chemical messengers that are produced by the body or manufactured synthetically and that travel through the bloodstream to their site of action. For example, thyroid hormone is naturally produced by most people; however, in some people the body produces insufficient amounts of thyroid hormone and they need supplemental thyroid to survive. In contrast, others may produce too much thyroid hormone, and then the thyroid gland needs to be suppressed. Both former President George H. W. Bush and his wife, Barbara Bush, had overactive thyroid gland, for which they were treated.

Adrenaline is a hormone that is naturally produced by the body, but in some cases, such as a severe allergic reaction, an injection of adrenaline or a similar substance is needed to supplement the sudden increase in demand for the body's adrenaline production to combat acute illness.

Insulin is a hormone that is produced by the pancreas and is required for glucose metabolism. A deficiency of insulin production leads to diabetes mellitus.

The key digestive hormones are cholecystokinin (CCK), gastrin, and secretin.

See also DIABETES MELLITUS; HORMONE THERAPY; SECRETIN.

hormone therapy Usually refers to the female hormones (estrogen or estrogen/progesterone combinations) that are given to women to resolve troubling symptoms of menopause; however, hormones may also be given as supplements for other conditions. Female hormones are also administered for the prevention of osteoporosis (the loss of bone density) to women who cannot tolerate the other drugs. Combination hormone replacement therapy increases the risk for the development of breast cancer, stroke and venous thrombosis.

Some people are deficient in thyroid hormone and need supplemental thyroid hormone to reach a normal level. Patients with type 1 diabetes are deficient in insulin and are treated with insulin injections, which they are trained to do themselves. Some men may become deficient in testosterone, which can be supplemented with testosterone hormone therapy. It is also true that women have a low level of testosterone present in their body, just as men have a low level of estrogen.

When female hormones are given, they are usually administered by a primary care physician or gynecologist. Other hormones, such as thyroid hormones or growth hormones, are likely to be monitored by an endocrinologist.

See also MENOPAUSE.

human immunodeficiency virus The virus (HIV) that leads to acquired immunodeficiency syndrome (AIDS). HIV is transmitted through sexual contact as well as through sharing of contaminated needles or through blood, such as in a blood transfusion from contaminated blood. Individuals who have HIV are at risk for development of CACHEXIA, a state in which weight loss and body wasting occur.

Once AIDS develops, the patient's immune system is compromised and the person has a high risk for the development of infections that may become fatal. Until recently, all HIV was uniformly fatal. However, today once HIV is diagnosed, patients are started on treatment against HIV to suppress it, and they may live for a long time. The famous basketball star Earvin "Magic" Johnson was diagnosed with HIV in the late 1980s and as of 2010 appeared to be doing extremely well with treatment.

See also KAPOSI'S SARCOMA.

Hymenolepis nana (H. nana) A dwarf tapeworm that infects individuals worldwide and is spread by bad or insufficient sanitation and poor personal hygiene. It is most common in Asia and Latin America, although it is also found among some low-income children in the United States. It is more commonly found among children than adults.

Infected individuals have abdominal pain, diarrhea, pruritus ani (itching at the anus), and poor appetite. Some patients experience sleep disorders, dizziness, and seizures. The diagnosis is made by finding *H. nana* eggs in the stool.

Those who have *Hymenolepis nana* are treated with praziquantel given in a single dose and repeated in 10 days, which is effective in 95 percent of the cases of patients infected with this tapeworm.

See also PARASITIC INFECTIONS.

hyperemesis gravidarum A condition of severe vomiting that usually occurs in the first trimester of pregnancy and is far more severe than the expected "morning sickness" that many pregnant women experience. The cause of hyperemesis gravidarum is unknown, although the condition is considered a pregnancy-associated LIVER disease. In extreme cases of the disease, hyperemesis gravidarum may cause patients to experience DEHYDRATION, MALNUTRITION, and even death. Most women with hyperemesis gravidarum recover in the second trimester of pregnancy.

An estimated 1 percent of all pregnant women experience hyperemesis gravidarum.

Symptoms and Diagnostic Path

In addition to the nausea and the severe vomiting that are characteristic of hyperemesis gravidarum, abdominal pain and mild JAUNDICE may be present. Many women with this condition also have GASTROESOPHAGEAL REFLUX DISEASE (GERD). Other symptoms and signs are as follows:

- dehydration
- loss of more than 5 percent of body weight
- abnormal liver enzyme values (in up to half of women who have hyperemesis gravidarum)

- hyperbilirubinemia (high level of bilirubin in the blood, which is found in about half of women who are hospitalized for hyperemesis gravidarum)

Physicians diagnose hyperemesis gravidarum on the basis of medical history, symptoms, and findings of a physical examination that is supplemented by laboratory tests, such as liver function tests. Blood levels may be abnormal among pregnant women with this condition, such as elevated levels of BILIRUBIN, alkaline phosphatase, and aminotransferases. Serum electrolytes (sodium, potassium, magnesium, etc.) may be abnormal as well.

Treatment Options and Outlook

Many women with hyperemesis gravidarum need to be hospitalized so that symptoms such as dehydration and electrolyte imbalance can be reversed with intravenous infusions of needed fluids. Pyridoxine (vitamin B$_6$), ginger, and antihistamines are commonly prescribed as a treatment. Antiemetic medications are also administered to stop vomiting, and GERD patients may need to take PROTON PUMP INHIBITOR medications, prokinetic drugs, or histamine-2 receptor blocker drugs.

Some patients may need total PARENTERAL NUTRITION (feeding through the veins). Most but not all women recover from hyperemesis gravidarum by the second trimester; in some it may last until the delivery. The goal of most physicians is to stabilize their condition until that time.

Risk Factors and Preventive Meausres

Pregnant women who are below the age of 25 years have a greater risk of development of hyperemesis gravidarum than older pregnant women. In addition, women who have had multiple pregnancies also have a greater risk. The cause of hyperemesis gravidarum is unknown, but psychogenic as well as hormonal factors and nutritional deficiencies have been implicated.

There are no known preventive measures.

See also LIVER ENZYMES/FUNCTION TESTS; NAUSEA AND VOMITING; PREGNANCY.

hypergastrinemia Excessively high blood level of gastrin, a gastrointestinal hormone that stimulates the secretion of gastric acid. Blood tests such as the serum gastrin level can determine whether patients are within the normal range; among patients who have fasted, serum gastrin levels are usually less than 100 pg/ml (picograms per milliliter).

If patients have a higher level of serum gastrin, they may have ZOLLINGER–ELLISON SYNDROME. They may also have renal insufficiency, PERNICIOUS ANEMIA, or a gastric outlet obstruction. Hypergastrinemia patients may also have MULTIPLE ENDOCRINE NEOPLASIA. If patients are taking high doses of proton pump inhibitor medications, the test result indicates hypergastrinemia that is medication induced, which is not considered a problem.

See also PROTON PUMP INHIBITORS.

hypoalbuminemia Below-normal level of albumin in the blood that is caused by liver disease, malnutrition, or severe kidney disease. Patients with kidney disease, especially nephrotic syndrome, excrete excessive amounts of protein in the urine, Hypoalbuminemia may result in fluid buildup in the body including swelling at the ankles and feet and in the abdomen (ASCITES). Individuals who have a low serum albumin level have a high risk for complications of any surgery.

See also ALBUMIN.

ileoanal pouch A pouch that comprises part of the small intestine and is connected to the anal canal. The procedure to create this pouch is usually done for ulcerative colitis patients. The ileoanal pouch is also known as the ileoanal reservoir. It is created in a process that is performed to remove the colon, the upper rectum, and most of the lower rectum. The surgeon then creates the ileoanal pouch from the small intestines so that it can hold the patient's stools, allowing continent function. Depending on how the pouch is constructed, it is sometimes called the J pouch, W pouch, or S pouch. This surgery is also performed in patients with familial adenomatous polyps. The pouch may become inflamed in some cases, a condition called POUCHITIS.

See also ULCERATIVE COLITIS.

imaging studies Radiologic diagnostic tests such as X-rays, computed tomography (CT) scans, nuclear scintigraphy (nuclear medicine scans) and magnetic resonance imaging (MRI) scans. Such tests are used to identify defects or diseases in the digestive system (as well as other systems). They are sometimes also used as part of therapy, for example, to assist a physician in performing a procedure such as a liver biopsy, PARACENTESIS, and drainage of an abscess. Radiologic imaging may be combined with endoscopic procedures, as in ERCP and endoscopic ultrasound.

See also ENDOSCOPY.

infants Babies may experience a broad range of digestive diseases and disorders, but of greatest concern are those illnesses that are severe or even life-threatening to the infant. Examples of such diseases and disorders include CELIAC SPRUE, food allergies, neonatal HEMOCHROMATOSIS (an iron overload in the blood of newborns), HIRSCHSPRUNG'S DISEASE, NECROTIZING ENTEROCOLITIS, and VITAMIN DEFICIENCIES. In addition, in some poor countries, untreated DIARRHEA and other infections may be sufficient to dehydrate and even kill some newborns.

See also FOOD ALLERGIES; DEHYDRATION; INTUSSUSCEPTION.

inflammatory bowel disease (IBD) A common disorder of the colon or the small intestine. It is often characterized by DIARRHEA, ABDOMINAL PAIN, BLEEDING, and other symptoms. The two primary types of illnesses that constitute chronic idiopathic inflammatory bowel disease are CROHN'S DISEASE and ULCERATIVE COLITIS. It may not be possible to determine the type of IBD in about 10 percent of cases; such cases are characterized as indeterminate.

Ulcerative colitis involves only parts of the colon and rectum, whereas Crohn's disease can involve any part of the gastrointestinal system from the mouth to the anus. As a result, the surgical removal of the colon and the rectum is curative for ulcerative colitis, whereas there is no known cure for Crohn's disease.

Inflammatory bowel disease patients can have the involvement of the organs outside the gut, such as eye problems (uveitis, episcleritis), arthritis, kidney stones, a skin rash such as erythema nodusum, autoimmune hepatitis, and PRIMARY SCLEROSING CHOLANGITIS. Individuals with inflammatory bowel disease also have an increased risk of development of COLORECTAL CANCER. In addition, researchers reporting their findings in 2000 in the *Annals of Internal Medicine* revealed that their patients with

IBD (more than 6,000 subjects) had a significantly increased risk of having osteopenia (low bone density) and a 40 percent greater risk of experiencing hip fractures than those without IBD. They also had a higher rate of other bone fractures.

Drugs used to treat IBD include aminosalicylates (Asacol®, Pentasa® Apriso®), corticosteroids (prednisone), Imuran®, Remicade®, Humira®, and methotrexate.

Although often confused with it, inflammatory bowel disease is not the same as IRRITABLE BOWEL SYNDROME (IBS), which is usually a condition of disturbed bowel habit (chronic CONSTIPATION or diarrhea or constipation that fluctuates with diarrhea) associated with abdominal pain. IBS does not cause any grossly evident damage to the colon; nor does it cause an increased risk of development of colorectal cancer. In contrast, IBD is manifested with visible damage to the involved portions of the small and/or the large intestine and may also affect other organs such as the skin, the eyes, the LIVER, the GALLBLADDER, and the joints.

See also CELIAC SPRUE.

interferon A substance that is naturally produced by the body and is useful in maintaining the body's immune defenses. It can also be given in the form of a drug to combat some kinds of infections and cancers. Some patients who have forms of hepatitis, primarily hepatitis B, C, and D, are treated with interferon. The pegylated form of interferon is a long-acting interferon that is required only once a week, in contrast to conventional interferon given to treat hepatitis C, which is administered three times a week.

Patients who have some other diseases, including melanoma, advanced renal (kidney) cancer, certain kinds of leukemia, and multiple sclerosis, are also treated with interferon.

See also HEPATITIS.

intussusception A very severe medical problem in which part of the intestines becomes wrapped up by another part, causing an intestinal obstruction and sometimes bleeding. Some cases are fatal, if not treated quickly. When it occurs, intussuscep-

tion is primarily a problem among infants ages three to five months old. Eighty percent of pediatric intussusceptions involve the ileum (the last part of the small intestine) and the colon. Infants who have this problem appear to be in abdominal distress. They vomit bilious material and have stools that resemble currant jelly.

In some cases, the baby has an intestinal defect, such as MECKEL'S DIVERTICULUM; in most cases, the cause of the intussusception is unknown.

Intussusception can also occur in adults; when it does, there is usually involvement of a distinct diseased part of the gut, and cancer occurs in up to one-half of these adults.

Some experts believe that respiratory adenovirus and rotavirus gastroenteritis can trigger intussusception. In one circumstance reported in 1999 in *Morbidity and Mortality Weekly Report,* a rotavirus vaccine that was given to infants apparently caused intussusception in some at a rate that was higher than was normally seen. The vaccine was withdrawn from the market.

Depending on the severity of the intussusception, some children can be treated with just an enema, whereas others will require hospitalization and may need surgery.

See also INFANTS.

Centers for Disease Control and Prevention. "Intussusception among Recipients of Rotavirus Vaccine—United States, 1998–1999." *Morbidity and Mortality Report* 48 (1999): 577–581.

Parashar, Umesh D., et al. "Trends in Intussusception-Associated Hospitalizations and Deaths among US Infants." *Pediatrics* 106, no. 6 (December 2000): 1,413–1,421.

iron A mineral that is necessary for health and in which some people may become deficient, as in iron deficiency anemia. The main role of iron is its involvement with the transport of oxygen throughout the body; iron is also an important part of many cell components as well as enzymes.

Heme iron and nonheme iron are the types of dietary iron. Foods that are rich in heme iron include cooked chicken liver, oysters, beef, turkey (dark turkey has a greater percentage of heme iron), and chicken. Foods that are rich in nonheme iron include soybeans, lentils, kidney beans, pinto beans, lima beans, spinach, grains, and fruit.

Risk Factors for Iron Deficiency

People who are at risk for development of iron deficiency include individuals in the following categories:

- people who have kidney failure on kidney dialysis, especially those who are receiving erythropoietin
- women who are *not* menopausal
- older INFANTS and toddlers
- people who have cancer
- patients who have chronic gastrointestinal BLEEDING that may be difficult to cure, such as that caused by abnormal blood vessels in the bowel wall and radiation proctitis

Signs of an iron deficiency include the following:

- chronic weakness and fatigue
- slower or worse performance at work or at school
- low body temperature
- increased numbers of infections, indicating a decreased immune function

Treatment of Iron Deficiency

Iron deficiency is usually treated with supplemental iron. Iron can be given orally or intravenously. Oral iron supplements may in some cases cause gastrointestinal problems, such as nausea and vomiting, and may cause either diarrhea or constipation. In patients for whom oral iron may cause problems, such as those who have inflammatory bowel disease, iron can be administered intravenously.

Excessive Levels of Iron

Most people do not have toxic levels of iron in their body unless they are taking high and unnecessary supplemental doses of iron and/or are otherwise susceptible to an iron overload state. Over-the-counter iron supplements should not be taken unless recommended by a physician. Women who

are postmenopausal rarely need to take iron supplements if they eat a well-balanced diet.

An iron overdose can be very dangerous in children. Even as little as one to three grams of iron can be fatal to a child weighing less than 22 pounds. For this reason, it is very important for people who take iron supplements and who have small children to keep the supplements securely capped and well out of reach of toddlers.

Some people suffer from a rare disease that causes an iron overload in the body called HEMACHROMATOSIS. They also have an increased risk of development of LIVER CANCER.

People who need frequent blood transfusions are also at risk for development of an iron overload problem.

Pregnant Women and Iron

Most women who are pregnant take vitamin pills with iron supplements to prevent anemia. Women who are anemic during PREGNANCY have an increased risk of having a baby who has low birth weight and/or is born prematurely. The mothers themselves are more likely to have complications from the delivery.

See also ANEMIA; VITAMIN DEFICIENCIES/EXCESSES.

iron deficiency anemia   See ANEMIA; IRON.

irritable bowel syndrome (IBS) A common chronic medical problem that is usually characterized by ABDOMINAL PAIN plus disturbance of bowel function, either CONSTIPATION or DIARRHEA, and sometimes by alternating conditions of both disorders. IBS is also also known as a spastic COLON. The colon of patients with IBS exhibits an abnormal pattern of colonic motility and contractions, although these findings are not consistent.

IBS is the most frequently diagnosed disease among patients seen by gastroenterologists in the United States.

IBS should not be confused with INFLAMMATORY BOWEL DISEASE (IBD), which is an intestinal inflammation that stems from either CROHN'S DISEASE or ULCERATIVE COLITIS. IBS is *not* associated with visible inflammation or cancer, and its presence does not increase the patient's risk of development of cancer. Some who are diagnosed with IBS may actually have other illnesses, such as CELIAC SPRUE or a small intestinal bacterial overgrowth, which should be treated if identified.

Irritable bowel syndrome can be very aggravating for the patients who have it, and some patients must change jobs because they must use the toilet frequently. However, despite the aggravation that IBS causes those who have it, the condition does not cause permanent grossly visible damage to either the colon or the digestive tract; nor does it appear to cause other diseases, although IBS patients have a lower quality of life and an increased risk for diagnosis with other medical problems, such as FIBROMYALGIA, a chronic muscle pain disorder as well as noncardiac CHEST PAIN; psychiatric disorders; and/or interstitial cystitis, a chronic spasming and irritation of the bladder.

It is unknown what causes IBS, although those with IBS appear to have a very sensitive colon that may react spasmodically to some triggers, such as some foods or medications. Chocolate is an apparent trigger for some patients with IBS; milk and fatty foods or tomatoes may induce spasms in others. Large meals may trigger IBS for some patients. Some doctors believe that women's reproductive hormones may play a role, because IBS symptoms often worsen during menstrual periods. In most instances, however, no single trigger for IBS is identified.

The presence of increased stress makes IBS symptoms more likely to occur, although stress does not cause IBS. (Stress often exacerbates many chronic conditions, such as headaches, arthritis, and back pain.) Recent studies suggest that the IBS may be preceded or precipitated by an intestinal infection, which normally would be self-limited, but the symptoms tend to persist in patients who are predisposed to development of IBS. A composite biopsychosocial model for causation of the disease has been proposed. This model includes the involvement at the brain and spinal cord, the gut, and environmental influences.

Symptoms and Diagnostic Path

Physicians report that IBS patients usually have abdominal pain plus disturbed bowel function in the form of diarrhea, constipation, or alternating diarrhea and constipation, a condition that has been present for at least three months in the past year. The pain of IBS lessens with defecation.

The presence of the following symptoms further supports the diagnosis:

- straining during BOWEL MOVEMENTS
- feelings of incompleteness after a bowel movement
- hard stools or loose and watery stools
- abdominal bloating

Irritable bowel syndrome is diagnosed on the basis of symptoms that patients report, as well as the absence of any other disorder that may explain the symptoms. ROME III criteria are used. Frequently, patients have a SIGMOIODOSCOPY or a COLONOSCOPY. The physician may take a biopsy specimen of the bowel during the procedure to exclude other causes of the symptoms. Physicians also rule out other possible diseases with laboratory tests, such as with a complete blood count and other common blood tests, such as a complete metabolic profile and thyroid function tests. The physician may also request a stool sample to analyze it for a possible PARASITIC INFECTION.

Treatment Options and Outlook

Patients who are diagnosed with IBS are often advised to keep a food diary as well as a stool diary, to help them note any apparent correlation between the day's events or the foods that they eat and subsequent symptoms. Some patients may benefit from avoiding caffeine and chocolate, as well as limiting their intake of fatty foods. Current guidelines suggest that increased FIBER intake is beneficial in IBS patients.

IBS is also treated with a variety of medications to help relax the bowel. Two drugs that are used to treat spasms are dicyclomine (Bentyl) and hyoscyamine sulfate (Levsin), both of which are anticholinergic agents. If patients are primarily troubled with diarrhea, other drugs, such as loperamide (Imodium), alosetron (Lotronex), diphenoxylate plus atropine sulfate (Lomotil), or cholestyramine resin, may be used. Alosetron, a drug that was formerly prescribed for IBS, was withdrawn from the market in 2000 after reports of severe constipation and several deaths. It was approved again in 2002 on a restricted basis by the Food and Drug Administration (FDA) for women with IBS who have severe diarrhea-predominant IBS that is not responsive to other treatments and is still used for this purpose in 2010.

Patients whose main problem is constipation may be given osmotic laxatives, such as magnesium hydroxide and lactulose. Polyethylene glycol solution may be used to flush out the stools. In 2002, the FDA approved tegaserod maleate (Zelnorm) for the short-term treatment of IBS among women whose primary problem is constipation. The drug was subsequently withdrawn from market because of an unacceptable side-effect profile. Lubiprostone (Amitiza®) is useful for chronic constipation and evidence suggests that it effective for IBS-constipation type.

Other types of drugs may be prescribed, such as low dosages of antidepressant medications. These drugs may help to calm patients, as well as help with sleep problems and relieve colonic cramping and spasms. Many patients actually do have depression and anxiety, although the dosages of these drugs are much lower than those normally used to treat depression or anxiety.

Some physicians have found that patients may improve with Chinese herbal medicine. In a study reported in a 1998 edition of the *Journal of the American Medical Association,* the researchers compared the results of patients in three groups. In one group, the patients were treated with individualized Chinese herbal formulations; in a second group, the patients were treated with a standard Chinese herbal formulation. Patients in the third group received a placebo (no drugs). The patients who received either form of the Chinese herbal formulations improved significantly compared to the patients receiving the placebo; however, in a follow-up that occurred 14 weeks after the end of the study, only the patients receiving the individualized Chinese herbal formulations maintained their improvement in their symptoms.

Peppermint and hypnotherapy has also been shown in controlled trials to be helpful for some patients with IBS. (See ALTERNATIVE MEDICINE.)

Risk Factors and Preventive Measures

IBS affects as many as 15 percent of adults at some point in their life; women have a greater risk of development of IBS than men. In Eastern cultures such as that in India, the prevalence of IBS is greater among men. Women who have been sexually or emotionally abused in the past appear to have an increased risk for development of irritable bowel syndrome.

Minocha, Anil, M.D., and David Carroll. *Natural Stomach Care.* New York: Penguin Putnam, 2003.

Minocha A., Abell T. L., Johnson, W. D., Wigington, W. C. "Racial Differences in Epidemiology of Irritable Bowel Syndrome Alone, Uninvestigated Dyspepsia Alone and the 'Overlap syndrome' among African Americans as Compared to Caucasians: A Population-Based Study." *Digestive Diseases and Sciences* 2,006, no. 51: 218–226.

ischemia A paucity or lack of blood supply that occurs because the blood supply is altogether blocked or because the blood supply is limited, a condition that can lead to tissue damage or death.

In mesenteric artery ischemia, the arteries that supply the blood to the intestines are narrowed or may undergo spasms. Mesenteric artery ischemia may be seen in patients with atherosclerosis and is more commonly found among smokers and individuals who have high cholesterol levels. Mesenteric venous thrombosis causes 5 to 15 percent of all mesenteric ischemia. Ischemic colitis occurs when a segment of the colon loses its blood supply. Abdominal pain upon eating occurs in patients with intestinal ischemia; they are afraid of eating and may lose weight.

Hepatic ischemia results from an inadequate blood supply to the LIVER, which causes damage or death to the liver cells. This condition, known as ischemic hepatitis or shock liver, can result from low blood pressure that results from abnormal heart rhythms, DEHYDRATION, severe bleeding, shock, or other causes. Most patients with shock liver recover unless the underlying condition persists.

Symptoms and Diagnostic Path

Indicators of intestinal or mesenteric ischemia are ABDOMINAL PAIN, NAUSEA AND VOMITING, and DIAR-

RHEA. Abdominal pain is usually disproportionate to the physical findings elicited by the physician on examination. Overt or occult (microscopic) blood is found in the stools. Since these are common symptoms of many other digestive problems, the physician must determine the diagnosis and treatment.

In hepatic ischemia, liver enzyme levels are elevated. These abnormal liver test findings and the liver itself usually return to normal rapidly if the underlying condition causing it is resolved. However, LIVER FAILURE may occur with hepatic ischemia, although it is very rare.

Laboratory tests may show an elevated white blood cell count when ischemia is the problem. An angiogram that uses dye injected into the arteries that supply the intestine will reveal whether there is an arterial blockage. If a narrowing is seen, it can be dilated. If a clot is identified, it can be dissolved with clot-busting drugs.

Treatment Options and Outlook

If there is spasm, a vasodilator drug is injected directly into the narrowed vessel to dilate it. However, sometimes test results are inconclusive and physicians must perform exploratory surgery to identify the cause of the problem. Computerized scanning (CT) is the test of choice to diagnose mesenteric venous thrombosis as the cause of mesenteric ischemia.

When surgery is performed, surgeons remove the dead part of the intestine and then reconnect the bowel to healthy tissue; however, in some cases, an osteomy is needed; in this procedure an opening is made and an external changeable pouch captures fecal matter. The pouch is periodically changed by the patient.

In chronic mesenteric ischemia, physicians remove any blockage in the arteries that connect to the intestines.

If the patient has acute mesenteric ischemia, this is a medical emergency.

The treatment of ischemic colitis is supportive, and most patients recover.

Treatment for hepatic ischemia is supportive; the patient maintains good hydration by intravenous fluids or blood transfusion and oxygenation, as well as by correcting any severe ANEMIA. Correction of the underying problem is done whenever possible, such as improving low blood pressure. Most patients recover completely from hepatic ischemia.

Risk Factors and Preventive Measures

In the digestive system, intestinal ischemia can be caused by a HERNIA that becomes entangled or by adhesions from prior surgeries that entrap the intestines with scar tissue.

jaundice Yellowing of the skin and eyes caused by an excessive level of bilirubin, a product of heme broken down by the liver. The condition is also known as hyperbilirubinemia. Jaundice may be a temporary problem faced by some newborn infants, who need pediatric treatment. It may also be a symptom of a serious liver disease, such as HEPATITIS or even CIRRHOSIS or PANCREATIC CANCER. The excessive hemolysis of red blood cells in hemolytic anemia is a non-liver-related cause of jaundice.

Any person whose skin appears more yellow than usual should consult a physician immediately for a medical evaluation. If the skin is bright yellow (for example, similar to a banana color), medical attention should be sought urgently. Note that yellow discoloration may also be seen in carotenemia (a high intake of vitamin A) and is best seen on the face, palms, and soles of the feet.

Newborn Infants with Jaundice

Sometimes newborn babies have jaundice that needs to be treated. Jaundice may not be apparent on the first one or two days after birth. It is important for an infant to be seen by a pediatrician within 24 to 48 hours after discharge if he or she is discharged from the hospital at any time before 48 hours after birth.

In one study of nearly 30,000 newborn INFANTS in Michigan, reported in a 1998 issue of *Pediatrics*, 127 babies had to be readmitted to the hospital in the first two weeks of their life to be treated for jaundice. In addition, researchers found several factors that caused infants to be more likely to need readmission, including discharge from the hospital within 72 hours of birth.

Maisels, Jeffrey M., and Elizabeth Kring. "Length of Stay, Jaundice, and Hospital Readmission." *Pediatrics* 101, no. 6 (June 1998): 995–998.

Kaposi's sarcoma Severe skin lesions of a low-grade vascular tumor that can occur in various parts of the body, including the digestive system which is involved in 40 to 80 percent of patients with AIDS. In the most extreme cases, Kaposi's sarcoma can result in gastrointestinal bleeding, which can rarely be fatal. It can also involve the respiratory system and the lymph nodes. Kaposi's sarcoma is caused by human herpesvirus 8 (HHV-8).

This condition was first described by the Hungarian dermatologist Moritz Kaposi in 1872. Variations of the condition that was described by Kaposi were subsequently identified; for example, a form of Kaposi's sarcoma was identified among homosexual men in New York in 1981.

Symptoms and Diagnostic Path

Trained physicians can usually identify the lesions of Kaposi's sarcoma by just looking at them. For example, the gastroenterologist recognizes the lesions in the gastrointestinal tract during ENDOSCOPY. Physicians can also test the blood of patients with skin lesions for the presence of antibodies against HHV-8 or Kaposi's sarcoma—associated herpesvirus (KSHV), which would be indirect evidence of an infection. A biopsy specimen of the skin lesions will confirm the presence of Kaposi's sarcoma.

The presence of Kaposi's sarcoma is declining; the reasons for this decline are not well known.

Treatment Options and Outlook

In patients with AIDS, treatment is based on the location of lesions and symptoms, CD4 cell count, and viral load. In the early stages, physicians concentrate on treating the symptoms and signs of Kaposi's sarcoma by shrinking the tumor to decrease swelling and to lessen psychological stress, as well as to prevent disease progression; for example, lesions can be removed with cryotherapy,

freezing them off the skin. Other local treatments that can control tumor growth include injections of chemotherapeutic drugs such as vinblastine into the lesion. In addition, radiation therapy, laser therapy, and topical applications of various drugs such as Panretin gel may be used.

More aggressive treatment is used in the following cases:

- The number of lesions increases to more than 25 lesions on the skin.
- Kaposi's sarcoma is extensive and is not responding to local therapy.
- There is severe swelling.
- Internal organs are involved, causing symptoms such as bleeding from the digestive system.

Patients may be treated with radiation therapy, chemotherapy, or a combination of radiation therapy and chemotherapy.

Risk Factors and Preventive Measures

Men have a greater risk for development of Kaposi's sarcoma than women by a ratio as high as 15 to one. ELDERLY Eastern European and Mediterranean men are at risk for Kaposi's sarcoma. Currently, Kaposi's sarcoma has been found in patients living in parts of Africa such as Uganda and Zambia. Gay men in the United States and other countries are at high risk for development of Kaposi's sarcoma. People at high risk for Kaposi's sarcoma include those who have acquired immunodeficiency syndrome (AIDS). In addition, organ transplantation recipients face an increased risk for Kaposi's sarcoma because of their impaired immune system.

There are no known preventive measures.

See also BLEEDING, GASTROINTESTINAL; INTERFERON.

L

Lactobacillus   Often considered to be one of the "friendly bacteria," *Lactobacillus* is a bacterium and the *Lactobacillus bulgaricus* is found in some products such as yogurt. (The other standard bacterium in yogurt is *streptococcus thermophilus*.) Sometimes patients who are taking antibiotics experience an imbalance because friendly bacteria are killed along with harmful bacteria. Such an imbalance of insufficient friendly bacteria can cause diarrhea and even severe colitis. The administration of some types of *Lactobacillus* has been shown to be helpful in certain forms of diarrhea.

Eating yogurt with live cultures or taking over-the-counter tablets containing such probiotic bacteria may help restore the normal ecological balance in the gut; however, patients should consult their physician to obtain treatment of their disorder and to determine whether they should take such probiotics as *Lactobacillus*. They should not self-medicate. You can identify the yogurt that contains live and active cultures by the Live Active Cultures seal on the container.

See also ALTERNATIVE MEDICINE; THRUSH.

lactose intolerance   A form of food intolerance; difficulty or inability related to digestion of the milk sugar (lactose) that is found in dairy products and in some other foods, which leads to the excessive production of fluid, GAS, cramps, and DIARRHEA. The problem may be mild, moderate, or severe, depending on the patient.

Lactose intolerance is the result of an enzyme deficiency of lactose in the patient. The deficiency or lack of the enzyme lactase is called alactasia, hypolactasia, and lactase deficiency. Some patients may exhibit symptoms of lactose intolerance without evidence of a lactase deficiency.

Often confused with a FOOD ALLERGY, lactose intolerance is instead actually an inability to digest lactose, and there is no involvement with the immune system at all, as there is in the case of a food allergy. Worldwide, as much as 75 percent of the global population may be lactose-intolerant. The prevalence of lactose intolerance also varies considerably within countries; for example, about 70 percent of the people in the southern part of India are lactose-intolerant, in contrast to about 25 percent of the population in the northern portion of India, who are lactose-intolerant.

Very few INFANTS are born lactose-intolerant. Most children up to the age of five years have the ability to tolerate lactose, but the level of their natural lactase enzyme starts to diminish in early childhood. For most people, lactose intolerance does not become a problem until they reach adolescence or adulthood.

Some children and adults acquire lactose intolerance as a result of a secondary medical problem, such as a severe gastrointestinal infection or other disease that damages the mucosa of the small intestines. In addition, chemotherapy or radiation therapy for cancer may also cause lactose intolerance. Some of the diseases or conditions that can cause secondary hypolactasia are:

- CELIAC SPRUE
- WHIPPLE'S DISEASE
- giardiasis
- CROHN'S DISEASE
- HUMAN IMMUNODEFICIENCY VIRUS
- ZOLLINGER-ELLISON SYNDROME

Symptoms and Diagnostic Path

The common symptoms of lactose intolerance are as follows:

- stomach cramps
- bloating of the stomach
- extreme gas
- frothy and watery stool after consumption of products that contain lactose (however, most who have lactase deficiency can tolerate about one glass of milk per day without problems)

If the physician or the patient suspects lactose intolerance to be a problem, the patient can have a hydrogen breath test and/or a blood test of the serum glucose level (both are administered after the patient consumes lactose), to confirm or refute the possible diagnosis. Some physicians also order biopsy examination of the small intestines to diagnose the level of lactase in the intestinal cells, although that test is performed only in research laboratories. Physicians who perform an intestinal biopsy may also be seeking to screen out other medical problems that may be causing malabsorption, such as celiac sprue.

Treatment Options and Outlook

Mild lactose intolerance can be managed with lactose-free products or supplemental lactase enzyme oral supplements, which are over-the-counter drugs such as LactAid and Lactase. These supplements may enable the patient who is moderately or severely lactose-intolerant to consume a glass of milk or several scoops of ice cream without incident.

In general, physicians do not advise lactose-intolerant patients to give up all dairy products because of concern that a calcium deficiency may develop. However, most lactose-intolerant patients should carefully monitor their consumption of dairy products. They may also need to take supplemental calcium to ensure a healthy intake. Some patients drink lactose-reduced milk.

Patients with lactose intolerance are also advised to eat other foods when they consume products with lactose, to diminish the overall effect of the lactose. Some foods that include lactose may be well tolerated, such as yogurt with active cultures in it. The reason for this is that the bacterial lactase breaks down the lactose, and thus, there is no remaining lactose to cause a reaction.

Milk and dairy products are not the only food items that include lactose, and patients who are extremely lactose-intolerant need to be aware of this fact. According to Dr. Swagerty and his colleagues in their 2002 article on lactose intolerance in *American Family Physician,* some products that include lactose are as follows:

- bread
- margarine
- breakfast cereals
- mixes for pancakes or cookies
- breakfast drinks
- salad dressings
- some candies
- packaged luncheon meats that are nonkosher
- some medications (patients should advise their pharmacists that they are lactose-intolerant)

Patients who have secondary lactose intolerance due to another medical problem may recover with treatment; for example, if patients have GIARDIASIS, which can cause a secondary lactose intolerance, then treatment with metronidazole (Flagyl) may resolve the problem. Patients who have lactose intolerance caused by excessive bacteria in the small bowel may improve after a course of antibiotics.

Risk Factors and Preventive Measures

Males and females are about equally likely to be lactose-intolerant.

There are racial differences among those who are lactose-intolerant. Asians (depending on ethnicity) have one of the greatest risk of lactose intolerance and they have a 30 to 95 percent intolerance rate. In the United States, Native Americans follow Asians in the percentages of those who are lactose-intolerant: an estimated 79 percent of Native Americans have this condition. Many African Americans (about 75 percent) are also lactose-intolerant. They are followed by Hispanics (about 50 to 75 percent are intolerant) and then by whites in the United States (a range of from 6 to 30 percent).

The only preventive measure is for those who know they are lactose intolerant to take remedies prior to consuming food that has lactose in it.

Srinivasan, R., and A. Minocha. "When to Suspect Lactose Intolerance." *Postgraduate Medicine* 105, no. 3 (1998): 109–123.

Swagerty, Daniel L., Jr., M.D., Anne D. Walling, M.D., and Robert M. Klein. "Lactose Intolerance." *American Family Physician* 65, no. 9 (May 1, 2002): 1,845–1,850.

laxatives and laxative abuse   Over-the-counter or prescribed medications taken by people who are constipated. In most cases, the individual has not had a bowel movement for two to three days or longer. The excessive use of laxatives may lead to DIARRHEA. Some patients may constantly use laxatives; this practice is called laxative abuse. Such laxative abuse may be present with factitious diarrhea. The long-standing use of certain laxatives may lead to *melanosis coli.*

There are various types of laxatives. Bulk laxatives (psyllium, methyl cellulose) increase the bulk of the stool and promote bowel movement. They should be taken with plenty of water and avoided by patients who have GASTROPARESIS and MEGACOLON. The bulk laxative is initially tried for CONSTIPATION. Other types of laxatives include stool softeners (docusate), stimulant cathartics (castor oil, bisacodyl, and senna), osmotic cathartics (Milk of Magnesia, lactulose, and sorbitol), and polyethylene glycol solutions (MiraLax). Phenolphthalein (Formerly in Ex-lax) has been withdrawn from the market because of increased risk for cancer. Lubiprostone (Amitiza®) is a prescription medication available for treatment of idiopathic chronic constipation. Laxatives with a high concentration of MAGNESIUM or phosphorus should be avoided by those who have kidney failure.

Extreme use of laxatives for the purpose of weight loss is considered laxative abuse. It is seen in some people who have ANOREXIA NERVOSA. Laxative abuse can also be found among some people who are chronically constipated or obsessed with the idea that they are "constipated," and have become dependent on laxatives in order to have regular bowel movements. Some patients with laxative abuse complain of "diarrhea." A search of the patient's room and a laxative screen test may be in order in some cases to look for laxative abuse.

Listeria monocytogenes   Common bacteria that cause food-borne illnesses. An infection with *Listeria* organisms is called listeriosis. According to the Centers for Disease Control and Prevention (CDC), about 1,700 severe cases of listeriosis are reported each year in the United States, and in these cases, as many as 450 patients die. In addition, listeriosis accounts for about 100 stillbirths each year.

When present, *Listeria* organisms may be found in such foods as coleslaw, luncheon meats, cold cuts, undercooked poultry, and dairy products. They are usually killed by cooking, or, in the case of dairy products, by pasteurization. The infection is treated with antibiotics. Epidemics may occur.

Symptoms and Diagnostic Path

People infected with *Listeria* organisms may experience fevers and chills and may believe that they have the flu. Some individuals experience stomach upset or gastroenteritis. The infection may occur in the brain (meningoencephalitis), and patients may have headaches, stiff neck, and even loss of balance and convulsions. Other sites that may be involved with infection include skin, eyes, joints (septic arthritis), lungs (pneumonia), LIVER (HEPATITIS), GALLBLADDER (CHOLECYSTITIS) and bones (osteomyelitis).

Since many of the symptoms of listeriosis are nonspecific, a precise diagnosis is made only by testing the blood or the cerebrospinal fluid of the patient. The cerebrospinal fluid is the fluid that bathes the brain and spinal cord. A magnetic resonance imaging (MRI) scan may also be helpful.

Treatment Options and Outlook

The infection is susceptible to many commonly used ANTIBIOTICS. In most cases, a combination of antibiotics, such as ampicillin or penicillin G plus gentamicin, is used.

Risk Factors and Preventive Measures

Most healthy people are unaffected by *Listeria* organisms; however, some groups of people are especially vulnerable to infection, particularly those in the following groups:

- pregnant women (who can transmit the illness to the fetus, potentially causing severe health problems)
- newborn babies
- ELDERLY individuals
- people who have a weakened immune system, such as those who have acquired immunodeficiency syndrome (AIDS) or have had organ transplantation
- cancer patients

Listeria infections can often be prevented by the following simple actions:

- washing hands before eating any ready-to-eat foods, such as cold cuts or deli-style meats
- avoiding soft cheese such as feta cheese and brie
- avoiding unpasteurized milk and unpasteurized cheese
- reading and heeding expiration dates of all food products
- reheating ready-to-eat foods such as hot dogs and cold cuts
- refrigerating perishable foods within two hours
- keep the refrigerator at 40°F or lower and the freezer at 0°F or lower

See also CONTAMINATED FOOD OR WATER.

liver A digestive and metabolic organ that is necessary to sustain life. The liver is essential for numerous important functions in the body, including the digestion, absorption, and assimilation of nutrients, the synthesis of the building blocks of the body such as proteins, glucose metabolism, and drug detoxification. (Many medications are metabolized by the liver.)

Hepatitis is a disease that attacks the liver, as are hepatocellular carcinoma and other forms of liver cancer. Chronic alcoholism or alcohol abuse can cause CIRRHOSIS of the liver, a condition of severe scarring. Nonalcoholic steatohepatitis (also known as nonalcoholic fatty liver disease) may also cause damage to the liver. SARCOIDOSIS, HEMATOCHROMATOSIS, and WILSON'S DISEASE can also be very harmful to the liver.

Some rare diseases that can cause damage to the liver are AMYLOIDOSIS, BUDD-CHIARI SYNDROME, CYSTIC FIBROSIS, alpha1-antitrypsin deficiency, PRIMARY SCLEROSING CHOLANGITIS, and glycogen storage disease. The acute fatty liver of pregnancy is a dangerous condition that some pregnant women experience.

If the liver fails because of severe disease or damage, the only way to continue to sustain a person's life in cases of advanced liver failure is through LIVER TRANSPLANTATION.

liver abscess Severe bacterial, fungal, or parasitic infection of the liver. Generally, CHOLANGITIS (inflammation of the bile duct) that is caused by a blockage of the bile duct by gallstones or tumors is the most frequent cause of liver abscess. A spreading of an abscess from APPENDICITIS or DIVERTICULITIS may also result in a liver abscess.

Signs and Symptoms

Patients who have a liver abscess experience abdominal pain, fever, sweating, nausea and vomiting, loss of appetite, and unintended weight loss. The physician's examination of the liver may find it swollen and tender.

Diagnosis and Treatment

Laboratory tests of patients with liver abscesses are nonspecific and reveal an elevated white blood cell count. Patients may have an elevated erythrocyte sedimentation rate of the blood and may also have elevated alkaline phosphatase levels. The ultrasound and computed tomography (CT) scan are usually required for diagnosis. In addition, a gallium scan and magnetic resonance imaging (MRI) scan may be helpful. An endoscopic retrograde cholangiopancreatography (ERCP) can help to delineate the cause of the liver abscess in some cases and can allow insertion of a biliary stent to hold the bile duct open if it is blocked.

Drainage of the abscess is frequently undertaken, and patients need to take antibiotics, such as penicillin or metronidazole. Treatment is usually long: it may take weeks to months, depending upon the patient's response, which is monitored clinically by the physician as well as with CT scans.

In some cases, a liver abscess is caused by *Entamoeba histolytica,* an amebic parasite that is found more commonly in developing countries as well as in areas with poor sanitation and overcrowding. Results of stool tests in such cases are rarely positive for the amoeba. The abscess can spread to the lungs and the heart and can cause even worse problems that are related to these organs. The diagnosis of *E. histolytica* abscess is helped by imaging tests such as the CT scan. Serology testing for antibodies against the ameba yields positive findings in most cases. Liver abscesses that are caused by *E. histolytica* can usually be resolved with metronidazole treatment, although occasionally drainage may also be necessary. The individual treatment of each patient must be decided by his or her doctor.

See also CAROLI'S DISEASE; ENDOSCOPY; LIVER.

Krige, J. E. J. "Liver Abscesses and Hydatid Diseases." *British Medical Journal* 322 (March 3, 2001): 537–540.

liver cancer   A malignant tumor that exists or originates in the LIVER, and that is frequently fatal, especially if it has spread from other parts of the body to the liver, rather than originating in the liver itself. According to the National Cancer Institute (NCI), there were 21,370 new cases of liver cancer in 2008 in the United States and 18,410 deaths. Unless the patient is a candidate for surgical removal of the cancerous part of the liver, he or she will not survive without a LIVER TRANSPLANTATION. In general, cancer of the liver is also considered along with cancer of the liver bile duct (bile duct cancer) as liver cancer.

There are several different types of liver cancer. Hepatocellular carcinoma (HCC) is the most common form of liver cancer, representing about 70 percent of all liver cancers. It is also known as "malignant hepatoma" or simply "hepatoma." HCC is usually associated with CIRRHOSIS of the liver,

stemming from chronic HEPATITIS B and C or from chronic alcoholism. (Chronic hepatitis B carriers may develop hepatoma without developing cirrhosis.) Hepatitis B and C are viruses that can be spread through blood products, sexual contact, or from sharing of needles used to inject drugs.

It is also possible for cancers arising in other parts of the body to spread to the liver, particularly cancers originating in the breast, colon, lung, pancreas, and stomach.

Of those liver cancer cases that are not hepatocellular carcinomas, the largest single cause, representing less than 10 percent of all liver cancers originating in the liver, are cholangiocarcinomas. These are cancers that develop in branches of the bile ducts from the liver. This form of cancer may be caused by liver parasites, especially in liver cancer victims in Southeast Asia. Patients with hepatitis C and/or PRIMARY SCLEROSING CHOLANGITIS are also at increased risk for this form of cancer.

Another form of liver cancer is angiosarcoma, which is a very rare cancer that can occur within the blood vessels of the liver. Angiosarcoma is associated with exposure to chemical carcinogens such as vinyl chloride and arsenic. Many patients have secondary or metastatic liver cancer, which means that their cancer originated elsewhere and spread to the liver.

Symptoms and Diagnostic Path

There are few or no symptoms in the early stages of liver cancer, when the disease might be treatable with surgical excision of the cancerous part of the liver. When symptoms occur, they may include the following:

- weight loss
- abdominal swelling
- APPETITE loss
- pain in the upper right abdomen
- yellow JAUNDICE of the skin or eyes
- darkened urine (caused by jaundice)
- NAUSEA AND VOMITING
- fever
- ASCITES (fluid buildup in the abdomen)

Liver cancer is diagnosed based on the patient's symptoms as well as on diagnostic tests, such as blood tests on a patient's liver function and a test for alpha-fetoprotein (AFP). High AFP blood levels could indicate liver cancer. CT scan is usually ordered. Doctors may also order a liver scan, a bone scan (in the event that the cancer may have spread to the bones), X-rays, and an ULTRASOUND. Magnetic resonance imaging (MRI) is also sometimes used. If cancer is present, these diagnostic imaging tools (MRI, CT, ultrasound) will also help the doctor to stage the cancer, which means to determine how severe the cancer is now.

A biopsy, which is the removal of a small amount of tissue to check for cancer, is usually used to definitively prove the presence of liver cancer, although in some cases, high alpha-fetoprotein laboratory tests and characteristic findings on a computed tomography (CT) scan may be considered adequate tools for diagnosis. Physicians may sometimes decide that the risks of performing a liver biopsy to the patient outweigh the benefits, because of the potential for fatal bleeding, and because of the risk of inadvertently spreading any existing cancer cells. Sometimes a diagnostic biopsy is obtained by the physician in exploratory surgery by using a laparoscope, a special device that can be inserted into a small incision in the abdomen, to visually inspect the liver and surrounding organs.

Treatment Options and Outlook

The prognosis is not good in most cases of liver cancer because the disease is frequently detected at a late stage. If only part of the liver is involved, as mentioned earlier, that part can be surgically removed in many cases. Liver cancer can also be treated with radiation and chemotherapy to extend the patient's life, although not to cure the liver cancer. Many patients with liver cancer are offered an opportunity to join a clinical trial, which is an ongoing study of diseases. Joining a clinical trial may enable patients to try drugs or treatments that are being tested and that are not available to the general public.

If the cancer has not spread beyond the liver, patients may be candidates for a liver transplantation, assuming that a donor liver can be located in time.

In the case of advanced cancer, patients are treated with radiation therapy or chemotherapy, and some patients will receive both forms of treatment. In 2008, the physician Lewis R. Roberts reported that the drug sorafenib showed promise in treating liver cancer, based on the Sorafenib Hepatocarcinoma Assessment Randomize Protocol (SHARP). This medication was approved by the Food and Drug Administration (FDA) to treat advanced renal-cell carcinoma (kidney cancer) in 2005 and hepatocellular carcinoma in 2007. Roberts cautions that patients taking sorafenib will need to be monitored to ensure they do not incur any extra risks; for example, patients with kidney cancer who took the drug developed a risk for hypertension and cardiovascular disease and other health issues. In addition, the drug is expensive, and according to Roberts, the cost in 2008 was about $5,400 per month in the United States.

Risk Factors and Preventive Measures

The presence of chronic hepatitis B or C is a risk factor for liver cancer. Some researchers believe that mutations in the hepatitis B virus may be the cause for an increased risk for liver cancer. In addition, the presence of cirrhosis of the liver is also a risk factor for liver cancer. Alcoholic and nonalcoholic fatty liver diseases as well as DIABETES MELLITUS are also risk factors. OBESITY and being overweight are also risk factors for developing and dying from liver cancer. People who are alcoholics with liver cirrhosis are at the greatest risk for developing liver cancer. Individuals with HEMOCHROMATOSIS, a disease of iron overload, are also at an increased risk for developing liver cancer.

Liver cancer occurs about four times more frequently among men than women. Age is another factor, and liver cancer is more common among people over the age of 55 to 60 years old. In the United States, African Americans and Hispanics have twice the risk of developing liver cancer as that experienced by whites. Some Asian groups have a high rate of incidence, and men who emigrated from Vietnam have a very high rate of occurrence, primarily because of the associated high rate of hepatitis in Vietnam.

In looking at the incidence of liver cancer by ethnicity in Los Angeles over the period 1988 to

1992, researchers considered trends and patterns among liver cancer patients, and they reported their findings in the 2001 issue of the *International Journal of Cancer*. The researchers found that white males in Los Angeles had a liver cancer rate of 2.9 per 100,000 people, followed by a rate of 5.1 for black men. The rate increased to 5.8 for Japanese men and 6.5 per 100,000 for Hispanic men. Chinese men had much higher rates of 16.1 per 100,000, and Korean men had the highest rates, which were 23.9 per 100,000.

Women also had an increased risk for liver cancer based on their ethnicity, but it was a much lower rate than found among men. For example, white women in Los Angeles had a rate of 1.1 cases of liver cancer per 100,000 women. The rate increased to 2.2 per 100,000 for black women. Again, the highest rates of liver cancer were found among Chinese women (4.4 per 100,000) and Korean women (5.5 per 100,000).

More recently a study published in a 2007 issue of the *Journal of the National Medical Association* reported that a screening of Asian Americans revealed that those ages 36 to 45 had a high rate of hepatitis B (9.1 percent). This high prevalence of hepatitis increases the risk of Asian Americans for developing liver disease and liver cancer. According to the authors, "In reducing liver cancer disparities as a result of HBV [hepatitis B], the experiences learned form this project render potential lessons of expanding the HBV prevention program to a wide scale, within or beyond [the] Asian-American community."

In very rare cases, liver cancer can be caused by aflatoxin, which is a substance that can occur in some forms of mold. The type of fungus that generates aflatoxin can sometimes be found on peanuts, corns, and nuts, and aflatoxin contamination is a serious problem in countries in Asia and Africa; however in the United States, the FDA prohibits the sale of foods that have high levels of aflatoxin.

A family history of liver cancer in other members also brings an increased risk for the development of liver cancer.

Hepatoma may be prevented in patients by avoiding the underlying conditions it is associated with, such as viral hepatitis B and C and treatment of chronic viral hepatitis if it has been con-tracted. Hepatitis B vaccination is now universally recommended.

See also ALCOHOL ABUSE AND ALCOHOLISM; HEMO-CHROMATOSOSIS; LIVER ENZYMES/FUNCTION; LIVER FAILURE; OBESITY.

Calle, Eugenia E., Ph.D., et al., "Overweight, Obesity, and Mortality from Cancer in a Prospectively Studied Cohort of U.S. Adults," *New England Journal of Medicine* 348, no. 17 (April 24, 2003): 1,625–1,638.

Hsu, Chiehwen, et al. "Reducing Liver Cancer Disparities: A Community-Based Hepatitis-B Prevention Program for Asian-American Communities." *Journal of the National Medical Association* 99, no. 8 (2007): 900–907.

Kukka, Christine, "Mutations in the Virus' Surface and Core Proteins Increase Risk of Liver Cancer." *HBV Journal Review* 6, no. 1 (2009): 1.

McGlynn, Katherine A., et al., "International Trends and Patterns of Primary Liver Cancer," *International Journal of Cancer* 94, (2001): 290–296.

Roberts, Lewis R. "Sorafenib in Liver Cancer—Just the Beginning." *New England Journal of Medicine* 359, no. 4 (July 24, 2008): 420–422.

liver enzymes/function tests Laboratory blood tests that are specifically helpful in identifying possible liver diseases because they provide markers of liver damage and, thus, they can lead the physician to further investigations of potential problems.

Elevated levels of serum aminotransferases (alanine aminotransferase [ALT]) and aspartine aminotransferase (AST), alkaline phosphatase, and gamma-glutamyltransferase may indicate possible liver disease. For example, above-normal levels of aminotransferase may indicate the presence of HEPATITIS B or C, HEMOCHROMATOSIS (iron overload), alcoholic hepatitis, or nonalcoholic steatohepatitis. Aminotransferases are also produced by the kidney and the muscles, and elevated levels may indicate a non-liver-related medical problem, such as kidney disorders, or muscle problems such as myoscitis, or even a prior period of excessive exercise. Above-normal levels of aminotransferase may also be caused by numerous medications or even by heart attack.

Elevated levels of alkaline phosphatase, another marker for liver disease, may indicate a bone disorder or a variety of cholestatic diseases, such as bile duct obstruction, choledocholithiasis, or PRIMARY BILIARY CIRRHOSIS; in some cases it may be medication induced (such as by chlorpromazine). It may also indicate the presence of SARCOIDOSIS or another granulomatous disease, such as TUBERCU-LOSIS. On occasion, high alkaline phosphatase level indicate the presence of advanced liver cancer.

As with conventional medications, herbal remedies, including chaparral, Chinese herbs, gentia, senna, and shark cartilage, may elevate liver enzyme level. Some illegal drugs, such as cocaine and anabolic steroids, can also raise an individual's liver enzyme level.

Beckingham, I. J., and S. D. Ryder. "Investigation of Liver and Biliary Disease." *British Journal of Medicine* 322 (January 6, 2001): 33–36.

Pratt, Daniel S., M. D., and Marshall M. Kaplan, M.D. "Evaluation of Abnormal Liver-Enzyme Results in Asymptomatic Patients." *New England Journal of Medicine* 342, no. 17 (April 27, 2000): 1,266–1,271.

liver failure Condition in which liver function is not present or is reduced significantly enough to cause severe problems. This is a life-threatening condition, and only LIVER TRANSPLANTATION can sustain life if the entire liver fails. The liver may fail because of medications, CIRRHOSIS, HEPATITIS, or other liver diseases, or from liver cancer.

In a study of 308 patients with liver failure reported in 2002 in *Annals of Internal Medicine,* overdose of acetaminophen was the most common cause of acute liver failure (representing 39 percent of all cases), followed by overdoses of or reactions to other drugs (13 percent), and infection with hepatitis A and B (12 percent). The survival rate for patients with acetaminophen-induced liver failure was 68 percent compared to only 25 percent survival rate of patients whose liver failed as a result of ingestion of other drugs. In addition, when the cause of the liver failure was unknown, only 17 percent of the patients survived. According to the researchers, "Acetaminophen overdose and idiosyncratic drug reactions have replaced viral hepatitis as the most frequent cause of acute liver failure."

Symptoms and Diagnostic Path

When the liver is failing, it can no longer function correctly or cannot function at all. Signs and symptoms of liver failure include the following indicators:

- jaundice (yellowed skin and eyes)
- enlarged fluid filled abdomen (ascites)
- extreme fatigue
- itching of the skin
- easy bruising and bleeding
- bleeding
- change in mental status (hepatic encephalopathy)

The diagnosis of liver failure is based on the patient's signs and symptoms as well as liver function laboratory test results. In severe cases, the presence of jaundice makes it clear that the patient has a liver disease, although jaundice in itself does not signify an irreversible liver failure.

In addition, the physician must rule out the presence of hepatitis, PANCREATIC CANCER, and other diseases that cause jaundice.

Treatment Options and Outlook

Treatment of liver failure is generally supportive plus the treatment of complications. Transplantation of a new liver is the only cure for advanced liver failure. A scoring system is generally used to triage the liver transplant candidates in order of severity. However, the patients who have fulminant liver failure receive the highest priority. Some very specialized intensive care facilities offer interim artificial support systems before liver transplantation; this practice is comparable to dialysis for kidneys that fail before a kidney transplantation can be accomplished.

An article in 2003 in the *Journal of the American Medical Association* described a review of 12 clinical trials of such interim bioartificial support systems. According to the authors, the meta-analysis of these trials revealed that such artificial support systems were successful in reducing the rate of death of liver failure by 33 percent.

According to the authors, "The objective of artificial and bioartificial support systems is to 'bridge' patients with liver failure to transplantation or recovery. Liver support must include removal of toxins, synthesis of products, and treatment of inflammation."

Risk Factors and Preventive Measures

Individuals who use acetaminophen to excess are at risk, as are those who abuse or are dependent on alcohol. Clearly, it is important to prevent overdosage of acetaminophen, since it is a common cause of liver failure. Other risk factors are the presence of hepatitis.

Kjaegard, Lise L., M.D., et al. "Artificial and Bioartificial Support Systems for Acute and Acute-on-Chronic Liver Failure." *Journal of the American Medical Association* 289, no. 2 (January 8, 2003): 217–222.

Ostapowicz, G., et al. "Results of a Prospective Study of Acute Liver Failure at 17 Tertiary Care Centers in the United States." *Annals of Internal Medicine* 137 (December 2002): 947–954.

liver transplantation   Replacement of a damaged liver with a donor liver from a recently deceased person or, in a very few cases, with the donated partial liver of a live person. Usually the patient has liver failure, often because of severe hepatitis or cirrhosis and is anticipated to die without transplantation. HEPATITIS C is the leading indication of liver transplantation in the United States.

Key Reasons for Liver Transplantation

In most cases of a need for a liver transplantation, the patient has extremely severe liver disease and the liver is failing as a result of hepatitis C, alcoholic liver disease, LIVER CANCER, or PRIMARY BILIARY CIRRHOSIS. Patients who have primary liver cancer (HCC) are usually not considered as candidates for liver transplantation if their tumor is larger than five centimeters in the case of a single lesion or there are more than three smaller tumor lesions because the cancer is likely to recur.

The signs suggesting the need for liver transplantation include recurrent episodes of bleeding esophageal or gastric varices (enlarged veins that usually occur in the esophagus or stomach), spontaneous bacterial peritonitis, refractory ASCITES, JAUNDICE, and encephalopathy. The model for end stage liver disease (MELD) is used to triage patients who have the greatest need for immediate transplantation.

Using Living Adult Donors

Some patients receive partial liver donations; this procedure is only performed at a few medical centers. The reason for the donation may be that the patient is on a waiting list for a liver transplantation and the family and friends fear that the patient will die before a donor is found; consequently, one of them donates part of his or her liver. Children who need liver donations receive a partial liver, but the practice of partial liver donation in adults is considered controversial. Adult LDLT has been declining since 2001 for a variety of reasons, including the possibility of the death of the donor. The one big advantage of LDLT in adults is that patients do not have to wait or die while waiting for transplantation.

Researchers reported on information they obtained on patients (donor and recipients) involved in adult-to-adult partial liver donations in 2003 in the *New England Journal of Medicine*. According to this study, most of the donors (74.4 percent) were related to the recipient. In 13.4 percent of the cases, friends donated part of their liver, and in 10.9 cases, the donors were spouses. In the remaining cases (1.3 percent) the donors were "good Samaritans" who were not relatives, friends, or spouses. In nearly all cases, the donors were screened by a hepatologist (medical liver expert), social worker, and a psychiatrist or psychologist before the procedure was approved and performed.

Among the donors, 14.5 percent had one or more complications of surgery, and 8.5 percent had to be rehospitalized because of complications from the procedure. A bile leak was the most common complication reported. Some patients needed blood transfusions or additional surgery. One donor died. The patients who received partial liver donations from live donors also had some complications: 22 percent had biliary complications, and 9.8. percent had vascular complications.

Immune System Rejection Problems

One key problem of liver transplantation (or any transplantation) is that the immune system rejects an organ from another person. To combat this rejection, patients must receive medications such as cyclosporine and tacrolimus to suppress their immune system; however, when the immune system is suppressed, the patient is more susceptible to infection as well as development of cancer and other complications. In addition, even with immune system-suppressing drugs, sometimes the immune system overcomes the effect and the transplanted organ is rejected.

lower gastrointestinal series X-rays taken of the lower part of the colon and the rectum; it is also called a barium enema. In the lower gastrointestinal series barium is introduced into the rectum in sufficient quantity to fill the entire colon so that the barium highlights the inside of the colon/rectum. Air may also be injected into the rectum to improve the visualization. In contrast to this test, an upper gastrointestinal series is the X-ray of the esophagus, stomach, and upper part of the small intestine. In that test, the patient drinks the barium and then X-rays are taken of the upper gastrointestinal tract. Similarly, the small bowel series examines the small intestines. Gastrogaffin is a water soluble contrast and can be used instead of barium in select cases; however, the pictures are not as good as the those seen with barium.

See also BARIUM STUDIES.

lymphoma A form of cancer that starts in the lymphatic system. The two key forms of lymphoma are Hodgkin's disease (HD) and non-Hodgkin's lymphoma (NHL). Non-Hodgkin's lymphoma may develop in the liver or other organs. About 7,400 people in the United States are diagnosed with Hodgkin's disease each year and about 57,000 with non-Hodgkin's lymphoma.

NHL may be considered indolent: that is, it is not curable with treatment, but at the same time, patients have a long survival period even if they are untreated for years. In contrast, the aggressive and the highly aggressive forms of lymphoma are curable, but patients with those forms of lymphoma can die quickly if they are untreated or do not respond to treatment.

Burkitt's lymphoma is a form of non-Hodgkin's lymphoma, first identified by David Burkitt in 1958, which is found in children as well as among acquired immunodeficiency syndrome (AIDS) patients. When diagnosed, it is often found in the digestive system.

The digestive system is frequently involved in non-Hodgkin's lymphoma, but it is rarely affected in Hodgkin's disease. For example, NHL may be seen in the stomach, the small or large intestine, or the liver. A computed tomography (CT) scan, barium studies, and/or an endoscopy with biopsy may be needed for diagnosis. Sometimes, lymphoma occurring outside the gut in the surrounding lymph nodes may cause an obstruction of the gut by extrinsic compression; for example, dysphagia (difficulty swallowing) may occur if the lymphoma surrounds the esophagus. In addition, the bowel may become obstructed if the lymphoma surrounds any loop of the bowel.

Mucosa associated lymphoid tissue (MALT) lymphoma is a specific form of lymphoma that frequently occurs in the gut. When it is found in the stomach, MALT lymphoma is frequently associated with a HELICOBACTER PYLORI infection. The eradication of the H. pylori can induce remission in the majority of these cases.

Risk Factors for NHL

According to Baris and Hoar Zahm in their 2000 article on the epidemiological characteristics of lymphomas in Current Opinion in Oncology, the key risk factor for NHL is immunosuppression, either primary or acquired. Lymphomas develop in as many as 25 percent of individuals with congenital immunosuppressive problems. The risk for development of lymphoma is greatest among individuals who have a first-degree relative (parent, child, or sibling) who has also been diagnosed with NHL. In addition, if a first-degree relative is diagnosed with leukemia or Hodgkin's disease, this diagnosis indicates an increased risk for NHL among other family members.

Individuals who have an acquired immune illness, such as AIDS, also face an increased risk of development of lymphoma.

Other individuals at risk for NHL development are those who are taking medications to suppress the immune system because they have received kidney, heart, or bone marrow transplantation. In one study of more than 18,000 patients worldwide who had had bone marrow transplantation, lymphomas developed in 78 patients compared to 1.5 cases in the general population.

Some infections increase the individual's risk of development of lymphoma; for example, infection with the Epstein-Barr virus increases the risk for Burkitt's lymphoma.

People who have some disorders have a greater risk for development of lymphoma, including individuals who have CELIAC SPRUE, DIABETES MELLITUS, rheumatoid arthritis, and Sjögen's syndrome. Some studies have also found a linkage between having malaria or tuberculosis and later diagnosis of NHL.

Individuals in some occupations appear to experience a greater risk of development of NHL, including farmers, pesticide workers, and some manufacturing workers. The exposure to pesticides appears to be the common denominator among these individuals.

Other workers are also at greater risk for NHL than most individuals, including employees in the rubber, petroleum refining, chemical, dry cleaning, and aircraft maintenance fields. Chronic exposure to organic solvents appears to be the factor that unites these workers. Laboratory technicians also face an increased risk of development of lymphoma.

See also MULTIPLE LYMPHOMATOUS POLYPOSIS.

Baris, Dalsu, M.D., and Sheilia Hoar Zahm. "Epidemiology of Lymphomas." *Current Opinion in Oncology* 12 (2000): 383–394.

Zebrack, Brad J., et al. "Psychological Outcomes in Long-Term Survivors of Childhood Leukemia, Hodgkin's Disease, and Non-Hodgkin's Lymphoma: A Report from the Childhood Cancer Survivor Study." *Pediatrics* 110, no. 1 (July 2002): 42–52.

magnesium An essential mineral needed by humans for many different biochemical reactions. Some researchers believe that a slightly low level of magnesium may result in migraine headaches and in many other symptoms, and supplemental magnesium has been used to treat acute migraine headaches.

Foods that are high in magnesium include wheat germ, almonds, pumpkin seeds, dry roasted cashews, nuts, cooked spinach, baked potato with the skin, peanut butter, chocolate bars, and bananas.

Magnesium is the key ingredient in many LAXA-TIVES that are given to treat constipation. Magnesium-containing antacids and laxatives should be avoided by patients who have renal failure.

Magnesium Deficiencies

A magnesium deficiency is more likely to occur in elderly individuals, although younger people may also become deficient. People who are taking diuretic drugs (water pills) are at risk for magnesium deficiency. Other groups of people who are at risk for magnesium deficiency include the following:

- people with poorly controlled diabetes
- people who are alcoholics or heavy drinkers
- people who take some anticancer drugs, such as Cisplatin
- people with gastrointestinal malabsorption disorders
- individuals with chronic vomiting and DIARRHEA

Indications of a severe magnesium deficiency include the following:

- seizures
- mental confusion
- appetite loss
- depression
- involuntary muscle contractions
- numbness and tingling
- abnormal heart rhythms

Low levels of magnesium can be present in the body despite normal serum levels. If individuals are deficient in magnesium, they should increase their dietary intake of foods that are rich in magnesium. They may also need to take magnesium supplements. If the magnesium level is dangerously low, the individual should be hospitalized to receive magnesium intravenously. A severe magnesium deficiency can be fatal.

Hypermagnesemia

Few people have toxically high levels of magnesium, but such toxicity can occur; for example, people who are taking large doses of laxatives are at risk for development of magnesium toxicity, as are those who have kidney failure.

High levels of magnesium may cause indicators ranging from sleepiness to coma as well as dizziness, muscle paralysis, slow heart, and heart blocks. People with toxic levels of magnesium may also have extremely low blood pressure (hypotension) and may also have breathing problems.

See also IRON; VITAMIN DEFICIENCIES/EXCESSES.

magnetic resonance cholangiopancreatography (MRCP) A noninvasive test that uses magnetic resonance imaging (MRI) technology to examine the pancreatic and bile ducts. The MRCP is noninvasive; however, it is a diagnostic procedure only, and consequently, physicians must perform endoscopic retrograde cholangiopancreatography (ERCP) if they wish to have subsequent access to the area to treat any abnormalities or blockages.

An MRCP may be used if a stone or a tumor in the bile duct or CHOLEDOCHAL CYSTS are suspected but not confirmed. It may also be a test that is used if the physician suspects CAROLI'S DISEASE or a patient has already undergone a failed ERCP.

In one study of patients with suspected choledo-cholithiasis, reported in the *Mayo Clinic Proceedings* in 2002, the researchers found that the MRCP was a useful tool in detecting risk for choledocholi-thiasis. Said the researchers, "Magnetic resonance cholangiopancreatography seems to be effective in diagnosing choledocholithiasis. It plays a funda-mental role in patients with a low or intermedi-ate risk of choledocholithiasis, contributing to the avoidance of purely diagnostic ERCP."

Calvo, M. M., et al. "Role of Magnetic Resonance Chol-angiopancreatography with Suspected Choledo-choli-thiasis." *Mayo Clinic Proceedings* 77, no. 5 (May 2002): 422–428.

major diagnostic tests for digestive diseases In diagnosing whether a person has a digestive dis-ease, and if so, which one is present, physicians need to rely upon key tests to aid them in their diagnosis of the underlying problem, including some invasive tests such as the ENDOSCOPY and noninvasive tests such as X-rays, ULTRASOUND, computerized tomography (CT) scans, and mag-netic resonance imaging (MRI) scans. Some tests combine two forms of testing, such as the endo-scopic ultrasound, which combines an invasive procedure with imaging technology.

Sometimes a test is performed because specific gastrointestinal symptoms are present. In other cases, a test is given when there are no symptoms but the individual is at risk for a disease because of age, a family, or past history for the disease or other factors. This is most often the case for the colonos-copy, which is frequently used as a screening test for COLORECTAL CANCER, even when no symptoms are present. (Often colorectal cancer has no symptoms, especially in the early stages.) In other countries, such as Japan, the upper endoscopy is commonly

used to screen for STOMACH CANCER, and thus, many cases that are present are detected and treated. This entry discusses these key diagnostic tools.

Endoscopic Procedures

Endoscopic procedures use a special device called the endoscope to view the gastrointestinal system internally, from the mouth and through to the anus. There are an estimated 1 million gastrointes-tinal endoscopies performed each year in the United States according to the National Institute of Diabe-tes and Digestive and Kidney Diseases (NIDDK). Such tests include the colonoscopy, the esopha-gogastroduodenoscopy (EGD), the endoscopic ret-rograde cholangiopancreatography (ERCP), the flexible SIGMOIDOSCOPY, and a procedure that is a kind of hybrid endoscopic/imaging test: the endo-scopic ultrasonography (EUS). In addition, wireless video camera technology uses a camera so tiny that it can be swallowed by the patient and the gastro-enterologist can view images as the camera travels through the gastrointestinal system.

Single- and double-balloon enteroscopy are a recent advancement that allows most if not all of the small bowel to be directly visualized by endos-copy. However, it is not available at many centers.

Colonoscopy The colonoscopy is the most fre-quently used endoscopic test in the United States, according to data from 2001–05 from the NIDDK and published in 2008. In their study of 885,593 endoscopic procedures performed on adults at 101 sites during this period, based on data from the Clinical Outcomes Research Initiative's National Endoscopic Database, the researchers analyzed data on 542,650 patients who had colonoscopies, followed by 270,957 patients who had an EGD, 55,708 who had a flexible sigmoidoscopy, 9,333 who had an ERCP and 6,945 who had an EUS procedure. (Note that according to the National Center for Health Statistics, 11.7 million people in the United States had a sigmoidoscopy or colonos-copy in 2006.)

As can be seen from this data, summarized in Table 1, the age group receiving the greatest percent-age of all the colonoscopies (32.9 percent) that were analyzed were patients ages 50 to 59 years, followed by those ages 60 to 69 years (18.4 percent). In con-sidering race/ethnicity alone, the overwhelmingly

TABLE 1: CHARACTERISTICS OF ENDOSCOPY SITES AND PERSONS UNDERGOING ENDOSCOPIC PROCEDURES, 2001–2005

	Colonoscopy	EGD	Flexible Sigmoidoscopy	ERCP	EUS
Number of patients	542,650	270,957	55,708	9,333	6,945
Number of practices	76	77	72	40	23
Number of sites	101	101	96	44	25
Site Characteristics (Percentage)					
Type of Endoscopy Site					
Community/HMO	78.1	72.8	58.5	40.1	2.9
Academic	11.3	14.6	16.6	41.1	66.5
VA/Military	10.6	12.6	24.9	18.8	30.6
Type of Facility					
Office	1.7	2.7	1.1	Less than 0.1	0
Hospital	40.9	49.7	51.3	96.7	100
Ambulatory Surgery Center	57.4	47.6	47.7	3.3	Less than 0.1
Patient Characteristics (Percentage)					
Age (years)					
20–29	1.7	4.6	5.6	9.2	2.3
30–39	4.0	9.4	8.6	10.3	5.3
40–49	11.7	17.4	12.2	14.1	13.1
50–59	32.9	23.1	34.6	19.3	24.3
60–69	25.6	19.5	19.8	16.5	24.1
70–79	18.4	17.5	13.6	18.3	22.8
80+	5.9	8.6	5.6	12.4	8.1
Race/Ethnicity					
Non-Hispanic White	85.9	81.3	78.2	72.0	86.9
Non-Hispanic Black	6.4	7.3	13.3	7.5	5.0
Asian/Pacific Islander	1.5	2.0	2.2	1.8	1.8
American Indian/ Alaska Native	0.8	1.2	0.9	6.0	0.4
Multiracial Non-Hispanic	0.2	0.2	0.6	0.3	0.3
Hispanic	5.3	8.0	4.8	12.4	5.6
Gender					
Female	49.6	51.4	41.0	52.0	40.7
Male	50.4	48.6	59.0	48.0	59.3

EGD = Esophagogastroduodenoscopy

ERCP = Endoscopic retrograde cholangiopancreatography

EUS = Endoscopic ultrasonography

Source: Adapted from Ruhl, Constance E., M.D., and James E. Everhart, M.D. "Indications and Outcomes of Gastrointestinal Endoscopy," edited by James E. Everhart, 125. *The Burden of Digestive Diseases in the United States*. Washington, D.C.: National Institute of Diabetes and Digestive and Kidney Diseases.

largest percentage was found among non-Hispanic whites, or 85.9 percent, followed not closely at all by 6.4 percent who were non-Hispanic blacks receiving colonoscopies. Males and females had colonoscopies at about the same rate. Most of the patients had their procedure at an ambulatory surgery center (57.4 percent), followed by a hospital (40.9 percent). See Table 1 for more details.

The colonoscopy has become a more popular procedure than in past years, and its use has increased by 63.4 percent, while the use of the flexible sigmoidoscopy decreased by about 60 percent, according to the NIDDK. This change has occurred as a result of the realization that because the colonoscopy covers the entire colon, it is generally a better procedure to use than the sigmoidoscopy.

The colonoscopy is also a very effective procedure at identifying disease in those with only a routine risk. For example, according to the research published in *The Burden of Digestive Diseases in the United States* in 2008, only 21.0 percent of 117,422 individuals with a routine risk and who received a colonoscopy had a normal examination with no findings. Nearly half (45.0 percent) had DIVERTICULOSIS, and more than a third (37.4 percent) had POLYPS, while 7.2 percent

had multiple polyps. Findings of problems with a flexible sigmoidoscopy among 55,708 patients had much lower rates of finding disease, possibly because the entire colon was not examined. See Table 2 for more details.

The bowel-cleansing preparation for the two procedures is different; while the colonoscopy requires a greater amount of laxatives to clean the entire colon, the flexible sigmoidoscopy can be accomplished by a couple of enemas administered right before the procedure. In addition, the colonoscopy is usually accomplished under sedation, whereas flexible sigmoidoscopy is done without sedation in most cases.

Individuals of all races should have screening colonoscopies as recommended by their physicians; however, it is particularly important for black men and women to have colonoscopies, based on recent data. A study of the prevalence of colon polyps that were detected by colonoscopy among black and white patients who had no symptoms, reported in 2008 in the *Journal of the American Medical Association,* revealed that both black men and black women who had colonoscopies had a significantly higher rate of having large polyps compared to both white males and females.

TABLE 2: COLONOSCOPY FINDINGS IN THE TOTAL POPULATION AND PERSONS AT ROUTINE RISK ONLY AND FLEXIBLE SIGMOIDOSCOPY FINDINGS, 2001–2005, PERCENTAGE

Finding	Colonoscopy		Flexible Sigmoidoscopy
	Total population (N =542,650)	Routine Risk Only (N =117,422)	N =55,708
Diverticulosis	42.8	45.0	22.3
Hemorrhoids	39.6	34.2	31.7
Polyp	35.9	37.4	16.2
Normal Exam/no findings	17.6	21.0	30.5
Polyp greater than 9 mm/Suspected malignant tumor	7.6	6.4	3.4
Multiple polyps	7.2	7.2	2.8
Mucosal Abnormality-Colitis	5.2	1.4	7.8
Tumor	1.2	0.4	0.9
Other finding	9.8	6.6	12.1

Source: Adapted from Ruhl, Constance E., M.D., and James E. Everhart, M.D "Indications and Outcomes of Gastrointestinal Endoscopy." In *The Burden of Digestive Diseases in the United States*, edited by James E. Everhart, 129. Washington, D.C.: National Institute of Diabetes and Digestive and Kidney Diseases.

The researchers stated, "In summary, we find that asymptomatic black men and women undergoing colonoscopy screening are more likely to have 1 or more polyps sized more than 9 mm compared with white individuals. The differences were especially striking among women. These findings emphasize the importance of encouraging all black men and women to be screening. We found that black women younger than 50 years have similar rates of polyps sized more than 9 mm compared with white men aged 50 to 59 years." The researchers recommended further study on these findings. African Americans with cancer are also likely to have advanced cancer on colonoscopy. As such, it is recommended that colonoscopy screening be initiated at 45 years of age for African Americans.

Esophogastroduodenoscopy (EGD)   The upper endoscopy, which has the official and very lengthy name of esophogastroduodenoscopy is frequently used as a diagnostic test or a screening test; it examines the esophagus, the stomach, and part of the duodenum, hence the name; for example, the EGD is used as a screening test to identify Barrett's esophagus in those patients with chronic, long-standing gastroesophageal reflux disease (GERD), unless they have had a previously normal EGD. It is also used to screen for stomach cancer in those individuals who are at risk. The EGD can also identify a gastrointestinal ulcer, such as a peptic or duodenal ulcer. This invasive test enables the physician to remove tissue for biopsy. It is also used to screen for esophageal varices in patients with liver cirrhosis.

According to *The Burden of Digestive Diseases in the United States*, of 270,957 EGDs performed on adults from 2001 to 2005, a large percentage (41.5 percent) of the 270,957 EGDs that were analyzed had normal findings. Of those with abnormal findings, the most common abnormal finding was a mucosal abnormality (38.8 percent), followed by hiatal hernia (33.4 percent) and esophageal inflammation (17.8 percent).

Among the symptoms experienced by patients who had EGDs in this analysis, the largest percentage (28.3 percent) were performed because of acid reflux symptoms/heartburn, followed by 27.7 percent that were performed for alarm symptoms, such as an unintended weight loss or vomiting.

TABLE 3: SYMPTOMATIC INDICATIONS FOR ESOPHAGASTRODUODENOSCOPY (EGD) N =-270,957, 2001–2005

Indication		Percentage
Symptoms	Reflux Symptoms/Heartburn	28.3
	Alarm Symptoms	27.7
	GERD	22.3
	Dyspepsia/Abdominal pain	21.6
	Dysphagia	20.5
	Bleeding cluster	20.4
	Abdominal pain/bloating	20.1
	Anemia	10.5
	Dyspepsia	9.7
	Nausea	6.7
	Vomiting	4.9
	Weight loss	4.0
	Chest pain	3.9
	Diarrhea	2.4
	Early satiety	1.3

Source: Adapted from Ruhl, Constance E., M.D., and James E. Everhart, M.D. "Indications and Outcomes of Gastrointestinal Endoscopy." In *The Burden of Digestive Diseases in the United States*, edited by James E. Everhart, 134. Washington, D.C.: the National Institute of Diabetes and Digestive and Kidney Diseases.

Other common symptoms that led to the EGD were signs of GERD (22.3 percent), dyspepsia/abdominal pain (21.6 percent), or DYSPHAGIA (20.5 percent). In addition, the EGD is used in cases of bleeding cluster, which refers to such issues as anemia, iron deficiency anemia, a positive fecal occult blood test or a suspected gastrointestinal bleed. (Together, these bleeding cluster issues represented 20.5 percent of the symptoms leading to an EGD). An emergency EGD may be needed in patients with gastrointestinal bleed or food impaction in the esophagus.

In other cases, the EGD is performed to determine how an individual who has been already diagnosed with a disease is doing, such as someone previously diagnosed with Barrett's esophagus or a gastric ulcer or gastric lymphoma/cancer. See Table 3 for further details.

Endoscopic Retrograde Cholangiopancreatography (ERCP)   The ERCP is an invasive endoscopic diagnostic test in which the gastroenterologist can visualize the bile ducts and the pancreatic ducts. It serves as a diagnostic and therapeutic purpose in biliary PANCREATITIS, and stones can be removed from the bile duct, thus benefiting pancreatitis in such cases. Pancreatic stones can also be removed and PANCREATIC CANCER as well as cholangiocarcinoma can be diagnosed by imaging and doing brushings/biopsies. In addition, it can also allow for the insertion of a biliary and pancreatic stent to hold the duct open when it is blocked or leaking.

If patients have consistently abnormal liver function blood tests that are of concern to the physician, the ERCP can determine if there are structural or functional abnormalities of the biliary system. According to data from the NIDDK, the age group of patients receiving the greatest numbers of ERCPs were ages 50 to 59 years (19.3 percent), followed by those ages 70 to 79 years (18.3 percent). See Table 1 for further details.

The papillotomy is an endoscopic procedure used to widen the papilla by making a cut so as to facilitate the removal of stones from the bile duct. It is a procedure performed during the ERCP.

Sometimes the noninvasive option of the magnetic resonance cholangiopancreatography (MRCP) is used as an alternative to the ERCP; however, this MRI test is only diagnostic, and thus, it cannot be used to take any treatment action, such as the biopsying of tissue, removal of cysts and so forth.

Flexible Sigmoidoscopy   The sigmoidoscopy is a diagnostic procedure in which the rectum and the lower part of the colon is examined with the use of a sigmoidoscope, a flexible tube measuring about 65 centimeters in length and which is inserted through the anus. This procedure is performed only after a couple of enemas to clean the lower bowel. Sometimes it is done "unprepped" or without enema cleaning. As seen from Table 1, most individuals undergoing a flexible sigmoidoscopy are in the 50–59-year-age range (34.6 percent), followed by those who are 60 to 69 years (19.8 percent).

Enteroscopy   The enteroscopy is an endoscopic examination of the small intestine. The endoscope (longer than the EGD scope) is inserted through the mouth and into the stomach and then is passed into the small intestine. Biopsies can be taken during the procedure. The enteroscopy examines the part of the small bowel that is beyond the reach of the EGD. Single- and double-balloon enteroscopy can further extend the reach of the endoscopic visualization of small bowel.

Endoscopic Ultrasound (EUS)   The endoscopic ultrasound combines the use of the endoscopy with the technology of ultrasound imaging. According to the National Commission on Digestive Diseases, endoscopic ultrasound has dramatically improved physicians' ability to view changes in the structure of the PANCREAS, and thus, they may be able to diagnose chronic pancreatitis early in the disease. The EUS is of benefit in staging esophageal, pancreatic, and rectal cancer.

With the endoscopic ultrasound, an ultrasound sensor is attached to the endoscope, which is then passed into the digestive tract, for example, into the stomach or the rectum, and images are then obtained for the gastroenterologist to analyze. It is important to note that while an ultrasound from outside the body is risk-free, the endoscopic ultrasound is associated with a significant risk for complications.

According to data analyzed by researchers for the NIDDK, individuals ages 50 to 59 years are the most likely to have an EUS (24.3 percent of all EUS procedures), followed by those ages 60 to 69 years (24.1 percent). As with all other endoscopic tests that were analyzed, the majority of those receiving the EUS are white (86.9 percent). Males represent 59.3 percent of all EUS procedures, and females represent 40.7 percent. Nearly all EUS procedures are performed in a hospital. (See Table 1 for further details.)

An ERCP as well as an EUS may be used to diagnose bile duct stones, pancreatitis, pancreatic cancer, and GALLBLADDER CANCER.

Chromoendoscopy   Chromoendoscopy is a procedure in which an endoscopy is performed, and in an additional step, a special dye is sprayed on the gastrointestinal wall at the area of interest, using a special spray catheter. The dye from the catheter allows the highlighting of abnormalities on the gastrointestinal wall that may have been ambiguous or otherwise have escaped detection. This procedure is not routinely performed as of this writing because of the lack of good studies showing whether using these special dyes produces better clinical outcomes than those using traditional endoscopy without the dyes.

Wireless Video Capsule Endoscopy   With wireless video capsule endoscopy, patients swallow a tiny camera that provides clear images of the gastrointestinal system as it passed through. Some experts use capsule endoscopy for an examination of the esophagus to screen for Barrett's esophagus as well as esophageal varices. According to the National Commission on Digestive Diseases in their 2009 report, this procedure has made great strides. Say the authors, "Development of the video capsule endoscope has revolutionized imaging of the small bowel mucosa and facilitated the evaluation of common disorders, such as Crohn's disease, idiopathic inflammatory diseases of the small bowel, and malignancy. Occult bleeding from the small bowel may now be identified, addressing a long-standing clinical dilemma prior to this technology."

The capsule endoscopy of the colon may supplant screening colonoscopy in the not too distant future.

X-Rays and Imaging Tests

X-rays and imaging tests can help considerably with diagnosis, although other more invasive tests and procedures are needed for treatment. Imaging tests are used for the diagnosis of cancers of the digestive system, such as the ultrasound, magnetic resonance imaging (MRI) scan and computerized tomography (CT) scan. Magnetic resonance cholangiopancreatography (MRCP) visualizes bile and the pancreatic duct.

Many different common and rare digestive diseases can be diagnosed with imaging studies; for example, with pneumatosis intestinalis, computed tomography (CT) scans is more effective at diagnosis.

Upper Gastrointestinal X-Ray   The upper gastrointestinal (GI) X-ray is a common diagnostic procedure in which the esophagus, stomach, and duodenum are all imaged after a person drinks contrast dye (such as barium) so that a physician can detect medical problems such as ulcers, stricture, cancer, and other diseases and conditions.

Magnetic Resonance Imaging (MRI)   The MRI is a noninvasive test. Magnetic resonance imaging (MRI) can help to identify many different forms of digestive cancers although it is not routinely used for this purpose.

Computerized Tomography (CT) Scan   Sometimes computerized tomography (CT) scans are used to assist physicians with their diagnoses of digestive issues; for example, a CT scan can help

with the diagnosis of pancreatitis, cholecystitis, and APPENDICITIS. CT scans can detect the presence of a liver abscess or a perforation, as well as nonalcoholic fatty liver disease. CT scans are also helpful in diagnosing mesenteric venous thrombosis. The CT scan can also identify some forms of cancer, such as pancreatic cancer. In addition, the CT scan can identify abdominal TUBERCULOSIS.

Ultrasound Imaging   The ultrasound is a noninvasive test (unless it is an endoscopic ultrasound). It uses sound waves to provide a view of the internal organs. It can identify most cases of gallstones. If patients have severe back pain and kidney problems are suspected, ultrasound may be used to help with diagnosis. Ultrasound is also used to diagnose problems with the pancreas and gallbladder.

Magnetic Resonance Cholangiopancreatography (MRCP)   The MRCP is a diagnostic noninvasive test that uses magnetic resonance imaging (MRI) technology to examine the pancreatic and bile ducts. An MRCP may be used if a stone or a tumor in the bile duct or CHOLEDOHAL CYSTS are suspected but not confirmed. It may also be a test that is used if the physician suspects CAROLI'S DISEASE, or when a patient has already undergone a failed ERCP.

Radionuclide Imaging   Radionuclide imaging is performed by the nuclear medicine department of the hospital, frequently a part of the radiology department. For example, a bleeding scan using a radionuclide material is performed when the source of gastrointestinal bleeding cannot be identified. The hepatobiliary iminodiacetic acid (HIDA) scan is used for diagnosing acute cholecystitis as well as possible leaks of the bile duct. Radionuclide imaging can also help distinguish between a hemangioma versus a tumor in the liver.

Barium Studies   BARIUM STUDIES involve the oral or rectal instillation of barium, a contrast dye that shows up under a fluoroscope. Barium studies are sometimes performed when a digestive disease is suspected and it is also a test to diagnose colorectal cancer; however a colonoscopy is a preferred test because with the colonoscopy, actions can be taken, such as removing polyps. In addition, biopsies cannot be taken during a barium study, which is a visual inspection only. If an abnormality is seen with a barium study, it is often followed up with an upper endoscopy or a colonoscopy. Barium studies are also useful to examine the patient's swallowing function.

Specialized Tests Not all tests are frequently given, as with the colonoscopy or the EGD. Some tests are ordered only in particular situations, such as with the electrogastrogram, BREATH TESTS, or MANOMETRY, topics discussed below.

Electrogastrogram The electrogastrogram is a procedure that measures gastric electrical activity. Similar to how the electrocardiogram studies the rhythms of the heart, the electrogastrogram can detect abnormally fast, slow, or irregular rhythms of the stomach. It can be a useful test in diagnosing GASTROPARESIS (slow stomach emptying). This test can be performed when patients are fasting and after they have consumed a meal.

Manometry Manometry is a diagnostic procedure that tests for resting pressure as well as for contractions and relaxations of the muscles of different parts of the digestive tube; for example, in esophageal manometry, the pressures in the esophagus and the upper and lower esophageal sphincters at rest and in response to swallowing are each measured with a specific type of catheter. The findings of this test may aid surgeons who are planning antireflux surgery on what kind of operation they should perform. Esophageal manometry is frequently used in patients with dysphagia and is an important for the diagnosis of achalasia. Anorectal manometry may be used in patients suffering from CONSTIPATION and fecal incontinence. High-resolution manometry is a recent advance in esophageal manometric technology.

Breath Tests Breath tests are generally tests that use the breath to test for the patient's digestive function and the presence of diseases. A breath test may be given to determine whether a person is infected with *Helicobacter pylori*, bacteria that are generally harbored within the stomach, when present in the body. After ingesting a specific meal labeled with a small amount of radioactivity, the patient breathes into a device, which measures the level of radioactivity released with radio-labeled carbon dioxide that is present in the breath. If the test result is positive for *H. pylori*, treatment is initiated.

Breath tests may also test for gastric emptying time, lactose intolerance, and small bowel bacterial overgrowth. Breath tests are also administered by police officials to individuals who are suspected of driving while they are under the influence of alcohol. The breath test reveals whether the driver has a level of alcohol that is above the allowable level in his or her state or at least above the 0.08 percent blood alcohol concentration, the nationwide standard.

See also CULTURES.

Everhart, James E., ed. *The Burden of Digestive Diseases in the United States.* Washington, D.C.: National Institute of Diabetes and Digestive and Kidney Diseases, 2008.

Lieberman, David A., M.D., et al. "Prevalence of Colon Polyps Detected by Colonoscopy Screening in Asymptomatic Black and White Patients." *Journal of the American Medical Association* 300, no. 12 (2008): 1,417–1,422.

U.S. Department of Health and Human Services. *Opportunities and Challenges in Digestive Diseases Research: Recommendations of the National Commission on Digestive Diseases.* Bethesda, Md.: National Institutes of Health, March 2009.

malabsorption syndrome A condition in which an individual's intestines are unable to absorb sufficient nutrients from food and leads to nutrient, vitamin, and mineral deficiencies.

Among causes of malabsorption are the following diseases or conditions:

- CROHN'S DISEASE
- CELIAC disease
- Chronic PANCREATITIS
- Extensive small bowel resection
- Overgrowth of bacteria in the small intestine
- WHIPPLE'S DISEASE

See also VITAMIN DEFICIENCIES/EXCESSES.

Mallory-Weiss syndrome A medical problem that some people with ALCOHOLISM experience, although not everyone who has Mallory-Weiss tear is an alcoholic. The primary symptom of Mallory-Weiss tear is internal bleeding (mild to heavy) in the area where the esophagus joins the stomach. It may be caused by vomiting and retching, which are common among people who are alcoholics. This vomiting or retching causes tears at the gastroesophageal junction and in turn causes bleeding. (However, about half of Mallory-Weiss syndrome patients do not have a history of prior vomiting or retching.)

Most Mallory-Weiss syndrome patients heal on their own; for others, cauterization hemoclip application and/or an injection of epinephrine into the damaged area through endoscopy is necessary to stop the hemorrhaging.

Mallory-Weiss syndrome is suspected clinically on the basis of a patient's history and is diagnosed with endoscopy.

See also NAUSEA AND VOMITING.

malnutrition/starvation   A serious condition in which nutritional intake is so low that if it is not corrected, an individual becomes sick and predisposed to many illnesses such as infection. The individual may also die. The condition may be caused by a famine, in which there is insufficient food for many people. It may also be caused by other problems, such as poverty or even by an elderly person's inability to feed him- or herself. In some cases, people who have eating disorders, such as anorexia nervosa, become malnourished and may actually starve to death. In other cases, malnutrition may be a result of a sickness, such as uncontrolled CROHN'S DISEASE and MALABSORPTION SYNDROME. Patients who are unable to be fed through the gut may need to receive PARENTERAL NUTRITION.

Although malnutrition is frequently seen in hospitalized patients, malnutrition due to a lack of sufficient food is not a common problem in the United States, Canada, and other developed countries.

See also BERIBERI; VITAMIN DEFICIENCIES/EXCESSES.

manometry   A diagnostic procedure that tests for resting pressure as well as for contractions and relaxations of the muscles of different parts of the digestive tube; for example, in esophageal manometry, the pressures in the esophagus and the upper and lower esophageal sphincters in both fasting and response to swallowing are each measured with a specific type of catheter. The findings of this test may aid surgeons in planning anti-reflux surgery on what kind of operation to perform.

See also ACHALASIA; HIRSCHSPRUNG'S DISEASE; MAJOR DIAGNOSTIC TESTS FOR DIGESTIVE DISEASES; ZENKER'S DIVERTICULUM.

Meckel's diverticulum   A congenital small pouch in the small intestine (similar to the appendix in the cecum) that is found in about 2 percent of all individuals. It is usually asymptomatic, but Meckel's diverticulum can cause or lead to an obstruction and to bleeding. This condition, which is frequently difficult to diagnose, is correctable with surgery.

See also ZENKER'S DIVERTICULUM.

medications for digestive diseases and disorders   There is a broad array of medications that are used to treat digestive diseases, including medications that are used for specific diseases, such as DIABETES MELLITUS, GASTROESOPHAGEAL REFLUX DISEASE (GERD), IRRITABLE BOWEL SYNDROME, CROHN'S DISEASE, or peptic ulcers, as well as medications that are primarily used to treat certain symptoms, such as antiemetics (antivomiting medications), ANTIBIOTICS (medications used to kill bacterial infections), laxatives used to treat constipation, and drugs in other categories. Sometimes medications that are taken for another illness affect the digestive system, such as antibiotics taken for an upper respiratory infection that cause diarrhea in the patient. This entry provides an overview of medications for specific diseases and specific symptoms that affect the digestive system.

Diarrhea

Antidiarrheal medications are available in both over-the-counter (OTC) and prescribed forms. Probably the most well-known OTC antidiarrheal is loperamide (Imodium). There are also prescribed antidiarrheal medications such as atropine sulfate (Lomotil). It is important to avoid taking too many antidiarrheal medications because their chronic use could lead to the development of constipation.

Note that if patients have loose stools in conjunction with bleeding and/or weight loss, they should always consult with their physicians to determine if there is a serious underlying disease that should be treated.

Diabetes Mellitus

The primary medications that are used to treat diabetes are drugs that decrease glucose production and circulation. Diabetes is managed primarily by medication and by nutritional adaptations. Individuals with type 1 (insulin-dependent) diabetes are treated with a variety of short-, medium-, and long-acting forms of insulin.

Individuals with type 2 diabetes are usually treated with oral agents, such as sulfonylureas medications, including glimepride (Amaryl), chlorpropamide (Diabinese), glyburide (Micronase), and glipizide (Glucotrol, Glucotrol XL). Those individuals with type 2 diabetes may also be treated with meglitinide drugs, including repaglinide (Prandin) or nateglinide (Starlix).

Biguanides are commonly-used medications for type 2 diabetes that decrease the glucose production of the liver. Medications in this class are various formulations of metformin (Glucophage, Glucophage XR, and Romet).

Thiazolidinediones (TZDs) are medications sometimes used by individuals with diabetes to help their bodies use the glucose more efficiently. These medications include such drugs as rosiglitazone (Avandia) and pioglitazone (Actos). In addition, alpha glucosidase inhibitor medications are sometimes prescribed by physicians to slow the digestion of carbohydrates, including such prescribed medications as acarbose (Precose) or miglitol (Glyset).

The DPP-4 inhibitor is a newer medication that is prescribed for type 2 diabetes. It affects both the alpha and beta cells in the PANCREAS that regulate glucose levels. The one DPP-4 inhibitor that has been approved by the Food and Drug Administration (FDA) as of this writing is sitagliptin (Januvia).

Infections

Antibiotic medications are frequently prescribed to treat bacterial infections; however, antibiotics can themselves cause gastrointestinal symptoms, such as loose stools, gastrointestinal upset, and sometimes colitis and gastrointestinal BLEEDING.

There are numerous antibiotics that may be prescribed for a wide variety of infections, and many of them affect the digestive system. If patients know that a particular antibiotic upsets their stomach, they should always advise the doctor ahead of time, who may be able to order a different antibiotic.

Patients should also advise their pharmacist of a past experience of an antibiotic that was very upsetting to the stomach because pharmacists are aware of the groupings of different antibiotics and can warn the patient that a newly prescribed antibiotic may cause similar side effects as what they have suffered in the past from a medication in the same classification of antibiotics.

Irritable Bowel Syndrome (IBS)

Medications are often prescribed to treat irritable bowel syndrome (IBS), including such drugs as antispasmodics like Bentyl, antidiarrheal agents like Imodium, and antianxiety medications like benzodiazepines (although they are often avoided by many physicians). Sometimes antidepressants are prescribed to treat patients with IBS, but they are usually given in dosages that would be too low to treat actual clinical depression. Antidepressants are also sometimes prescribed for patients with noncardiac CHEST PAIN and other chronic PAIN syndromes.

Lubiprostone (Amitiza) is a medication that is used for constipation-predominant irritable bowel syndrome. Some data suggests that gut selective antibiotics also have a beneficial role in IBS.

Peptic Ulcers

Ulcers are primarily caused by an infection with HELICOBACTER PYLORI or by the use of nonsteroidal anti-inflammatory drugs (NSAIDs). Acid blocking agents are used to help the stomach heal, and these medications are also used to treat people with chronic gastroesophageal reflux disease. Histamine-2 receptor blockers (H2 blockers) are one type of medication that is used to treat ulcers as well as GERD. H2 blockers are available in both OTC and prescribed form. Some examples of H2 blockers that are available as of this writing include Zantac, Pepcid, and other brands.

Medications in the PROTON PUMP INHIBITOR class are more potent than H2RAs and are more commonly used than H2RAs. Some examples of medications which are proton pump inhibitors and are currently available as of this writing are omeprazole (Prilosec), lansoprazole (Prevacid), rabeprazole (Aciphex), pantoprazole (Protonix), and esomeprazole (Nexium). Prilosec is also available over the counter as well as in generic form (omeprazole). In addition, the cause of the ulcer needs to be treated. For example, the treatment of the bacterium *Helicobacter pylori* (*H. pylori*) involves a combination of multiple medications like antibiotics and PPIs. Prevpac is one example of such a dosepak.

Categories of Medications

Medications are divided into different categories, such as antiemetics, antispasmodics, and so forth.

Antiemetics   Antiemetics are prescribed or over-the-counter drugs that are taken to prevent NAUSEA AND VOMITING. Commonly used examples are promethazine (Phenergan) and prochlorperazine (Compazine). Newer and more potent antiemetics include ondansetron (Zofran) and granisetron (Kytril). Among alternative medicines, ginger is a popular remedy for the nausea and vomiting of pregnancy, since most physicians are reticent about prescribing medications to pregnant women.

Antispasmodics   Antispasmodics are drugs that limit or stop intestinal muscle spasms, such as dicyclomine (Bentyl), hyoscyamine (Levsin), and a medication that is a combination of atropine, hyoscyamine, scopolamine, and phenobarbital (Donnatal).

Corticosteroids   Corticosteroids (also often referred to as STEROIDS) are medications that are prescribed for some illnesses characterized by excessive inflammation, such as CROHN'S DISEASE, ULCERATIVE COLITIS, autoimmune hepatitis, and rheumatoid arthritis. They are often taken orally or intravenously, but steroids can also be used in the form of enemas, topical ointments and creams to treat such problems as colitis, HEMORRHOIDS, and pruritus ani (itching of the rectal area). The long-term use of steroids has serious potential side effects, including a change in the body shape and structure (such as the development of a plump and moonlike face), osteoporosis, diabetes, as well as immunosuppression.

Physicians taper the dose of the steroid to the lowest possible level as soon as possible, since the side effects are both dose- and duration-related. Steroids are also synthesized inside the body. Some people take steroids for body-building reasons; this is not medically advisable because of the many negative consequences that can ensue. In addition, those who abuse steroids often take high dosages that are not medically approved.

Immunosuppressive Medications   In addition to corticosteroids, individuals with Crohn's disease may need to take immunosuppressive medications such as azathioprine or 6-mercaptopurine (6-MP). Also, anyone who has had an organ transplant of any type, such as a LIVER TRANSPLANTATION, pancreas transplant, or a kidney transplant needs to take an immunosuppressive medication for life. These drugs block an immune reaction against the transplanted organ inside the body. Immunosuppressive medications may also cause such side effects as nausea and vomiting and diarrhea, and they may also lower the patient's resistance to infection or even to cancer.

Prokinetics   Prokinetics are medications in a class of prescribed medications that enhance motility in the gut. They were formerly popular in the use of treating patients with GERD. These drugs are also known as promotility medications because they speed stomach emptying and/or transit through the gut. The drugs are useful for those who have GASTROPARESIS and intestinal pseudo-obstruction.

In 2000, cisapride (Propulsid), a very popular medication at that time, was virtually withdrawn from the market in the United States by the Food and Drug Administration (FDA) because some patients who had used cisapride became sick or they died of cardiac ailments. On a restricted basis today, physicians may currently continue to prescribe cisapride to some patients who do not respond to other medications; however, patients who have heart problems cannot take this drug; nor should those who are taking some antibiotics or antidepressants because of problems with adverse drug reactions. Cisapride is widely available outside the United States.

The other primary prokinetic drug is metoclopramide (Reglan). Because metoclopramide has many side effects, especially on the brain, many physicians avoid prescribing this drug whenever possible. Domperidone, another prokinetic drug, is sold in some pharmacies where it is actually compounded by the pharmacist. Domperidone is similar to metoclopramide, but without many of its side effects on the brain. Since it is not widely available, many patients buy their domperidone over the Internet from other countries, although the legality of such actions is questionable. It should also be noted that erythromycin, in addition to its antibiotic function, also has prokinetic activity. However, the effects of erythromycin are short-lived, lasting no more than a few weeks.

Proton Pump Inhibitors Proton pump inhibitors are medications in a class of medications that are given to people who suffer from chronic heartburn, also known as gastroesophageal reflux disease and/or to patients who have either stomach or duodenal ulcers. Drugs in this class are more potent inhibitors of stomach acid than are the histamine-2 receptor blockers, such as rantidine (Zantac) or cimetidine (Tagamet). The reduced acid secretion in the stomach due to these drugs allows time for healing. Proton pump inhibitors (PPIs) are also prescribed for individuals who have ZOLLINGER-ELLISON SYNDROME.

See also ADAPTATIONS TO DAILY LIVING AND LIFE-STYLE FACTORS; ELDERLY; MAJOR DIAGNOSTIC TESTS FOR DIGESTIVE DISEASES.

megacolon Very enlarged large intestine (colon), which may cause abdominal distension, NAUSEA AND VOMITING, as well as CONSTIPATION. Megacolon may be caused by impaired PERISTALSIS, the wavelike process that moves digesting food and waste through the digestive system. Megacolon may also be caused by an inflammation or blockage stemming from a tumor or volvulus (a type of obstruction that occurs when the gut twists, producing obstruction as well as interruption of the blood supply to the region). A diatrizoate meglumine (Gastrografin) enema or colonoscopy may be ordered to exclude a blockage. In the case of an acute megacolon, decompression of the colon can be carried out, for example, by colonoscopy, in order to reduce the risk of perforation. A gastrogaffin enema or colonoscopy can also remove the obstruction caused by volvulus.

men and digestive diseases Digestive ailments that occur in adult males. In many cases, men and women have about an equal risk of development of digestive diseases and disorders; however, some higher risks are based on gender. For example, men have a much greater risk of cancer of the esophagus than women. Similarly, they are more likely to have KAPOSI'S SARCOMA (15 men to one woman). Men also have a higher risk of CIRRHOSIS of the liver, liver cancer, stomach cancer, alcoholic pancreatitis, and HEMOCHROMATOSIS than women. In contrast, women have a higher risk for development of GALLSTONES, gallbladder cancer, HIRSCHSPRUNG'S DISEASE, IRRITABLE BOWEL SYNDROME (IBS), and WATERMELON STOMACH.

See also ESOPHAGEAL CANCER; GALLBLADDER CANCER; LIVER CANCER; STOMACH CANCER.

Ménétrier's disease A rare disease that is characterized by large reddened folds of gastric tissue inside the stomach. It is also known as hypoproteinemic hypertrophic gastropathy. This disease causes a depletion of the stomach glands and the acid-producing cells, as well as a loss of proteins from the stomach wall. Ménétrier's disease also increases the risk of STOMACH CANCER. It is not known what causes this disease. It may involve transforming growth factor-alpha (TGf-alpha), which increases gastric mucous production and inhibits acid secretion. Association with cytomegalovirus infection is seen in childhood Ménétrier's.

Symptoms and Diagnostic Path

Ménétrier's disease patients experience the following symptoms:

- appetite loss
- pain in the upper middle of the abdomen
- NAUSEA AND VOMITING, including vomiting of blood
- ulcerlike pain that occurs after eating
- fluid buildup in the body, resulting in swelling
- bleeding

Gastric acid secretion may be low or normal. Gastrin levels may be increased. The diagnosis of Ménétrier's disease is based on the patient's symptoms and signs as well as the results of X-rays, ENDOSCOPY, and biopsy of tissue from the stomach.

Treatment Options and Outlook

A variety of medications have been used to treat Ménétrier's disease, including anti-ulcer medications, but the results have been inconsistent. Patients are also placed on a high-protein diet. Patients who have *HELICOBACTER PYLORI* infection require ANTIBIOTICS to eradicate the infection.

Octreotide may help to reduce protein loss. In some severe cases of Ménétrier's disease, surgery to remove part or all of the stomach is required.

Risk Factors and Preventive Measures

Ménétrier's disease is more common in men than women and usually presents between ages 30 and 60. There are no known preventive measures.

menopause The time of life in a middle-aged or older woman (usually in her 40s or older) when hormonal balance changes. She ceases to menstruate and other body and hormonal changes occur. These changes can also affect the digestive system; for example, calcium absorption may be reduced during menopause, thus increasing the risk for osteoporosis (bone density loss). Diseases such as HEMOCHROMATOSIS (iron overload) may become unmasked when the blood loss due to menstruation ceases. Older women are also more likely to have problems with OBESITY.

Some women who experience difficult problems with menopause, such as hot flashes, insomnia, and mood swings, take hormone replacement therapy to resolve these problems. They may take combination therapy (estrogen and progesterone) or may take estrogen only. Studies released in 2002 reported on potential health problems associated with combination therapy, such as an increased risk of heart disease and breast cancer. Women should consult their own physician to obtain individualized advice on dealing with menopausal medical problems that they experience.

See also HORMONE THERAPY.

mesenteric circulation Blood supply to and drainage from the large intestines and the stomach. In mesenteric artery ISCHEMIA, arteries that supply the blood to the intestines may be narrowed. In extreme cases, the blood flow is completely blocked, because of a thrombosis or an embolism. If the blockage is not cleared, it can be fatal to the patient.

Patients who have problems with mesenteric circulation experience abdominal pain that is usually disproportionate to the physical findings. Bleeding may be present. Patients with colonic ischemia (ischemic colitis) primarily have bleeding or bloody diarrhea. Patients with atherosclerosis are at risk for mesenteric artery ischemia. Elderly individuals also have an increased risk for vascular problems of the bowel and the digestive system.

The treatment depends upon the type of disorder involved and may include observation, medications, angioplasty, or surgery.

See also ISCHEMIA; VASCULITIS, SMALL VESSEL.

microlithiasis Gallstones that are so small that they may not be detectable as discrete stones in imaging studies. The stones are usually less than five millimeters in diameter. Most patients who have such small stones do not have any symptoms; however, some do experience pain. In some cases, microlithiasis can lead to pancreatitis.

On an ultrasound, microlithiasis may appear as "biliary sludge," or a suspension of fluid that contains tiny crystals or granules of stone. The presence of biliary sludge is more commonly found among patients who are receiving total parenteral nutrition. If patients have repeated attacks and biliary sludge is identified, physicians may determine that cholecystectomy (the surgical removal of the gallbladder) is the best treatment.

See also CHOLECYSTITIS; GALLSTONES; PANCREATITIS; PARENTERAL NUTRITION.

migrating motor complex (MMC) A complex sequence of myoelectrical gastrointestinal events in the fasting state involved in the propelling of the contents of the gut downward. Myoelectric patterns of the gut are divided into two distinct parts: fasting and feeding. Migrating motor complex occurs during the fasting phase of digestion.

In the fasting phase, the electro muscular activity of the gastrointestinal system is relatively quiet. The only exception to this quiet is the occurrence of periodic waves of electrical and muscular activity that causes propagation of the luminal contents of the gut. This is called the migrating myoelectric complex (MMC), which often begins in the esophagus or stomach and may transmit regular contractions for variable distances through the stomach and the small intestine and even into the colon.

MMC starts about four to six hours after a meal is consumed, and it occurs throughout the day in the fasting state, including during sleep. This cycle usually occurs about every 90 to 120 minutes.

Phases of Migrating Motor Complex

There are four phases of migrating motor complex. In the first phase, there is little motor activity; it is often called the quiescent (quiet) phase. In phase II, a series of seemingly random and erratic contractions occur. Then in phase III, continuous and intense bursts of contractions occur. Phase IV is a transition between phase III and phase I. The entire cycle of phases I through IV takes one to two hours, affecting the entire digestive system. The MMCs perform a "housekeeping" function by clearing the intestines of cellular and useless bacterial debris. When eating occurs, the MMC is interrupted by a burst of chaotic contractions, and the fed phase of myoelectric activity then starts.

After Eating Occurs

During and soon after a meal, when a person is in the "fed" state, the kinetics of the system change drastically. It is then primarily a mixing flow, as opposed to a migrating motor, that propels the luminal contents downward.

The stomach in the fed state provides regular contractions, usually at a maximum of three contractions per minute. These contractions perform the functions of both mixing and propagation, for example, emptying of small particles from the stomach and into the small intestine. The fed phase of myoelectric activity usually lasts two to three hours postprandially (after a meal); then the fasting phase resumes.

See also DIGESTION AND ABSORPTION.

milk–alkali syndrome A condition of very high calcium blood level that is caused by a combination of an excessive amount of both milk and calcium-containing antacids plus alkaline antacids. Milk–alkali syndrome was once very common, when antacids alone were used to treat ulcers. Then this treatment declined, as did milk–alkali syndrome. However, the incidence of milk–alkali syndrome is again rising, because of an increased emphasis on calcium intake for the prevention of osteoporosis as well as the increased availability of calcium-containing antacids. Milk–alkali syndrome occurs predominantly among women.

In past years, before it was known that nearly all ulcers are caused by either HELICOBACTER PYLORI bacteria or chronic consumption of NONSTEROIDAL ANTI-INFLAMMATORY DRUGS (NSAIDs), many patients used very high doses of antacids and some physicians also believed that milk had a soothing influence on the medical problem. As a result, some patients experienced milk–alkali syndrome. However, patients today who do not see a doctor for chronic digestive disorders, such as ulcer or heartburn, and who attempt to treat themselves by using high doses of over-the-counter antacids and drinking large quantities of milk are still at risk for development of milk–alkali syndrome.

Milk–alkali syndrome can cause calcium deposits in the kidneys, which are seen in computed tomography (CT) scans, magnetic resonance imaging (MRI) scans, X-rays, or ULTRASOUND of the kidneys.

In severe cases (which are rare), the kidney is damaged and the patient may experience kidney failure and require dialysis or kidney transplantation.

Symptoms and Signs

Most milk–alkali syndrome patients have acute symptoms, although some may remain asymptomatic. The acute form of the syndrome occurs after about one week of self-treatment with milk and antacids; patients report nausea, vomiting, weakness, and mental changes. Kidney failure may also occur. Stopping the milk and antacids resolves the problem.

In its subacute or intermediate form, milk–alkali syndrome is called Cope's syndrome. It occurs after months to years of intermittent treatment. Kidney function may not always return to normal, even after stopping both milk and antacids.

The chronic form of milk–alkali syndrome is called Burnett's syndrome. Burnett's syndrome patients have a long-standing history of treatment; they report increased thirst and urination, muscle aches, and itchy skin. They may have calcium deposits in the eyes and kidneys. Their kidney function does not return to normal after stopping of the treatment that caused the milk–alkali syndrome.

See also ULCERS, PEPTIC.

multiple endocrine neoplasia (MEN)   A genetic condition that causes hyperactivity of the endocrine organs and results in endocrine cancers, such as thyroid cancer and tumors of the adrenal gland, pituitary, and parathyroid glands.

If one family member is diagnosed with multiple endocrine endoplasia (MEN), all first-degree relatives (parents, siblings, and children) should be tested for this condition.

MEN is categorized into MEN I and II. In MEN I, patients are at risk for multiple tumors, starting with the parathyroids, then the pancreas and pituitary, whereas in MEN II, the thyroid, parathyroid, and adrenals may be involved. MEN II is further classified into MEN IIa and IIb, depending on the clinical presentation of the condition.

ZOLLINGER-ELLISON SYNDROME, also known as gastrinoma, is a pancreatic tumor that leads to a severe peptic ulcer disease that is caused by the body's overproduction of gastrin from a tumor in the pancreatic islet cells. It may occur sporadically or can result from MEN I.

Treatment of MEN is usually a combination of medical and surgical therapies, depending upon the site involved and the symptoms of the disease.

See also ULCERS, PEPTIC.

Brandi, Maria Luisa, et al. "Guidelines for Diagnosis and Therapy of MEN Type 1 and Type 2." *Journal of Clinical Endocrinology & Metabolism* 86, no. 12 (2001): 5,658–5,671.

Wynbrandt, James, and Mark D. Ludman. *The Encyclopedia of Genetic Disorders and Birth Defects.* 2d ed. New York: Facts On File, 2000.

multiple lymphomatous polyposis (MLP)   A rare form of gastrointestinal non-Hodgkin's lymphoma that occurs primarily among middle-aged to elderly individuals. It occurs more commonly among men than among women. Multiple lymphomatous polyposis (MLP) is considered as the intestinal form of Mantel cell lymphoma.

Patients with multiple lymphomatous polyposis (MLP) have ABDOMINAL PAIN as well as DIARRHEA, which may be bloody. The colon and the rectum are involved in about 90 percent of cases of MLP and show numerous POLYPS of varying sizes. Involvement of the ESOPHAGUS is unusual, whereas total gut involvement is rare. Usually chemotherapy is administered.

MLP is generally thought of as an incurable disease, with a median survival of three to five years. Aggressive chemotherapy followed by stem cell transplantation improves survival. A 60 percent five-year survival rate has been reported with some treatment regimens. In one study of 31 patients with multiple lymphomatous polyposis, reported in a 1997 issue of *Gastroenterology,* the prognosis for patients was improved with high-dose radiochemotherapy and stem cell autotransplantation.

myotomy   A surgical procedure in which the muscle layer of the digestive tube is cut, for example, when a patient suffers from ACHALASIA. Then a Heller's myotomy is performed to allow the lower esophageal sphincter to stay open so that food can pass from the esophagus into the stomach. Similarly, a myotomy may be carried out for infantile pyloric hypertrophic stenosis, to relieve gastric outlet obstruction. This is called Ramstedt pyloromyotomy.

See also ESOPHAGITIS; GASTROESOPHAGEAL REFLUX DISEASE.

narcotic bowel syndrome A medical problem that is caused by the chronic and long-term use of opiate painkillers that physicians have prescribed for patients who have a variety of painful medical problems. It is worth noting that United States comprises less than 5 percent of the world's population, but it uses 80 percent of the world's opioids.

Symptoms and Diagnostic Path

Narcotic bowel syndrome is characterized by the following symptoms and signs:

- severe constipation
- NAUSEA AND VOMITING
- excessive GAS, which leads to abdominal bloating
- abdominal pain
- weight loss

Patients may also appear to have intestinal obstructions, although no obstruction is present (intestinal pseudo-obstruction).

Physicians may suspect the presence of narcotic bowel syndrome if a patient has been taking large doses of narcotics for pain relief for two weeks or more, although not all patients who use narcotics experience this medical problem. X-rays of the abdomen show dilated loops of the small and large bowels, with a lot of stool and air but no evidence of any obstruction.

A chronic or increasing dose of narcotics leads to persistence or worsening of symptoms.

Treatment Options and Outlook

Effective treatment frequently involves a biopsychosocial approach. In most cases, narcotic bowel syndrome patients need to stop taking narcotics, although they should consult the physician about slowly tapering off the drug to prevent a severe withdrawal reaction. Naltrexone is a medication that is frequently used as part of a narcotic detoxification program.

During the initial withdrawal from the narcotic, patients may also experience vomiting, DIARRHEA, and cramps, which can be reduced by taking clonidine. For patients who have an absolute requirement for the continued use of narcotics (such as those who have severe cancer pain), metoclopramide and laxatives may be tried. Narcotic bowel syndrome can be treated successfully in most cases.

Risk Factors and Preventive Measures

Patients who are chronic users of opioids are at risk for the development of narcotic bowel syndrome. Avoidance of narcotics is a preventive measure, although patients in severe chronic pain may need narcotics.

See also CONSTIPATION; LAXATIVES AND LAXATIVE ABUSE; MEDICATIONS FOR DIGESTIVE DISEASES; PAIN.

Gwinnell, Esther, M.D., and Christine Adamec. *The Encyclopedia of Drug Abuse*. New York: Facts On File, 2008.

nausea and vomiting Nausea is a subjective complaint that may be described as the feeling or sensation that immediately precedes vomiting. Patients may say that they are about to vomit or may describe themselves as "sick to the stomach" or feeling "queasy." Vomiting is a physical event, involving the rapid, forceful expulsion of the gastric contents from the stomach and up and out of the mouth. Nausea may also precede vomiting that is followed by retching, which creates abdominal pressure to cause further vomiting.

Just as with nausea, retching may occur alone, without actual vomiting of the stomach contents. Similarly, vomiting need not be preceded by nausea.

Vomiting is different from regurgitation, which is a passive phenomenon of the backward flow of the esophageal or gastric contents out of the mouth, such as regurgitation of the stomach contents including the acid in GASTROESOPHAGEAL REFLUX DISEASE (GERD).

Rumination, on the other hand, is the effortless regurgitation of recently ingested food, which is then followed by rechewing and reswallowing. No nausea or retching occurs in rumination. Although rumination is usually seen in developmentally disabled patients or in those who have psychiatric problems, it may also occur among some patients without such problems.

Nausea and vomiting may accompany relatively minor viruses and illnesses. They are often also symptoms present in the first trimester of pregnancy.

Persistent nausea and vomiting may indicate a serious illness, such as a form of ulcer or cancer or one of many different digestive diseases; however, often nausea and vomiting are signs that are present in common gastrointestinal infections that resolve themselves within a day or two.

If nausea and vomiting become severe, patients are in danger of dehydration and electrolyte imbalances and may require hospitalization. The treatment of nausea and vomiting is directed at identifying the cause and relieving the symptoms. Drugs used to treat nausea and vomiting include metoclopramide (Reglan), promethazine (Phenergan), granisetron (Kytril), and ondansetron (Zofran).

See also CANCERS OF THE DIGESTIVE SYSTEM; RUMINATION SYNDROME.

necrotizing enterocolitis   A severe form of colon inflammation in which all or part of the colon is damaged by severe inflammation and infection. This rare condition, which occurs primarily in underweight newborn infants, is due to a combination of factors, including prematurity, milk feeding, poor blood circulation, infection, and impaired immune defenses. Necrotizing enterocolitis may also occur in adults who are immune suppressed, especially after chemotherapy for cancer treatment.

Treatment for necrotizing enterocolitis includes antibiotics, bowel rest, PARENTERAL NUTRITION, and sometimes surgery.

nerve block   A procedure involving the injection of a medication, usually a local anesthetic, to produce short-term pain relief or of a chemical, such as phenol or alcohol, to disrupt the nerve over a longer term. A nerve block is usually injected at the site of a nerve to stop the nerve from functioning, and it is used to stop severe chronic pain. For example, nerve blocks are used for the pain of Herpes zoster, chronic PANCREATITIS, and cancer.

neurotransmitters   Chemicals that act as chemical messengers inside the nervous system, including the brain, spinal cord, and nerves. The part of the nervous system that involves the gut is known as the enteric nervous system. Serotonin and norephinephrine are two of the numerous neurotransmitters in the body, and their actions depend upon the organ, nerves, and nerve cells that are involved. In the gut, the neurotransmitters participate in the regulation of peristalsis (the wavelike movements that push food through the gastrointestinal system), gut immune function, and intestinal secretions.

nocturnal acid breakthrough   A controversial digestive problem that is faced by some people who also have GASTROESOPHAGEAL REFLUX DISEASE (GERD), in which there is a surge of stomach acid production leading to ACID REFLUX in the middle of the night, usually when the person is asleep. This may occur despite patients' taking the standard doses of acid blocker medications to block acid production overnight. In considering the problem, doctors ask patients questions about the timing of their acid-related symptoms, and physicians may also prescribe additional doses of the acid blockers in the evening or recommend additional medications at bedtime. Doctors may also recommend over-the-counter drugs to supplement the acid blocker medications that patients already use.

As in any case of GERD, patients are also usually urged to avoid foods such as orange juice, chocolate, and cola drinks, especially before going to bed at night. GERD patients should not go to bed for at least two to four hours after eating their evening meal. They should also sleep on the left side, and with the head of the bed elevated.

nonalcoholic steatohepatitis (NASH; nonalcoholic fatty liver disease (NAFLD)) An illness that is characterized by an enlarged liver that is caused by the accumulation of fat in the LIVER and may be associated with inflammation and scarring (fibrosis) and, in some cases, even with CIRRHOSIS. Nonalcoholic steatohepatitis (NASH), which is also called nonalcoholic fatty liver disease (NAFLD), was first described in 1980 by physicians at the Mayo Clinic, although its clinical significance was not appreciated until the 1990s. The disease has also previously been called "fatty liver hepatitis," "alcohol-like liver disease," pseudoalcoholic hepatitis and, among patients who have diabetes, "diabetes hepatitis."

Although NASH does not lead to significant medical symptoms or problems in most patients, it may in the long run in some cases lead to liver cirrhosis and even to LIVER FAILURE. Predicting in which patients the condition will progress to cirrhosis and in which it will not is difficult.

It is unknown how many people in the United States and other countries have NASH. It is the most common liver disease in the United States. It is believed to affect 20 to 40 percent of the general population in the United States, whereas 5 to 30 percent people may be affected in the Asia-Pacific region. It also occurs more commonly among men. It is the most common liver disorder seen in adolescents. In the majority of cases, patients are between 40 and 60 years old. It is more common among Hispanics followed by Caucasians and then African Americans.

The precise cause of NASH remains to be determined, but insulin resistance appears to be a key factor. The disease may be associated with many different conditions. About 70 to 100 percent of NASH patients are overweight. As many as 35 to 75 percent of NASH patients may have DIABETES MELLITUS. Medications may also induce the disease, including such drugs as aspirin, estrogens, calcium channel blockers, glucocorticoids, synthetic estrogens, methotrexate, tetracycline, tamoxifen, amiodarone, and some antiviral agents as well as some pesticides.

The disease is also associated with extremely rapid weight loss, as well as with bariatric surgery to treat OBESITY, and with gallbladder and pancreatic surgery, HUMAN IMMUNODEFICIENCY VIRUS (HIV), small intestinal DIVERTICULOSIS, and total PARENTERAL NUTRITION. It is also associated with overexposure to some environmental toxins, such as phosphorus, toxic mushrooms, organic cleaning solvents, and oil-based chemicals.

Symptoms and Diagnostic Path

There are usually few or no symptoms or signs of nonalcoholic fatty liver disease. Some patients may feel some pain in the right side at the location of the liver, and others complain of tiredness.

Physicians perform a physical examination, noting the enlarged liver that is seen in nonalcoholic fatty liver disease. Blood tests show mild to moderate elevations of liver enzymes (aspartate aminotransferase [AST] and alanine aminotransferase [ALT]) levels. Other blood tests may be done to exclude other causes of abnormal liver enzyme level, such as viral hepatitis.

An ULTRASOUND reveals the excessive fat of the liver. However, the ultrasound may not provide information on inflammation and scarring and does not distinguish NASH from other diseases that may be similar. CT scan and magnetic resonance imaging (MRI) can also help to determine the presence of nonalcoholic fatty liver disease. However, imaging studies cannot show the extent of damage to the liver, which can only be determined by liver biopsy.

It is controversial whether a liver biopsy should be performed in all cases. The liver biopsy can definitively confirm the presence of nonalcoholic fatty liver disease, assuming that alcohol has been excluded as a factor by the taking of a medical history. Liver biopsy may be deferred by the doctor, pending a therapeutic trial of weight loss.

Treatment Options and Outlook

Treatment is usually directed to the associated problems; for example, if the patient is obese, the liver test findings may improve with weight loss.

Diabetes patients should be treated with medications to achieve optimal glucose level control. Some improvement may also occur if patients with diabetes improve their blood sugar level, maintaining the level at as close to normal as possible.

It is best to prevent very rapid weight loss with this disease because sudden major weight loss can also cause NASH. Adults should lose no more than 1,600 grams (3.5 pounds) per week, and ideally no more than one to two pounds per week, and children with NASH should lose about 500 grams per week.

There are no medications definitively proved to effectively treat nonalcoholic fatty liver disease, as of this writing. Physicians frequently recommend medications such as ursodeoxycholic acid, vitamin E supplements, and trimethylglycine (Betaine). Metformin and pioglitazone have been recommended for their insulin-sensitizing effects. Treatment of the cause, especially lifestyle changes, should be the primary focus.

The biopsy findings are similar for NASH and alcoholic hepatitis, although NASH patients lack a history of significant alcohol consumption. The prognosis is different in the two conditions. In about 40 to 50 percent of alcoholic hepatitis patients, cirrhosis develops over a period of seven years; in 8 to 26 percent of NASH patients, cirrhosis develops over the same period.

Risk Factors and Preventive Measures

Conditions that are commonly associated with nonalcoholic steatohepatitis are obesity, type 2 diabetes, and hyperlipidemia. Some children diagnosed with this medical problem have type 1 (insulin-dependent) diabetes. The excessive weight of the patient is generally centered on the abdomen, among obese people who also have nonalcoholic steatohepatitis, and thus, they are "apple"-shaped rather than "pear"-shaped. Diabetes, obesity, and hyperlipidemia patients are frequently labeled as having insulin resistance syndrome.

There appears to be a genetic risk for the disease, although little is known about the genetic transmission, and it has simply been observed that the condition seems to "run in families."

See also BARIATRIC SURGERY; HEPATITIS; LIVER ENZYMES/FUNCTION TESTS; STEATORRHEA.

Angulo, Paul, M.D. "Nonalcoholic Fatty Liver Disease." *New England Journal of Medicine* 346, no. 16 (April 18, 2002): 1,221–1,231.

nonerosive reflux disease (NERD) Gastroesophageal reflux disease (GERD) with an absence of esophagitis (inflammation of the esophagus). About half of GERD patients have no esophagitis. Patients with nonerosive reflux disease (NERD) have normal endoscopy results but still have GERD which can be confirmed by esophageal biopsy. They must be diagnosed based on their symptoms with or without esophageal biopsy and treated with the same medications and lifestyle recommendations as GERD patients.

See also GASTROESOPHAGEAL REFLUX DISEASE.

nonsteroidal anti-inflammatory drugs (NSAIDs) Over-the-counter and prescribed medications that are taken to decrease the pain and inflammation that are caused by illnesses such as arthritis or muscle pain. They are also used for menstrual cramps. Aspirin is used to protect against heart attack and stroke. Stomach distress, gastritis, and even ulcers are often side effects of use of these medications. In a small number of patients, these side effects can lead to life-threatening gastrointestinal bleeding.

The side effects of NSAIDs can be particularly risky for individuals who are 65 years and older, who may have many medical problems and may also may be taking a wide variety of medications. Patients who are elderly or have a history of severe heart disease, prior ulcers, or prior gastrointestinal bleeding and who have chronic pain that would normally be relieved by an NSAID should take, in addition to the NSAID, a medication protective against its ulcerogenic effects, such as misoprostol (Cytotec) or a proton pump inhibitor medication. Alternately, a cyclooxygenase-2 (COX-2) inhibitor has lower gastrointestinal toxicity. Other popular COX-2 inhibitors such as rofecoxib (Vioxx) and valdecoxib (Bextra) were withdrawn from the market because of the potentially increased risk for heart attack and stroke. Some high risk patients may be prescribed prophylactic medication (misoprostol or a proton pump inhibitor) even when taking COX-2 inhibitors.

See also PAIN; PROSTAGLANDINS; PROTON PUMP INHIBITORS; ULCERS, PEPTIC.

nonviral liver disease A liver ailment that is not caused by a virus, such as HEPATITIS, or by CIRRHOSIS, that results from alcoholism. Examples of nonviral liver diseases are HEMOCHROMATOSIS (iron overload), WILSON'S DISEASE (copper overload), PRIMARY BILIARY CIRRHOSIS, NONALCOHOLIC STEATO-HEPATITIS (NASH), autoimmune hepatitis, and LIVER CANCER.

See also ALCOHOL ABUSE AND ALCOHOLISM.

obesity Excessive weight for one's height, which is an increasing health problem in the United States, Canada, and many other developed nations and even among people in many developing countries. Obesity increases the risk for many diseases and disorders, including type 2 diabetes, GALLSTONES, heart disease, and many other illnesses. Obesity is also linked to ESOPHAGEAL CANCER and colon cancer as well as cancer of the breast and kidney. According to the Centers for Disease Control and Prevention (CDC), in considering all adults ages 18 and older in the United States, 26.1 percent of this population was obese in 2008. In their 2009 article on obesity and genetics in *Nature Reviews Genetics*, Andrew J. Walley and colleagues state that if the current trends continue, then half of the population in the United States will be obese by 2030.

In their 2009 report on obesity, *F AS IN Fat*, the Robert Wood Johnson Foundation reported that adult obesity rates have doubled since 1979, and childhood obesity rates have tripled since that time. Federal data also reveals that the number of obese adults is greater than 25 percent in most states. In addition, in six states (Alabama, Mississippi, Oklahoma, South Carolina, Tennessee, and West Virginia), the rate of obesity is 30 percent or greater for all residents. In only one state, Colorado, are fewer than 20 percent of the adults obese. (Rates are higher among blacks and Hispanics; see Table 2.)

Individuals with higher levels of BODY MASS INDEX are less likely to be satisfied with their body size, according to research by Rachel A. Millstein, et al., published in *Medscape Journal of Medicine* in 2008. According to their telephone survey of 9,740 adults nationwide in the United States, dissatisfaction was also correlated with attempts to lose weight among both men and women. The researchers found higher levels of body dissatisfaction among women than men. White women were most likely to be dissatisfied, and black and Latina/Hispanic female adults had a lower rate of dissatisfaction. This was true even though blacks and Hispanic females are more likely to be obese than white females.

According to the researchers, "This study of adult Americans showed that women were around twice as likely as men to be dissatisfied with their body size. Having worse general health and a higher BMI were factors associated with dissatisfaction, and dissatisfaction differed by race/ethnicity among women."

In the United States as well as in many other countries, obesity is defined in terms of the individual's body mass index (BMI): people are obese when they have a body mass index that is equal to or greater than 30 kilograms per square meter (meters of height squared, or the number multiplied times itself). BMI is usually expressed without units, for example, a person is said to have a BMI of 30 or another number. The BMI is based on a mathematical formula of the person's body weight divided by the square of his or her height. Simply put, it is body weight in kg/height in m^2. In order to compute the actual BMI in inches, an individual can take his or her own weight in pounds, multiply that number by 704.5, and then divide the result by his or her height in inches. That number is then divided *again* by the height in inches to determine the numerical BMI. However, most people simply view a chart of their height and weight to look up their individual BMI.

Individuals who have a BMI that lies between 25 and 29 are considered to be overweight, but they are not regarded as obese. As mentioned earlier, a BMI of 30 or more indicates obesity.

TABLE 1: BMI AND OVERWEIGHT AND OBESITY

BMI	Weight Status
Less than 18.5	underweight
18.5 to 24.9	normal weight
25.0 to 29.9	overweight
30.0 to 39.9	obese
40.0 and greater	morbidly obese

(This information is summarized in Table 1.) In addition, individuals who have a BMI of 40 or greater are considered to be morbidly obese; they are at an especially high risk for the development of diabetes, hypertension, and heart disease.

According to a 2009 issue of *Morbidity and Mortality Weekly Report*, rates of obesity vary by race and ethnicity, and the rate of obesity is the highest among blacks (35.7 percent), followed by Hispanics (28.7 percent), and then whites (23.7 percent). There are also some significant gender differences which vary by race and ethnicity; for example, among whites, men are more likely to be obese than women, but among Hispanics and blacks, it is women who are more likely to be obese than men. The difference is particularly pronounced among blacks, in which case 39.2 percent of adult females are obese compared to the significantly lower rate of 31.6 percent of adult males.

See Table 2 for further racial breakdowns by the area of the country and by race and ethnicity, and see Table 3 for a state-by-state breakdown. As can be seen from Table 2, the rates of obesity are highest for most groups in the South and Midwest and lowest in the West.

As can be seen from Table 3, the greatest percentage of obese white (30.2 percent) individuals resided in West Virginia, while the greatest percentage of obese blacks (45.1 percent) were found in Maine. Among Hispanics, the greatest percentage of obese Hispanics (36.7 percent) resided in Tennessee. The lowest percentage of obese individuals among whites (9.0 percent) were in the District of Columbia. Among blacks, the lowest percentage of obesity (23.0 percent) was in New Hampshire. Among Hispanics, the lowest rate was 21.0 percent in Maryland.

Obesity is sometimes associated with psychiatric disorders; for example, many obese individuals have problems with depression or anxiety disorders, and some obese children and adults also have attention deficit/hyperactivity disorder, in which they behave impulsively, have difficulty planning and fail to pay attention to what is going on around them. As a result, they may forget to plan meals and then become hungry and consequently impulsively overeat calorie-laden fast foods that they purchase.

Another important issue is that of abdominal obesity, or an obese person who is an "apple" shape rather than a "pear" shape. Many people who are obese carry much of their weight in their abdomen rather than in their hips. Yet studies have shown that abdominal obesity (the apple shape) greatly

TABLE 2: PREVALENCE OF OBESITY AMONG ADULTS, BY BLACK/WHITE RACE OR HISPANIC ETHNICITY, CENSUS REGION AND SEX, 2006-2008, BY PERCENTAGE

Census Region	White, non-Hispanic (n = 900,629)	Black, non-Hispanic (n = 84,838)	Hispanic (n = 63,825)
Both sexes	23.7	35.7	28.7
Men	25.4	31.6	27.8
Women	21.8	39.2	29.4
Northeast			
Both sexes	22.6	31.7	26.6
Men	25.0	26.5	26.9
Women	20.0	36.1	26.0
Midwest			
Both sexes	25.4	36.3	29.6
Men	27.0	32.1	29.7
Women	23.8	40.1	29.2
South			
Both sexes	24.4	36.9	29.2
Men	26.3	32.6	28.3
Women	22.5	40.6	29.7
West			
Both sexes	21.0	33.1	29.0
Men	22.1	34.1	27.3
Women	19.8	32.0	30.4

Source: Adapted from Centers for Disease Control and Prevention. "State-Specific Prevalence of Obesity Among Adults—United States, 2007." *Morbidity and Mortality Weekly Report* 57, no. 28 (July 17, 2009): 741.

TABLE 3: STATE BY STATE PERCENTAGE OF ADULTS CATEGORIZED AS OBESE, BY BLACK/WHITE RACE OR HISPANIC ETHNICITY, UNITED STATES, 2006-2008, BY PERCENTAGE

State	White, non-Hispanic	Black, non-Hispanic	Hispanic
Alabama	27.3	40.4	29.0
Alaska	25.0	30.8	30.8
Arizona	21.7	35.9	31.4
Arkansas	27.1	37.6	25.5
California	19.8	34.3	29.2
Colorado	16.2	26.2	25.1
Connecticut	19.9	31.2	24.6
Delaware	24.3	39.2	29.0
District of Columbia	9.0	32.9	22.6
Florida	20.9	35.1	26.0
Georgia	23.5	36.0	26.1
Hawaii	16.4	26.0	26.7
Idaho	23.6	Unknown	28.7
Illinois	23.4	33.3	30.7
Indiana	26.1	35.7	26.6
Iowa	25.5	35.7	27.5
Kansas	25.7	39.8	31.7
Kentucky	27.4	38.5	27.0
Louisiana	24.9	35.9	24.4
Maine	23.6	45.1	27.8
Maryland	22.4	34.0	21.0
Massachusetts	20.0	30.0	27.1
Michigan	26.2	37.4	31.2
Minnesota	24.3	32.5	27.9
Mississippi	27.6	40.4	26.0
Missouri	26.5	36.1	28.8
Montana	21.0	Unknown	22.9
Nebraska	25.7	35.9	29.0
Nevada	22.8	28.7	29.1
New Hampshire	22.9	23.0	32.3
New Jersey	21.9	33.0	24.1
New Mexico	19.5	31.9	27.6
New York	22.8	29.7	27.1
North Carolina	24.9	38.8	25.3
North Dakota	25.1	Unknown	31.9
Ohio	26.6	42.5	25.9
Oklahoma	27.3	32.7	30.7
Oregon	24.6	41.6	23.0
Pennsylvania	25.0	36.5	31.3
Rhode Island	20.1	30.1	26.0
South Carolina	25.1	38.8	27.0
South Dakota	25.3	Unknown	28.6
Tennessee	27.0	38.0	36.7
Texas	23.5	37.8	32.3
Utah	22.6	34.9	21.6
Vermont	21.2	Unknown	24.4
Virginia	23.6	34.5	24.7
Washington	24.0	29.7	29.9
West Virginia	30.2	36.3	26.1
Wisconsin	24.5	36.4	27.3
Wyoming	22.5	36.9	28.6

Source: Adapted from Centers for Disease Control and Prevention. "State-Specific Prevalence of Obesity Among Adults—United States, 2007." *Morbidity and Mortality Weekly Report* 57, no. 28 (July 17, 2009): 742.

increases the risk of the development of diabetes, hypertension, and other medical problems.

In a related issue, some researchers believe that the waist-hip ratio is a better predictor than the body mass index of poor health or even mortality among obese people when abdominal obesity is the problem. In one study, reported in 2000 in *Archives of Internal Medicine*, the researchers compared the waist-to-hip ratio of deceased subjects with their body mass index to determine which measure was ultimately a better predictor of death among obese individuals. They found that the waist-hip ratio was a significantly better predictive measure.

The Stigmatization of Obese Individuals

Some studies indicate that obese people are often stigmatized and blamed for their obesity. They may be labeled with such pejorative terms as *lazy, unmotivated, idle,* and so forth—even by physicians. In a study by Melanie Jay and colleagues and reported in 2009 in *BMC Health Services Research*, the authors surveyed 399 doctors in the fields of pediatrics, internal medicine, and psychiatry on their attitudes toward individuals who were obese, and 40 percent of the doctors reported a negative response toward obese patients. Forty-five percent of the physicians said that they had a negative reaction to the appearance of an obese patient, and this response did not differ by specialty. In addition, 25 percent said that they felt uncomfortable when examining an obese patient and that they had difficulty empathizing with a patient who was obese.

The researchers also found that doctors with more years since their medical school training had a lower positive outcome expectancy and a higher negative outcome expectancy toward their patients than did younger doctors.

According to the researchers, "We have at least two possible explanations for this. First, physicians may become disillusioned with years of attempted treatment of obese patients in the face of modest weight loss or even weight gain. Second, obesity management training may be different for recent graduates who practice in an era in which it is widely accepted that even modest weight loss should be considered a successful outcome."

In an article by Rebecca M. Puhl and Chelsea A. Heuer on the stigmatizing of the obese, published in a 2009 issue of *Obesity*, the researchers reported considerable stigma. The authors reported:

> The prevalence of weight discrimination in the United States has increased by 66% over the past decade, and is comparable to the rate of racial discrimination, especially among women. Weight bias translates into inequities in employment settings, health-care facilities, and educational institutions, often due to widespread negative stereotypes that overweight and obese persons are lazy, unmotivated, lacking in self-discipline, less competent, non-compliant, and sloppy. These stereotypes are prevalent and are rarely challenged in Western society, leaving overweight and obese persons vulnerable to social injustice, unfair treatment, and impaired quality of life as a result of substantial disadvantages and stigma.

Reasons for Increased Levels of Obesity in the U.S.

Obviously obesity is caused by Americans eating many more calories than they expend every day and also by exercising less than in past years, but researchers actively debate why so many Americans are obese in comparison to recent past years. Some experts believe it is because many people live far more sedentary lives than did individuals in past years. Others say that Americans eat greater and often "super-sized" portions of fast foods than in past years.

Cultural or racial/ethnic issues may play a role; for example, eating large quantities of food may be seen as normal among some groups, whereas the same heavy portions (as well as the types of foods) would be viewed as excessive by other groups.

There may be fewer opportunities to exercise for some groups, or it might even be unsafe to travel to areas where individuals could engage in sports, such as cities that have high crime rates. In addition, in significant contrast to 20 years ago, more people today rely upon motorized vehicles rather than bicycles (or walking) to transport them to work, shopping, and other places where they travel.

Obesity and Disease

As mentioned, obesity causes or contributes to the development of many serious and chronic digestion-related illnesses, such as some forms of cancer, as well as diabetes, gallstones, and NONALCOHOLIC STEATOHEPATITIS (NASH). The risk for other nondigestive illnesses, such as hypertension, heart disease, kidney disease, arthritis, sleep disorders, and stroke, are also significantly increased among those who are obese. Obesity also increases the risk for heart failure.

Diabetes and Obesity   The risk in obese people for the development of type 2 diabetes is very well documented by many researchers. An article in a 1999 issue of *Diabetes Care* reported on a study in which researchers followed nearly 7,000 men with no diabetes history over 12 years. During that time, 237 of the men developed type 2 diabetes. The researchers found that a weight gain greater than 10 percent was significantly associated with the development of diabetes.

According to the researchers: "This study confirms the critical importance of overweight and obesity, particularly of long duration, in the development of type 2 diabetes. The data support current public health recommendations to reduce the risk of type 2 diabetes by preventing weight gain in middle-aged men who are not overweight and by encouraging weight loss in overweight and obese men." (Of course, obese and overweight women should also lose weight because they too are at risk for type 2 diabetes. The study emphasized weight loss among obese men because the subjects were males.)

Cancer and Obesity   Obesity apparently also increases the risk of development of different types of cancer, such as COLORECTAL CANCER. A 2003 study by researchers published in the *New England Journal of Medicine* attributed 14 percent of the cancer deaths in men and 20 percent in women in part to either overweight or obesity. Many of the cancers that subjects died of were digestion-related cancers, and the risk of death of these cancers increased proportionately with the patient's body mass index. (See also CANCERS OF THE DIGESTIVE SYSTEM.)

Causes of Obesity

In most cases, the basic and obvious cause of obesity is overeating combined with insufficient physical activity; however, rarely, there are other prevailing causes, such as hypothyroidism (low thyroid level), Cushing's syndrome, and other serious medical problems. Some endocrinological researchers believe that there may be a link between problems with obesity and blood levels of cortisol, a hormone that is secreted by the adrenal glands, and research is ongoing.

Recent research indicates that some adults with attention deficit/hyperactivity disorder (ADHD) are obese, possibly because of poor impulse control. In some studies, when adults with ADHD are treated, they lose a significant amount of weight. For example, a study by L. D. Levy, J. P. Fleming and D. Klar, reported in a 2009 issue of the *International Journal of Obesity*, found that when newly diagnosed adults were treated for their ADHD with stimulants, they lost about 36 pounds, compared to a weight gain of about seven pounds in the control group of untreated adults with ADHD.

The researchers said the initial effect of the medication was to reduce appetite, but that appetite suppression diminished and disappeared over two months. What happened was that individuals taking medication became much more aware of their own internal mental state and thus they obtained better control over their eating.

According to the authors, "Our subjects reported that they experienced the greatest reduction in calorie intake because the medication reduced restlessness, fatigue and anxiety, and thus diminished the chronic use of food to assuage those feelings. Binge eating diminished very substantially or stopped altogether and impulsivity in food selec-

tion was curtailed. They reported that they were much more aware of internal cues of hunger and fullness and could act on those feelings, often for the first time."

Some of the subjects had never noticed satiety (feeling full) before taking medications for ADHD.

Emotional Issues Some doctors and therapists believe that obesity is both a maladaptive behavior and a response to stress. It may also be a learned behavior, based on childhood experiences; for example, perhaps cake or cookies were used as a reward by parents as well as a comfort food for distressing events. This learned behavior may become incorporated into the patient's basic habits, and overeating may continue to be a pattern when the person is struggling with problems or celebrating successes. Patients may need to resolve their underlying emotional conflicts and fully explore these issues before they can successfully lose a significant amount of weight.

Genetics and Obesity Obesity may be caused by a genetic problem; research on an association is ongoing. According to authors Walley, Asher, and Froguel, there are many theories to explain obesity but little consensus. Some exceptions exist, however. For example, it is known that the melanocortin 4 receptor (MC4R), as well as brain-derived neurotrophic factor (BDNF), are each linked to an inherited risk for obesity. According to Walley and colleagues, other recently identified related candidate genes for obesity include the following:

- ENPP1 (Ectonucleotide pyrophosphatase/phosphodiesterase 1)
- PCSK1 (Proprotein convertase subtilisin/kexin type 1)
- NAMPT (Nicotinamide phosphoribosyltransferase, a genetic risk for severe obesity)
- LMNA (Lamin A/C)
- GHSR (Growth hormone secretagogue receptor)
- SOCS1 (Suppressor of cytokine signaling 1)
- KLF7 (Kruppel-like factor 7)
- DLK1 (Delta-like homologue 1)
- CNR1 (Cannabinoid type 1 receptor)
- NPY2R (Neuropeptide Y receptor Y2)

Disabilities and Obesity

Some studies have shown that individuals who are disabled are more likely to be obese. In a study reported in a 2002 issue of the *Journal of the American Medical Association*, the researchers analyzed subjects who had a variety of disabilities, including blindness or severe difficulties with sight, deafness or impaired hearing, and inability to walk without difficulty. The researchers found that nearly 25 percent of the disabled individuals were obese, compared to 15.1 percent of individuals without disabilities who were obese.

Some patients who are ill or disabled may find it very difficult to obtain opportunities for sufficient exercise. Their physician may also feel sorry for them or not wish to take the time to help them create a plan of exercise that is within the scope of their abilities. Such a plan is important because patients can become even less active and more obese, worsening a disability, in a vicious cycle.

Psychiatric Disorders and Obesity

Researchers have found that both overweight and obesity are associated with psychiatric disorders, and the greater the individual's BMI, the greater the risk for depression, anxiety disorders, and personality disorders, as well as alcohol use disorders. According to Nancy M. Petry and colleagues in their 2008 article in *Psychosomatic Medicine*, the specific anxiety disorders linked to overweight and obesity were generalized anxiety disorder, panic disorder, and specific phobia.

Children and Obesity

Many children and adolescents in the United States and other countries have problems with obesity, and some are morbidly obese. Often they have parents and other family members who are obese, although this is not always the case. It is very important that parents and others help children overcome their problems with obesity to prevent a lifelong problem of obesity; however, at the same time, it is also important to prevent the stigmatizing of children who are overweight or obese.

According to the CDC, overweight children are defined as those with a BMI at or above the 85th percentile for children their own gender and age and lower than the 95th percentile. Children are defined as obese when they are at or above the 95th percentile.

A study of Pima children in Arizona reported in 2002 in *Pediatrics* indicated that they have a greater obesity problem than other children. (The Pima are noted for their severe problems with obesity and with the highest rate of type 2 diabetes worldwide.) The researchers found that prominent factors for obesity were a low rate of participating in sports and a higher rate of watching television than those of peers.

The prevalence of obesity among children has increased markedly since the period 1976 to 1980, when 5 percent of children ages two to five years were obese, to the rates 2003 to 2006, when 12.4 percent of children two to five years were obese. Rates of obesity have also increased among children of all ages, according to the CDC, based on data from the National Health and Nutrition Examination Survey (NHANES). The most recent survey as of this writing was for 2003–06. (See Table 4.) As can be seen from Table 4, the rates of obesity among adolescents more than tripled, from 5 percent over the period 1976 to 1980 to 17.6 percent during the period 2003 to 2006.

The rates of obesity are particularly high among adolescent black and Mexican American boys and girls; for example, 22.1 percent of Mexican American adolescents were obese in 2003–06. (See Table 5.) Among girls, rates were very high among black adolescent girls, and 27.7 percent were obese. (See Table 6.)

TABLE 4: PREVALENCE OF OBESITY AMONG U.S. CHILDREN AND ADOLESCENTS AGES 2–19 YEARS

	NHANES II 1976–1980	NHANES III 1988–1994	NHANES 1999–2002	NHANES 2003–2006
Ages 2–5	5%	7.2%	10.3%	12.4%
Ages 6–11	6.5%	11.3%	15.8%	17.0%
Ages 12–19	5%	10.5%	16.1%	17.6%

Source: Adapted from: Centers for Disease Control and Prevention. "Prevalence." Available online. URL: http://www.cdc.gov/obesity/childhood/prevalence.html

TABLE 5: ADOLESCENT BOYS: PREVALENCE OF OBESITY BY RACE/ETHNICITY (AGES 12–19 YEARS)

	NHANES III 1988–1994	NHAMES 2003–2006
Non-Hispanic white	11.6%	17.3%
Non-Hispanic Black	10.7%	18.5%
Mexican American	14.1%	22.1%

Source: Adapted from: Centers for Disease Control and Prevention. "Prevalence." Available online. URL: http://www.cdc.gov/obesity/childhood/prevalence.html

Diagnosing and Treating Obesity

Some doctors specialize in assisting patients with weight loss, but most patients who try to lose weight see an internist or a general practitioner. Most doctors can readily identify obesity on the basis of a patient's weight and body mass index. Treatment is far more difficult. Many physicians believe that chronic obesity is a very complex problem. For a normal-weight or slightly overweight person who gains five or 10 pounds, eating less and exercising more to lose the weight are relatively simple. However, for an obese person who needs to lose 50 pounds or more, that task is far more daunting for both the patient and the physician.

Dieting Attempts   Millions of dollars are spent each year by individuals seeking an easy and quick way to lose a lot of weight, including money spent on DIET DRUGS and other weight loss items, as well as purportedly easy-to-use exercise devices. Some patients use hypnotherapy to lose weight.

Medications for weight loss are recommended for patients with a BMI of greater than 30 or greater than 27 if they have obesity-related prob-

TABLE 6: ADOLESCENT GIRLS: PREVALENCE OF OBESITY BY RACE/ETHNICITY

	NHANES III 1988–1994	NHANES 2003–2006
Non-Hispanic white	7.4%	14.5%
Non-Hispanic black	13.2%	27.7%
Mexican American	9.2%	19.9%

Source: Adapted from: Centers for Disease Control and Prevention. "Prevalence." Available online. URL: http://www.cdc.gov/obesity/childhood/prevalence.html

lems for which conservative management with diet and exercise have failed. Weight loss medications should not be used by children or by the ELDERLY (older than age 65 years); nor should they be used by women who are pregnant or those who are breastfeeding. Individuals who have pulmonary hypertension, uncontrolled systemic hypertension, or unstable heart disease should also avoid diet drugs.

Orlistat (Xenical) prevents the digestion of fat in the gut, and thus, reduces its absorption in the body. A side effect of this drug is fecal incontinence. This drug is also available in an over-the-counter form under the brand name Alli. Sibutramine (Meridia) is a prescribed drug that increases norepinephrine and serotonin at the nerve terminals, reduces food intake, and may increase body metabolism.

At best, orlistat or sibutramine produce a 10 percent weight loss in subjects with a slowed level of weight loss thereafter, according to Samuel Klein, associate editor for nutrition in a 2005 article for *Gastroenterology*. Phentermine is another diet drug, but phentermine is approved by the Food and Drug Administration (FDA) only for short-term use. Some researchers have used off-label medications to treat obesity, such as the antiseizure drug topiramate (Topamx), reporting mixed success.

Others such as Gadde, et al., reporting on their findings in the *International Journal of Obesity* in 2006, have used medications such as atomoxetine (Strattera), a nonstimulant medication that is approved to treat adult ADHD, to treat obesity and have found modest success.

Weight Reduction Surgery   Some obese individuals choose to have weight reduction surgery, also known as BARIATRIC SURGERY, although this procedure is considered controversial by some physicians because of the serious health risks associated with this surgery as well as potential postsurgical risks. In addition, some patients lose weight but subsequently begin an overeating pattern, sometimes gaining as much weight as was lost with the surgery.

Surgery can be an effective method for weight control for highly motivated patients who maintain their motivation and compliance with physician postoperative requirements. Bariatric surgery is indicated for patients who have a BMI that is greater than 40 or for patients whose BMI exceeds 35 and is associated with obesity-related conditions that are also present (such as diabetes or hypertension).

The weight reduction operations that are commonly used by bariatric surgeons include Roux en-Y (the gastric bypass or RYGB) the biliary-pancreatic diversion (duodenal switch) and the laparoscopic adjustable lap band (Lap-Band) and these procedures can be performed laparoscopically. The gastric bypass is superior to the Lap-Band in producing sustained weight loss among morbidly obese patients.

See also EXERCISE; GHRELIN; YO-YO DIETING.

Centers for Disease Control and Prevention. "Differences in Prevalence of Obesity among Black, White, and Hispanic Adults—United States, 2006–2008." *Morbidity and Mortality Review* 58, no. 27 (July 17, 2009): 740–744.

———. "U.S. Obesity Trends." Available online. URL: http://www.cdc.gov/obesity/data/trends.html. Accessed July 21, 2009.

Cortese, Aamuele, et al. "Attention-Deficit Hyperactivity Disorder (ADHD) and Obesity: A Systematic Review of the Literature. *Critical Reviews in Food Science and Nutrition* 49 (2008): 524–537.

Gadde, K.M., et al. "Atomoxetine for Weight Reduction in Obese Women: A Preliminary Randomised Controlled Trial." *International Journal of Obesity* 30 (2006): 1,138–1,142.

Gilsen Tsai, Adam, M.D., and Thoams A. Wadden. "Systematic Review: An Evaluation of Major Commercial Weight Loss Programs in the United States." *Annals of Internal Medicine* 142 (2005): 56–66.

Jay, Melanie, et al. "Physicians' Attitudes about Obesity and Their Associations with Competency and Specialty: A Cross-sectional Study." *BMC Health Services Research* 2009. Available online. URL: http://www.biomedcentrl.com/1472-6963/9/106. Accessed July 19, 2009.

Klein, Smauel. "Does Paying for Obesity Therapy Make Cents?" *Gastroenterology* 128 (2005): 530.

Levi, Jeffrey, et al. *F as in Fat: How Obesity Policies Are Failing in America*. Washington, D.C.: Robert Wood Johnson Foundation, 2009.

Levy, L. D., J. P. Fleming, and D. Klar. "Treatment of Refractory Obesity in Severely Obese Adults Following Management of Newly Diagnosed Attention Deficit Hyperactivity Disorder." *International Journal of Obesity* 33 (2009): 326–334.

Millsten, Rachel A., et al. "Relationships between Body Size Satisfaction and Weight Control Practices among US Adults." *Medscape Journal of Medicine* 10, no. 5 (2008). Available online. URL: http://www.pubmedcentral.nih.gov/articlerender.fcgi?artaid=2438482. Accessed July 21, 2009.

Petry, Nancy M., et al. "Overweight and Obesity Are Associated with Psychiatric Disorders: Results from the National Epidemiologic Survey on Alcohol and Related Conditions." *Psychosomatic Medicine* 70 (2008): 288–297.

Puhl, Rebecca M., and Chelsea A. Heuer. "The Stigma of Obesity: A Review and Update." *Obesity* 17, no. 5 (2009): 841–964.

Simon, Gregory E., M.D., et al. "Association between Obesity and Psychiatric Disorders in the US Adult Population." *Archives of General Psychiatry* 64 (2006): 824–830.

Walley, Andrew J., Julian E. Asher, and Philippe Froguel. "The Genetic Contribution to Non-Syndromic Human Obesity." *Nature Reviews Genetics* 10 (2009): 431–442.

occult gastrointestinal bleeding Microscopic or "hidden" (not visible to the naked eye) gastrointestinal bleeding that may indicate the presence of medical problems or diseases, such as ulcers and COLORECTAL CANCER. This bleeding is not usually noticed by the patient but is sufficient to be detected in specific tests for occult blood. Fecal occult bleeding may be an indication of the presence of colorectal cancer, which should be ruled out.

Other diseases that may produce occult gastrointestinal bleeding include the following:

- CROHN'S DISEASE
- WATERMELON STOMACH
- TUBERCULOSIS enterocolitis
- PARASITIC INFECTIONS
- CELIAC DISEASE
- ULCER
- ESOPHAGITIS
- colitis
- telengiectasia (abnormal blood vessels in the gut that may bleed slowly or heavily)

In addition, use of some medications can cause occult bleeding, such as chronic use of aspirin or nonsteroidal anti-inflammatory drugs (NSAIDs).

Testing for Occult Bleeding

Most physicians recommend that individuals who are age 50 and older have an annual fecal occult blood test (FOBT) to check for microscopic blood in the stool. In this test, the person smears a small sample of feces on a card to be tested in a laboratory for blood by adding a chemical reagent to the card. A change of color to blue indicates the presence of blood. A negative FOBT result does not entirely rule out cancer, but screening by using this noninvasive test has been shown to decrease the rate of colorectal cancer mortality. Only a colonoscopy can rule out colorectal cancer. Note, however, that no test is perfect and, rarely, cancers can be missed even during colonoscopy.

Some patients are resistant to performing this test, finding it repugnant, and sometimes physicians have had considerable difficulty convincing patients to comply with this test requirement.

See also COLORECTAL CANCER; GUAIAC; NONSTEROIDAL ANTI-INFLAMMATORY DRUGS .

Rockey, Don C., M.D. "Occult Gastrointestinal Bleeding." *New England Journal of Medicine* 341, no. 1 (July 1, 1999): 38–46.

Ogilvie's syndrome   An extreme dilation of the right side of the colon when no obstruction is present. Sometimes the whole colon may be involved. The syndrome is also known as acute colonic pseudoobstruction. This condition was first described by Dr. Ogilvie in 1948. Ogilvie's syndrome may occur among hospitalized patients who have experienced recent surgery, trauma, or a severe infection.

Ogilvie's syndrome patients experience nausea, vomiting, and abdominal distention with constipation. The diagnosis is based on the patient's medical history and a physical examination, plus the results of X-rays.

Treatment for this medical problem involves identification and correction of the cause, if possible, for example, treatment of an existing infection or correction of any fluid and electrolyte abnormalities. A nasogastric tube with or without a rectal tube may be placed for suctioning air from the gastrointestinal system.

In one study of patients with an acute form of Ogilvie's syndrome who were treated with the medication neostigmine, reported in a 1999 issue of the *New England Journal of Medicine,* the patients responded well and the colon rapidly downsized to normal. Erythromycin has also been used with beneficial results by Ogilvie's syndrome patients.

If conservative measures fail, Ogilvie's syndrome patients are treated with decompression done by colonoscopy, or, in some cases, by cecostomy by the surgeon. Major abdominal surgery may rarely be required.

See also FLUID AND ELECTROLYTE BALANCE.

Ponec, Robert J., M.D., Michael D. Saunders, M.D., and Michael B. Kimmey, M.D. "Neostigmine for the Treatment of Acute Colonic Pseudo-Obstruction." *New England Journal of Medicine* 341, no. 3 (July 15, 1999): 137–141.

oral cancer   Malignant tumor of the mouth, the oropharynx (the part of the throat that is in the back of the mouth), the lips, the lining inside the lips and cheeks, the floor of the mouth that lies under the tongue, the tongue itself, and the tonsils. Oral cancer is the sixth most common cancer worldwide. Most oral cancers are squamous cell carcinomas rather than adenocarcinomas. According to the National Cancer Institute, an estimated 22,900 new cases of oral cancer were diagnosed in 2008, and 5,390 people died of oral cancer in 2008. According to the National Institutes of Health, oral cancer represents about 8 percent of all cancers. If the cancer is diagnosed early, the cure rate is about 75 percent.

Symptoms and Diagnostic Path

An oral cancer may occur without symptoms in the early stages. Symptoms that may occur (at any stage) include the following:

- a sore throat that does not heal
- DYSPHAGIA or odynophagia (difficulty or pain with swallowing or trouble with moving the tongue or the jaw)
- changes in the sound of the voice
- ear pain in one ear with no hearing loss

- a sore in the mouth or on the lip or another area of the oral cavity that does not heal
- a lump on the mouth
- white or red patchy areas on the gums, tongue, or lining of the mouth

Note: These symptoms may also occur with other diseases, and only a physician can diagnose an oral cancer. Often, however, it is the dentist who first notices possible signs of oral cancer, and then refers the patient back to his or her physician for evaluation.

If physicians suspect the presence of an oral cancer, on the basis of a patient's symptoms and/or the appearance of the oral cavity or mouth, they refer the patient to either an oral surgeon or an ear, nose, and throat specialist. The expert performs a biopsy, which is the removal of a small amount of tissue, to check for cancer.

If cancer is found, then the cancer is staged. The pathologist who analyzed the biopsy result and the doctor (who may order other tests) will determine how advanced the cancer is and how aggressively it is growing. Dental X-rays and X-rays of the head, neck, and chest can help in staging the cancer. The physician may also order a computed tomography (CT) scan, ULTRASOUND, or magnetic resonance imaging (MRI) scan to obtain more information about the tumor. The positron emission tomography (PET) scan may also be used to detect early stages of oral cancer. These tests may help doctors to determine the location and size of the tumor and to detect whether cancer has spread (metastasized) to other parts of the body.

Treatment Options and Outlook

The treatment depends on how advanced the cancer is and whether it has spread beyond the oral cavity. Regardless of the treatment chosen, doctors may advise patients to have any needed dental work performed first, because having it done later may be too difficult.

The treatment for oral cancer may include surgery, radiation therapy, or both. Chemotherapy is another treatment option. In addition to the surgeon and the oncologist (cancer doctor), physicians also often recommend that patients receive treatment by other specialists, such as a dentist or a plastic surgeon (because surgery may cause facial deformities). A dietitian may also be consulted because surgery and the cancer itself may make eating difficult.

Many physicians recommend that the patient get a gastrostomy tube placed so that the patient may be fed directly into the stomach through this tube in the likely event that the treatment causes problems with swallowing. In many cases, the swallowing improves after the treatments are over and the gastrostomy can be removed.

Patients with advanced oral cancer may be treated with chemotherapy, which is the administration of cancer-killing drugs. Patients who have advanced oral cancer are also often offered an opportunity to join a clinical trial. In clinical trials, physicians test experimental medications and other therapies on people who have specific diseases and medical problems. These drugs and treatments are generally not available to patients unless they are enrolled in clinical trials.

Studies done worldwide suggest that screening for oral cancer performed by primary care providers helps identify a large number of at-risk individuals and that early detection and treatment has the potential to reduce overall mortality.

According to the National Institute of Dental and Craniofacial Research, individuals who have been diagnosed with oral cancer should ask their physician the following questions:

- What is the stage of the disease? Has the cancer spread? If so, where?
- What are my treatment choices? Which do you recommend for me? Will I have more than one kind of treatment?
- What are the expected benefits of each kind of treatment?
- What are the risks and possible side effects of each treatment? How will treatment affect my normal activities? Will I be given anything to control side effects?
- How long will treatment last?
- Will I have to stay in the hospital?
- What is the treatment likely to cost? Is this treatment covered by my insurance plan?

- Would a clinical trial (research study) be appropriate for me?

If surgery is recommended to treat the oral cancer, the NCI recommends that patients ask their physician the following questions before having the surgery:

- What kind of operation do you recommend for me?
- Do I need any lymph nodes removed? Why?
- How will I feel after the operation? How long will I be in the hospital?
- What are the risks of surgery?
- Will I have trouble speaking, swallowing, or eating?
- Where will the scars be? What will they look like?
- Will I have any long-term effects?
- Will I look different?
- Will I need reconstructive or plastic surgery? If so, when can that be done?
- Will I lose my teeth? If so, can they be replaced? How soon?
- Will I need to see a specialist for help with my speech?
- When can I get back to my normal activities?
- How often will I need checkups?
- Would a clinical trial be appropriate for me?

If radiation therapy is recommended, the doctor may use either external radiation from a machine or implanted radiation that is used internally. With external radiation, the patient goes to a clinic or hospital once or twice a day for about five to seven days over a period of several weeks. With implant radiation, the implanted material is placed internally with needles, seeds, or thin plastic tubes while the patient is hospitalized for several days. The implants are usually removed before the patient is discharged from the hospital. Some patients receive both internal and external radiation.

Radiation can also cause serious tooth decay, and it may help to rinse the mouth out several times a day with a solution of ¼ teaspoon of baking soda and ⅛ teaspoon of salt, dilated in warm water and followed by a plain water rinse. Radiation therapy can also cause changes in taste and smell, and it can affect the thyroid gland and the sound of the individual's voice.

The NCI recommends that the patient with oral cancer ask the physician the following questions before having radiation therapy:

- Which type of radiation therapy do you recommend for me? Why do I need this treatment?
- When will the treatments begin? When will they end?
- Should I see my dentist before I start treatment? If I need dental treatment, how much time does my mouth need to heal before radiation therapy starts?
- What are the risks and side effects of this treatment? What can I do about them?
- How will I feel during therapy?
- What can I do to take care of myself during therapy?
- How will my mouth and face look afterward?
- Are there any long-term effects?
- Can I continue my normal activities?
- Will I need a special diet? If so, for how long?
- How often will I need checkups?
- Would a clinical trial be appropriate for me?

If the patient needs chemotherapy, which is the use of anticancer drugs that kill the cancer cells, the chemotherapy drugs are generally injected in the case of oral cancer. The NCI suggests patients who are recommended chemotherapy ask their doctor the following questions before treatment with chemotherapy starts:

- Why do I need this treatment?
- Which drug or drugs will I have?
- How do the drugs work?
- Should I see my dentist before I start chemotherapy? If I need dental treatment, how much time does my mouth need to heal before the chemotherapy begins?

- What are the expected benefits of the treatment?
- What are the risks and possible side effects of treatment? What can I do about them?
- When will treatment start? When will it end?
- Will I need to stay in the hospital? How long?
- How will treatment affect my normal activities?
- Would a clinical trial be appropriate for me?

Risk Factors and Preventive Measures

According to the National Cancer Institute, oral cancer is most common among people age 40 years and older, and it is about twice as common in adult males. SMOKING greatly increases the risk of the development of oral cancers, as does the use of smokeless (chewing) tobacco or pipe tobacco, and an estimated 80 percent of all oral cancers are attributed to smoking.

Chronic or heavy alcohol use, poor oral hygiene, and immune suppression in organ transplantation patients can also lead to oral cancers. When individuals both smoke and consume alcohol regularly, their risk for development of oral cancer is greatly increased. The deleterious effect of alcohol combined with smoking is synergistic; the risk of developing head and neck cancer is an estimated 200 times greater for heavy smokers and drinkers.

Chronic and heavy sun exposure may cause cancer of the lip, as may pipe smoking.

Preventive measures include ending a smoking habit and using sunscreen if the individual is exposed to the sun. Lip balm that contains sunscreen should be used.

National Institute of Dental and Craniofacial Research, National Cancer Institute. *What You Need to Know about Oral Cancer*. Bethesda, Md.: National Institutes of Health, September 2003.

outlet obstruction   A blockage that prevents the normal flow of digestive juices or the outflow of solids such as food or fecal matter; for example, in gastric outlet obstruction, food contents are prevented from passing in an antegrade fashion from the stomach to the intestine by a blockage of the pylorus. Gastric outlet obstruction may be due to a complication of an ulcer or cancer.

See also GALLSTONES; POLYPS.

pain Mild, moderate, or severe discomfort. Because of its importance in patient management pain is now called the fifth vital sign by many. Pain may be acute: generally short-term pain lasts several minutes, hours or as long as a day. For many patients, pain is chronic: the person experiences continuous or intermittent pain that may increase and decrease in severity.

Pain varies not only in intensity, but in its very nature. For example, pain may be stabbing or burning. It may also feel like dull or stronger pressure. For this reason, physicians usually ask patients to describe *how* the pain feels, as well as specifically which area hurts.

Rating the Pain

In the United States, many physicians ask patients to rate their pain on a scale of one to 10: one is the mildest pain that they have experienced and 10 is the worst they can imagine ever feeling. This subjective rating helps doctors to know how severe the patient considers his or her own pain and aids the physician in determining the treatment: the type of drug to use, the dosage, and so forth. For patients who cannot use such ratings, such as children or those who have trouble with the scale, doctors may show a series of simple drawings of a person in pain and ask the patient to select which drawing illustrates his or her pain.

Causes of Pain

There are many causes of pain, ranging from organ damage or injury due to infection, to inflammation and other causes. Sometimes pain is caused by a disease, such as an ulcer or appendicitis. Sometimes it is difficult for the doctor to determine the underlying cause of the pain, even with results of laboratory tests or findings of imaging studies such as magnetic resonance imaging (MRI) or computed tomography (CT) scans.

Determining the source of pain can be challenging in some cases. One reason for this is that sometimes pain is *referred:* stemming from one part of the body but actually experienced as pain elsewhere. Heart pain may be experienced as pain in the chest, arms, or other locations, such as the upper abdomen. Some people who think they are having a heart attack may be experiencing severe heartburn or ulcer. On the other hand, they may also be having a heart attack, and sometimes even a physician has difficulty in determining the difference without testing.

Purpose of Pain

Pain is necessary to life, because it is the body's warning system of a problem. Without pain, severe injuries would be unnoticed and could ultimately lead to death.

It can be hard to understand the purpose of chronic pain; pain may stem from an untreated or insufficiently treated ailment, such as GASTRO-ESOPHAGEAL REFLUX DISEASE, an ULCER or CROHN'S DISEASE. Sometimes physicians cannot determine the exact cause of pain and can only treat the pain and other related symptoms the patient experiences.

Treatment of Pain

When individuals have severe acute pain, in addition to their need for the underlying problem to be diagnosed and treated, they may require strong painkilling drugs, such as meperidine (Demerol) or morphine. The use of Demerol is declining because of its toxicity. Over-the-counter medications such as acetaminophen (Tylenol) or ibuprofen (Advil) may be sufficient to manage the pain that is less severe.

If the pain is a chronic problem that has occurred for weeks, months, or even longer, the doctor may prescribe a variety of different analgesic medications. For example, if the physician believes that the pain is inflammatory in nature (as in rheumatoid arthritis), he or she may prescribe nonsteroidal anti-inflammatory drugs (NSAIDs).

If chronic pain is severe, the doctor may prescribe narcotics, such as oxycodone or a codeine-based drug. In the United States, narcotics are medications that are *scheduled,* or controlled by the Drug Enforcement Administration. The federal government requires that careful records be kept on such drugs by both physicians and pharmacies, and there are both federal and state laws governing the prescribing of narcotic painkillers.

A key reason for these laws is that some people abuse painkilling drugs, taking them to obtain an artificial high or using excessively high doses. Another reason is that these drugs can be physically and psychologically addicting, and physicians need to maintain a careful watch over their patients who take them. Sometimes patients become dependent on such narcotics and may develop severe constipation, abdominal distention, and other symptoms associated with narcotic bowel syndrome. Physicians who are pain specialists are best at managing chronic pain, especially when narcotics are needed.

See also NARCOTIC BOWEL SYNDROME; NONSTEROIDAL ANTI-INFLAMMATORY DRUGS ; PROSTAGLANDINS.

pancreas A large combined exocrine–endocrine gland that secretes digestive juices, including enzymes that help to digest foods. The endocrine function of the pancreas involves secretion of the hormone insulin in the bloodstream. Endocrine glands produce hormones. An exocrine gland secretes through ducts, such as the digestive juices secreted by the pancreas.

Major medical diseases of the pancreas include pancreatitis (inflammation of the pancreas) and pancreatic cancer. Diabetes mellitus occurs when the pancreas secretes too little insulin for the metabolism of glucose or the body is unable to respond to all the insulin that is produced, as in insulin resistance.

See also; DIABETES MELLITUS; PANCREATIC CANCER; PANCREATITIS.

pancreatic cancer Malignancy of the pancreas, a pear-shaped organ that is about six inches long and is surrounded by the stomach and intestines in close proximity to the spleen, the liver, and the GALLBLADDER. The PANCREAS produces insulin, which controls the blood sugar level. The pancreas also generates pancreatic juices, which help to digest food. When cancer is diagnosed in the pancreas, it usually appears in the head of the pancreas (75 percent of the time); it appears in the body or tail of the pancreas in the remaining cases. Most forms of pancreatic cancer start in the ducts carrying the pancreatic juices.

According to Ahmedin Jemal and colleagues in *CA: A Cancer Journal for Clinicians,* there were an estimated 42,470 new cases of pancreatic cancer in 2009 in the United States, including 21,050 males and 21,050 females with this disease. In addition, there were an estimated 35,240 deaths from pancreatic cancer in 2009, including 18,030 men and 17,210 women who died. Pancreatic cancer represents 3 percent of the top 10 new cases of cancer in both women and men. In addition, pancreatic cancer represented 6 percent of all cancer deaths among men and women. (Lung cancer is the number one cancer killer among both men and women.) Pancreatic cancer is one of the most lethal form of cancers, and the majority of people diagnosed with this disease die within 12 months. The five-year survival rate is less than 5 percent among patients who are diagnosed with pancreatic cancer, largely because symptoms are not apparent until the disease can no longer be treated because it has spread to other organs. Actor Patrick Swayze and columnist William Safire both died of pancreatic cancer in 2009. Supreme Court Justice Ginsburg underwent surgery for pancreatic cancer in 2009, and is alive as of this writing in 2010. Neuroendocrine tumor in the pancreas has a better prognosis. Apple founder and CEO Steve Jobs was diagnosed with this type of cancer, and he subsequently had LIVER TRANSPLANTATION for the metastatic disease.

Symptoms and Diagnostic Path

Most patients have no symptoms until the disease is very advanced. The most common symptom is abdominal pain, which may radiate into the patient's back.

Other symptoms of pancreatic cancer are as follows:

- DIARRHEA
- a yellowish tinge to the skin and the whites of the eyes (JAUNDICE)
- abdominal and upper back pain or discomfort
- appetite loss
- unintended weight loss
- NAUSEA AND VOMITING
- weakness
- very dark (cola-colored) urine
- pale, chalky stool
- itchy skin

The doctor who suspects that a patient may have pancreatic cancer orders blood tests involving the liver, as well as imaging studies. Laboratory tests reveal an increased level of bilirubin, a substance that is produced by the liver. Normally, bilirubin travels from the liver to the gallbladder to the intestine. However, when a bile duct is blocked by a tumor in the pancreas, bile cannot be normally excreted through the bile ducts; thus the bilirubin may accumulate instead in the blood and consequently, bilirubin levels are elevated in the blood and urine. This accumulation of bilirubin causes the yellow skin color that is characteristic of jaundice. Stools, on the other hand, appear pale and chalky because of the ABSENCE of bile. Blood levels of tumor marker CA-19-9 are usually but not always elevated in pancreatic cancer. The use of genetic markers in diagnosis (such as mutations of the *K-ras* gene and p53 tumor suppressor gene) is investigational as of this writing.

Other diagnostic tests that are commonly ordered by most physicians when they are suspicious of the presence of pancreatic cancer are computed tomography (CT) testing and/or magnetic resonance imaging (MRI), as well as ULTRASOUND imaging or other tests to help with diagnosis. An endoscopic retrograde cholangiopancreatography (ERCP) (an endoscope test of the bile ducts and the pancreas) and an endoscopic ultrasound study (EUS) may also be undertaken.

Ultimately, a biopsy determines whether pancreatic cancer is present. The biopsy or brushings may be performed by inserting a needle through the abdomen or inserting an endoscope in the throat for performing an ERCP or EUS. Doctors seek to determine whether the cancer has spread to any neighboring organs, such as the gallbladder or even farther afield, such as to the kidney or the bones. CT scans, an endoscopic ultrasound (EUS), and MRI scans can also help doctors to determine the size of the primary tumor and to pinpoint its exact location. If endoscopic ultrasound is available, it may further help doctors to diagnose and stage pancreatic cancer. In the case of a typical finding on imaging studies when a lesion is deemed to be surgically resectable, the surgeon may proceed directly to surgery without undertaking a biopsy.

Treatment Options and Outlook

Most patients with pancreatic cancer are treated by a gastroenterologist, as well as by an oncologist (cancer specialist), and by surgeons as well as by their regular physicians. The most common and effective treatment for pancreatic cancer is surgery to remove part of the pancreas and the surrounding tissue, including parts of the stomach and the small intestine, a procedure that is known as the Whipple resection; however, this surgery is very complex, and to date, the prognosis for patients remains poor, despite surgical advances.

Doctors may also use radiation therapy to irradiate the cancerous area or chemotherapy to destroy the cancer cells.

As of this writing, many doctors offer patients whose cancer is surgically nonresectable participation in a clinical trial, in which they will receive medication or treatment that is otherwise not available to them because it has not yet been approved for general public use.

Risk Factors and Preventive Measures

Age is a key risk factor for pancreatic cancer, and most people in whom this disease develops are older than 60 years. The presentation of painless jaundice with weight loss in an ELDERLY individual is an ominous sign.

Some health habits can increase the risk for the development of pancreatic cancer, and SMOKING is a known risk factor. Smokers who stop smoking may decrease their risk for pancreatic cancer within several years.

Other risk factors for developing pancreatic cancer are as follows:

- a family history of pancreatic cancer (the disease is more likely if a parent or sibling has had pancreatic cancer)

- the presence of chronic PANCREATITIS (an inflammation of the pancreas)

- A diagnosis of diabetes, especially long-standing type 2 diabetes. Some studies suggest that diabetes may be a consequence of pancreatic cancer. A new onset of diabetes in a thin older adult suggests the possibility of underlying pancreatic cancer and should be screened as such.

- chronic occupational exposure to some chemicals, such as exposure to petrochemicals

- having had a partial gastrectomy (stomach surgery)

- Having had a cholecystectomy may be a risk factor although this is a controversial risk factor.

- HELICOBACTER PYLORI infection in the stomach increases the risk.

- A diet very high in fat and meat consumption; in contrast, fruit/vegetable consumption is believed to be a protective factor against the development of pancreatic cancer; however the data is conflicting.

- Individuals with blood group A, AB, or B are at greater risk for pancreatic cancer compared to blood group O.

- An association between pancreatic cancer and exposure to hepatitis B has also been reported.

Data on the role of coffee and alcohol as well as aspirin intake in the pathogenesis of pancreatic cancer is conflicting. The optimal screening strategy for screening for pancreatic cancer in high-risk individuals remains to be established. Usually a screening program is started at the age of 35 years in patients with hereditary pancreatitis. In patients with a family history of pancreatic cancer, it begins 10 years before the age at which pancreatic cancer was first diagnosed in family members, and a spiral CT and endoscopic ultrasound (EUS) are recommended as screening tools.

See also LIVER ENZYMES/FUNCTION TESTS.

Jemal, Ahmedin, et al. "Cancer Statistics, 2009." *CA: A Cancer Journal for Clinicians* 59 (2009): 225–249. Available online. URL: http://caonline.amcancersoc.org/cgi/reprint/59/4/225?ijkey=b939af835bcd5e227911f9c2e179a4502a3fe4f7. Accessed August 18, 2009.

pancreatic cholera A condition of diarrhea, hypokalemia (a potassium deficiency), and a neuroendocrine tumor of the pancreas. The diarrhea causes a loss of fluids and electrolytes from the intestine and is severe and watery. It is caused by an excessive secretion of vasoactive intestinal peptide (VIP) from the tumor, which is usually located in the pancreas. Pancreatic cholera is also known as Verner-Morrison syndrome, named for Verner and Morrison, who described the condition in 1958.

The treatment of pancreatic cholera involves preventing fluid and electrolyte depletion, as well as controlling the diarrhea and the tumor. The treatment of choice for controlling the diarrhea is octreotide. Some patients need a combination of a corticosteroid drug and octreotide. The surgical excision of the tumor may be an option in selected cases. Patients may also be treated with interferon alfa.

In contrast to treatment of many cases of pancreatic cancer, aggressive treatment of pancreatic cholera can often be lifesaving. The five-year survival rate is 90 percent, and the 10-year survival rate is 25 percent. Survival rate is better in cases of small tumors and tumors that have not spread.

See also PANCREAS; PANCREATIC CANCER; PANCREATITIS.

pancreatic insufficiency A condition in which the PANCREAS does not make enough digestive enzymes for the normal digestive process. In the most severe cases, pancreatic insufficiency leads to malabsorption, in which the nutrients are not digested and, therefore, cannot be absorbed from the small intestine. Clinically significant pancreatic insufficiency usually does not occur until about 80 to 90 percent of the pancreas is destroyed or nonfunctional.

Symptoms and Diagnostic Path

The symptoms and signs of pancreatic insufficiency include fatty and loose stools, vitamin deficiencies, and unintended weight loss. Some patients have muscle cramps and abdominal pain. The diagnosis of pancreatic insufficiency is based on the patient's clinical signs, a physical examination, and laboratory tests.

Treatment Options and Outlook

Patients who are diagnosed with pancreatic insufficiency are given pancreatic enzyme supplements, and they are also advised to consume a low-fat diet. Patients who drink are advised to avoid all alcohol, especially since alcohol exacerbates PANCREATITIS and may worsen the pancreatic insufficiency. Patients who develop diabetes due to chronic pancreatitis would need to be treated appropriately.

Risk Factors and Preventive Measures

Pancreatic insufficiency is seen in patients who have chronic pancreatitis or CYSTIC FIBROSIS. Sometimes DIABETES MELLITUS may also occur in association with pancreatic insufficiency. Chronic pancreatis can be prevented by not drinking alcohol if the pancreatitis is alcohol-related. Cholecystectomy is preventive if it is due to gallstones.

See also ALCOHOL ABUSE AND ALCOHOLISM; CROHN'S DISEASE; MALABSORPTION SYNDROME; PANCREATIC CANCER; ULCERS, PEPTIC.

pancreatitis   Painful and acute or chronic inflammation of the PANCREAS, which may be caused by disease, stones that are blocking the bile duct, pancreatic tumors, or a chronic illness that has caused damage to the pancreas. Sometimes a physical trauma, such as a blunt trauma to the abdomen, causes pancreatitis. In about 10 percent of acute cases of pancreatitis, patients become severely ill and are at risk for death.

Chronic ALCOHOL ABUSE is one of the two common causes of pancreatitis. An estimated 80 percent of all cases of pancreatitis are due to either gallstones or alcoholism. In addition, an estimated 85 different medications, particularly sulfa drugs, metronidazole, and valproic acid, can induce pancreatitis. The presence of high triglyceride blood levels (hypertriglyceridemia) is another cause of pancreatitis among patients.

Rarely, hypercalcemia, which is a condition of excessively high blood levels of calcium that is frequently caused by hyperparathyroidism, causes pancreatitis. A penetrating peptic ulcer is another rare cause of pancreatitis.

Symptoms and Diagnostic Path

Patients report severe pain and NAUSEA AND VOMITING. They may enter a hospital emergency room for treatment of their symptoms.

Laboratory tests are performed in cases of suspected pancreatitis. If pancreatitis is present, blood levels of pancreatic enzymes (such as amylase and lipase) are usually elevated. Normal levels of pancreatic enzymes cannot exclude pancreatitis, but they make it less likely. An ULTRASOUND of the GALLBLADDER is also done, to check for gallstones. A computed tomography (CT) scan may be ordered to assess the severity of the pancreatitis and to look for complications.

Chronic pancreatitis can be diagnosed with a plain X-ray of the abdomen if pancreatic calcifications are visible or with endoscopic retrograde cholangiopancreatography (ERCP) or an endoscopic ultrasound procedure that uses endoscopic ultrasonography. This procedure usually follows a CT scan of the pancreas. Normal findings on imaging studies do not exclude chronic pancreatitis but make it less likely.

Treatment Options and Outlook

Chronic pancreatitis patients may have reduced levels of the pancreatic enzymes that are needed for digestion and may require exogenous enzyme supplementation. Some may develop DIABETES MELLITUS. Surgery is required in some cases of acute and chronic pancreatitis.

The treatment of pancreatitis involves control of the symptoms, such as control of pain with analgesics (painkilling medications). It also includes treatment of the causes/complications of the pancreatitis, such as infections or other medical problems. For example, if gallstones have caused the pancreatitis, they are removed, along with the gallbladder. If alcoholism appears to be the primary cause, the patient is urged to refrain from drinking all alcohol and is warned about the consequences of failure to comply with the recommendation, which are more attacks of pancreatitis and a shortened life span. If medications appear to be the cause of pancreatitis, they are discontinued. If high triglyceride levels are the cause, the patient is instructed on how to change his or her diet, and appropriate medications are prescribed.

Risk Factors and Preventive Measures

Patients who are at highest risk for development of pancreatitis include the following groups:

- patients who have abused alcohol for several years
- patients who have gallstones
- patients who have a family history of pancreatitis
- patients who have acquired immunodeficiency syndrome (AIDS)
- patients who have hypertriglyceridemia (high blood levels of triglycerides)

Avoiding alcohol is the only known preventive measure.

See also HEPATITIS; HEREDITARY PANCREATITIS; ULCERS, PEPTIC.

papillotomy   An endoscopic procedure used to widen the papilla by making a cut so as to facilitate the removal of stones from the bile duct. This procedure is performed during ENDOSCOPIC RETROGRADE CHOLANGIOPANCREATOGRAPHY (ERCP). The ERCP alone is considered a diagnostic test; the papillotomy is regarded as more invasive and is used for therapeutic purposes. Early ERCP and endoscopic papillotomy are beneficial in the case of acute biliary pancreatitis. However, patients who do not have biliary obstruction do not benefit from the procedure.

According to a study published in 1997 in the *New England Journal of Medicine,* patients who have acute biliary pancreatitis but do not have obstructive jaundice do not benefit from this procedure. In this study, of the 126 patients in the ERCP group, some had severe complications, including death in the case of 14 patients, during the course of three months. Among the 112 subjects who were in the conservative treatment group, seven died during the same period.

Although the overall complication rates for both groups of patients were similar, the group who had the invasive procedure experienced more severe complications. Concluded the researchers, "Our controlled, randomized trial of early ERCP and papillotomy in patients with acute biliary pancreatitis demonstrated that patients without biliary obstruction or biliary sepsis did not benefit from these interventions."

See also ENDOSCOPIC RETROGRADE CHOLANGIOPANCREATOGRAPHY; GALLSTONES; PANCREATITIS.

Folsch, Ulrich R., M.D., et al. "Early ERCP and Papillotomy Compared with Conservative Treatment for Acute Biliary Pancreatitis." *New England Journal of Medicine* 336, no. 4 (January 23, 1997): 237–242.

paracentesis   A procedure in which a needle is inserted into the abdomen to remove excess fluid that has been caused by ASCITES. The most common cause of ascites is liver cirrhosis. The extracted fluid is analyzed for abnormalities to determine the cause of the ascites as well as to see whether any infection is present. In some cases, there may be so much fluid in the abdomen that it causes the patient difficulty with breathing. In such cases, a therapeutic large-volume paracentesis is performed by removing several liters of fluid (as many as 10 to 20 liters) to ease the patient's breathing difficulties. Paracentesis is usually a relatively risk-free procedure, and complications are uncommon. However, death may occur rarely as a complication of the procedure.

See also ALCOHOL ABUSE AND ALCOHOLISM; CIRRHOSIS.

Minocha, A. "A Fatal Case of Paracentesis." *American Journal of Gastroenterology* 94 (1999): 856.

parasitic infection   An illness that is caused by a nonbacterial and nonviral organism, such as by an *Entameba histolytica* (AMEBIASIS), an *Enterobius* (pinworm), or a hookworm, tapeworm, round-worm, or another parasite. The diagnosis may be made by a variety of laboratory tests, such as tests of the blood or stool, depending on the parasite. Medications can usually cure or at least improve the condition in most instances.

See also CHAGAS' DISEASE; CHOLANGITIS; CRYP-TOSPORIDIUM PARVUM; DIARRHEA; DIGESTION AND ABSORPTION; DIGESTIVE ENZYMES; EOSINOPHILIC GAS-TROENTERITIS; FAILURE TO THRIVE; IRRITABLE BOWEL SYNDROME; LIVER ABSCESS; OCCULT GASTROINTESTINAL BLEEDING; TRICHINOSIS.

parenteral nutrition Provision of food through a tube that is connected to a catheter that is inserted into the veins. Thus, nutrition is introduced directly into the blood rather than taken by mouth or by a tube into the stomach or small intestine. Parenteral nutrition is used when the person is too ill to have oral nutrition or an abnormality of the gastroin-testinal system makes it difficult or impossible for the person to eat normally or to handle nutrients fed into the gut, such as an intestinal obstruction. Long-term parenteral nutrition may lead to compli-cations, such as catheter sepsis, venous thrombosis, and NONALCOHOLIC STEATOHEPATITIS/NONALCOHOLIC FATTY LIVER DISEASE.

See also ENTERAL NUTRITION; FEEDING TUBE.

pasteurization A food processing procedure that removes microbes that can cause disease. Pasteuri-zation improves the quality of food by making it safer and by prolonging its shelf life. The process was named after Louis Pasteur, a 19th-century researcher who discovered that beer and wine could be preserved by heating them to below the boiling point, then rapidly cooling them.

Pasteurization techniques were later used to eradicate the bacteria in milk, cheese, and other products, which are heated and then cooled rapidly. For example, the pasteurization of milk removes an estimated 97 to 99 percent of such bacteria as *Myco-bacterium tuberculosis*, SALMONELLA, and *Streptococcus* species.

The temperature and duration used in pasteuri-zation vary by product; for example, milk must be heated to 63°C for 30 minutes or to 72°C for 16 seconds, then rapidly cooled. Ice cream must be heated to 69°C for 30 minutes or 80°C for 25 sec-onds. The addition of other products, such as sugar or chocolate, changes both the temperature and duration requirements.

See also CONTAMINATED FOOD OR WATER.

peritonitis A dangerous and possibly life-threat-ening infection of the peritoneum, which is the lining that protects the internal abdominal organs. Individuals who have peritonitis require antibiot-ics and hospitalization, and, depending upon the cause of the peritonitis, may need surgery. Those who have a weakened immune system, such as liver CIRRHOSIS patients, are at risk for contracting peritonitis.

pernicious anemia A major cause of vitamin B_{12} deficiency. Pernicious anemia as a cause should be excluded in all cases of vitamin B_{12} deficiency, since 75 percent of the cases of this deficiency are caused by pernicious anemia. Pernicious anemia is an autoimmune attack on gastric intrinsic factor, which is a chemical that is necessary for the absorp-tion of vitamin B_{12}. The lack of functional intrinsic factor contributes to vitamin B_{12} deficiency. Perni-cious anemia also causes atrophic gastritis, which causes decreased production of intrinsic factor, thereby further exacerbating the condition. There is also an increased risk for gastric cancer associated with pernicious anemia.

There are numerous other causes of vitamin B_{12} deficiency, such as Crohn's disease, HELICOBACTER PYLORI infection, HUMAN IMMUNODEFICIENCY VIRUS (HIV) infection, the chronic use of proton pump inhibitors (PPIs) or an inherited disorder.

Symptoms and Diagnostic Path
The symptoms and signs of pernicious anemia vary; they may include numbness and tingling in the hands and feet, weakness, as well as mood swings and memory loss. If the illness is untreated for years, it may also produce irreversible nerve damage.

If a deficiency is suspected, laboratory tests may be done to confirm it. A deficiency of vitamin B_{12}

is characterized by large red blood cells (macrocytosis). Anti-intrinsic factor antibodies are present in most patients and are confirmatory. A Schilling test confirms the diagnosis but is unavailable in most of the United States.

Treatment Options and Outlook

A pernicious anemia-related vitamin B_{12} deficiency is treated with either injections of vitamin B_{12} or, in some cases, high doses of oral tablets of vitamin B_{12}. It can also be given sublingually (under the tongue) or in the form of nasal sprays, but the extent of B_{12} absorption for these forms is not reliable.

Risk Factors and Preventive Measures

Pernicious anemia is a common problem, especially among ELDERLY subjects. In fact, some older individuals are misdiagnosed with Alzheimer's disease or dementia when their true medical problem is actually a vitamin B_{12} deficiency.

Pernicious anemia is more common in women than in men (4.1 percent of women versus 2.1 percent of men). It is rare among Hispanic and Asian Americans.

See also ANEMIA; VITAMIN DEFICIENCIES/ EXCESSES.

Peutz-Jeghers syndrome A hereditary disorder that is characterized by the presence of intestinal POLYPS and skin lesions. This syndrome is mapped to chromosome l9pl3.3. Patients with Peutz-Jeghers syndrome are also at an increased risk for the development of intestinal cancers, as well as PANCREATIC CANCER, lung cancer, breast cancer, uterine cancer, ovarian cancer, and testicular cancer. For Peutz-Jeghers syndrome patients, the risk of dying of cancer approaches 45 to 50 percent by the age of 60 years. The syndrome was named after J. L. A. Peutz, a Dutch physician who first described it in 1921. Dr. Jeghers, an American doctor, provided further details in 1944, and the condition was subsequently named after both men.

The polyps that are characteristic of this syndrome usually begin to develop in childhood, although the newborn infant may also have the identifiable black frecklelike lesions on the body, especially on and around the lips and the mouth, that are characteristic of this disease.

Symptoms and Diagnostic Path

Peutz-Jeghers syndrome patients may have frequent attacks of mild to severe abdominal pains. As mentioned, they also have polyps of the gastrointestinal tract, which are benign, usually multiple, and of variable size. The polyps may be present in the stomach and the small and/or large intestine and can lead to intestinal blockage as well as to gastrointestinal BLEEDING. Only a minority of these polyps (1 to 13 percent) become cancerous. However, the syndrome is associated with an increased risk of gastrointestinal as well as nongastrointestinal tumor malignancies and the risk of cancer is about 50 percent by the age of 60.

The diagnosis is made by observing the classic skin/buccal lesions (blue-gray to brown in color) varying from one to five mm in size and by finding polyps in the gut. They can be distinguished from freckles by the fact that freckles are absent at birth and do not occur in the mouth. The doctor orders a colonoscopy and upper ENDOSCOPY, as well as a small bowel endoscopy or X-ray to look for these polyps. If polyps are found, they are excised, especially the large ones, while biopsies may be taken from the small polyps. Genetic testing is available at specialized centers; however, a negative genetic test does not exclude the diagnosis.

Treatment Options and Outlook

Periodic surveillance by colonoscopy and upper endoscopy is recommended for those who have Peutz-Jeghers syndrome, as well as a surveillance for breast and testicular tumors.

Risk Factors and Preventive Measures

Patients develop Peutz-Jeghers syndrome because of a genetic risk. There are no known preventive measures.

See also SIGMOIDOSCOPY.

Wynbrandt, James, and Mark D. Ludman. *The Encyclopedia of Genetic Disorders and Birth Defects.* 3d ed. New York: Facts On File, 2008.

physical activity See EXERCISE; OBESITY.

pica A strange desire or compulsion to eat non-food items, such as paper, clay, laundry detergent, baking soda, or dirt, a compulsion that lasts for at least a month. Pica may stem from iron deficiency ANEMIA. Sometimes pica for ice, or papophagia, may be seen even when patients are not anemic, and even in such cases, patients often respond promptly to treatment with IRON.

Although actual pica may develop during pregnancy, food cravings, such as the intense desire to eat pickles or other foods, are not a form of pica; eating nonfood is true pica.

Pica may sometimes be associated with a psychotic disturbance, such as schizophrenia or another severe emotional disorder. Pica is also behavior that is sometimes exhibited by mentally retarded adults.

It is unknown how many children and adults have pica and why it occurs.

Some preschool children experience a form of pica in that they consume paper or paint chips. (This is not the same type of behavior as when infants put virtually everything into their mouth in an exploration phase.) Eating paint chips can cause lead poisoning and lead to irreversible brain damage to the child.

It is important that parents and other caregivers monitor the behavior of young children because it is impossible to predict which children will exhibit pica (unless they have already been known to have such symptoms in the past). The child exhibiting pica should be corrected and kept away from the desired nonfood as much as possible.

pneumatosis intestinalis (PI) A condition of digestive gas that is found inside the wall of either the COLON or the small intestine. It is known by various names including pneumatosis cystoides intestinalis, intramural gas, pneumatosis coli, pseudolipomatosis, intestinal emphysema, bullous emphysema of the intestine, and lymphopneumatosis It is not a disease per se, but rather a manifestation of some disorder. It may be seen in infants or adults. Among infants with PI, most have NECROTIZING ENTEROCOLITIS, although some infants and children may have very severe gastroenteritis.

Symptoms and Diagnostic Path

Most patients have no symptoms or signs. Usually the signs and symptoms of PI, if any are present, pertain to the underlying disorder involved. When the condition occurs in the small intestine and symptoms result, patients may have NAUSEA AND VOMITING, unintended weight loss, DIARRHEA, and abdominal pain. When PI is present in the colon and symptoms occur, patients may have diarrhea, abdominal pain, enlarged abdomen, and CONSTIPATION.

Generally, pneumatosis intestinalis is identified in plain X-rays of the abdomen; however, computed tomography (CT) scans are more effective at diagnosing PI. The condition may also be diagnosed during a routine SIGMOIDOSCOPY or colonoscopy. A magnetic resonance imaging (MRI) scan can also reveal gas inside the bowel wall.

Treatment Options and Outlook

The treatment involves the treatment of the underlying disorder. If patients are not symptomatic and there is no apparent emergency, physicians may decide to continue to observe the condition over time and prescribe no medication or treatment. The condition may also resolve on its own. If patients do have symptoms, some physicians treat them with hyperbaric oxygen; others treat with ANTIBIOTICS, particularly metronidazole, for as long as three months.

Some patients may need surgery; most do not. Surgery is indicated, however, if the patient experiences an obstruction or a perforation of the intestine or the colon. The puncture of these gas-filled lesions can be accomplished during an ENDOSCOPY for patients who are otherwise symptomatic but are poor candidates for surgery.

Risk Factors and Preventive Measures

Among adults, pneumatosis intestinalis more commonly appears from about age 50 to 80 years. Although it can be benign, it may be associated with serious intestinal conditions such as bowel ischemia and infarction.

polyps Nodule or mushroomlike growths that are usually benign but may sometimes become cancerous if they are not removed in a timely fashion. Polyps are most frequently found in the colon and can be detected and removed by a physician while a patient is having a COLONOSCOPY. If they are not removed, these polyps may become cancerous within the colon in about 10 years; however, not all polyps are precancerous; nor do all become cancerous.

Most polyps do not cause symptoms; however, large polyps may cause abdominal pain and gastrointestinal bleeding. Colon cancer screening is generally recommended for average-risk patients after the age of 50 years so that physicians can look for precancerous polyps and remove any they find.

See also COLORECTAL CANCER.

portal circulation The transmission of blood from the portal vein, which accounts for 75 percent of the blood flow to the liver. The portal vein is formed by the union of the superior mesenteric vein from the intestines and the splenic vein from the spleen. In some cases, the resistance to the blood flow in the portal vein is increased, resulting in increased portal pressure; which is also known as portal hypertension, for example, in liver cirrhosis or a blockage in the portal or splenic vein by a clot that leads to elevated pressure in the portal vein.

See also CIRRHOSIS; LIVER.

pouchitis A complication of some surgeries involving the formation of an artificial reservoir for stool from the small intestine, particularly the ileal pouch created in ileoanal anastomosis, an operation used for patients who have ULCERATIVE COLITIS.

The symptoms of pouchitis are bloody stools, an increased frequency and urgency of defecation, and fever and lethargy. Pouchitis may be acute or chronic, and it can usually be treated with metronidazole. ANTIBIOTICS have been used to treat pouchitis, as well as corticosteroids and aminosalicylate enemas. If medications are not effective, patients may need additional surgery.

See also INFLAMMATORY BOWEL DISEASE; ULCERATIVE COLITIS.

pregnancy Period during which a human fetus grows inside a woman for approximately nine months. In the early part of pregnancy (the first trimester, or first three months), many women experience nausea and some also experience periodic vomiting as well. In an extreme and unusual case, the vomiting and dehydration become dangerous and life-threatening, as with HYPEREMESIS GRAVIDARUM.

As many as 75 percent of all pregnant women may also experience GASTROESOPHAGEAL REFLUX DISEASE. Women in their third trimester may experience digestive problems such as CONSTIPATION, because of hormonal influences as well as the pressure of the growing fetus on the internal organs. The liver can also be affected by diseases that are unique to pregnancy, such as the acute fatty liver of pregnancy and other syndromes that may be life-threatening.

See also NAUSEA AND VOMITING.

primary biliary cirrhosis (PBC) A progressive liver disease that mainly affects women and can lead to LIVER FAILURE.

The illness is apparently caused by an immunological defect, and both genetic and environmental factors have been implicated. Primary biliary cirrhosis (PBC) is unique among autoimmune diseases because it never occurs in childhood, and it is also rare in young adults. Many primary biliary cirrhosis patients also have another autoimmune disease, such as rheumatoid arthritis, SCLERODERMA, or thyroid disease (hypothyroidism), or other illnesses, such as CREST SYNDROME. Patients who have primary biliary cirrhosis have liver inflammation and scarring as well as damaged intrahepatic bile ducts, which ultimately lead to liver cirrhosis and liver failure.

Symptoms and Diagnostic Path

Patients with primary biliary cirrhosis may have no symptoms or signs in the early stages of the illness, or they may have some vague indicators, such as fatigue and pruritus (itching of the skin). The pruritus may become severe, with no apparent cause, and sometimes patients who have not been diagnosed with primary biliary cirrhosis are sent to dermatologists for diagnosis and treatment.

As the disease progresses further, the patient's liver becomes enlarged (hepatomegaly). Many patients have pain on the right upper quadrant of the body.

About a third of patients who have this illness also have an enlarged spleen, particularly as the disease progresses. Some patients have JAUNDICE in the early stages, and many are jaundiced at the later stages of the illness. Patients with advanced primary biliary cirrhosis may also have edema (water retention) and ASCITES. Some patients experience unintended weight loss.

According to experts, there are usually four stages of primary biliary CIRRHOSIS, and cirrhosis is clearly apparent in the fourth stage. It is possible, however, to see several different stages at the same time in different parts of the patient's liver.

Routine liver enzyme and function tests may help the physician to suspect the problem. Patients who have primary biliary cirrhosis have elevated blood levels of alkaline phosphaste and gammaglutamyltransferase. Another test, the antimitochondrial antibody test, has a positive result in nearly all (95 percent) of patients who have this condition. Blood cholesterol level is also usually mildly to significantly elevated in primary biliary cirrhosis patients.

Doctors should carefully question patients about the medications that they take, because a wide variety of medications can cause fatigue, pruritus, and other signs that are also characteristic of primary biliary cirrhosis.

Physicians usually order an ULTRASOUND of the patient's liver to look for any other causes of liver disease. In some cases, however, a computed tomography (CT) scan may be needed; in others, an ENDOSCOPIC RETROGRADE CHOLANGIOPANCREATOGRAPHY (ERCP) is required to determine the cause of abnormal liver test findings. A liver biopsy specimen is usually taken to make the diagnosis.

Treatment Options and Outlook

Much of the treatment is directed at the complications or associations of PBC such as pruritus, MALABSORPTION SYNDROME, and hypothyroidism. There is no medical cure for primary bihiary cirrhosis, but medications may help treat the symptoms. Ursodiol is the most commonly used medication. It helps relieve symptoms and slows the progression of the disease, and it has essentially no significant side effects. Physicians may also try such medications as colchicine and methotrexate although that is controversial. A combination of ursodiol plus colchicine may be superior to either drug alone, However, most patients eventually experience liver failure, and the only known cure is a LIVER TRANSPLANTATION.

Risk Factors and Preventive Measures

Nearly 95 percent of primary biliary cirrhosis patients are females, and most of them are between 30 and 65 years old. The disease is rare: It has an estimated incidence of 3.9 to 15 individuals per million. It is found among women of all races worldwide. There is an apparent genetic risk, and individuals in families in which parents or siblings have the disease have a significantly increased risk of development of primary biliary cirrhosis.

There are no known preventive measures.

See also LIVER; LIVER ENZYMES/FUNCTION TESTS.

primary sclerosing cholangitis A severe and chronic liver disease that involves inflammation and scarring of the bile ducts of the LIVER. These ducts can become so narrow that they are blocked and cannot effectively transport bile out of the liver. With this increasing bile buildup, frequent infections occur, and the liver becomes damaged. The cause of primary sclerosing cholangitis (PSC) is unknown; it may be caused by an infection of the bile duct. Some experts believe that it may be an autoimmune disease.

Symptoms and Diagnostic Path

The key indicators of primary sclerosing cholangitis are JAUNDICE, intermittent fevers, pruritus (itching of the skin), and fatigue. Because these symptoms occur in many different illnesses, physicians must rule out other causes. PSC can lead to GALLSTONES, CHOLANGITIS, and cholangiocarcinoma (cancer of the GALLBLADDER). ULCERATIVE COLITIS that is associated with PSC may lead to colon cancer.

Primary sclerosing cholangitis is diagnosed through the injection of dye into the bile ducts, followed by X-rays known as ENDOSCOPIC RETROGRADE

CHOLANGIOPANCREATOGRAPHY (ERCP). The MRCP scan is a valuable adjunct.

Treatment Options and Outlook

The treatment primarily deals with symptoms; for example, patients are given ANTIBIOTICS to treat infections and/or medications to control itching. They may also take vitamin supplements if they are deficient in vitamins. The most common vitamin deficiencies of primary sclerosing cholangitis patients are of vitamins A, D, and K.

Some physicians treat patients with ursodiol, which is also used to treat PRIMARY BILIARY CIRRHOSIS patients; however, while this may improve symptoms, the efficacy of this medicine in improving the outcome has not been proved in primary sclerosing cholangitis.

If the bile ducts are severely blocked, an ERCP with PAPILLOTOMY and even surgery may be indicated. If patients experience LIVER FAILURE, the only cure is LIVER TRANSPLANTATION.

Risk Factors and Preventive Measures

Most primary sclerosing cholangitis patients are 30 to 60 years old, and the majority are male. The majority of primary sclerosing cholangitis patients (75 percent) have INFLAMMATORY BOWEL DISEASE (IBD). CROHN'S DISEASE and ulcerative colitis are the two forms of an inflammatory bowel disease.

IBD and PSC may have the same or similar underlying cause like an autoimmune disease; however other factors (e.g. genetics, infection, ischemia) may be involved as well since the two diseases may occur without the presence of other or at different times during life. PSC can occur long after colectomy for ulcerative colitis. Similarly, the onset of ulcerative colitis may follow a liver transplantation for PSC. Also, it should also be pointed out that primary sclerosing cholangitis develops in only a minority (less than 5 percent) of inflammatory bowel disease patients.

progressive familial intrahepatic cholestasis A group of inherited disorders that are characterized by defects in bile secretion that often appear in infancy or early childhood and are associated with growth failure and severe liver disease.

Progressive familial intrahepatic cholestasis type I, also known as Byler disease or Greenland familial cholestasis, is associated with a defect on chromosome 18q21. Another form is progressive familial intrahepatic cholestasis type II, which occurs primarily in families in Europe and the Middle East. It is caused by a defect in chromosome 2q24. In addition, a third form, progressive familial intrahepatic cholestasis type III, appears to be caused by mutations in a protein that is known as multidrug resistance protein-3-P-glycoprotein (PGY-3 or MDR-3). Physicians can treat the symptoms of familial intrahepatic cholestasis, but there is little else that they can do.

Another form of familial intrahepatic cholestasis is benign recurrent intrahepatic cholestasis (BRIC). This condition manifests itself in adolescence or early adulthood, with episodic symptoms and signs of poor appetite, itching, weight loss, and malabsorption. The episodes may last weeks to months, followed by complete normalization. There is no specific treatment for BRIC, and treatment is directed to the symptoms. Liver transplantation is not undertaken because the disease is episodic and nonprogressive in nature.

See also LIVER; LIVER FAILURE; LIVER TRANSPLANTATION.

prokinetics A class of prescribed medications that was formerly popular in the use of treating patients with GASTROESOPHAGEAL REFLUX DISEASE (GERD). These drugs are also known as promotility medications because they speed stomach emptying and/or transit through the gut. The drugs are useful for those who have GASTROPARESIS and intestinal pseudoobstruction.

In 2000 cisapride (Propulsid), a very popular medication, was virtually withdrawn from the market in the United States by the Food and Drug Administration (FDA) because some patients who used cisapride became sick or died of cardiac ailments. On a restricted basis, physicians may currently continue to prescribe cisapride to some who do not respond to other medications; however, patients who have heart problems cannot take this drug; nor should those who are taking some antibiotics or antidepressants because of problems with adverse drug reactions. Cisapride is widely available outside the United States.

The other primary prokinetic drug is metoclopramide (Reglan). Because metoclopramide has many side effects, especially on the brain, many physicians avoid prescribing this drug whenever possible. Domperidone, another prokinetic drug, is sold in some pharmacies where it is compounded by the pharmacist. It is like metoclopramide, but without many of its side effects on the brain. Erythromycin, in addition to its antibiotic function, has prokinetic activity. However, its effects are short-lived, lasting no more than a few weeks.

See also ACID REFLUX; HYPEREMESIS GRAVIDARUM; PROTON PUMP INHIBITORS.

Minocha, Anil, M.D., and Christine Adamec. *How to Stop Heartburn: Simple Ways to Heal Heartburn and Acid Reflux.* New York: John Wiley & Sons, 2001.

prostaglandins Specialized products of arachidonic acid metabolism that are synthesized in many tissues of the body and that have a short half-life. They act locally close to the site of production in a variety of ways. There are various kinds of prostaglandins with different functions, such as prostaglandin D_2 (PGD_2) and PGE_2, that act as short-term hormones close to the area where they are synthesized. They are not stored; instead, they are released on an as-needed basis.

Prostaglandins are involved in regulating the kidney function, blood pressure, the production of blood clots, the functioning of the uterus and ovaries, and the generation or inhibition of pain and inflammation. They are also involved in erectile function.

NONSTEROIDAL ANTI-INFLAMMATORY DRUGS (NSAIDs) inhibit the production of prostaglandins, thus reducing inflammation; however, they also often cause damage to the gastric mucosa. Cyclo-oxygenase-2 (COX-2) inhibitor medications such as rofecoxib (Vioxx) and valdecoxib (Bextra) were developed to decrease inflammation and at the same time reduce toxicity to the gastrointestinal system. However, Vioxx and Bextra were withdrawn from the market due to increased risks. COX-2 inhibitors may cause some harm to the stomach, although usually less than is caused by an NSAID.

See also PAIN.

proton pump inhibitors A class of medications that are given to people who suffer from chronic heartburn, also known as GASTROESOPHAGEAL REFLUX DISEASE, and/or to patients who have stomach or duodenal ulcers. Drugs in this class are more potent inhibitors of stomach acid than are the histamine-2 receptor blockers such as ranitidine (Zantac) or cimetidine (Tagamet). The reduced acid secretion in the stomach due to these drugs allows time for healing. Proton pump inhibitors (PPIs) are also prescribed for individuals who have ZOLLINGER–ELLISON SYNDROME. As of this writing, the available PPIs include omeprazole (Prilosec), lansoprazole (Prevacid), rabeprazole (Aciphex), pantoprazole (Protonix), and esomeprazole (Nexium). Dexlansoprazole (Kapidex) is a new PPI as of this writing. Prilosec and Zegenid are also available over the counter.

See also ACID REFLUX; NONSTEROIDAL ANTI-INFLAMMATORY DRUGS ; ULCERS, PEPTIC.

radiation injury   Damage to the body that occurs as a result of radiation therapy for cancer or radiation from another source. Radiation can harm the digestive system, causing problems with the colon and other parts of the gastrointestinal tract. Digestive symptoms may appear several years after radiation exposure. Patients who have radiation enteritis may experience diarrhea and gastrointestinal bleeding, as well as strictures. They may also have esophageal strictures that cause swallowing problems or intestinal strictures that cause bowel obstructions.

radiation therapy   Radiotherapy that is given to individuals who have digestive cancers (and other forms of cancer), in an attempt to destroy cancer cells. In some cases, the cancer may be too far advanced for the patient to be cured, but radiation therapy may prevent the cancer from spreading farther for some period, thus extending the individual's life by months or even by years and/or improving his or her quality of life. Sometimes radiation is also given to alleviate pain. Radiation therapy may also be used to shrink an otherwise nonresectable tumor to a resectable one in order to attempt curative surgery. Radiation treatments are overseen by radiation oncologists.

Depending on the type of cancer, some patients may receive implanted radiation therapy, whereas others need to go to a facility three or four times a week for several weeks to receive treatment from equipment that beams the radiation directly at the body part that is cancerous.

In some cases, patients may receive chemotherapy (cancer-killing drugs) at the same time as they are having radiation treatments. In other cases, chemotherapy is used separately.

See also RADIATION INJURY.

Roux-en-Y stasis syndrome   A condition that may occur after gastric surgery, which includes chronic nausea, vomiting, and abdominal pain along with a bloated feeling, especially one that occurs after eating meals.

In Roux-en-Y stasis syndrome, motility is slowed in the stomach as well as in the small intestine, resulting in stasis of food. Treatment is difficult. The Roux limb, which is less than 45 centimeters in size, reduces the probability of occurrence of this disorder. Patients who have predominant gastric stasis may improve after a subtotal GASTRECTOMY. Medical treatment for Roux-en-Y stasis syndrome involves hydration (provision of fluids) and treatment with antiemetics such as promethazine (Phenergan) and ondansetron (Zofran), as well as with prokinetic agents, such as metoclopramide (Reglan) and domperidone (Motilium).

In one study, reported in 1998 in *Archives of Surgery,* patients who had severe symptoms of Roux-en-Y stasis syndrome improved significantly with intravenous administration of erythromycin, which, in addition to its antibiotic effect, has prokinetic action.

Petrakis, John, M.D., et al. "Enhancement of Gastric Emptying of Solids by Erythromycin in Patients with Roux-en-Y Gastrojejunostomy." *Archives of Surgery* 133, no. 7 (July 1998): 709–714.

rumination syndrome   A behavioral disorder that is an effortless regurgitation of recently eaten food, which is then followed by the patient's rechewing and then reswallowing the food. No nausea or retching is involved. It is unclear by what mechanism the food is regurgitated.

The behavior usually occurs at every meal and has been described as "meal in, meal out, day in, day out" behavior. Although rumination is usually seen only in some developmentally disabled children or among subjects who have psychiatric problems, it may also occur in some patients without such problems. Patients report that the food tastes good and is just like the food that was swallowed. The patient experiences no nausea, although belching may precede the rumination.

Some patients may experience weight loss. Some patients spit out the ruminated food, and others reswallow it, especially depending on the social situations.

This behavioral disorder is treated with reassurance, behavioral therapy, and explanations to the patient and to the family as well.

See also BELCHING; NAUSEA AND VOMITING.

S

saliva/salivary problems Saliva is the substance that is formed in the mouth, especially when a person eats, and helps to lubricate as well as partially break down food. Saliva is secreted by the salivary glands. There are three major salivary glands: the parotid, submandibular, and sublingual glands. Causes of insufficient salivation include Sjögren's syndrome, anxiety, and use of many different antidepressant drugs, anticholinergic medications (phenothiazines), and diuretics.

Salmonella Bacteria that can cause minor to life-threatening diarrheal illness in children and adults. According to the Centers for Disease Control and Prevention (CDC) in Atlanta, Georgia, Salmonella refers to a group of microscopic organisms or bacteria that pass from the feces of people or animals to other people or animals. The CDC reports that *Salmonella* commonly appears in the intestines of birds, reptiles, and mammals, and it can live in water and soil for months. The infection that *Salmonella* organisms cause is called salmonellosis. About 400 people die every year from acute salmonellosis in the United States, according to the CDC. As of this writing, the most recent case of *Salmonella* contamination was reported in peanut butter distributed to nine states through food service providers.

Salmonella organisms are the most common cause of food-borne illnesses in the world and are often spread in contaminated food that was prepared by people who did not wash their hands after using the toilet. According to the CDC, there are about 40,000 cases of salmonellosis reported each year in the United States; however, because milder cases are often not reported to health officials, the incidence may be 30 or more times greater than this figure.

All clinically important Salmonella are classified into one species *Salmonella choleraesuis*. The most common types of *Salmonella* bacteria in the United States are *Salmonella* serotype typhimurium and *Salmonella* serotype enteritidis. However, there are many other types of *Salmonella*; for example, *Salmonella* Saintpaul caused a reported 57 cases of salmonellosis in New Mexico and Texas from April through June 2008, and was spread by contaminated raw red tomatoes. Also in 2008, 51 people in 16 states were infected with *Salmonella* litchfield, spread by infected cantaloupes from Honduras. In addition, *Salmonella* agona was spread through contaminated Malt-O-Meal unsweetened puff rice cereals in 2008, infecting 28 people in 15 states.

In addition to being spread by individuals who prepared food that they contaminated, *Salmonella* organisms are also transmitted by individuals who handle infected pet reptiles, especially turtles, lizards, and snakes.

Typhoid fever is caused by a form of *Salmonella* (*Salmonella enterica serotype typhi* and *serotype paratyphi*), but this form of infection is uncommon in the United States, Canada, and other developed countries and is usually seen among travelers and immigrants. It is usually spread by contaminated water, especially after natural disasters such as earthquakes or floods, when the normal water systems are disrupted and the sewer systems overflow. Other modes include contact with an acutely infected patient, a chronic carrier, or contaminated food.

About 400 cases of typhoid fever occur each year in the United States according to the *Travelers' Health Yellow Book* published by the CDC. Most of these individuals were recent travelers to developing countries. Worldwide, there are about 22 million cases of typhoid fever each year and 200,000 people die of the illness. Individuals who plan to travel to other countries with a risk for typhoid fever can be immunized against the disease in advance. However, according to the CDC, typhoid vaccines are not 100 percent effective, and travelers should still take precautions in what they eat and drink.

Symptoms and Diagnostic Path

According to the CDC, the most frequently occurring symptoms of a *Salmonella* infection are DIARRHEA, fever, and abdominal cramps. These symptoms occur within 12 to 72 hours from the time of infection. The infected individual may also have NAUSEA AND VOMITING.

The physician may suspect a *Salmonella* infection on the basis of symptoms and may order an analysis of the stools to confirm the diagnosis. Blood cultures may be done as well.

With typhoid fever, the key symptoms are a very high fever (103 to 104 degrees Fahrenheit), as well as headache, rash, lethargy, and a lack of appetite.

Treatment Options and Outlook

Most people with nontyphoidal *Salmonella* infection recover without any medications within five to seven days. As such, they are treated with fluids and electrolytes during the acute period. However, if doctors believe that the infection has spread to the blood, ANTIBIOTICS are prescribed because such infection can be dangerous and sometimes even fatal. Patients involved in food handling occupations and health-care workers should remain at home while recovering from the symptoms.

Patients with typhoid fever are frequently treated with a fluoroquinolone such as Cipro®. Without treatment, the illness lasts for three to four weeks, and death rates range from 12 percent to 30 percent.

Most individuals recover completely from nontyphoidal *Salmonella* infections, but it may be several months before normal bowel habits occur. In some cases of *Salmonella* infection, the bacteria may cause the development of a chronic condition that is known as reactive arthritis (formerly known as Reiter's syndrome), which can lead to arthritis, painful urination due to urethritis (inflammation of the urethra, the tube that carries urine) and painful red eye due to uveitis.

Researchers have discovered that some *Salmonella* strains are resistant to antibiotics; for that reason, it is increasingly important that government agencies be vigilant and that consumers follow simple techniques that can help prevent the transmission of *Salmonella* infections.

Risk Factors and Preventive Measures

Children have the greatest risk for contracting salmonellosis, especially children who are younger than age five, and who are about five times more likely to be infected than individuals in other age groups. Children are also the most likely to develop severe infections, as are the ELDERLY and those with weak immune systems.

Salmonellosis occurs more commonly in the summer than in the winter.

There are no vaccines to prevent *Salmonella* infection other than the typhoid vaccine for *S. serogroup Typhi*. Although it is not possible to wipe out all *Salmonella* bacteria, many infections can be prevented through simple actions; for example, if a restaurant patron receives undercooked meat, it should always be sent back to the kitchen for further cooking.

Examples of good preventive actions against *Salmonella* infection are the following:

- washing hands immediately after handling reptiles
- washing hands immediately after handling raw poultry or raw eggs
- washing food surfaces that have had contact with uncooked poultry or eggs
- cooking eggs and poultry thoroughly
- washing hands after any contact with pets or with animal feces (such as after cleaning out the cat litter box)
- drinking only pasteurized milk
- avoiding foods that include raw eggs, such as found in raw cookie dough and homemade salad dressing
- avoiding foods prepared by a person infected with any form of *Salmonella*

See also CONTAMINATED FOOD OR WATER.

Center for Food Safety and Applied Nutrition. *Safe Handling of Raw Produce and Fresh-Squeezed Fruit and Vegetable Juices*. Food and Drug Administration. Undated. Available online. URL: http://www.cfsan.fda/gov/~dms/prodsafe.html. Downloaded June 12, 2008.

Centers for Disease Control and Prevention. *Travelers' Health: Yellow Book*, Chapter 4. Prevention of Specific Infectious Diseases. Available online. URL: http://www.cdc.gov/travel/yellowBookCh4-Typhoid.aspx. Downloaded June 12, 2008.

Franko, Kantle. "Salmonella Prompts Peanut Butter Recall." Associated Press, January 11, 2009. Available online. URL:http://news.yahoo.com/s/ap/20090111/ap_on_re_us/salmonella_outbreak_recall. Accessed January 12, 2009.

White, David G., et al. "The Isolation of Antibiotic-Resistant *Salmonella* from Retail Ground Meats." *New England Journal of Medicine* 345, no. 16 (October 18, 2001): 1,147–1, 154.

sarcoidosis   A systemwide disease with symptoms that are sometimes similar to those that are found among TUBERCULOSIS patients. In contrast to that of tuberculosis, the cause of sarcoidosis is unknown. It is not an infection, although some experts believe that sarcoidosis may be environmentally triggered by an exposure to antigens or metal dusts. No single genetic or environmental cause has been established to date for sarcoidosis, despite extensive investigations.

Symptoms and Diagnostic Path

The symptoms and signs of sarcoidosis depend on the organ involved, and there may be no symptoms or mild to severe symptoms. The most common sites beyond lungs include the skin, eyes, joints, PANCREAS, heart, kidney, and nervous system. Sarcoidosis causes skin lesions and lymph node enlargements and fibrosis of the lungs. Fever, weight loss, joint pains, and lack of appetite are common problems.

The LIVER is almost always involved, and many patients have an enlarged liver. Stomach, intestines, and colon may also occasionaly be involved. The disease can also affect the eyes, causing cataracts, glaucoma, blurred vision, and abnormal amounts of tears, caused by ophthalmic lesions produced by the disease. Sarcoidosis may lead to blindness.

A variety of skin rashes may also occur. In addition, the heart and brain may be involved. Some patients experience excessive absorption of calcium, which may ultimately lead to kidney failure.

The key symptoms are fatigue, fever, weight loss, and lack of appetite. Most patients also have chronic respiratory symptoms as well. In about half the cases, the diagnosis may be detected on a routine chest X-ray.

During the physical examination, and with laboratory as well as imaging studies, the physician notes changes to the lungs, skin, heart, liver, and eyes. The chest X-ray finding is abnormal in 90 percent of patients with sarcoidosis. An ophthalmologic examination reveals eye changes that have been caused by sarcoidosis.

Sarcoidosis is definitively diagnosed with a biopsy. Chest X-rays are also indirectly needed for diagnosis. Tuberculosis and fungal infections should be excluded as part of the diagnosis.

Treatment Options and Outlook

Patients who have few or no symptoms do not require any treatment. Most symptomatic patients with widespread involvement, including of the heart, brain, and eyes, as well as those who have hypercalcemia and respiratory problems, are treated with corticosteroid drugs such as prednisone. Some patients who are not responding to prednisone are treated with methotrexate. Some patients, especially those who have disfiguring skin conditions, are treated with antimalarial agents such as hydroxychloroquine.

Some sarcoidosis patients are very ill and may require lung or heart transplantation.

Risk Factors and Preventive Measures

Most people diagnosed with sarcoidosis are younger than age 40. The disease is more commonly found among American blacks, and to a lesser extent, among northern Europeans. In the United States, the incidence is about 35.5 per 100,000 blacks. Among whites in the United States, the incidence is about 10.9 per 100,000. Experts estimate the lifetime risk of sarcoidosis for blacks at 2.4 percent and at less than 1 percent (0.85) percent for whites. The symptoms are also often more severe among blacks who have the disease, There are no known gender differences in the incidence of sarcoidosis.

There appears to be a genetic risk for the disease because sarcoidosis occurs more commonly in identical twins than in fraternal twins. In addition, family members of people who have sarcoidosis have a higher risk of development of the disease. There appear to be racial disparities among people who are at risk for development of sarcoidosis; for example, when sarcoidosis is identified in a black family, as many as 19 percent of other members are diagnosed with the disease. When it is found in a white family, only about 5 percent of other members have sarcoidosis.

There are no known preventive measures.

Schilling test A laboratory test used for detecting a cobalamin (vitamin B_{12}) deficiency that is caused by the decreased absorption of this vitamin, as seen in PERNICIOUS ANEMIA and in MALABSORPTION SYNDROME. The test is performed by oral administration of radiolabeled cyano-cobalamin followed by an intramuscular injection of cobalamin. A 24-hour urine sample is then collected. A low percent excretion of radiolabeled cobalamin suggests cobalamin malabsorption, due to pernicious anemia or other causes of intestinal malabsorption.

If this stage of the test is abnormal, further stages of the test are performed to precisely define the cause of B_{12} deficiency; for example, to distinguish from intrinsic factor deficiency due to pernicious anemia from intestinal malabsorption. The Schilling Test is not available in most centers in the United States.

scleroderma A condition that affects the connective tissues as well as the nerves and muscles, causing a hardening and tightening of the skin and affecting the digestive system as well. It may cause difficulty in swallowing (DYSPHAGIA), large diverticula (pockets in the small intestine and the COLON), slow gut movements leading to CONSTIPATION, and other medical problems. Scleroderma can affect organs throughout the body. For example, it can impair the ESOPHAGUS, causing not only dysphagia but also GASTROESOPHAGEAL REFLUX DISEASE

(GERD). Some scientists estimate that as many as 165,000 people in the United States have systemic scleroderma.

The disease can also cause swollen puffy skin as well as contractures of the hands, wrists, and elbows. Men who have scleroderma may experience erectile dysfunction.

Scleroderma may be an autoimmune disorder, although researchers are not certain of the cause of this condition. There is a complex yet poorly understood interplay among immunological events, fibrogenic fibroblast cells, and the blood vessels in various parts of the body.

Symptoms and Diagnostic Path
The most common sign is thick and hardened skin, particularly on the face. Sometimes cosmetics can conceal scleroderma. Patients may have limited skin involvement restricted to the hands, and to a lesser extent, the face and neck. Others may have involvement of different organs in the body such as heart, lungs, kidneys, joints, etc.

A scleroderma diagnosis is based on the signs and symptoms of the patient, in addition to the results of blood and imaging studies.

Treatment Options and Outlook
The symptoms are treated by physicians who are specialists in the field; for example, gastroenterologists treat dysphagia, GERD, GASTROPARESIS, intestinal pseudoobstruction, constipation, and fecal incontinence, and rheumatologists treat problems with the joints or muscles. A dermatologist may be consulted for skin problems. Scleroderma can also affect the heart and kidneys, and thus, referrals to a cardiologist and nephrologist may also be needed.

Scleroderma patients who have gastrointestinal problems are often advised to eat small and frequent meals and to avoid fatty foods. They are also advised to raise the head of their bed to prevent the problems associated with gastroesophageal reflux disease. Patients may need ANTIBIOTICS to treat small-intestine bacterial overgrowths that cause DIARRHEA and MALABSORPTION SYNDROME.

Risk Factors and Preventive Measures
Scleroderma is much more commonly found among women than among men; women have

scleroderma at about seven to 12 times the rate of men, according to the National Institutes of Health. It is more commonly found among people of European descent and is found infrequently among African Americans. There are no known preventive measures.

See also ACID REFLUX; CREST SYNDROME; DIVERTICULOSIS; PRIMARY BILIARY CIRRHOSIS; SKIN DISEASES AND DIGESTIVE SYSTEM.

secretin   A natural hormone that causes the release of pancreatic juice. In physiologic doses, this hormone also inhibits stomach acidity and motility. In pharmacologic doses, secretin increases gastrointestinal motility as well as bile flow to the intestines.

Secretin has also been artificially synthesized and is used in some procedures done on patients for digestive problems. It is used for the diagnosis of PANCREATIC INSUFFICIENCY as well as of a pancreatic tumor that is known as gastrinoma or ZOLLINGER–ELLISON SYNDROME.

At one point, parents of children who had autism, a severe psychiatric disorder, believed that infusions of secretin would improve the children's condition. This belief was based on anecdotal findings that some autistic children improved after abdominal surgery in which secretin was used by physicians. Subsequent studies have proved that secretin is neither a cure nor a treatment for children or adults who have autism.

Sandler, Adrian D., M.D., et al. "Lack of Benefit of a Single Dose of Synthetic Human Secretin in the Treatment of Autism and Pervasive Development Disorder." *New England Journal of Medicine* 341, no. 24 (December 9, 1999): 1,801–1,806.

selenium   A trace mineral in the human body that is also an antioxidant (cancer fighter). Epidemiologic data suggests a beneficial role for selenium in reducing cancer mortality. Selenium is needed for healthy functioning of the thyroid gland and the immune system. Selenium is found in the soil and has a high concentration in northern Nebraska and North and South Dakota, where many residents have the highest concentrations of selenium in

the United States. For adults, the recommended requirement of selenium is 70 micrograms per day for men and 55 micrograms per day for women.

Foods that are rich in selenium include the following:

- Brazil nuts
- canned tuna
- beef or calf liver
- cod cooked in dry heat
- enriched boiled noodles
- oven-roasted turkey breast
- enriched elbow macaroni
- spaghetti with meat sauce

Deficiency of Selenium

Most people in the United States and Canada are not deficient in selenium. In some parts of China and Russia, selenium deficiency is very common. There are no obvious specific symptoms or signs of a selenium deficiency; however, such a deficiency can be detected by a blood test for selenium levels.

Patients who are deficient in selenium may have arthritis, decreased immune function, heart failure, and increased susceptibility to cancer. In China, patients deficient in selenium may have Keshan disease, which causes cardiac dysfunction. It can be prevented but not cured by selenium supplements. There is a direct correlation between selenium deficiency and a reduction in CD4 cell counts (the lower the count, the lower the immune function) in patients infected with the human immunodeficiency virus (HIV).

Other people who are at risk for development of a selenium deficiency include the following categories of individuals:

- People relying solely on intravenous (IV) nutrition because their digestive system is malfunctioning (selenium can be added to the IV drip). Newer trace-element solutions for total parenteral nutrition (TPN) contain selenium
- People who have had serious gastrointestinal surgery, such as having half or more of their small intestine removed
- People who have Crohn's disease

Excessive Levels of Selenium

It is also possible to have too much selenium in the body. Selonisis occurs when selenium is consumed in high doses of greater than 900 micrograms per day. This condition is extremely rare, and the only reported cases have occurred in people who were taking selenium supplements that included an excessive level of selenium, the result of a mistake by the selenium seller. The Institute of Medicine has reported that the maximal amount of selenium that any adult should take is 400 micrograms per day; the usual supplemental dose is fifty to 200 micrograms per day.

The key symptoms of selenium excess are as follows:

- hair loss
- skin rash
- gastrointestinal upset
- mild nerve damage
- white blotchy fingernails
- altered mental status

See also ALTERNATIVE MEDICINE; ANTIOXIDANTS.

Shigella Common bacteria that cause DYSENTERY in humans worldwide. In the United States alone, there are about 14,000 cases of shigellosis (infection with *Shigella* organisms) diagnosed each year, according to the Centers for Disease Control and Prevention (CDC), but it is anticipated that there may actually be as many as 280,000 and as high as 450,000 actual case of shigellosis that occur each year in United States. There is a high risk of outbreaks of shigellosis in some facilities, such as day care centers and psychiatric institutions.

The bacteria may be spread by person-to-person contact or in contaminated food prepared by food workers who did not wash their hands after using the toilet. The bacteria can also be spread through other means, such as swimming in a pool or lake contaminated by the bacteria passed through fecal contamination or by drinking contaminated water. The most common form of *Shigella* bacteria in the United States, Canada, and other developed countries is *Shigella sonnei*, which is also written as

S. sonnei. This form of *Shigella* is responsible for an estimated over two-thirds of all shigellosis, according to the division of food-borne, bacterial, and mycotic diseases section of the Centers for Disease Control and Prevention (CDC). According to the CDC, *Shigella flexeneri* is responsible for nearly all other infections with *Shigella*.

Symptoms and Diagnostic Path

The severity of symptoms varies and some people have no symptoms. Symptoms usually occur from one to seven days after the person is infected; once they have begun, symptoms may last as long as five to seven days. The most common symptoms of shigellosis are as follows:

- fever
- bloody or watery DIARRHEA (about 10 stools, but there may be as many as 100 or more per day although of small volume)
- NAUSEA AND VOMITING
- ABDOMINAL PAIN

Children younger than two years with shigellois may have seizures with high fevers. In addition, young girls may develop vaginitis or vulvovaginitis with or without diarrhea.

Rarely, hemolytic-uremic syndrome may occur especially in infants and young children and result in renal failure.

Shigella infection is usually suspected because of a patient's symptoms. The diagnosis is confirmed with the results of stool tests. The illness resolves in about seven days in most cases; thus, doctors may just advise certain adult patients to wait for the body to recover on its own.

Treatment Options and Outlook

Physicians prescribe ANTIBIOTICS for patients with severe symptoms, as well as for food handlers, health-care workers, ELDERLY people, and immune-suppressed individuals, kids in day-care, and those requiring hospitalization for severe symptoms. Antibiotics such as trimethoprim sulfamethoxazole (Bactrim) or ciprofloxacin (Cipro) may be prescribed in adults. Treatment of mild cases in case of kids who have recovered is controversial, while symptomatic cases are usually treated as soon as disease is suspected.

Most people recover completely from a *Shigella* infection; however, some individuals have bowel problems for months afterward. Shigellosis may cause severe complications such as proctitis (inflammation of the rectum), bowel obstruction or perforation, bacteremia (bacterial spread to the blood), MALNUTRITION, DEHYDRATION, and seizures. In some cases, these complications may be life-threatening.

In other cases, such as with infection with *S. fiexneri*, the condition may worsen and reactive arthritis also known as Reiter's syndrome, a medical problem that may lead to chronic arthritis and to painful urination (urethritis) may develop.

Risk Factors and Preventive Measures

Small children are at risk for shigellosis. In addition, men having sex with other men have an increased risk for shigellosis flexneri.

To prevent *Shigella* infection, the following steps are recommended:

- Individuals should drink only water that they know is safe. Any unreliable water should be chlorinated.
- Anyone who prepares food should wash the hands with soap after using the toilet or changing a baby's diapers.
- People who prepare food should wash their hands with soap before preparing food (even if they have not just used the toilet).
- Strict refrigeration and proper cooking of food are important.
- Children should be trained to wash their hands after using the toilet, to lower the risk of their spreading disease to themselves and others.
- Swimmers should avoid swallowing swimming pool, pond, or lake water, which may be contaminated with *Shigella* organisms.

The spread may be controlled in school or day care by eliminating water play areas.

Patients with active *Shigella* infection and employed in daycare setting should refrain from going to work until the diarrhea is resolved and stool cultures are negative.

See also CONTAMINATED FOOD OR WATER; PARASITIC INFECTIONS; TRAVEL.

Division of Foodborne, Bacterial and Mycotic Diseases. *Shigellosis.* Available online. URL: http://www.cdc. gov/nczved/dfbmd/disease_listing/shigellosis_gi.html. Downloaded June 13, 2008.
Keene, William E., et al. "A Swimming-Associated Outbreak of Hemorrhagic Colitis Caused by *Escherichia coli* O157:H7 and *Shigella sonnei.*" *New England Journal of Medicine* 331, no. 9 (September 1, 1994): 579–584.

short bowel syndrome   A malabsorption condition in which the patient has difficulty absorbing nutrients after a large part of the small intestine has been removed as a treatment for CROHN'S DISEASE, CANCER, enterocolitis, or other medical conditions. It is also known as short gut syndrome.

Some signs and symptoms of short bowel syndrome are diarrhea, unintended weight loss, and weakness. Patients who have extensive short bowel removal need PARENTERAL NUTRITION. Small intestinal transplantation is an option, especially for patients who are not candidates for receiving long-term parenteral nutrition.

sigmoidoscopy   A procedure in which the rectum and the lower part of the colon is internally examined with a sigmoidoscope. A sigmoidoscope is a flexible tube, measuring about 65 centimeters. This procedure is performed to detect the presence of colorectal cancer, POLYPS, and other diseases and abnormalities. The procedure is usually performed after the rectum and lower colon have been evacuated with a couple of enemas given about 30 minutes to an hour before the procedure. Whereas sigmoidoscopy examines only a part of a colon, COLONOSCOPY, a much more comprehensive procedure, inspects the entire colon. It is an outpatient procedure and sedatives are usually not administered.

See also COLORECTAL CANCER.

skin diseases and digestive system   Some skin disorders and infections can cause minor or long-standing harm to the digestive system; for example, staphylococcal infection can cause nausea and vomiting and may worsen in rare cases. CELIAC SPRUE is associated with dermatitis herpetiformis; hyperpigmentation of skin is seen in WHIPPLE'S DISEASE. Pemphigus vulgaris may involve the esophagus, causing dysphagia (difficulty in swallowing food) and odynophagia (painful swallowing). Pyoderma gangrenosum and erythema nodosum may be seen in INFLAMMATORY BOWEL DISEASE. HEPATITIS C is associated with porphyria cutanea tarda and mixed CRYOGLOBULINEMIA.

See also SCLERODERMA; *STAPHYLOCOCCUS.*

sleep A period of unconsciousness during which the body relaxes, dreams, and replenishes itself. Sleep is important for the individual's overall well-being. A lack of sleep can moderately or severely affect digestion, as well as affecting other body processes.

Sometimes medical problems prevent sleep or impair an individual from obtaining sufficient sleep; for example, individuals who have GASTROESOPHAGEAL REFLUX DISEASE may have troubled sleep. Pain and irritation due to ulcers or DIARRHEA caused by INFLAMMATORY BOWEL DISEASE may waken a person in the middle of the night, thus preventing or impairing normal sleep. Sleep patterns are also often disturbed among IRRITABLE BOWEL SYNDROME (IBS) patients.

See also ULCERS, PEPTIC.

small intestine A key organ in the digestive system, where most of the digestion and absorption of nutrients and fluids occur. The small intestine starts at the pylorus and includes the duodenum, the jejunum, and the ileum. It ends at the ileocecal valve, where the ileum opens into the cecum, the first part of the large intestine (colon).

small intestine cancer Malignancy of the small intestine, also known as the small bowel. The small intestine connects the stomach to the large intestine. According to the National Cancer Institute, there are five types of cancers that may occur in the small intestine, including adenocarcinoma, sarcoma, carcinoid tumors, gastrointestinal stromal tumors, and lymphomas. In recent years, carcinoids have surpassed adenocarcinomas as being the most commonly occurring small intestinal malignancy. Adenocarcinoma is a cancer that originates in the glandular cells of the small intestine that secrete a variety of substances. These cells do not need to be part of a gland, as long as they have secretory functions. The word *sarcoma* is derived from the Greek word *sarx*, which means "flesh"). It is a cancer of the connective or supportive tissue as well as the soft tissues

Sarcoma is a cancer that has its onset in the connective tissue of the small intestine. A carcinoid tumor is a slow-growing form of cancer. A gastrointestinal stromal tumor is a form of soft tissue sarcoma. Lymphoma is a cancer that originates in the immune system cells.

Small intestine cancer is rare, and according to the National Cancer Institute, there were an estimated 6,100 new cases in the United States in 2008 and 1,110 deaths. In contrast, the cancer of colon is much more prevalent. The discrepancy has been attributed to liquid stool and a lower bacterial load in the small intestine along with the rapid transit of intestinal contents through the small intestine into the colon.

According to federal data on cancer statistics from the Surveillance Epidemiology and End Results (SEER) organization, the median age of diagnosis for small intestine cancer was 67 years over the period 2001 to 2005, and the median age of death from this form of cancer was 71 years.

Symptoms and Diagnostic Path
Some possible symptoms and signs of cancer of the small intestine may include the following:

- unintentional weight loss
- blood in the feces
- middle abdominal pain or cramps
- a lump in the abdomen

If the physician suspects that any form of small intestine cancer may be present, he or she will perform a physical examination and take a medical history. Laboratory tests may help reveal if there is a potential problem. Other tests such as computerized tomography (CDT) scan of the abdomen may be performed, as may an upper ENDOSCOPY, small bowel enteroscopy, or ileoscopy which can enable the doctor to visualize the small intestine and get biopsy tissue sample. Small bowel enteroscopy helps visualize areas of small bowel beyond the reach of EGD. More recently, single- and double-balloon enteroscopy have emerged as tests to visualize the small bowel in its entirety. Capsule endoscopy involves swallowing a capsule type device fitted with a camera and takes tens of thousands of images over several hours and helps visualize small bowel without an endoscopy. A lymph node biopsy may be performed.

The doctor may also perform a laparoscopy or exploratory laporotomy, which allows the doctor to check for disease and also to obtain tissue to be biopsied for cancer. Resection may be done based on diagnosis.

Treatment Options and Outlook

As with most forms of cancer, treatment usually includes the surgical removal of the malignancy, and it may also include chemo-radiation therapy depending on type and characteristic of the cancer. If the cancer has spread to other parts of the body, the patient may be treated with chemotherapy, which involves drugs that are specifically designed to destroy the cancer. Sometimes radiation therapy is used to help control pain.

The outlook depends on the type of cancer that is identified and whether it has metastasized (spread) to other parts of the body; for example, if the cancer has spread, the prognosis is poorer than if the cancer is localized. In addition, the outlook depends on whether the cancer can be removed completely with surgery, as well as whether the cancer is newly diagnosed or a recurring malignancy. The outlook may be more positive with newly diagnosed cancer although recurrent cancer may also be treatable, depending on the particular case and its circumstances.

Risk Factors and Preventive Measures

Some individuals have a higher risk for the development of small intestine cancer than others; for example, individuals with CROHN'S DISEASE

TABLE: INCIDENCE OF SMALL INTESTINE CANCER IN THE UNITED STATES BY RACE AND GENDER, 2001–2005

Race/Ethnicity	Male	Female
All Races	2.2 per 100,000 men	1.6 per 100,000 women
White	2.1 per 100,000 men	1.5 per 100,000 women
Black	3.8 per 100,000 men	2.7 per 100,000 women
Asian/Pacific Islander	1.4 per 100,000 men	0.7 per 100,000 women
Hispanic	1.6 per 100,000 men	1.1 per 100,000 women

Adapted from Cancer, Small Intestine, Surveillance Epidemiology and End Results. Available online. URL: http://seer.cancer.gov/statfacts.html/smint.html. Downloaded January 29, 2009.

OR CELIAC DISEASE have a higher risk for developing small intestine cancer. In addition, those with familial adenoma polyposis (FAP) have an increased risk, compared to others. A high-fat diet also increases the risk for cancer of the small intestine. Other factors implicated as risk factors include alcoholism and increased intake of red and processed meats. Data is conflicting in regard to role of SMOKING and obesity.

In considering demographic factors, according to SEER, males have a higher incidence for small intestine cancer than females, particularly black males and females. (Incidence refers to newly diagnosed cases in a year.) For example, among black males, 3.8 men of every 100,000 black males develop small intestine cancer, compared to all races of 2.2 men per 100,000. In the case of black females, 2.7 per 100,000 women develop the disease, compared to 1.6 per 100,000 women of all races and ethnicities. Asians and Pacific Islanders have the lowest risk for developing this form of cancer among all ethnicities and racial groups. (See table.)

The five-year survival rate from small intestine cancer was 57.8 percent for all individuals, based on SEER data for the period 1996 to 2004. When considering both race and gender, the survival rates were as follows: 59.2 percent for white males, 60.3 percent for white females, 48.2 percent for black males, and 53.7 percent for black females.

smoking Inhalation of tobacco smoke, usually through cigarettes, but also through cigars or pipes. Smoking is extremely harmful to the body over the long term. Many people start smoking as adolescents because their friends smoke and/or they think smoking impresses others. Then they become addicted to the nicotine in tobacco and find stopping smoking extremely difficult. According to the National Center for Health Statistics, 80 percent of all smokers smoke every day.

Whereas smoking was once believed to enhance digestion, researchers have subsequently discovered that smoking seriously impedes digestion, and this habit can also cause many chronic and long-term serious digestive diseases and cancers. The Centers for Disease Control and Prevention (CDC) estimates that about 440,000 deaths in the United States each year can be directly attributed to smoking.

Risk Factors for Smokers

According to a report that was released by the National Center for Health Statistics in 2003 on cigarette smoking among adults in 1997–98, about 24 percent of all adults who are 18 and older in the United States are smokers. Men are slightly more likely to smoke than women: about 28 percent of men in the United States smoke, versus 22 percent of women.

In considering racial differences among those who smoke, about 25 percent of white adults smoke and about 26 percent of black non Hispanics do. Among Hispanic adults, about 19 percent are smokers. Asians and Pacific Islanders are the least likely to smoke: about 14 percent are smokers.

Marital status also has an impact on whether people smoke: for example, 21 percent of married adults in the United States smoke, versus 36 percent of adults who are either divorced or separated and 40 percent of adults who live with a partner to whom they are not married.

Generally, smokers are less educated than non-smokers, and the incidence of cigarette smoking steadily declines with education. About 34 percent of adults who have less than a high school diploma smoke, compared to only 8 percent with a master's degree, doctorate, or medical degree. Among women, about 30 percent with less than a high school diploma smoke, compared to about 8 percent who have an advanced degree.

An individual's income level is also directly related to whether he or she smokes. Men with an income below the poverty level are nearly twice as likely to smoke (38 percent) as men in the highest-income group (20 percent). Income clearly affects whether women smoke as well: about 31 percent of women with income below the poverty level smoke, compared to 16 percent at the highest income level.

Health Problems Caused or Worsened by Smoking

A large number of cases of oral and lung cancer are attributable to smoking. Smoking is also linked to anal cancer, bladder cancer, esophageal cancer, pancreatic cancer, and cervical cancer. It may also contribute to colorectal cancer and kidney cancer.

Smoking does not cause DIABETES MELLITUS, but it makes controlling the disease much more difficult. Smoking also worsens GASTROPARESIS, or slowed stomach emptying. Smoking increases the risk for development of cardiovascular disease. In addition, healing in CROHN'S DISEASE patients is difficult for those who continue to smoke.

The harmful effects of active smoking (smoking by an individual) can also be documented in cases of passive smoking (being in the presence of another person who smokes). Paradoxically, however, smoking apparently has a preventive or beneficial effect on ULCERATIVE COLITIS. In fact, when used as a medication, nicotine has been shown to be of therapeutic benefit in this disorder.

Smoking Cessation Methods

Physicians urge their patients to stop smoking immediately, regardless of their health status. It is even more imperative for ill patients to stop smoking. Some patients are successful with nicotine replacement drugs, in the form of oral tablets and skin patches. Nasal sprays and inhalers are being tested. The goal is to start at one dose of nicotine and gradually taper. The risk of complications is higher if the patient continues to smoke while also using nicotine patches.

Some patients use bupropion (Zyban), a drug that helps suppress the desire for nicotine in some individuals. Alternative methods of quitting smoking include acupuncture and hypnotherapy.

A major problem that many smokers face, in addition to their own addiction, is that they may associate frequently with other smokers among their family members and friends. These other individuals may refrain from urging the smoker to continue smoking, but when he or she observes constant smoking, quitting becomes much more difficult. In addition, many smokers associate certain cues with smoking, such as smoking after a meal. Asking to be seated in the nonsmoking section of a restaurant may help to break that association, and choosing to eat at a different time or changing the place at home where the food is consumed may help extinguish other smoking cues.

See also ANAL CANCER; ESOPHAGEAL CANCER; ORAL CANCER; PANCREATIC CANCER.

Blackwell, D. L., J. G. Collins, and R. Coles. "Summary Health Statistics for U.S. Adults: National Health Interview Survey, 1997." National Center for Health Statistics. *Vital Health Statistics* 10, no. 205 (2002).

Schoenborn, Charlotte A., Jackline A. Vickerie, and Patricia M. Barnes. Division of Health Interview Statistics. "Cigarette Smoking Behavior of Adults: United States, 1997–1998." *Advance Data from Vital and Health Statistics* no. 331 (February 7, 2003).

sphincter   Specialized muscle tissue that allows for opening and closing. The lower esophageal sphincter is a muscle that allows opening between the esophagus and the stomach. There is also a sphincter between the stomach and duodenum (the pyloric sphincter or just the pylorus). The sphincter of Oddi involves the confluence of the common bile duct and the pancreatic duct as they enter the wall of the duodenum. An anal sphincter, which is made up of internal and external anal components, allows regulation of defecation.

Staphylococcus   Ubiquitous bacteria that are even found on the skin and anterior nares of healthy adults, it may be spread in food by preparers who fail to wash their hands. "Staph" infections can cause severe nausea and vomiting and abdominal cramps within one to six hours of consuming infected food. Fever and diarrhea may also occur in a small number of cases. In most cases of *Staphylococcus* infection, patients recover within two to three days.

Staphylococcus infections can be prevented by infected people's washing their hands before preparing food. Since most people infected with *Staphylococcus* bacteria do not know that they are infected, everyone should wash their hands before food preparation, to be on the safe side.

It should also be noted that *Staphylococcus* infections can occur in the blood (bacteremia), the heart (endocarditis), and prosthetic joints. Staphylococcal scalding skin syndrome is a deadly disease, which is treated with methicillin or vancomycin. Another severe illness that is caused by *Staphylococcus* bacteria is staphylococcal toxic shock syndrome.

See also CONTAMINATED FOOD OR WATER; SKIN DISEASES AND DIGESTIVE SYSTEM.

steatorrhea   High levels of fat that are found in the stool due to malabsorption, which may indicate the presence of a disease, such as chronic PANCREATITIS, CELIAC SPRUE, WHIPPLE'S DISEASE, small intestinal bacterial overgrowth, or ZOLLINGER-ELLISON SYNDROME.

steroids   Drugs that are prescribed for some illnesses characterized by excessive or uncontrolled inflammation, such as CROHN'S DISEASE, ULCERATIVE COLITIS, autoimmune hepatitis, and rheumatoid arthritis. They can also be used in the form of enemas, topical ointments and creams to treat such problems as colitis, hemorrhoids, pruritus ani and anal FISSURES. The long-term use of steroids has serious side effects, including a change in the body shape and structure (such as the development of a plump and moonlike face), osteoporosis, DIABETES MELLITUS, and immunosuppression. Thus, physicians taper the dose of the steroid to the lowest possible level as soon as possible, since the side effects are both dose- and duration-related. Steroids are also synthesized inside the body. Some people take steroids for body-building reason; this is not medically advisable because of negative consequences.

stomach   Key organ of the digestive system, lying between the esophagus and the small intestine. Digestion of proteins begins in the stomach. The stomach breaks food down into small particles about one to two millimeters in size before allowing them to proceed to the small intestine for further digestion and absorption. Hydrochloric acid produced in the stomach kills many infectious organisms that are consumed with food. There are a wide variety of diseases and disorders that can occur in the stomach, such as ulcers, CANCER, and GASTROPARESIS (slow stomach emptying).

See also STOMACH CANCER; ULCERS, PEPTIC.

stomach cancer   A malignancy that is found in the stomach, a major organ of the digestive system. It is also known as gastric cancer. Most stomach cancers are adenocarcinomas. According to the National Cancer Institute, 21,500 new cases of stomach cancer were diagnosed in 2008 in the United States, and there were an estimated 10,800 deaths from stomach cancer in the United States in 2008.

Early gastric cancer is diagnosed when the cancer remains within the superficial layers of the stomach wall. Advanced gastric cancer is cancer that has spread deep beyond the stomach's submucosal layer. Most people in North America (80 to 95 percent) who are diagnosed with stomach cancer have advanced gastric cancer. However, in contrast, about 30 percent of Japanese people who are diagnosed with gastric cancer have early gastric cancer. The difference occurs because Japanese undergo screening for gastric cancer on a regular basis, whereas it is not done in the United States because of the low incidence.

Some studies indicate that the common stomach bacterium *Helicobacter pylori* may be implicated in some cases of gastric cancer because some clinical studies have demonstrated that people who are infected with *H. pylori* have two to six times the risk of development of stomach cancer than do others. *H. pylori* is the same bacterium that causes most peptic ULCERS.

A study of 1,246 Japanese patients with *H. pylori* and 280 patients who were *not* infected was reported in a 2001 issue of the *New England Journal of Medicine*. All of the subjects had duodenal ulcers, gastric ulcers, or other stomach problems. In about 3 percent of the *H. pylori* group stomach cancer developed, but it developed in none of the uninfected persons in the control group. As a result, researchers concluded that *H. pylori* was implicated in gastric cancer.

Symptoms and Diagnostic Path
Patients who have stomach cancer may have a few nonspecific or no symptoms in the early stages. If symptoms do occur, they may be vague or easily ignored by the patient, and sometimes by the physician. Some symptoms that may occur with stomach cancer are the following:

- abdominal pain or discomfort
- weight loss
- chronic indigestion or HEARTBURN
- NAUSEA AND VOMITING
- ulcer-like pain
- CONSTIPATION OR DIARRHEA
- extremely bloated feeling after eating
- appetite loss
- gastrointestinal BLEEDING
- DYSPHAGIA (difficulty in swallowing)
- early satiety (sensation of being very full soon after starting to eat)
- excessive BELCHING
- weakness and fatigue
- vomiting of blood or presence of blood in the stool

Important note: not everyone who has these symptoms has stomach cancer; such symptoms may indicate a temporary gastric problem or another health problem altogether. However, people with such symptoms should consult their physician for a complete physical examination and should also have any diagnostic tests that the doctor recommends.

An upper gastrointestinal X-ray of both the ESOPHAGUS (the food tube leading to the stomach) and the stomach can help by highlighting the stomach to detect possible tumors. The patient swallows liquid barium (which tastes like chalk), so that the stomach and esophagus can be seen on a fluoroscope and any serious abnormalities can often be detected.

An ENDOSCOPY is another procedure in which a special tube is passed through the mouth and into the esophagus and then the stomach. Using this device, the doctor can see inside the stomach and can remove tissue for biopsy. The endoscopy is preferred to the upper gastrointestinal (GI) X-ray test because the doctor can obtain a biopsy specimen with the endoscopy. If cancer is present, a biopsy (removal of tissue for examination by a pathologist) also helps the doctor to determine how aggressive the cancer is at the time of the biopsy. Staging of the tumor is important because it helps the doctor determine the treatment to recommend. A chest X-ray or preferably chest CT scan plus an abdominal CT scan are usually done as part of staging and treatment planning. Endoscopic ultrasound may help in select cases. A preoperative staging laparoscopy is recommended in many patients. The role of the positron emission tomography (PET) scan is evolving with gastric cancer.

Most countries, including the United States, rely on the Tumor-Node-Metastasis (TNM) system of staging all forms of cancer. This system uses various tests and parameters to evaluate the depth of the tumor invasion into the stomach wall (T), whether it has advanced into the lymph nodes (the N part of the TNM system), and whether it has spread beyond the stomach, or metastasized ($M0$ or $M1$).

Routine screening for stomach cancer is not recommended in the United States. Periodic upper endoscopy (EGD) can be offered to patients who are at higher risk for gastric cancer.

Treatment Options and Outlook

Patients with stomach cancer may be treated with surgery, chemotherapy, and radiation treatment.

Surgery The most common form of treatment for stomach cancer is surgery, in which the surgeon removes all or part of the stomach (a gastrectomy or partial gastrectomy). At least 80 percent of patients have an advanced case of stomach cancer at the time of diagnosis, and curative surgery is not indicated in those cases; however, palliative surgery (surgery that is performed not to cure the patient, but to alleviate the symptoms) may be done to relieve obstructions.

A gastrectomy is a major operation. Patients may need to change their diet considerably and permanently after the surgery. Patients who have had total gastrectomy often also need injections of vitamin B_{12} because they can no longer absorb the vitamin naturally through the food that they eat.

Some patients who have had gastric surgery may experience DUMPING SYNDROME, a condition that occurs when the food enters the small intestine too quickly. The primary symptoms of dumping syndrome are weakness, dizziness, palpitations, sweating, cramps, nausea, as well as vomiting that occurs shortly after eating. Chronic diarrhea is another complication experienced by patients who have had a gastrectomy. Eating smaller and more frequent meals may help resolve this problem, as well as avoiding foods high in sugar content.

Some patients with early gastric cancer may benefit from endoscopic mucosal resection (removal of tumor during endoscopy) rather than undergoing gastrectomy.

Chemotherapy Another treatment option for some forms of stomach cancer is chemotherapy. Cancer-killing drugs for stomach cancer patients may be administered in oral form or by injection, depending on the particular patient and the treatment regimen. Chemotherapy may cause NAUSEA AND VOMITING, as well as hair loss, which side effects usually end when the chemotherapy is completed.

Radiation therapy RADIATION THERAPY is another treatment for some cases of stomach cancer. High-energy rays are directed at the cancerous part of the body. An appropriate time frame for radiation therapy is best determined by the radiation oncologist (the cancer radiotherapy doctor). Radiation therapy patients may experience nausea and vomiting, and the irradiated area may become reddened and sore. Patients receiving radiation therapy may also be very fatigued and have diarrhea.

Risk Factors and Preventive Measures

Age is a key risk factor, and most stomach cancer patients are older than age 50. Gender is another risk factor: Most stomach cancer victims are male in a ratio of about 1.7 males to 1.0 female. Race is also a risk factor for stomach cancer: African Americans have about a 1.5 higher risk of development of stomach cancer than whites. There may also be a genetic risk involved in stomach cancer, although research continues on that subject to identify the chromosomal location of the gene that triggers stomach cancer; however, it is known that those with a family history of stomach cancer have a two to three times greater risk of development of stomach cancer. The emperor Napoleon, his father, and his grandfather all died of gastric cancer.

The risk for stomach cancer is increased two- to threefold among patients who have PERNICIOUS ANEMIA; in a small fraction of these patients stomach cancer will develop.

The use of tobacco increases the risk of the development of gastric cancer, and tobacco users have a 1.5 to three times greater risk of development of stomach cancer than nonusers.

Other risk factors include the following:

* presence of MÉNÉTRIER'S DISEASE
* individuals with Type A blood
* those with deficiencies of vitamins A, C, E, beta-carotene; SELENIUM; or FIBER
* people who eat diets that are rich in fava beans as well as heavy consumption of salted, pickled, or smoked foods; dried fish; and cooking oil (Note: a diet rich in fiber, milk, fresh fruits especially citrus, and vegetables leads to a *decreased* risk for stomach cancer). Cooked vegetables are not as beneficial as uncooked vegetables.
* individuals with a low socioeconomic status
* individuals who have had gastric POLYPS in the past
* patients who have had stomach surgery
* patients with *H. pylori* infection
* *SMOKING*
* Epstein-Barr virus

Preventive measures against stomach cancer include immediately ending a smoking habit.

Mayne, Susan T., et al. "Nutrient Intake and Risk of Subtypes of Esophageal and Gastric Cancer," *Cancer Epidemiology, Biomarkers Prevention* 10 (October 2001): 1,055–1,062.

Uemura, Naomi, M.D., et al. "*Helicobacter Pylori* Infection and the Development of Gastric Cancer." *New England Journal of Medicine* 345, no. 11 (September 13, 2001): 784–789.

stress Emotional or psychological strain. Stress can greatly affect digestion, slowing it down. Some people who are under stress may have diarrhea. In addition, people who are experiencing severe stress often engage in either overeating, which may lead to obesity, or undereating. Often stress does not cause diseases (such as GASTRO-ESOPHAGEAL REFLUX DISEASE, ulcers, or many other digestive disorders) but considerably exacerbates already-existing ailments. Relaxation therapy or hypnotherapy may be helpful to alleviate stress. Some patients improve with psychotherapy. Therapists should understand that the painful condition may improve but may not completely resolve with therapy alone.

Another form of stress is the physical stress of a severe illness that occurs among patients who are admitted to the intensive care units of hospitals, such as patients who have a serious head injury, severe burns, and so forth. In such cases, ulcers in the stomach may occur, and they may bleed. Such stress-induced ulcers can be prevented by use of acid blocking medications (such as ranitidine [Zantac] or famotidine [Pepcid]) by individuals who are at high risk for development of such ulcers.

See also ULCERS, PEPTIC.

stricture An abnormal narrowing of the lumen in the hollow tube of the digestive system. It is also called stenosis especially when the narrowing involves the junction of two different parts of the digestive tube; for example, pyloric stenosis is a narrowing of the pylorus between the stomach and the duodenum. In the esophagus a stricture may develop as a result of long-standing ACID REFLUX, and this stricture may cause difficulty with swallowing. A stricture may develop in the intestines as a result of CROHN'S DISEASE or RADIATION THERAPY.

Strictures may be minor and asymptomatic or may cause pain and even completely block the hollow tube of the digestive tract. Strictures can be treated by dilation during endoscopy or by surgery called stricturoplasty. In another surgical option the narrowed segment is excised and the normal lumens are hooked back at both ends.

taste impairments Difficulties or inabilities to taste normal flavors. A total loss of taste (ageusia) is rare. Taste is important for enjoying food, but it is also a gatekeeper to what is consumed. It is also a protective factor in some cases; for example, spoiled food or milk tastes unpleasant, and thus, people who have normal taste capacity do not eat or drink it.

Hypogeusia is a below-average ability to detect tastes. It may be caused by illness or by medications. Dysgeusia is taste distortion or phantom taste (tasting of something that is not present). Aliageusia is an unpleasant taste of food or fluids that are normally pleasant.

Aging affects the sensation of taste, and many ELDERLY people have impaired ability to taste, which may affect their appetite and even cause weight loss. Other causes of taste dysfunctions are infections, ACID REFLUX, gastritis, and exposure to chemicals such as mercury, copper, zinc, chromium, and lead. Some medications can affect the ability to taste such as the antibacterial drug ciprofloxacin (Cipro) and some blood pressure and chemotherapy drugs. Lithium can cause dysgeusia. Irradiation in head and neck surgery may impair the ability to taste.

See also APPETITE.

thrombosis, mesenteric venous A blood clot in the veins of the intestines, which is the cause of 5 to 15 percent of the incidences of mesenteric ISCHEMIA. This form of thrombosis may be a mild, chronic, or severe acute problem. In the most extreme case, a mesenteric venous thrombosis can cause intestinal gangrene. It can also recur.

Sometimes this medical problem is caused by another illness or by a medication or another known cause, and if so, it is said to be secondary mesenteric venous thrombosis. If the cause is unknown, it is deemed to be a primary mesenteric venous thrombosis. A cause can be determined in about 75 to 90 percent of patients who have a mesenteric venous thrombosis.

If the mesenteric venous thrombosis worsens, it can lead to PERITONITIS, a life-threatening condition requiring hospitalization.

Symptoms and Diagnostic Path
Mesenteric venous thrombosis patients may or may not have abdominal pain, depending on the severity and chronicity of their condition. If pain is present, it is usually concentrated in the middle part of the abdomen. Other symptoms and signs which may occur include the following:

- NAUSEA AND VOMITING
- loss of APPETITE
- DIARRHEA
- presence of either frank or occult blood in the stools

Laboratory tests and plain X-rays do not aid the physician in his or her diagnosis of mesenteric venous thrombosis. Computed tomography (CT) is the preferred test to identify this medical problem; CT scan can accurately pinpoint the presence of mesenteric venous thrombosis in the majority of cases. Sometimes the condition is diagnosed on a CT scan done for an unrelated problem. Acute cases with peritoneal signs may be diagnosed and treated at exploratory laparotomy. Angiography may be performed; it also allows for the administration of vasodilator drugs, if needed.

Treatment Options and Outlook

Once the condition has been diagnosed, patients with acute cases without peritoneal signs may be observed without treatment, others may be treated with clot-busting drugs (thrombolytics), and/or anticoagulants such as heparin and warfarin (Coumadin). This therapy may last six months or longer, or it may be lifelong for some patients, such as those who have an inherited disorder that has led to mesenteric venous thrombosis. Some patients also require surgery, with or without bowel resection, particularly if bowel infarction is suspected or if they have peritonitis.

The underlying cause of the thrombosis, such as an abdominal infection or cancer, should also be treated. The prognosis is good for most patients, with the exception of those who have cancer.

Risk Factors and Preventive Measures

The following individuals have an increased risk for mesenteric venous thrombobis. Those who:

- have an inherited blood clotting disorder
- have cancer
- have portal hypertension
- use oral contraceptives

Kumar, Shaji, M.D., Michael G. Sarr, M.D., and Patrick S. Kamath, M.D. "Mesenteric Venous Thrombosis." *New England Journal of Medicine* 345, no. 23 (December 6, 2001): 1,683–1,688.

thrush A yeast infection that often occurs in the mouth and is more common among infants and small children than in people of other ages. Thrush is common among immune-suppressed individuals, such as acquired immunodeficiency syndrome (AIDS) patients. Patients with diabetes are at higher risk for developing thrush. The chronic use of antibiotics may sometimes cause thrush. Medications such as nystatin can usually clear up minor infections. In more serious cases, stronger drugs like Diflucan may be needed. Some physicians may recommend the use of probiotics.

See also ANTIBIOTICS; *LACTOBACILLUS;* YEAST.

thyroid disease Generally either an excessively low or excessively high level of circulating thyroid hormone, which affects the entire metabolism and directly affects a person's energy level, appetite, mood state, and many other aspects of an individual's life. However, thyroid disease may be seen in the presence of normal levels of thyroid hormone.

Many thyroid diseases are autoimmune disorders; for example, Hashimoto's thyroiditis is an autoimmune disorder that causes hypothyroidism, and Graves' disease is an autoimmune disorder that causes hyperthyroidism. In both of these diseases, the individual may have a visibly enlarged gland (goiter). However, the symptoms and signs of thyroid disease, especially when it is mild, may not be clearly detectable to the layperson or even to a physician. Instead, abnormal thyroid levels are often found through a blood test of a patient's thyroid stimulating hormone (TSH) level. The TSH is a test often administered as part of a general physical examination for employment, life or disability insurance, or another purpose, such as excluding thyroid disease as a cause of constipation.

Other thyroid diseases include thyroid cancer and thyroid nodules that may be benign or cancerous.

In general, women have a greater risk for development of thyroid diseases than men. Outside the United States and Canada, shortages of iodine in the diet can sometimes cause thyroid disease. Exposure to excessive radiation of the neck or head may also induce thyroid disease.

Symptoms and Signs

People who are low in thyroid hormone level (hypothyroid) may be sluggish, have a puffy face and dry skin, and become cold (cold intolerance) very readily. They experience constipation and may have unexplained weight gain. In contrast, hyperthyroidism patients are more active, may have diarrhea, and may sometimes even seem manic.

Individuals with hyperthyroidism often experience heat intolerance and heavy sweating, moist skin, and unexplained weight loss despite a normal or even high appetite. Paradoxically, however, some individuals who have hypothyroidism may lose weight and some patients who have hyperthyroidism may gain weight. Symptoms and signs of thyroid disease also vary with age; for example, the symptoms and signs are far more subtle in elderly individuals than they are among younger or middle-aged adults.

Diagnosis and Treatment

The physician diagnoses thyroid disease on the basis of the patient's symptoms and signs as well as on thyroid hormone blood levels. Thyroid hormone levels are easily tested with the TSH blood test, which has a normal range of about 0.3 to 3.0 mU/l (milliunits per liter) as indicated by 2003 guidelines of the Amercian Academy of Clinical Endocrinologists (AACE).

In this test, *above-normal* blood levels indicate hypothyroidism. (One might think that high levels indicate hyperthyroidism, but the reverse is actually true). Thus, TSH greater than 3.0 indicates hypothyroidism. The higher the value, the more severe the degree of hyperthyroidism; consequently, a level of 10.0 indicates a more severe hypothyroid condition than one of 4.0. Conversely, *below*-normal blood levels, levels less than 0.3, indicate hyperthyroidism.

Low levels of thyroid hormone can be treated with supplemental dosages of thyroid hormone. Usually physicians start a patient at a low dosage of thyroid medication and then retest the patient two to four weeks later to see whether his or her level is in the normal range. If the patient is still hypothyroid, the physician increases the dosage.

If the patient's levels of thyroid hormone are excessively high, physicians may administer medication to decrease the levels. Sometimes radiation is used to destroy the thyroid gland. President George H. W. Bush received radioactive iodine for treatment of his hyperthyroidism. In some cases, a partial thyroidectomy is indicated.

travel   Many people experience digestive diseases while away from their home, especially when they travel to other countries, or travelers may be diagnosed with such illnesses after their return home. Most people recover from these illnesses, although some individuals become chronically ill, and others become extremely ill and die.

Diarrhea is the most common form of digestive disease that travelers experience, and it is so common that "traveler's diarrhea" is a universally recognized problem. Interestingly, when people from other countries visit the United States and Canada, they may have diarrhea as well, although to a lesser degree. One underlying problem is the difference in water, and sometimes the difference in food is a factor as well. Another potential problem is that people may be infected by microbes that are unusual in their country of origin and thus have inadequate immunities to these particular germs. Most traveler's diarrhea is short-lived. Medications such as ciprofloxacin (Cipro) help relieve it. Prophylactic antibiotics for travel abroad are not routinely recommended.

Travelers to foreign countries may also be susceptible to infection with viral hepatitis (hepatitis A) caused by conditions of poor sanitation. CHOLERA may also be seen as part of epidemics in overcrowded conditions when the sanitation system breaks down, for example, where there are floods, large fairs, and so forth.

See also CONTAMINATED FOOD OR WATER; DIARRHEA; HEPATITIS; PASTEURIZATION.

Ryan, Edward T., M.D., and Kevin C. Kain, M.D. "Health Advice and Immunizations for Travelers." *New England Journal of Medicine* 342, no. 23 (June 8, 2000):1,716–1,725.

Ryan, Edward T., M.D., Mary E. Wison, M.D., and Kevin C. Kain, M.D. "Illness after International Travel." *New England Journal of Medicine* 347, no. 7 (August 15, 2002): 505–516.

trichinosis   Also known as trichinellosis, it is an infection with *Trichinella* species, the parasite that can be ingested in the cyst form by eating infected uncooked or undercooked pork, sausage, wild game, or other contaminated foods. Cows are herbivorous, i.e. they do not consume meat. As such, beef is less likely a source of the parasite unless it becomes contaminated, with *Trichinella* larvae from pork during processing. Several species of *Trichinella* are recognized to infect humans, and *T. spiralis* is the most common.

In his 2001 article in *Archives of Internal Medicine,* Jan V. Hirschmann speculates that the composer Mozart died of a trichinosis infection in 1791. Trichinosis, stated Hirschmann, caused death within weeks of infection in past centuries, and caused "fever, rashes, and edema without dyspnea [shortness of breath]. Limb pain and swelling from muscle inflammation and vascular damage are common, prominent findings." According to Hirschmnn, Mozart apparently ate pork 44 days before he became ill. (Others, however, have speculated that Mozart died of kidney failure caused by complications from a strep throat.)

In the United States today, trichinosis is very rare, primarily because of laws on meat packing and food preparation as well as public education on the necessity of cooking meats such as pork. (No one should eat pork as a sushi dish.)

When humans eat infected meat containing the encysted larvae of the worms, the gastric acid and pepsin in the digestive system cause the larvae to be released. They then enter the small intestine and mature into adulthood.

After about a week, the fertilized female worms release their larvae. The adult worms burrow through the intestinal wall and enter the bloodstream. They then spread in the body and attach themselves to the muscles of the host. Sometimes the parasite does not encyst. This is especially likely with *Trichinella pseudospiralis*. During the muscle phase, symptoms include muscle pain, fatigue, and weakness that may last months to years. Other symptoms may include skin rash, cough, shortness of breath, difficulty in swallowing, and headaches.

Symptoms and Diagnostic Path

Symptoms depend upon the number of larvae ingested and may be subclinical, mild, or severe. Trichinosis patients exhibit some symptoms and signs that are common to many other digestive diseases and disorders, including the following:

- DIARRHEA
- NAUSEA AND VOMITING
- fatigue
- fever
- ABDOMINAL PAIN
- headaches

- aching joints
- pruritis (itching skin)
- hemorrhages
- swelling of the eyes
- muscle pain
- weakness
- difficulty in swallowing
- cough

The abdominal symptoms caused by trichinosis infection usually occur within a day or two after the patient is infected. Other symptoms may appear within two weeks to two months of the time of infection. Some patients have mild symptoms, and others are severely ill, depending on the number of worms ingested in the contaminated meat. The heart, lungs, and brain may also be involved.

Some patients who have traveled to other countries and eaten uncooked or undercooked meat may contract trichinosis. Physicians should ask patients who have digestive symptoms about their TRAVEL to other countries in the past year or so. If the doctor suspects trichinosis, he or she orders laboratory tests; for example, tests may reveal an eosinophil count that is high. Serum muscle enzymes (creatine kinase and lactate dehydrogenase) may be elevated. Serologic tests for antibody levels are reliable; however they do not correlate with severity of disease, and they may not yield positive findings for at least three weeks after infection. A muscle biopsy is the test of choice for trichinosis.

Treatment Options and Outlook

Most patients have spontaneous resolution of their problems and do not require specific treatment. Analgesics and antipyretics may be used in mild cases. For patients who have symptoms, especially symptoms involving the heart, respiratory muscles, or central nervous system, corticosteroids such as prednisone and antiparasitic drugs such as mebendazole or albendazole are generally prescribed.

Risk Factors and Preventive Measures

To prevent potential trichinosis infection, all meat should be thoroughly cooked. Even the meat that is fed to pigs or other animals should be cooked, to prevent contamination from animal to human. Microwaving or marinating infected meat does not kill the worms. Instead, the meat must be cooked until either the meat juices run clear or the internal temperature of the meat is 77°C. Smoking or salting meat does not kill the worms. Freezing at -15°C for three weeks in a home freezer will also generally kill larvae of most species.

See also PARASITIC INFECTIONS.

tropical sprue   A digestive disorder that is characterized by intestinal abnormalities as well as by a reduction in carbohydrate-digesting enzymes. This causes an impaired carbohydrate digestion plus the malabsorption of all types of nutrients from ingested foods. In most patients, ANEMIA develops as a result of tropical sprue. The cause of tropical sprue is unknown but is presumed to be infectious in origin.

Symptoms and Diagnostic Path

Patients who have tropical sprue have such symptoms as DIARRHEA, cramps, fatigue, and weight loss. Physicians diagnose tropical sprue on the basis of medical history as well as information about areas where patients have lived or traveled to an endemic area (an area where tropical sprue is known to occur). Rarely, the disease may not manifest for months to years after traveling back from an endemic area. The stools are checked to exclude other infections, such as AMEBIASIS or GIARDIASIS, and determine that excess fat is present in the stools. Laboratory test results show macrocytic anemia. D-xylose test, which measures absorption of a type of sugar, is positive.

Other illnesses such as acquired immunodeficiency syndrome should be excluded as the cause of patients' complaints. Although the finding is nonspecific, ENDOSCOPY and a small intestinal biopsy is performed to confirm the diagnosis of tropical sprue. The colon may rarely be involved. CELIAC SPRUE should be excluded since it may have similar clinical features as well as endoscopic and biopsy findings.

Treatment Options and Outlook

Patients with anemia due to tropical sprue are treated with the administration of vitamin B$_{12}$ and folic acid. Folic acid administration improves most symptoms, although intestinal abnormalities may persist. Prescribing broad-spectrum antibiotics, such as tetracycline taken for three to six months and given in combination with folic acid, is an effective treatment, although 20 percent of patients may experience reinfection or relapse.

Risk Factors and Preventive Measures

Tropical sprue affects people who live in Central America, Asia, and the West Indies, as well as travelers to these areas.

tuberculosis   A chronic infection of *Mycobacterium tuberculosis*, this bacterium was first discovered by Robert Koch in 1882, and World TB Day is observed on March 24 each year, the date that Koch made his discovery. According to the Centers for Disease Control and Prevention (CDC), there were a reported 12,898 cases of tuberculosis in the United States in 2008, the lowest number of cases since national reporting started in 1953, when there were 84,304 people with TB in the United States.

TB rates are highest among African Americans, who represent 43 percent of all cases in the United States, followed by whites (33 percent). Many people in the United States with tuberculosis were born in other countries, and the CDC reports that foreign-born individuals have a rate of tuberculosis that is nearly 10 times that of individuals born in the U.S. In addition, foreign-born individuals represented 59 percent of all tuberculosis cases in 2008, according to the CDC.

Individuals born in some parts of the world have a higher likelihood of infection with tuberculosis, such as those from Latin America, the Caribbean, Africa, Asia, eastern Europe, or Russia.

Tuberculosis is passed through the air by a person with TB who coughs or sneezes. The CDC reports that TB is *not* passed by kissing someone infected with TB, nor is it passed by sharing drinking containers or eating utensils. Neither is it spread from shaking someone's hand or touching a toilet seat.

Some people have a latent form of TB, and they have no symptoms and do not feel sick. They can-

TABLE 1: DIFFERENCE BETWEEN LATENT TB INFECTION AND ACTIVE TB DISEASE

Person with Latent TB Infection	Person with Active TB Disease
Does not feel sick	Usually feels sick
Has no symptoms	Usually has symptoms that may include: • a bad cough that lasts 3 weeks or longer • pain in the chest • coughing up blood or sputum • weakness or fatigue • weight loss • no appetite • chills • fever • night sweats
Cannot spread TB to others	May spread TB to others
Usually has a positive skin test or positive TB blood test	Usually has a positive skin test or positive TB blood test
Has a normal chest X-ray and a negative sputum smear	May have an abnormal chest X-ray or positive sputum smear or culture
Should consider treatment for latent TB infection to prevent active TB disease	Needs treatment for active TB disease

Source: National Center for HIV/AIDS, Viral Hepatitis, STD, and TB Prevention, Division of Tuberculosis Elimination. Questions and Answers about Tuberculosis. 2009. Available online. http://www.cdc.gov/tb/publications/faqs/pdfs/qa.pdf.

not pass TB to others, but they usually do have a positive reaction to a TB skin test. They may later develop an active TB infection. See the table for a comparison of the person with latent TB and active TB.

An airborne disease, tuberculosis is contracted by contact with people who have active symptoms, especially coughing and sneezing. A chance encounter with a person who has TB is unlikely to cause tuberculosis; however, frequent or prolonged contacts, such as the contacts that family members or hospital workers experience, significantly raise the risk of contracting tuberculosis. In recent years, an attorney who was infected with tuberculosis flew across continents despite knowing that he had disease and he had to be quarantined by the U.S. government for a period of time.

Most people with tuberculosis have an inactive form of the disease, and only an estimated one in 10 patients infected with tuberculosis has an active and symptomatic form of the disease. As a result, many people who have tuberculosis never know that they have it, unless they are tested for it.

Symptoms and Diagnostic Path
People who have an active form of tuberculosis may have a chronic cough and may cough up blood. In addition, they may be fatigued, lose their APPETITE, and lose weight. They may also experience night sweats and fevers. Many patients, especially those who are in the early stages of the disease or have an inactive form of TB, have no symptoms at all.

Digestive involvement in tuberculosis may take the form of tuberculous peritonitis, ileocecal tuberculosis, or tuberculosis of the lymph nodes in the abdomen that surround the gut.

A skin test, the purified protein derivative (PPD) test, is usually used to check for tuberculosis and evaluated 48 to 72 hours later. It is a screening test that yields both false positive and false negative findings.

To determine whether a patient actually has tuberculosis when the individual tests positive with the skin test, a chest X-ray is needed, along with a complete medical history. Serial sputum examinations are done to check for tuberculosis involving the lungs. In patients who have tuberculosis that involves the digestive system, the chest X-ray and sputum tests may have negative results. Colonoscopy with ileoscopy, small bowel follow-through, and computerized tomography (CT) scans also help aid with the diagnosis of abdominal tuberculosis.

There are also special blood tests to determine whether TB is present. A whole-blood interferon (IFN)-gamma release assay (IGRA) is now available in the for detection of latent tuberculosis infection (QuantiFERON-TB Gold, QFT) and is being used by most hospitals in lieu of PPD. QuantiFERON-TB Gold has largely replaced the TB skin test.

Treatment Options and Outlook

If the patient's TB skin test result is positive, but active TB is not confirmed, patients may be given preventive medications to lower the risk of tuberculosis. These patients are treated with the drug isoniazid for six to nine months. Unfortunately, HEPATITIS is a common side effect of this drug, and the risk increases with age. Patients taking isoniazid must also completely abstain from using all alcohol to prevent damage to the liver.

Patients who have active TB take a combination of three to four medications, such as isoniazid, rifampin, pyrazinamide, and ethambutol.

Some patients with TB have extensively drug-resistant TB (XDR TB). This form of TB is resistant to most medications. Treatment for such patients is over a longer period, and they have a greater risk of dying from TB. Foreign-born people with a previous history of TB are more likely to have multidrug resistance or a resistance to isoniazid alone. As can be seen from Table 2, there were 686 individuals with no prior history of TB who were resistant to

TB medications, including 4.4 percent of U.S.-born patients and 9.4 percent of foreign-born patients who were resistant to isoniazied. In addition, 98 individuals were resistant to both isoniazid and rifampin, including 20 patients born in the United States and 78 born in other countries.

One problem with treating tuberculosis is that patients may be resistant to taking medication, in part because of potential side effects. However, the medication must be taken for at least six months in order to treat the infection. Some public health departments provide the medication and watch the patient take the drug to make sure it is taken.

Acquired immunodeficiency syndrome (AIDS) patients can contract an opportunistic form of tuberculosis caused by *Mycobacterium avium intracellulare* (MAI), which can be widespread in the body, including in the LIVER. Treatment of MAI is unsatisfactory.

Individuals being treated for TB should notify their physician immediately if they have any of the

TABLE 2: TUBERCULOSIS CASES AND PERCENTAGES, BY RESISTANCE TO ISONIAZID OR MULTIDRUG RESISTANCE IN PERSONS WITH NO PREVIOUS HISTORY OF TB, 1993–2007

	Resistance to Isoniazid						Resistance to Isoniazid and Rifampin					
	Total cases		U.S.-born		Foreign-born		Total cases		U.S.-born		Foreign-born	
Year	Number	%	Number	%	Number	%	Number	%	Number	%	Number	%
1993	1399	8.4	804	6.8	579	12.4	407	2.5	301	2.6	103	2.2
1994	1360	8.3	711	6.5	635	12.0	353	2.2	238	2.2	110	2.1
1995	1174	7.3	555	5.4	618	11.0	254	1.6	169	1.6	85	1.5
1996	1137	7.4	495	5.2	639	11.3	207	1.3	105	1.1	101	1.8
1997	1079	7.5	435	5.0	640	11.2	155	1.1	76	0.9	79	1.4
1998	1013	7.5	367	4.8	644	11.3	132	1.0	55	0.7	76	1.3
1999	899	7.1	283	4.0	614	11.0	127	1.0	39	0.6	88	1.6
2000	891	7.5	268	4.4	620	11.0	120	1.0	38	0.6	82	1.5
2001	806	7.0	243	4.4	562	9.6	118	1.0	34	0.6	84	1.4
2002	823		206	4.1	616	10.8	130	1.2	36	0.7	94	1.7
2003	821		215	4.5	603	10.4	92	0.9	24	0.5	68	1.2
2004	802		213	4.5	589	10.2	102	1.0	26	0.6	76	1.3
2005	764		188	4.3	571	10.1	98	1.0	19	0.4	78	1.4
2006	764		170	4.2	592	10.4	94	1.0	17	0.4	77	1.4
2007	686		165	4.4	520	9.4	98	1.1	20	0.5	78	1.4

Adapted from Centers for Disease Control and Prevention. *Reported Tuberculosis in the United States, 2007.* Atlanta, Ga: Centers for Disease Control and Prevention, September 2008, 22.

following symptoms, which may be side effects to their TB medications:

- fever
- rash
- aching joints
- aches or tingling in fingers or toes
- changes in eyesight, such as blurring
- changes in hearing, such as ringing in the ears
- dizziness
- bruising
- easy bleeding when cut
- decreased or absent appetite
- numbness or tingling around the mouth
- yellow skin or eyes (JAUNDICE)

Risk Factors and Preventive Measures

ELDERLY people and babies and young children have a greater risk for developing TB if infected because their immune system is not as strong as older (or younger) individuals. Individuals who are homeless or who have been incarcerated have an increased risk for contracting TB.

Some individuals have a greater risk for contracting TB than others, including those in the following groups:

- individuals with HIV
- those who have been infected with TB in the past two years
- those who abuse alcohol or inject illegal drugs
- those who not treated correctly for a past TB infection

People who have been recently exposed to tuberculosis, as well as other groups, including the following, are at risk and should be tested for tuberculosis:

- employees of health-care facilities that treat tuberculosis patients
- immigrants from countries with a high rate of tuberculosis
- people who have HIV
- people who have kidney failure
- patients on immunosuppressive therapy
- patients who are malnourished

Robison, Valerie, et al. Centers for Disease Control and Prevention. *Reported Tuberculosis in the United States, 2007.* Atlanta, Ga: Centers for Disease Control and Prevention, September 2008.

Centers for Disease Control and Prevention. "Trends in Tuberculosis—United States, 2007." *Morbidity and Mortality Weekly Report* 57, no. 11 (March 21, 2008): 281–285.

ulcerative colitis A chronic disease that causes sores and inflammation of the COLON. Ulcerative colitis is one of the two medical problems that constitute INFLAMMATORY BOWEL DISEASE (IBD); the other is CROHN'S DISEASE. (Patients must have only one of these diseases to have IBD. Both do not occur simultaneously although the type of IBD may be indeterminate in 10 to 15 percent of the cases.)

The inflammation in the rectum/colon causes it to bleed and to empty frequently; bowel movements are more frequent than is normal and are usually loose, bloody stools.

The cause of ulcerative colitis is unknown; it may be linked to an immune system abnormality. It is not caused by a FOOD ALLERGY or sensitivity, although foods may trigger symptoms. Stress does not cause ulcerative colitis but may worsen the symptoms of the condition.

Ulcerative colitis increases the risk for development of COLORECTAL CANCER, and as a result, patients who have long-standing disease need a periodic colonoscopy to look for any early signs of cancer. The frequency of the colonoscopy is determined by the patient's physician but may be every one to two years or more often.

Symptoms and Diagnostic Path

Most patients with ulcerative colitis have bloody DIARRHEA and ABDOMINAL PAIN, often on the left side. Other signs and symptoms that may occur are as follows:

- loss of appetite and unintended weight loss
- fatigue
- fecal incontinence (accidents)
- rectal bleeding
- loss of nutrients and body fluids

Ulcerative colitis may cause or be associated with other medical problems, such as arthritis, liver disease, osteoporosis (low bone density), ANEMIA, PRIMARY SCLEROSING CHOLANGITIS, and pyoderma gangrenosum.

The physician takes a complete medical history and performs a physical examination. Laboratory tests such as complete blood count are frequently ordered to test for anemia or for a high white blood cell count indicating infection and/or inflammation.

The doctor also frequently orders testing of a stool sample, particularly for bloody diarrhea, in order to rule out infection as the cause of the diarrhea. In addition, a colonoscopy with biopsy is required to establish a diagnosis, so that a visual inspection of the colon can be made and the doctor can check for ulcers or inflammation.

Some patients have relatively mild symptoms, whereas ulcerative colitis is a severe and disabling condition for others. Some patients experience spontaneous (even without medications) remission of ulcerative colitis for periods lasting months or years, although no one knows why the disease eventually recurs.

Ulcerative colitis is different from Crohn's disease, but differentiating them in a patient can be difficult in about 10 to 15 percent of the cases; such cases are labeled indeterminate colitis. The perinuclear antineutrophil cytoplasmic antibody (pANCA) is seen in about two-thirds of patients with ulcerative colitis and about 10 to 20 percent of patients with Crohn's disease. In contrast, the anti–*Saccharomyces cereviciae* antibody (ASCA) is positive in about two-thirds of patients with Crohn's disease and about 10 percent of patients with ulcerative colitis. Using the two tests in combination may distinguish ulcerative colitis from Crohn's disease in patients with indeterminate colitis. The role of other antibodies like anti-Omp C antibody is evolving.

In general, according to Ghosh and colleagues in 2000 in *British Medical Journal,* ulcerative colitis patients are not smokers (or are former smokers), whereas Crohn's disease patients frequently smoke. SMOKING appears to be protective against ulcerative colitis, whereas it tends to delay healing in Crohn's disease. Ulcerative colitis patients frequently do not have osteopenia (low bone density) when they are diagnosed, in contrast to patients who have Crohn's disease. In ulcerative colitis, the problem is usually restricted to the colon; in Crohn's disease, any part of the entire gut (the ESOPHAGUS, the stomach, the small intestine, the colon, rectum, and anal canal) may be affected.

There are other differences: Ulcerative colitis patients usually do not have STRICTURES or FISTULAS in the bowel, and granulomas on biopsy and their presence suggests the diagnosis of Crohn's disease. The rectum is almost always involved in ulcerative colitis (95 percent of the cases) but is rarely involved in Crohn's disease (5 percent of cases).

Treatment Options and Outlook

Antibiotics usually do not help patients who have ulcerative colitis, although they may improve the condition of patients who have Crohn's disease. Ulcerative colitis patients are cured of this illness by surgery to remove the colon and rectum, whereas Crohn's disease frequently recurs after surgery.

Lifestyle changes Physicians may ask people who have ulcerative colitis to keep a food diary to help determine whether particular foods trigger a worsening of the illness. For many people with ulcerative colitis, spicy foods or the lactose in milk can exacerbate illness; other foods may be the cause for others. If specific foods that aggravate the condition can be identified, patients can actively avoid them.

Some patients may need psychological support, including from mental health professionals, because the disease may seem to overpower their life. Patients who seek help from mental health professionals should be sure to work only with psychologists or psychiatrists who understand the medical aspect of ulcerative colitis and recognize

that although stress can make the condition worse, it does not cause it. Thus, psychological counseling alone cannot cure ulcerative colitis, although it may help patients to learn to accept their condition and deal better with stress.

Interestingly, however, in the cotton top tamarin monkey, an animal model of ulcerative colitis, colitis rarely occurs when the animal lives freely in the jungle, and in most cases occurs in animals that are in captivity. The stress of captivity may be involved.

Medications can help Many ulcerative colitis patients are treated with drugs such as sulfasalazine (Azulfidline), which combines a sulfonamide (sulfapyridine) and aminosalicylate (ASA). Other patients are given drugs in the form of 5-aminosalicylic acid (5-ASA) without the sulfonamide (mesalamine [Asacol or Pentasa]). 5-ASA is also available as a rectal enema. Some patients are treated with corticosteroids, such as prednisone or hydrocortisone, which may be given as a pill, intravenously, or in an enema. Doctors hesitate to prescribe corticosteroids for an extended period because of the many side effects they can cause, such as hypertension, increase of facial hair, change in body shape and structure, osteoporosis, weight gain, and mood swings. Use of immunosuppressants such as azathiorine or 6MP can help in treatment. Biologics such as infliximab (Remicade) and Humira are also useful in treatment.

Surgery sometimes is necessary If ulcerative colitis is very severe, causing severe bleeding and/or extreme weight loss, physicians may decide that the best treatment for an individual patient is surgical removal of the colon and rectum in order to achieve a cure. According to the National Institutes of Health, up to 40 percent of all patients with ulcerative colitis eventually need surgery because of severe bleeding, colonic rupture, or other serious conditions caused by the disorder. A colectomy is also performed if cancer or a precancerous lesion is found during a colonoscopy.

The surgery requires ileostomy, or the creation of a stoma, an opening to the outside, through which the fecal contents pass into a pouch that the patient empties regularly. Presently, many surgeons create a reservoir or a pouch (artificial rectum) from the small intestine and hook it up to the anal canal so that the patient can have continued bowel movements instead of an ileostomy. Inflammation of the pouch is known as POUCHITIS.

Risk Factors and Preventive Measures

People of any age can have ulcerative colitis, but the illness is more commonly found among people between the ages of 15 and 30. There is a second increase in the 50s and 60s. According to the National Institutes of Health, both men and women can have ulcerative colitis. One study, reported in a 2001 issue of the *New England Journal of Medicine,* found that people who had an appendectomy before age 20 had a significantly reduced risk of later development of ulcerative colitis; the reason for the reduced risk is not known. Several other studies, including one by Minocha (1997), have shown similar results in the United States.

See also APPENDICITIS; FISH OIL.

Andersson, Roland E., M.D., et al. "Appendectomy and Protection against Ulcerative Colitis." *New England Journal of Medicine* 344, no. 11 (March 15, 2001): 808–814.

Ghosh, Subrata, Alan Shand, and Anne Ferguson. "Ulcerative Colitis." *British Medical Journal* 320 (April 22, 2000): 1,119–1,123.

Minocha, Anil, and C. A. Raczkowski. "Role of Appendectomy and Tonsillectomy in Pathogenesis of Ulcerative Colitis." *Digestive Disease Sciences* 42 (1997): 1,567–1,569.

ulcer, peptic A break of the lining of the stomach or duodenum that causes mild, moderate, or severe PAIN. Some ulcers are painless, especially among patients who are taking NONSTEROIDAL ANTI-INFLAMMATORY DRUGS (NSAIDs) or STEROIDS. An ulcer may occur in the stomach (gastric ulcer) or in the duodenum (duodenal ulcer).

If an ulcer becomes very severe, it can produce bleeding, and ulcers constitute about 50 percent of all the causes of cases of upper gastrointestinal BLEEDING. In addition to causing possibly life-threatening bleeding in the most extreme case, an ulcer can also be life-threatening when it is perforated and when the food, acid, and bacteria from the stomach or duodenum are spilled into the peritoneum, the lining of the abdominal cavity.

Patients who have perforation need both emergency hospitalization and surgery.

Most peptic ulcers (about 60 to 90 percent) are caused by *HELICOBACTER PYLORI* bacteria; some ulcers are caused by medications, particularly nonsteroidal anti-inflammatory drugs (NSAIDs) given to treat arthritis and other chronic ailments. *H. pylori* is seen more often with duodenal ulcers than with gastric ulcers. Complicated ulcers (with bleeding and perforation) are more likely to be caused by NSAIDs.

For about a century and until the early 1990s, most physicians throughout the world believed that ulcers were caused by increased acid, stress, or diet and, consequently, urged patients to relax and prevent stress and/or to change their diet. In 1982, the Australian physicians Marshall and Warren insisted that *H. pylori* was the cause of most cases of gastritis and ulcers. They were ridiculed for years and finally proved right and awarded the Nobel Prize for their discovery. The presence of HP results in production of increased gastric acid in patients with duodenal ulcers. Paradoxically, in some cases HP may cause decreased gastric acidity.

Symptoms and Diagnostic Path

The key symptom of an ulcer is pain in the upper abdominal area, which is often said to be a gnawing type of pain. Other indicators of a peptic ulcer are as follows:

- NAUSEA AND/OR VOMITING
- loss of APPETITE
- unintended weight loss
- upper ABDOMINAL PAIN that occurs two to five hours after eating a meal when the stomach is empty but acid is secreted in the case of duodenal ulcer. While the stomach empties in two to three hours, food-stimulated acid secretion continues for 3–5 hours.
- upper abdominal pain that occurs in the night, when the stomach is empty but acid secretion is maximal, in the case of a duodenal ulcer
- upper abdominal pain that occurs shortly after eating, causing a fear of eating, as found with a gastric ulcer and the pain may not be relieved by antacids
- pain that is relieved by eating and/or by use of antacids

Patients who experience gastrointestinal bleeding may feel weak and lethargic and sometimes may even pass out. If gastrointestinal bleeding is severe, blood may appear in the patient's vomit or stools. Patients may bleed without a prior history of any significant abdominal pain or discomfort.

It is also true that ulcers may be totally silent. In addition, the predictability of whether a person has an ulcer on solely clinical grounds is poor.

Emergency Symptoms Some symptoms and signs of an ulcer are emergency indicators that the patient needs to see a physician as soon as possible. The reason for the urgency is that these symptoms may indicate perforation, bleeding, or an obstruction of the stomach. These symptoms include the following:

- black, tarry stools (melena)
- sudden sharp and persistent pain in the stomach that is worse with movement
- vomit that includes blood or has a coffee grounds appearance
- weakness and dizziness
- persistent vomiting, especially vomiting of undigested food ingested several hours or a day earlier

An ulcer is diagnosed on the basis of a patient's symptoms and the findings of the physical examination, along with the results of such tests as an upper gastrointestinal series (barium X-ray) and/or an esophagogastroduodenoscopy (EGD). Clinically distinguishing gastric from duodenal ulcer often yields an inaccurate diagnosis. In addition, less than 25 percent of patients who have classic symptoms of ulcer disease are found to have an ulcer when they have endoscopy (EGD) or upper gastrointestinal X-ray.

If an ulcer is seen on an upper gastrointestinal barium X-ray, doctors may still use EGD, especially in the case of gastric ulcer, in order to take a biopsy specimen during the procedure, in order to make sure that there is no cancer. In some cases, as in the case of an obstruction or perforation, a computed tomography (CT) scan or magnetic resonance imaging (MRI) scan may be indicated.

Treatment Options and Outlook

Once an ulcer has been identified, the patient is usually given acid blocking medications so that the damaged tissue can have a chance to heal. Common histamine-2 blockers include cimetidine (Tagamet), ranitidine (Zantac), famotidine (Pepcid), and nizatidine (Axid). Common PROTON PUMP INHIBITORS (PPIs) that physicians may prescribe include omeprazole (Prilosec), pantoprazole (Protonix), rabeprazole (Aciphex), lansoprazole (Prevacid), and esomeprazole (Nexium). Generic and over-the-counter formulations are now available for some of these products.

Some physicians also treat their peptic ulcer patients with mucosal protective drugs such as sucralfate (Carafate), which are as effective as H-2 blockers. PPIs are superior to H-2 blockers in their efficacy.

Rarely, ulcer patients require surgery, particularly in cases of complicated ulcers (with perforation, obstruction, and bleeding) and of ulcers that are refractory (do not respond) to medical treatment.

When **H. Pylori** *May Be Causing the Ulcer* When a patient is found to have an ulcer through EGD or physicians suspect that *H. pylori* is causing the ulcerlike symptoms, they can test for *H. pylori* with BREATH TESTS, a stool test, or blood tests. Doctors can also take tissue samples during an ENDOSCOPY to test for the presence of *H. pylori*. If tests identify that *H. pylori* is present, then physicians use antibiotic treatment to eradicate the bacteria. *H. pylori* is a very resistant organism, and multiple ANTIBIOTICS are required.

Usually a three-drug regimen for two weeks is recommended to eradicate *H. pylori*. Most medication regimens have either metronidazole (Flagyl) or clarithromycin (Biaxin) or both. "Dosepaks" such as Prevpac and Helidac enhance compliance. (A dosepak includes two or more medications in one package, with days and times marked appropriately and in order, to help patients remember to take all their medicine.) PPIs also have actions against *H. pylori* and are part of many regimens, including Prevpac. A variety of four-drug regimens have been advocated to treat refractory *H. pylori* and include antibiotics such as Levaquin.

When NSAIDS May Be the Cause When physicians know that patients are taking nonsteroidal anti-inflammatory drugs (NSAIDs) for medical problems, they may assume that an ulcer was caused by the NSAID and treat the patient accordingly. In addition to prescribing acid blocking medication to heal the ulcer, they may choose to reduce the dosage of the NSAID or try another medication such as a COX-2 inhibitor that is less harmful to the stomach and/or the duodenum. However, the use of COX-2 inhibitors has come under fire in recent years, and most of them (e.g. Vioxx) have been withdrawn from the market because of complications. The risks of NSAIDs causing a bleeding peptic ulcer increases with the use of corticosteroids or anticoagulants, a history of peptic disease, and older age.

Another course of action is to continue the NSAID and at the same time prescribe preventive antiulcer medications for those who are at risk for the development of ulcers. In research reported in 2002 in the *Archives of Internal Medicine*, the researchers studied 537 patients who did not have *H. pylori* but were long-term NSAID users and also had peptic ulcers in the past, as verified through endoscopies. The patients took their NSAID medication. One group of subjects were given misoprostol four times a day. Another group was given 15 mg of lansoprazole (Prevacid), a proton pump inhibitor medication, once a day, and a third group was given a higher dosage of lansoprazole (30 mg). The fourth group was given a placebo (no medication). The subjects were later evaluated on whether an ulcer developed after eight weeks and after 12 weeks.

The researchers found that most patients who took the misoprostol were ulcer-free (93 percent), followed by those who took proton pump inhibitors. In contrast, 82 percent of the patients taking 30 mg of lansoprazole were ulcer-free, and 80 percent of those taking 15 mg of lansoprazole had no ulcer at the end of the study. Among the placebo group, 51 percent were ulcer-free; thus, in almost half of the patients ulcers developed.

It would initially seem evident that misoprostol is the best ulcer preventive. However, misoprostol has many side effects, such as abdominal pain and DIARRHEA, and thus, there is less compliance in using medication among patients; for example, more than 90 percent of those in the placebo group

and the lansoprazole group took their medication as directed, compared to only 73 percent of patients in the misoprostol group. When those factors were considered, misoprostol and the proton pump inhibitor performed about the same in preventing the development of ulcers.

Considering Cyclooxygenase-2 (COX-2) Inhibitors Another class of anti-inflammatory medication is the COX-2 inhibitor, which includes medications such as celecoxib (Celebrex). Rofecoxib has been tested to determine whether it is less likely to cause peptic ulcers than NSAIDs among patients who need to reduce the inflammation of arthritis.

According to information reported in 1999 in the *Journal of the American Medical Association*, arthritis patients who were treated with rofecoxib had a significantly lower risk of development of peptic ulcers than patients taking the classic NSAIDs such as ibuprofen, diclofenac, or nabumetone. (However, the risk is not zero, and some patients have ulcers when taking COX-2 inhibitor medications.) Valdecoxib (Bextra) is another COX-2 inhibitor that had prescribed by physicians. As mentioned above, most of COX-2 inhibitors, including Bextra® and Vioxx, have been withdrawn from the market.

If patients have a bleeding ulcer caused by NSAIDs, the medication is usually stopped immediately. In fact, it is best that such patients stop taking NSAIDs permanently. Alternatively, if they must continue to take an NSAID, they are preferably treated with adjunctive treatment with misoprostol or a PPI medication such as lansoprazole (Prevacid®) or esomeprazole (Nexium®).

If Surgery Is Needed Sometimes the ulcer is so severe (refractory or complicated) that surgery must be performed. The type of surgery depends upon the nature of the problem, for example, whether it is bleeding, perforation, obstruction, or a medically refractory ulcer. Surgeons may perform a vagotomy, in which the vagus nerve is severed to reduce acid secretion. In other cases, surgeons may need to perform an antrectomy of the last part of the stomach that is involved in acid secretion.

A third type of surgery that may be performed is the pyloroplasty, which enables the surgeon to dilate the opening to the small intestine. Gastrojejunostomy, hooking up of the stomach through a new surgically created opening to the distant part of the small bowel (the jejunum), is also frequently performed. The operation to treat the ulcer frequently involves various combinations of the aforementioned surgical techniques.

Risk Factors and Preventive Measures

Some studies have shown that when only the population of patients who are age 65 and older are considered, medications are responsible for up to 50 percent of peptic ulcers. In one study, reported in a 2001 issue of the *Journal of the American Medical Association,* when ELDERLY patients were screened for *H. pylori* and if positive, treated, there was no reduction in the rate of repeat hospitalizations for ulcers. In contrast, patients who took NSAIDs and were counseled that the drugs could cause ulcers *did* have a decreased subsequent rate of hospitalization. The researchers concluded that NSAIDs play a large role in the development of peptic ulcers among older individuals.

Effects of Stress Are Present   Stress, although it does not cause ulcer, may worsen the symptoms of an existing ulcer. SMOKING also exacerbates ulcer symptoms. Some physicians point out that in some extreme cases of stress, such as in war, earthquake, or another severe event, the event has been followed by an increase in the incidence of peptic ulcers in the population affected by the event. Physicians emphasize that although stress does not usually cause ulcers, stress may cause or exacerbate ulcer symptoms in some cases. In fact, hypnotherapy has been shown to be an effective remedy in the prevention of relapse of peptic ulcer disease, although it is not widely accepted or routinely recommended.

Other Diseases Can Increase the Risk For Ulcers   It is also true that some illnesses, such as ZOLLINGER-ELLISON SYNDROME, may cause ulcers among some patients who are diagnosed with this disease. Patients with CROHN'S DISEASE may develop ulcers in stomach or duodenum.

Some studies have shown a higher incidence of ulcers among men; for example, in the Finnish Twin Cohort, which studied thousands of twins who were born before 1958, the incidence of ulcers was 6.2 percent among men and only 2.8 percent among women. However, other studies have indicated virtually no gender difference in individuals who are at risk for development of peptic ulcers. The Finnish Twin Cohort study also found other factors among patients that increased their risk for development of ulcers, including high stress, as well as smoking among men and long-term use of analgesics (painkillers) among women.

In the United States, the numbers of men and women with peptic or stomach ulcers are about equal.

Refractory Ulcers   Some patients have an ulcer that is not responsive to the usual treatments. A study of risk factors associated with refractory peptic ulcers (ulcers resistant to treatment) was reported in 1995 in *Gastroenterology.* The researchers found that the risk factors for refractory ulcers included an earlier onset of development of ulcer, a longer history of symptoms caused by the ulcer, and more frequent incidences of relapses from the ulcer. In addition, the patients who had a refractory ulcer were more likely to smoke during the refractory period, and presumably the smoking caused an impairment of the healing process.

About 40 percent of the patients with refractory ulcers were abusing nonsteroidal anti-inflammatory drugs (NSAIDs): This one factor alone accounted for the greatest risk for development of a refractory ulcer.

See also BLEEDING, GASTROINTESTINAL; HISTAMINE-2 BLOCKERS; MULTIPLE ENDOCRINE NEOPLASIA (MEN); PANCREATITIS; STOMACH CANCER.

Brock, Jane, M.D., M.S.P.H. "Process of Care and Outcomes for Elderly Patients Hospitalized with Peptic Ulcer Disease: Results from a Quality Improvement Project." *Journal of the American Medical Association* 286, no. 16 (October 24/31, 2001): 1,985–1,993.

Colgan, S. M., B. B. Faragher, and P. J. Whorwell. "Controlled Trial of Hypnotherapy in Relapse Prevention of Duodenal Ulceration." *Lancet* (June 11, 1988): 1,299–1,300.

El-Serag, Hashem B., M.D., et al. "Prevention of Complicated Ulcer Disease among Chronic Users of Nonsteroidal Anti-inflammatory Drugs: The Use of a Nomogram in Cost-Effectiveness Analysis." *Archives of Internal Medicine* 162 (October 14, 2002): 2,105–2,110.

Graham, David Y., M.D., et al. "Ulcer Prevention in Long-Term Users of Nonsteroidal Anti-inflammatory Drugs." *Archives of Internal Medicine* 162 (January 28, 2002): 169–175.

Minocha, Anil, M.D., and Christine Adamec. *How to Stop Heartburn: Simple Ways to Heal Heartburn and Acid Reflux.* New York: John Wiley & Sons, 2001.

Räihä, Ismo, M.D., et al. "Lifestyle, Stress, and Genes in Peptic Ulcer Disease: A Nationwide Twin Cohort Study." *Archives of Internal Medicine* 158 (April 13, 1998): 698–704.

ultrasound An imaging procedure that uses sound waves to provide a view of internal organs. The procedure may be performed from outside the body, by touching a sensor to the body, or the sensor may be attached to a scope, such as an endoscope, to provide an internal view.

Ultrasound is used to diagnose inflammation, cancer spread, or other abnormalities of the digestive organs, such as the liver, pancreas, gallbladder, and stomach, as well as other abdominal organs, such as the ovaries and the uterus. It may also be used with procedures that are performed by gastroenterologists or surgeons, such as the endoscopic ultrasound, wherein the ultrasound sensor is attached to the endoscope, which is then passed into the digestive tract, for example, into the stomach or the rectum, and images are then obtained from a closer distance. While an ultrasound from outside the body is risk-free, the endoscopic ultrasound is associated with significant risk for complications.

Ultrasound is also used to monitor the fetus during PREGNANCY and to check the heart and blood vessels.

See also IMAGING STUDIES; MAJOR DIAGNOSTIC TESTS FOR DIGESTIVE DISEASES.

upper gastrointestinal X-ray See MAJOR DIAGNOSTIC TESTS FOR DIGESTIVE DISEASES.

vasculitis, small vessel   Inflammation of the blood vessel walls, a condition that can lead to a variety of illnesses in various parts of the body, including the digestive system. Vasculitis may cause a decreased blood supply to the intestines, resulting in abdominal pain and a lack of appetite.

Various forms of vasculitis are recognized. CHURG–STRAUSS SYNDROME is a form of small-vessel vasculitis first described in 1951. Mixed cryoglobulinemia is another example of small-vessel vasculitis.

Medications may cause vasculitis, particularly drugs such as penicillamine, hydralazine, quinolones, minocycline and sulfonamides.

In the early stages of vasculitis, patients may experience flulike symptoms of aches and pains in their joints and fever. Different vessels may be affected, including vessels in the gut, the kidneys, and the respiratory tract. Patients may also have skin lesions and nodules.

vitamin deficiencies/excesses   An imbalance of levels of vitamins in the body, including a lack of needed vitamins as well as an excessive or even toxic level of vitamins (hypervitaminosis).

Vitamin A and Carotenoids

Vitamin A affects vision. It also helps the body to maintain the lining of the intestinal tract, the eyes, the urinary tract, and the respiratory tract. In addition, vitamin A is involved in the immune system in fighting off infections. Carotenoids are provitamins that are easily converted to vitamin A. Although there are numerous carotenoids, beta-carotene is the most active, and many others serve as antioxidants. Foods that contain vitamin A or provitamin A carotenoids include eggs, whole milk, liver, cheddar cheese, carrots, green vegetables, and orange fruits. Many prepared foods are also fortified with vitamin A.

Deficiencies of Vitamin   A few people in the United States have a deficiency of vitamin A, but many children in poor countries suffer from dietary deprivation and lack a sufficient store of vitamin A; that lack can cause blindness. In the United States, night blindness is an early indicator of a deficiency of vitamin A. Sometimes vitamin A deficiency can develop as a result of CELIAC SPRUE, CYSTIC FIBROSIS, and intestinal infections.

Alcoholism can cause vitamin A deficiency, and vegetarians who do not eat eggs or dairy products may experience vitamin A deficiency. Deficiencies in vitamin A translate into difficulty in fighting infection.

Some doctors in the United States are concerned by subclinical (slightly low, so that patients do not have symptoms) levels of vitamins, especially among growing children. Children at particular risk for subclinically low levels of vitamin A include the following groups:

- poor children, including those living at or below the poverty level
- children who have emigrated from countries where there are known deficiencies of vitamin A
- children who have been diagnosed with disease of the LIVER, PANCREAS, or intestines
- children who have difficulty in digesting or absorbing fat
- children who have received inadequate health care

Hypervitaminosis Vitamin A   It is also possible to have too much vitamin A, and excessive levels of vitamin A can cause increased pressure in the brain, vomiting, and yellowing of skin. Babies born to pregnant women who have overly high levels of vitamin A can have birth defects.

Hypervitaminosis vitamin A can occur in a short period (days) if a person ingests an excessive amount of this vitamin. The key signs of toxic levels of vitamin A include the following:

- headache
- weakness
- joint pains
- NAUSEA AND VOMITING
- blurred vision
- poor muscle coordination

Because these signs and symptoms are also characteristic of many other diseases, the physician must obtain a complete medical history. Patients should cooperate by reporting all drugs that they take, especially over-the-counter vitamins or herbal preparations.

Vitamin B₆

The human body needs vitamin B_6 for a variety of functions, including maintaining red blood cells, assisting function of both the immune system and the nervous system, and converting tryptophan (a natural amino acid) into serotonin. It is also needed to maintain normal blood sugar (glucose) levels. Vitamin B_6 is used as a treatment for the nausea and vomiting of PREGNANCY.

Vitamin B_6 is found in beans, cereals, fish, meats, poultry, and some fruits and vegetables. Good sources of vitamin B_6 are potatoes, bananas, chicken breast, lean pork loin, cooked rainbow trout, sunflower seeds, canned tuna, avocado, creamy peanut butter, and lima beans.

Deficiencies of Vitamin B₆ Most people in the United States and other developed countries are not deficient in vitamin B_6. However, some older individuals, particularly those age 65 and older, may have low levels of this vitamin, primarily because of poor diet. Individuals at risk include those who have MALABSORPTION SYNDROME, alcoholics, and women who are using oral contraceptives.

Physical indicators of a deficiency of vitamin B_6 include the following signs and symptoms:

- sore tongue (glossitis)
- skin inflammation (dermatitis)
- depression
- confusion
- convulsions
- ANEMIA

Because these signs can indicate many other medical problems, patients must be evaluated by their physician. If a deficiency is diagnosed, individuals may be given supplements.

Vitamin B₆ Hypervitaminosis It is also possible to have excessive levels of vitamin B_6 if taking megadoses of the vitamin over long period. The recommended daily allowance (RDA) of vitamin B_6 is 2 mg/day for adult males and 1.6 mg/day for adult females. Adults should avoid taking more than 100 mg of this vitamin per day. Toxicity occurs when doses of 250 mg per day or more are taken for several months, which can cause patients to suffer dizziness and nerve damage, creating problems related to walking and various sensations of touch, pain, and temperature. It is, however, rare. Most patients who are taking supplemental vitamin B_6 improve, but may not recover completely, when they stop using it.

In the past, some health books have recommended that people who have carpal tunnel syndrome take supplements of vitamin B_6. Data related to whether vitamin B_6 can help improve carpal tunnel syndrome or asthma are controversial at best since most data suggests it is ineffective. Large doses should be avoided since some individuals have experienced nerve damage (neuropathy) after taking high doses of this vitamin over the long term.

Some women who have premenstrual syndrome have taken vitamin B_6 to alleviate symptoms, but there is limited clinical evidence that this vitamin improves symptoms, particularly among patients who have depression. There is evidence that high doses are toxic to women who have taken the vitamin for this purpose. Overall, there does not appear to be beneficial effect of this vitamin in patients with depression except in premenopausal women.

Vitamin B₁₂

Vitamin B_{12} is important for the nerve cells and the blood. Foods that are high in vitamin B_{12} include the following: cooked liver, fortified breakfast cereals, cooked rainbow trout, cooked beef, cooked haddock, breaded or fried clams, breaded or fried oysters, canned white tuna, milk, and yogurt.

Deficiencies in Vitamin B₁₂ Deficiencies of vitamin B_{12} are rare because it is stored in the liver and the stores can last up to 10 years. The most common deficiency of vitamin B_{12} is due to PERNICIOUS ANEMIA, in which a substance normally produced in the stomach and needed for absorption of vitamin B_{12} (intrinsic factor) is absent. People who have pernicious anemia need intramuscular shots of this vitamin throughout their life. For others deficient in B_{12}, oral, sublingual, or nasal administration may be undertaken, especially after the B_{12} levels have normalized with parenteral administration.

People who have digestive disorders may also have a deficiency of vitamin B_{12}, such as those who have celiac sprue or a chronic inflammation of the stomach or small intestine called CROHN'S DISEASE. People who have had gastric surgery may also become deficient in vitamin B_{12}.

Sometimes older people (individuals who are age 65 and older) have a deficiency of vitamin B_{12}. Vegetarians who avoid fish, eggs, or milk can also have deficiency. People who are deficient in this vitamin may need to take supplements and increase their intake of foods that are rich in vitamin B_{12}.

Experts report that most people are not harmed by high doses of this vitamin; however, people should consult their physician before adding vitamin B_{12} supplements to their diet.

Vitamin E

Vitamin E is a powerful antioxidant, or cancer fighter, in the body. It protects against free radicals that can harm the cells. Vitamin E is found in green leafy vegetables, nuts, and vegetable oils. Some foods that are high in vitamin E are eggs, meat, wheat germ oil, almonds, safflower oil, turnip greens, mangoes, peanuts, and broccoli.

Vitamin E supplementation does not appear to have a role in the prevention or treatment of cancers, cardiovascular and cerebrovascular disease, dementia, and retinopathy of prematurity. Its role in Alzheimer's disease, tardive dyskinesia, and macular degeneration is controversial. In addition, vitamin E supplementation does not benefit healthy children or adults. However, vitamin E has been found to be beneficial in nonalcoholic fatty liver disease.

Deficiencies of Vitamin E Vitamin E deficiencies are rare in people worldwide. They can develop when people have disorders of fat metabolism. It has also been found in very low birth-weight INFANTS, weighing three-and-a-half pounds or less at birth. Others who may be deficient in vitamin E include those who have the following:

- cystic fibrosis
- Crohn's disease
- some forms of chronic liver disease
- pancreatic insufficiency

Some people have a rare hereditary fat metabolism disorder that is called abetalipoproteinemia, which makes their body unable to absorb adequate amounts of vitamin E or fat. They need prescribed vitamin E supplements. Ataxia with vitamin E deficiency (AVED) is a genetic defect in the alpha-tocopherol transfer protein (A-TTP).

A person deficient in vitamin E may experience muscle weakness, impaired vision, drooping eyelids, speech difficulty, and other neurological problems. He or she also has abnormal breakdown of red blood cells.

Excessive Levels of Vitamin E Clinical studies have not tested the effects of very high doses of vitamin E, which generally are not recommended. Doses up to 800 IU per day appear to be safe. High doses, especially in excess of 1,200 IU per day, may cause bleeding problems because high doses of vitamin E supplements may interfere with the absorption of vitamin K, which is needed for synthesis of clotting factors. As a result, anyone taking blood thinner drugs should not also take high doses of vitamin E. In addition, no one should take vitamin E supplements (or any other supplements) without checking with his or her physician to make sure that such supplements will not be harmful. Other symptoms of toxicity include DIARRHEA and headache.

The United States National Academy of Sciences Food and Nutrition Board recommends 15 mg of dietary alpha-tocopherol units (22 IU of "natural-source" vitamin E (RRR-alpha-tocopherol or 33 IUs of the synthetic form) per day for adults. Patients with vitamin E deficiency require large doses of up to 200 IU/kg/day. Up to 400 IU/day of vitamin E supplements may be safe for most people, although this data has been questioned. The Institute of Medicine, a Washington, D.C., organization that performs studies for federal government agencies, has set an upper level of vitamin E at 1,000 mg of supplemental alpha-tocopherol (approximately 1,500 IU of natural source or 1,100 IU of synthetic vitamin E) per day.

Vitamin D

Vitamin D helps the body to maintain normal levels of calcium and phosphorus. The body uses sunshine to make vitamin D and obtains it from foods that are consumed. Many foods are fortified with vitamin D. Few foods except for fortified ones have high vitamin D content and include eggs and fatty fish. Foods high in vitamin D include cod liver oil, cooked salmon, cooked mackerel, sardines, eels, and milk (nonfat, reduced fat, or whole milk).

Deficiencies of Vitamin D People can become deficient in vitamin D if they have little or no sunlight exposure. In some people the body cannot absorb vitamin D from the gastrointestinal tract. Sometimes the kidney is unable to produce 1, 25 (OH) 2-vitamin D. The most commonly known deficiencies of vitamin D are rickets and osteomalacia. Rickets is a childhood disease caused by a vitamin D deficiency, which causes weak bones and skeletal abnormalities. Osteomalacia, which causes muscle and bone weakness, is the disease in adults caused by vitamin D deficiency. Vitamin D deficiency is being called a "silent epidemic" by some.

People older than age 50 have a greater risk of being deficient in vitamin D than do younger individuals, and consequently, they may need to take supplemental vitamin D. People who may become deficient in vitamin D include the following groups:

- people who have Crohn's disease
- individuals who have kidney disease
- people who have celiac sprue
- individuals who have liver disease
- people who have pancreatic enzyme deficiency
- elderly individuals

A minimum of 200 IU (5 micrograms) daily of vitamin D per day is recommended However, due to potentially harmful subclinical vitamin D deficiency, higher vitamin D intakes are frequently recommended especially in pregnant and geriatric population. A dosage of 800 IU (20 micrograms) daily is beneficial for the prevention and treatment of osteoporosis. The "tolerable upper intake level" for vitamin D is 50 micrograms (2000 IU) daily for healthy adults and children 1 to 18 years.

Hypervitaminosis Vitamin D It is also possible to have too much vitamin D. It is almost impossible to have toxic levels of vitamin D through diet alone. Most people who have an excessively high level are taking supplements. Vitamin D excess can cause the following problems:

- nausea and vomiting
- CONSTIPATION
- increased thirst and urination
- itching
- weakness
- poor APPETITE
- weight loss
- mental confusion

The treatment of hypervitaminosis of vitamin D employs discontinuation of vitamin D, a low-calcium diet, and acidification of urine. Sometimes corticosteroids (such as prednisone) are prescribed.

See also IRON; MAGNESIUM; SELENIUM.

watermelon stomach   A rare condition of upper gastrointestinal bleeding that causes the stomach lining to have a characteristic endoscopic appearance of parallel red sores that form stripes similar to the striped pattern that is found on a watermelon. The red stripes represent abnormal blood vessels. The condition is also known as gastric antral vascular ectasia (GAVE). Most who have watermelon stomach are ELDERLY females (older than 65 or 70 years old). Watermelon stomach is a form of a malformation of blood vessels. Bleeding may be slow occult (microscopic) or overt; if it is untreated, the condition can lead to anemia and even vomiting of blood. Sometimes watermelon stomach is also associated with cirrhosis or scleroderma.

GAVE is formally diagnosed with an endoscopy. The diagnosis may be confirmed on histopathology and endoscopic ultrasound. In addition, when GAVE is present, the patient's stool specimens may test positive for occult bleeding. Occasionally, patients need blood transfusions. Patients who have watermelon stomach may be treated with cautery or laser therapy, and most need repeated procedures over time. Surgery may be needed for refractory cases. Some patients have been treated with female hormone replacement therapy (estrogen/progesterone).

See also ENDOSCOPY; OCCULT GASTROINTESTINAL BLEEDING.

Wernicke's encephalopathy   A condition that constitutes a medical emergency, which is caused by a severe deficiency of thiamine (vitamin B1), along with a continued intake of carbohydrates. It is also often brought on by chronic ALCOHOLISM. The condition was named after Carl Wernicke, a German neurologist.

Patients who are on prolonged vitamin-free intravenous nutrition, as after surgery, or who are engaging in fad diets are also at risk for development of Wernicke's encephalopathy. This condition is also called cerebral BERIBERI; it is precipitated by an acute deficiency as well as the acute or already chronic deficiency of thiamine. Typically, it occurs when glucose is administered to an alcoholic who is already deficient in thiamine, further depleting the body of thiamine.

Wernicke's encephalopathy causes a malfunction of the central nervous system, leading to balance disorder, severe confusion, and disorders of the eye movements. It may progress to coma and death.

Treatment requires intravenous or intramuscular administration of thiamine for prolonged periods. Recovery is not always complete; some symptoms start to improve within a few hours of treatment, and others may take a few months to improve. Wernicke's encephalopathy can be fatal.

See also VITAMIN DEFICIENCIES/EXCESSES.

O'Brien, Robert, Morris Chafetz, M.D., and Sidney Cohen, M.D., eds. *The Encyclopedia of Understanding Alcohol and Other Drugs.* New York: Facts On File, 1999.

Whipple's disease   An extremely rare systemwide bacterial infection that was first described in the medical literature in 1907 by a medical missionary, George Whipple. (About 30 cases per year are reported worldwide.) The disease is caused by the bacterium *Tropheryma whippelii*. These bacteria invade the gut wall, blood vessels, COLON, LIVER, brain, heart, lung, synovium, kidney, bone marrow, and skin.

Despite considerable difficulty, scientists were able to culture this infection; its cultivation was reported in 2000 in the *New England Journal of Medicine*.

Symptoms and Diagnostic Path

The most common symptoms found among patients with Whipple's disease are

- chronic weight loss
- arthralgias (joint pains)
- ABDOMINAL PAIN
- DIARRHEA
- ANEMIA
- hyperpigmentation
- abnormal rhythmic movements of the eyes and jaws

Diarrhea may be absent in a small number of patients making the suspicion for diagnosis difficult. Other symptoms that have been seen in some patients with Whipple's disease include the following:

- hypotension (low blood pressure)
- fever
- swollen lymph nodes
- shortness of breath

Patients may also exhibit a wasting away, or CACHEXIA, such as occurs in other diseases, such as acquired immune deficiency syndrome and in advanced stages of cancer.

Because it is so rare, and the symptoms are so diverse and nonspecific, physicians may initially have difficulty in diagnosing Whipple's disease. However, the diagnosis can be easily made by a microscopic view of a biopsy tissue sample from the small intestine. Special tests using polymerase chain reaction (PCR) may be able to identify the infection in the future. Other conditions that may mimic Whipple's disease and need to be considered in differential diagnosis include hyperthyroidism, connective tissue disorders, INFLAMMATORY BOWEL DISEASE, and AIDS.

Treatment Options and Outlook

Most Whipple's disease patients are treated with long-term ANTIBIOTICS for a year or more, though they start to feel better within a few days. The disease relapses after discontinuation of treatment in 17 to 35 percent of cases.

Risk Factors and Preventive Measures

When found, the disease has usually been diagnosed in middle-aged or older men. There are no known preventive measures.

Raoult, Didier, M.D., et al. "Cultivation of the Bacillus of Whipple's Disease." *New England Journal of Medicine* 342, no. 9 (March 2, 2000): 620–625.
Swartz, Morton N., M.D. "Whipple's Disease—Past, Present, and Future," *New England Journal of Medicine* 342, no. 9 (March 2, 2000): 648–650.

Wilson's disease An unusual genetic disease in which the body retains toxically high levels of copper, primarily in the LIVER and brain; it is also known as hepatolenticular degeneration. The neurologist Samuel Alexander Kinnier Wilson first described the disease in 1912, and it was subsequently named after him. Wilson's disease is found among men and women in all racial and ethnic groups. The symptoms are usually first identified in childhood or adolescence but may be missed altogether till old age.

Experts estimate that Wilson's disease occurs in about one in 100,000 births, although it may be underdiagnosed. Some experts believe the true incidence is actually one in 30,000 births.

The cause of Wilson's disease is a genetic defect found on chromosome 13 involving copper transporting protein in the liver. This results in decreased transport of copper from the liver into bile, thus leading to copper excess in the liver.

Symptoms and Diagnostic Path

Some Wilson's disease patients may appear healthy; their illness draws attention when they are found to have abnormal liver test results on routine testing. Children and adolescents who have Wilson's disease usually have liver problems, whereas adults experience neuropsychiatric disorders, such as tremors, rigidity, difficulty with speaking and walking, and drooling.

A classic sign of Wilson's disease is found in the eye: a rusty brown ring in the cornea that is caused by the accumulation of copper. This sign, called the Kayser-Fleischer ring, is usually seen by an ophthalmologist, using a procedure called a slit lamp examination. Rarely, the sign may be visible to the naked eye. However, this sign may not be present, especially in an early stage of the disease. Another problem is that observing it may be difficult to impossible in a routine physical examination of individuals who have brown eyes.

Other symptoms of hepatic disease caused by Wilson's disease include the following:

- APPETITE loss
- dark urine
- JAUNDICE

As the disease progresses, indicators of advanced disease are found. Some symptoms of neuropsychiatric problems are:

- slurred speech
- tremors
- double vision
- DYSPHAGIA (difficulty with swallowing)
- spastic movements

Some Wilson's disease patients may present for the first time with a life-threatening fulminant hepatic failure; such patients require LIVER TRANSPLANTATION on an emergency basis.

Wilson's disease can be a very difficult disease to diagnose because it can mimic symptoms of CIRRHOSIS and HEPATITIS due to different causes, as well as a wide variety of diseases of the brain, liver, blood, and kidneys (such as kidney stones). In addition, some individuals diagnosed with schizophrenia, a severe psychiatric disease, may actually have Wilson's disease. Patients with psychotic disorders should be screened for Wilson's disease because medications given to treat psychosis may worsen the illness and not resolve the psychotic behavior.

Testing includes serum ceruloplasmin, 24 hour urinary copper, slit lamp exam of the eyes, and liver biopsy. Screening of family members of patients diagnosed with Wilson's disease may be undertaken.

Treatment Options and Outlook

If Wilson's disease is diagnosed in the early stages, patients can be treated with medications called chelators, which combine with metals and decrease copper accumulation in the body. Treatment is aimed at removing the excess copper and preventing it from reaccumulating. Thus, people who have Wilson's disease must take these drugs for the rest of their life; those who stop treatment may worsen rapidly.

The most commonly used chelators are D-penicillamine and trientine. Trientine has a favorable side-effect profile and is preferred by many. For the prevention of reaccumulation, lower doses of these chelators or, alternatively, ZINC may be used. If the disease is diagnosed in a later stage, patients with severe liver damage may need a liver transplantation to save their life.

Risk Factors and Preventive Measures

Wilson's disease is a genetic disorder. There are no preventive measures.

See also HEMOCHROMATOSIS; LIVER ENZYMES / FUNCTION TESTS.

women and digestive diseases Although both men and women have a variety of digestive diseases and disorders, women are more likely to have some illnesses, such as GALLSTONES, GALLBLADDER CANCER, HIRSCHSPRUNG'S DISEASE, IRRITABLE BOWEL SYNDROME (IBS), PRIMARY BILIARY CIRRHOSIS, and WATERMELON STOMACH. In contrast, men have a much greater risk of development of KAPOSI'S SARCOMA than women (15 men to one woman). Men also have a higher risk of cirrhosis of the liver, esophageal cancer, liver cancer, stomach cancer, alcoholic pancreatitis, and hepatocelluclar carcinoma.

yeast See *CANDIDA;* THRUSH.

yo-yo dieting The process of frequently gaining and losing significant amounts of weight (20 pounds or more in a short period, such as a month or less). It is also known as weight cycling. Some experts believe that individuals who repeatedly gain and lose large amounts of weight are at risk for development of some illnesses, such as gallbladder disease, hypertension, and high cholesterol levels. That conclusion is controversial, and firm data about the harmful effects of yo-yo dieting are lacking.

Obese individuals should try to lose weight; a slow, steady weight loss of several pounds per month is recommended by most physicians. Rapid weight loss can cause development of GALLSTONES as well as NONALCOHOLIC STEATOHEPATITIS/NONALCOHOLIC FATTY LIVER DISEASE.

See also DIET DRUGS; OBESITY.

Z

Zenker's diverticulum   A pouch that forms in the ESOPHAGUS due to evagination from a defect in the hypopharynx in a natural area of weakness known as "Killian's hiatus." This evagination (protrusion of a layer of the esophagus) occurs due to the high pressures on the weakened area occurring due to abnormal esophageal motility, shortening of the esophageal tube, or problems associated with the opening of the upper esophageal sphincter. GASTROESOPHAGEAL REFLUX DISEASE may also be a contributing factor. (More than one diverticulum are diverticula.) A second diverticulum is present in 1 to 2 percent of all cases.

Named after Albert Zenker, a German physician and pathologist who described the problem in 1877, these diverticula constitute about two-thirds of all esophageal diverticula.

Symptoms and Diagnostic Path

Zenker's diverticulum does not always cause symptoms or signs. It can result in bad breath (halitosis) as well as regurgitation of food. The regurgitation can be frightening because it is more likely to occur when the patient is lying down and can lead to aspiration and pneumonia in some patients. Zenker's diverticulum patients may also experience difficulty with swallowing (DYSPHAGIA). Some patients report a bad taste in the mouth and a feeling of something stuck in the throat. Patients may also have neck pain, and some experience weight loss. Zenker's diverticulum can even cause cancer in the pouch. An ulcer in the diverticulum and bleeding due to retained medications such as aspirin may occur.

Physicians identify Zenker's diverticulum through barium swallow. Some physicians use MANOMETRY to measure esophageal pressures. Physicians may also use an upper ENDOSCOPY.

Treatment Options and Outlook

Patients who have symptomatic Zenker's diverticula usually need surgery. Procedures using an endoscope may be performed in some centers.

Risk Factors and Preventive Measures

Men are two to three times more likely to have Zenker's diverticula, and generally they are found among ELDERLY individuals age 70 years and older. There are no preventive measures.

See also MECKEL'S DIVERTICULUM.

Overbeck, J. J. van. "Pathogenesis and Methods of Treatments of Zenker's Diverticulum," *Otology, Rhinology, Laryngology* 112, no. 7 (July 2003): 583–593.

zinc   An essential mineral that is involved in more than 100 enzyme systems and that helps promote numerous important biochemical reactions in the human body. The body contains about 2 to 3.0 grams of zinc. Zinc is also important in providing support to the immune system, healing wounds, and maintaining the senses of smell and taste. Zinc is essential for normal growth during childhood and adolescence and for fetal growth during pregnancy.

Foods that are high in zinc include the following items: shellfish, oysters, whole-grain cereals, lean cooked beef shank (leg meat), lean cooked beef chuck, lean cooked pork shoulder, roasted chicken leg meat, and legumes. Zinc supplementation is useful in treating WILSON'S DISEASE, in which there is an overload of copper. Zinc prevents copper absorption and/or promotes copper excretion into the feces, and hence is useful for treatment of Wilson's disease. Chronic high doses of zinc supplementation may cause copper deficiency.

Deficiencies of Zinc

In most cases, a person's daily diet provides sufficient amounts of zinc. (The recommended daily allowance for adults per the Institute of Medicine is 11 mg per day for men and 8 mg per day for nonpregnant women; the RDA increases to 11 mg/d during PREGNANCY and 12mg/d during lactation.) Others recommend 15 to 18 mg/d for all adults. Some people have a zinc deficiency. People who are at most risk for a zinc deficiency include the following groups:

- vegetarians
- ELDERLY people
- individuals who have liver disease
- alcoholics
- people who have CROHN'S DISEASE or short bowel syndrome
- people who have chronic DIARRHEA
- patients on total PARENTERAL NUTRITION without adequate zinc supplementation

Pharmacologic doses of zinc supplementation may help increase linear growth and weight gain in INFANTS and enhance immune function of the elderly; they are also beneficial in cases of preterm labor, premature birth, prolonged labor, intrapartum hemorrhage, and low sperm counts. It has been found to be helpful in preventing respiratory infections and diarrhea as well as possibly reducing mortality. Before anyone takes a zinc supplement, he or she should consult a physician to ensure that it is really necessary.

Signs of a zinc deficiency include the following:

- impaired taste
- impaired immunity
- skin rash
- impaired wound healing
- delayed growth of a child
- loss of hair
- diarrhea
- sterility and impotence
- APPETITE loss
- night blindness

Toxic Levels of Zinc

It is possible for individuals to take too much zinc. It is virtually impossible to attain toxic levels in the diet, but a zinc overdose may occur when people take zinc supplements in excessive amounts. Excessive levels of zinc may cause NAUSEA AND VOMITING and may impair important metabolic functions in the body. In addition, they may lead to copper deficiency.

See also VITAMIN DEFICIENCIES/EXCESSES.

Zollinger-Ellison syndrome A medical condition that is characterized by digestive problems, such as peptic ULCERS, DIARRHEA, and ABDOMINAL PAIN. This syndrome was first described by D. Zollinger and Ellison in 1955.

Individuals who have Zollinger-Ellison syndrome have tumors (called gastrinomas) that secrete a hormone called gastrin, which in turn leads to the excessive secretion of digestive acid (hydrochloric acid). Tumors may be single or multiple and are frequently present in the gastrinoma triangle which is bordered by the head of the pancreas and duodenum, but they may also occur in the stomach, bones, ovaries, LIVER, heart or abdominal lymph nodes. The gastrinoma may be benign or cancerous (localized or metastatic), with an associated spread to other organs, such as the liver and the bones. About one-third of the tumors are metastatic at the time of diagnosis. In about 25 percent of cases, the disease is associated with MULTIPLE ENDOCRINE NEOPLASIA type 1 (MEN-1), a genetic syndrome that is characterized by tumors of the pituitary and parathyroid glands, in addition to the gastrinomas frequently seen in the PANCREAS.

Symptoms and Diagnostic Path

Symptoms of this medical condition include abdominal pain, diarrhea, and high amounts of fat found in the patient's stool (steatorrhea). As many as 90 percent of these patients have peptic ulcer disease.

Patients are suspected to have Zollinger-Ellison syndrome on the basis of symptoms of abdominal pain and/or diarrhea, with the associated finding of atypical peptic ulcer disease and/or MALABSORPTION SYNDROME. However, less than 1 percent of peptic ulcer patients have Zollinger-Ellison syndrome.

Once this medical problem is suspected, the physician orders testing of serum level of the hormone gastrin in a fasting state, which may be complemented by testing after stimulation injection of secretin, another hormone. Hydrochloric acid levels of the stomach can also be measured; they are abnormally high among Zollinger-Ellison syndrome patients.

After the diagnosis, the physician orders tests such as radionuclide somatostatin scan and/or computed tomography (CT) scan to localize the gastrinoma. An endoscopic ultrasound is also helpful.

Treatment Options and Outlook

Acid suppression with PROTON PUMP INHIBITOR medications is required for these patients, in order to suppress the effects and complications of excess acid secretion. In sporadic cases, the tumor is usu-ally a single one, and there is no spread to distant organs such as the liver or bones, surgery is the treatment of choice. In individuals who have metastatic disease (in which the cancer has spread), chemotherapy may be employed. Palliative surgery (to relieve pain) may also be chosen by the physician. Surgery is not recommended in patients with gastrinoma as part of MEN.

Risk Factors and Preventive measures

Zollinger-Ellison syndrome usually is diagnosed when an individual is between 20 and 50 years, although it may also be seen in children as well as elderly adults.

Wynbrandt, James, and Mark D. Ludman. *The Encyclopedia of Genetic Disorders and Birth Defects.* 2d ed. New York: Facts On File, 2000.

APPENDIXES

APPENDIX I
NATIONAL ORGANIZATIONS

AARP
601 E Street NW
Washington, DC 20049
(202) 434-2277
(888) 687-2277 (toll-free)
http://www.aarp.org

Administration on Aging
Department of Health and Human Services
200 Independence Avenue SW
Washington, DC 20201
(202) 619-0724
http://www.aoa.gov

Agency for Healthcare Research Quality (AHRQ)
Publications Clearinghouse
540 Gaither Road
Rockville, MD 20850
(301) 427-1364
http://www.ahrq.gov

Alagille Syndrome Alliance
10500 SW Starr Drive
Tualatin, OR 97062
(503) 885-6455
http://www.alagille.org

Alcoholics Anonymous
Grand Central Station
P.O. Box 459
New York, NY 10163
http://www.alcoholics-anonymous.org

Alliance for Aging Research
2021 K Street NW
Suite 305
Washington, DC 20006
(202) 293-2856
http://www.agingresearch.org

Alpha-1 Foundation
2937 Southwest 27th Avenue
Suite 302
Miami, FL 33133
(877) 228-7325
http://www.alphaone.org

American Academy of Allergy, Asthma and Immunology
611 East Wells Street
Milwaukee, WI 53202
(414) 272-6071
(800) 822-2762 (toll-free)
http://www.aaaai.org

American Academy of Family Physicians (AAFP)
11400 Tomahawk Creek Parkway
Leawood, KS 66211
(800) 274-2237 (toll-free)

American Academy of Ophthalmology
P.O. Box 7424
San Francisco, CA 94120
(415) 561-8500
http://www.aao.org

American Academy of Pediatrics
141 Northwest Point Boulevard
Elk Grove Village, IL 60007
(847) 434-4000
http://www.aap.org

American Anorexia Bulimia Association
165 West 46th Street, #1108
New York, NY 10036
(212) 575-6200

American Association for Diabetes Educators
100 West Monroe Street

4th Floor
Chicago, IL 60603
(800) 338-3633
http://www.aadenet.org

American Association for Higher Education
One Dupont Circle
Suite 360
Washington, DC 20036
(202) 293-6440
http://www.aahe.org

**American Association for the Study of Liver
  Diseases (AASLD)**
1729 King Street
Suite 200
Alexandria, VA 22314
(703) 299-9766
http://www.aasld.org

**American Association of Clinical
  Endocrinologists**
1000 Riverside Avenue
Suite 205
Jacksonville, FL 32304
(904) 353-7878
http://www.aace.com

**American Association of Poison Control
  Centers**
3201 New Mexico Avenue
Suite 330
Washington, DC 20016
(202) 362-7217
http://www.aapcc.org

**American Autoimmune Related Diseases
  Association**
22100 Gratiot Avenue
East Detroit, MI 48021
(586) 776-3900
http://wwvv.aarda.org

American Behçet's Disease Association
P.O. Box 19952
Amarillo, TX 79114
(800) 723-4238 (toll-free)
http://www.behcets.com

American Board of Medical Specialties
47 Perimeter Center East
Suite 500

Atlanta, GA 36346
(800) 776-2378 (toll free)

American Board of Pediatric Surgery
1601 Dolores Street
San Francisco, CA 94110
(415) 826-3200

American Cancer Society
1599 Clifton Road NE
Atlanta, GA 30329
(404) 320-3333
(800) 277-2345 (toll-free)
http://www.cancer.org

**American Celiac Society Dietary Support
  Coalition**
P.O. Box 23455
New Orleans, LA 70183–0455
(504) 737–3293
http://www.americanceliacsociety.org

American Chronic Pain Association
P.O. Box 850
Rocklin, CA 95677
(916) 632-0922
http://www.theacpa.org

American College of Gastroenterology
P.O. Box 342260
Bethesda, MD 20827–2260
(301) 263–9000
http://www.acg.gi.org

**American College of Physicians, American
  Society of Internal Medicine (ACP-ASIM)**
190 North Independence Mall West
Philadelphia, PA 19106
(215) 351-2400
(800) 523-1546 (toll-free)
http://www.acpoline.org

American College of Sports Medicine
P.O. Box 1440
Indianapolis, IN 46206
(317) 637-9200

American College of Surgeons (ACS)
633 North Saint Clair Street
Chicago, IL 60611
(312) 202-5000
http://www.facs.org

American Diabetes Association (ADA)

1701 North Beauregard Street
Alexandria, VA 22311
(703) 549-1500
(800) 232-3472 (toll-free)
http://www.diabetes.org/

American Dietetic Association

120 South Riverside Plaza
Suite 2000
Chicago, IL 60606–6995
(312) 899-0040
(800) 877-1600 (toll-free)
http://www.eatright.org

American Gastroenterological Association (AGA)

National Office
4930 Del Ray Avenue
Bethesda, MD 20814
(301) 654-2055
http://www.gastro.org

American Heart Association/American Stroke Association

7272 Greenville Avenue
Dallas, TX 75231
(800) 242-8721 (toll-free)
http://www.americanheart.org

American Hemochromatosis Society

4044 West Lake Mary Boulevard, #104
PMB 416
Lake Mary, FL 32746–2012
(407) 829-4488
(888) 655-4766 (toll-free)
http://www.americanhs.org

American Hospital Association (AHA)

One North Franklin
Chicago, IL 60606
(312) 422-3000
http://www.aha.org

American Institute for Cancer Research

1759 R Street NW
Washington, DC 20009
(202) 328-7744
(800) 843-8114 (toll-free)
http://www.aicr.org

American Liver Foundation

75 Maiden Lane
Suite 603
New York, NY 10038
(212) 668-1000
(800) 465-4837 (toll-free)
http://www.liverfoundation.org

American Lung Association

1740 Broadway
New York, NY 10019
(212) 315-0870
http://www.lungusa.org

American Medical Association

515 North State Street
Chicago, IL 60610
(312) 464-5000
http://www.ama-assn.org

American Motility Society

45685 Harmony Lane
Belleville, MI 48111
(734) 699-1130
http://www.motilitysociety.org

American Nurses Association

600 Maryland Avenue SW
Suite 100 West
Washington, DC 20024
(800) 274-4262
http://www.nursingworld.org

American Pancreatic Association

P.O. Box 14906
Minneapolis, MN 55414
(612) 626-9797
http://www.american-pancreatic-association.org

American Partnership for Eosinpohilic Disorders

3419 Whispering Way Drive
Richmond, TX 77469
(713) 498-8216
http://www.apfed.org
mail@apfed.org

American Pharmacists Association

2215 Constitution Avenue NW
Washington, DC 20037
(202) 628-4410
http://www.pharmacist.com

American Porphyria Foundation
4900 Woodway
Suite 780
Houston, TX 77056–1837
(866) APF-3635
(713) 266-9617
http://www.porphyriafoundation.com

American Psychiatric Association
1000 Wilson Boulevard
Suite 1825
Arlington, VA 22209
(703) 907-7300
http://www.psych.org

American Society for Metabolic and Bariatric Surgery
100 SW 75th Street
Suite 201
Gainesville, FL 32607
(352) 331-4900
http://www.asbs.org

American Society for Gastrointestinal Endoscopy (ASGE)
1520 Kensington Road
Suite 202
Oak Brook, IL 60523
http://www.asge.org

American Society for Parenteral and Enteral Nutrition (ASPEN)
8630 Fenton Street
Suite 412
Silver Spring, MD 20910
(301) 587-6315
http://www.nutritioncare.org

American Society of Abdominal Surgeons
1 East Emerson Street
Melrose, MA 02176
(781) 665-6102
http://www.abdominalsurg.org

American Society of Colon and Rectal Surgeons (ASCRS)
85 West Algonquin Road
Suite 550
Arlington Heights, IL 60005
(847) 290-9184
http://www.fascrs.org

American Society of Human Genetics
9650 Rockville Pike
Bethesda, MD 20814
(301) 634-7300
http://www.ashg.org

Association of Gastrointestinal Motility Disorders, Inc. (AGMD)
(formerly American Society of Adults with Pseudo-Obstruction, Inc.)
AGMD International Corporate Headquarters
12 Roberts Drive
Bedford, MA 01730
(781) 275-1300
http://www.agmd-gimotility.org

Autosomal Recessive Polycystic Kidney Disease & Congenital Hepatic Fibrosis Alliance
P.O. Box 70
Kirkwood, PA 17536
(717) 529-5555
http://www.arpkd.org

Cancer Research Foundation of America
1600 Duke Street
Suite 110
Alexandria, VA 22314
(703) 836-4412
(800) 227-2732 (toll-free)
http://www.preventcancer.org

Carcinoid Cancer Foundation, Inc.
The Carcinoid Cancer Foundation, Inc.
333 Mamaroneck Avenue, # 492
White Plains, NY 10605
(914) 683-1001
(888) 722-3132 (toll-free)

Celiac Disease Foundation
13251 Ventura Boulevard, #1
Studio City, CA 91604
(818) 990-2354
http://www.celiac.org

Celiac Sprue Association USA
P.O. Box 31700
Omaha, NE 68131–0700
(877) CSA-4CSA
http://www.csaceliacs.org

Centers for Disease Control and Prevention (CDC)
1600 Clifton Road NE
Atlanta, GA 30333
(800) 311-3435
http://www.cdc.gov

Centers for Medicare and Medicaid Services
7500 Security Boulevard
Baltimore, MD 21244
(800) 633-4227 (toll-free)
http://www.cms.hhs.gov

Colorectal Cancer Network
P.O. Box 182
Kensington, MD 20895
(301) 879-1500
http://clickonium.com/colorectal-cancer.net/html/

Crohn's & Colitis Foundation of America
386 Park Avenue South
17th Floor
New York, NY 10016
(212) 685-3440
(800) 932-2423 (toll-free)
http://www.ccfa.org

Cushing's Support and Research Foundation, Inc.
65 East India Row, #22B
Boston, MA 02110
(617) 723-3824
http://csrf.net/

Cyclic Vomiting Syndrome Association
CVSA USA/Canada
3585 Cedar Hill Road NW
Canal Winchester, OH 43110
(614) 837-2586
http://www.cvsaonline.org

Diabetes Action Research and Education Foundation
426 C Street NE
Washington, DC 20002
(202) 333-4520
http://www.diabetesaction.org

Diabetes Exercise and Sports Association
8001 Montcastle Drive
Nashville, TN 37221

(800) 898-4322 (toll-free)
http://www.diabetes-exercise.org

Digestive Disease National Coalition
507 Capitol Court NE
Suite 200
Washington, DC 20002
(202) 544-7497
http://www.ddnc.org

Disability Rights Education and Defense Fund, Inc.
221 Sixth Street
Berkeley, CA 94710
(510) 644-2555
(800) 348-4232 (toll-free)
http://www.dredf.org

Family Caregiver Alliance
180 Montgomery Street
Suite 1100
San Francisco, CA 94104
(415) 434-3388
http://www.caregiver.org

Food Allergy & Anaphylaxis Network
11781 Lee Highway
Suite 160
Fairfax, VA 22033–3309
(800) 929-4040 (toll-free)
http://www.foodallergy.org

Food and Drug Administration (FDA)
5600 Fishers Lane
Rockville, MD 20857
(888) 463-6332 (toll-free)
http://www.fda.org

Food and Nutrition Information Center
National Agricultural Library
10301 Baltimore Boulevard
Room 105
Beltsville, MD 20705
(301) 504-5414

Gastro-Intestinal Research Foundation
70 East Lake Street
Suite 1015
Chicago, IL 60601–5907
(312) 332-1350
http://www.girf.org

The Genetic Alliance
4301 Connecticut Avenue NW
Suite 404
Washington, DC 20008
(202) 966-5557
http://www.geneticalliance.org

Gluten Intolerance Group of North America (GIG)
31214 124th Avenue SE
Auburn, WA 98092
(253) 833-6655
http://www.gluten.net

Hepatitis B Coalition/Immunization Action Coalition
1573 Selby Avenue
Suite 234
St. Paul, MN 55104
(651) 647-9009
http://www.immunize.org

Hepatitis B Foundation
3805 Old Easton Road
Doylestown, PA 18902
(215) 489-4900
http://www.hepb.org

Hepatitis Foundation International
504 Blick Drive
Silver Spring, MD 20904
(301) 622-4200
(800) 891-0707 (toll-free)
http://www.hepfi.org

Human Growth Foundation
997 Glen Cove Avenue
Suite 5
Glen Head, NY 11545
(800) 451-6434
http://www.hgfound.org

Huntington's Disease Society of America
505 Eighth Avenue
Suite 902
New York, NY 10018
(800) 345-4372 (HDSA) (toll-free)
http://www.hdsa.org

International Association for Medical Assistance to Travelers
1623 Military Road
Suite 279
Niagara Falls, NY 14304
(716) 754-4883
http://www.iamat.org

International Foundation for Functional Gastrointestinal Disorders, Inc.
P.O. Box 170864
Milwaukee, WI 53217-8076
(414) 964-1799
(888) 964-2001 (toll-free)
http://www.iffgd.org

Iron Disorders Institute
2722 Wade Hampton Boulevard
Suite A
Greenville, SC 29615
(864) 292-1175
http://www.irondisorders.org

Iron Overload Diseases Association, Inc.
P.O. Box 15857
North Palm Beach, FL 33416
(561) 586-8246
http://www.ironoverload.org

Juvenile Diabetes Research Foundation (JDF) International
120 Wall Street
New York, NY 10005
(800) 533-2873 (toll-free)
http://www.jdf.org

MedicAlert Foundation International
2323 Colorado Avenue
Turlock, CA 95832
(888) 633-429 (toll-free)
http://www.medicalalert.org

National Association of Anorexia Nervosa and Associated Disorders
P.O. Box 7
Highland Park, IL 60035
(847) 831-3438
http://www.anad.org

National Association of Nutrition and Aging Service Programs
1612 K Street NW
Suite 400

Washington, DC 20006
(202) 682-6899
http://www.nanasp.org

National Cancer Institute
6116 Executive Boulevard
Room 3036-A
Bethesda, MD 20892
(800) 422-6237 (toll-free)

National Center for Complementary and Alternative Medicine (NCCAM)
9000 Rockville Pike
Bethesda, MD 20892
(888) 644-6226 (toll-free)
http://www.nccam.nih.gov

National Center for Health Statistics
3311 Toledo Road
Hyattsville, MD 20782
(800) 232-4636 (toll-free)
http://www.cdc.gov/nchs

National Coalition for Cancer Survivorship (NCCS)
1010 Wayne Avenue
Suite 770
Silver Spring, MD 20910
(888) 650-9127
http://www.canceradvocacy.org

National Council on Aging
1901 L Street NW
4th Floor
Washington, DC 20036
(202) 479-1200
(800) 424-9046 (toll-free)
http://www.nooa.org

National Diabetes Information Clearinghouse
1 Diabetes Way
Bethesda, MD 20892
(800) 438-5383 (toll-free)
http://www.ndep.nih.gov

National Digestive Diseases Information Clearinghouse
2 Information Way
Bethesda, MD 20892
(800) 891-5389 (toll-free)
http://digestive.niddk.nih.gov

National Dissemination Center for Children and Youth with Disabilities
P.O. Box 1492
Washington, DC 20013
(800) 695-0285 (toll-free)
http://www.nichcy.org

National Eating Disorders Organization
603 Stewart Street
Suite 803
Seattle, WA 98101
(206) 382-3587
http://www.nationaleatingdisorders.org

National Family Caregivers Association
10400 Connecticut Avenue
Suite 500
Kensington, MD 20895
(301) 942-6430
http://www.nfcacares.org

National Foundation for Celiac Awareness
P.O. Box 544
Ambler, PA 19002
(215) 325-1306
http://www.celiaccentral.org

National Health Information Center (NHIC)
Department of Health and Human Services
P.O. Box 1133
Washington, DC 20013
(800) 336-4797 (toll-free)
http: //www.health.gov/NHIC

National Heart, Lung and Blood Institute Information Center
31 Center Drive
MSC 2486
Building 31, Room 5A48
Bethesda, MD 20892
(301) 592-8573
http://www.nhlbi.nih.gov/health/infoctr.index.htm

National Institute of Arthritis and Musculoskeletal and Skin Diseases (NIAMS)
One AMS Circle
Bethesda, MD 20892
(301) 495-4484
http://www.niams.nih.gov

National Institute of Diabetes and Digestive and Kidney Diseases

National Institutes of Health
31 Center Drive
MSC 2560
Building 31, Room 9A06
Bethesda, MD 20892
(301) 496-3583
http://ww2.niddk.nih.gov

National Institute of Mental Health (NIMH)

Public Inquiries
6001 Executive Boulevard
Room 8184, MSC 9663
Bethesda, MD 20892
(301) 443-4513
http://www.nimh.nih.gov

National Institutes of Allergy and Infectious Diseases

6610 Rockledge Drive
MSC 6612
Bethesda, MD 20892
(866) 284-4107
http://www3.niad/gov

National Kidney Foundation, Inc.

30 East 33rd Street
New York, NY 10016
(800) 622-9010 (toll-free)
http://www.kidney.org

National Organization for Rare Disorders (NORD)

55 Kenosia Avenue
Danbury, CT 06813
(203) 744-0100
http://www.rarediseases.org

The National Pancreas Foundation

364 Boylston Street
4th Floor
Boston, MA 02116
(866) 726-2737
http://www.pancreasfoundation.org

National Women's Health Information Center

8270 Willow Oaks Corporation Drive
Fairfax, VA 22031
(800) 994-9662 (toll-free)
http://www.womenshealth.gov

Nevus Outreach, Inc.

600 SE Delaware Avenue
Suite 200
Bartlesville, OK 74003
(918) 331-0595
http://www.nevus.org

North American Menopause Society (NAMS)

P.O. Box 94527
Cleveland, OH 44101
(440) 442-7550
http://www.menopause.org

North American Society for Pediatric Gastroenterology, Hepatology, and Nutrition

NASPGHAN
P.O. Box 6
Flourtown, PA 19031
(215) 233-0808
http://www.naspghan.org

Office of Dietary Supplements

National Institutes of Health
6100 Executive Boulevard
Room 3B01, MSC 7517
Bethesda, MD 20892
(301) 435-2920
http://ods.od.nih.gov/

Office of Minority Health Resource Center

P.O. Box 37337
Washington, DC 20013
(800) 444-6472 (toll-free)
http://www.omhrc.gov

Oley Foundation for Home Parenteral and Enteral Nutrition (HOmePEN)

Albany Medical Center
214 Hun Memorial
MC-28
Albany, NY 12208
(518) 262-5079
(800) 776-6539 (toll-free)
http://www.oley.org

Overeaters Anonymous World Services

P.O. Box 44020
Rio Rancho, NM 87124
(505) 891-2664
http://www.oa.org

Pancreatic Cancer Action Network
2141 Rosecrans Avenue
Suite 7000
El Segundo, CA 90245
(877) 272-6226
http://www.pancan.org

Pediatric/Adolescent Gastroesophageal Reflux Association (PAGER)
P.O. Box 486
Buckeystown, MD 21717–0486
(301) 601-9541
http://www.reflux.org

Pull-thru Network
2312 Savoy Street
Hoover, AL 35226-1528
(205) 978-2930
http://www.pullthrough.org

Reach Out for Youth with Ileitis and Colitis, Inc.
84 Northgate Circle
Melville, NY 11747
(631) 293-3102
http://www.reachoutforyouth.org

Scleroderma Foundation
300 Rosewood Drive
Suite 105
Danvers, MA 01923
(978) 463-5843
http://www.scleroderma.org

Scleroderma Research Foundation
220 Montgomery Street
Suite 1411
San Francisco, CA 94104
(415) 834-9444
http://www.srfcure.org

Social Security Administration (SSA)
Office of Public Inquiries
Windsor Park Building
6401 Security Boulevard
Baltimore, MD 21235
(800) 772-1213 (toll-free)
http://www.ssa.gov

Society for Neuroscience
1121 14th Street NW
Suite 1010

Washington, DC 20005
(202) 962-4000
http://www.sfn.org

Society for Surgery of the Alimentary Tract, Inc.
900 Cummings Center
Suite #221-U
Beverly, MA 01915
(978) 927-8330
http://www.ssat.com/

Society of Gastroenterology Nurses and Associates (SGNA)
401 North Michigan Avenue
Chicago, IL 60611
(800) 245-7462 (toll-free)
http://www.sgna.org/

Substance Abuse and Mental Health Services Administration (SAMHSA)
SAMHSA's Health Information Network
P.O. Box 2345
Rockville, MD 20847-2345
(800) 729-6686 (toll-free)
http://www.samhsa.gov

TOPS Club (Take Pounds Off Sensibly)
4575 South Fifth Street
Milwaukee, WI 53207
(414) 482-4620
http://www.tops.org

Transplant Recipient International Organization (TRIO)
2100 M Street NW, #170-353
Washington, DC 20037-1233
http://www.trioweb.org

United Ostomy Association, Inc.
P.O. Box 66
Fairview, TN 37062-0066
(800) 826-0826 (toll-free)
http://www.uoaa.org

Weight-Control Information Network
National Institute of Diabetes and Digestive and Kidney Diseases (NIDDK)
1 WIN Way
Bethesda, MD 20892
(202) 828-1025
http://win.niddk.nih.gov/

Wilson's Disease Association
1802 Brookside Drive
Wooster, OH 44691
(888) 264-1450 (toll-free)
http://www.wilsonsdisease.org

World Health Organization (WHO)
    Headquarters
Avenue Appia 20
1211 Geneva 27
Switzerland
+41-22-791-2111
http: //www.who.int

Organizations in Canada

Canadian Celiac Association
5170 Dixie Road
Suite 204
Mississauga, ON L4W 1E3
(800) 363-7296 (toll-free)
http://www.celiac.ca/

Canadian Liver Foundation
2235 Sheppard Avenue East
Suite 1500
Toronto, ON M2J B5B
(800) 563-5483 (toll-free)

APPENDIX II
STATE HEALTH DEPARTMENTS IN THE UNITED STATES

ALABAMA

Alabama Department of Public Health
RSA Tower
201 Monroe Street
Suite 914
Montgomery, AL 36104
(334) 206-5300
http:/ /www.adph.org

ALASKA

Department of Health and Social Services
350 Main Street
P.O. Box 110601
Juneau, AK 99811
(907) 465-3030
http://hss.state.ak.us/commissioner

ARIZONA

Arizona Department of Health Services
150 North 18th Avenue
Phoenix, AZ 85007
(602) 542-1025
http://www.azdhs.gov

ARKANSAS

Arkansas Department of Public Health
4815 West Markham Street
Little Rock, AR 72205
(501) 661-2000
http://www.healthyarkansas.com

CALIFORNIA

California Department of Public Health
P.O. Box 997410
Sacramento, CA 95899
(916) 558-1784

COLORADO

Colorado Department of Public Health and Environment
4300 Cherry Creek Drive South
Denver, CO 80246
(303) 692-2000
http://www.cdphe.state.co.us

CONNECTICUT

Connecticut Department of Public Health
410 Capitol Avenue
Hartford, CT 06134
(860) 509-8000
http://www.ct.gov.dph/site/default.asp

DELAWARE

Delaware Department of Health and Social Services
Division of Public Health
1901 North DuPont Highway
Main Building
New Castle, DE 19720
(302) 255-9040
http://dhss.delaware.gov/dhss

DISTRICT OF COLUMBIA

Department of Health
825 North Capitol Street NE
Washington, DC 20002
(202) 442-5955
http://dchealth.dc.gov/doh/site/default.asp

FLORIDA

Florida Department of Health
4052 Bald Cypress Way
Bin A00
Tallahassee, FL 32399
(850) 245-4444
http://www.doh.state.fl.us

GEORGIA

Georgia Department of Community Health
Division of Public Health
2 Peachtree Street NW
Atlanta, GA 30303
(404) 657-2700
http://health.state.ga.us

HAWAII

Hawaii State Department of Health
1250 Punchbowl Street
Honolulu, HI 96813
(808) 586-4400
http://hawaii.gov/health

IDAHO

Idaho Department of Health & Welfare
450 West State Street
10th Floor
Boise, ID 83720
(208) 334-5500
http://healthandwelfare.idaho.gov

ILLINOIS

Illinois Department of Public Health
535 West Jefferson Street
Springfield, IL 62761
(217) 782-4977
http://www.idph.state.il.us

INDIANA

Indiana State Department of Health
2 North Meridian Street
Indianapolis, IN 46204
(317) 233-1325
http://www.in.gov/isdh

IOWA

Iowa Department of Public Health
321 East 12th Street
Des Moines, IA 50319
(515) 281-7689
http://www.idph.state.ia.us

KANSAS

Kansas Department of Health and Environment
Curtis State Office Building
1000 Southwest Jackson
Topeka, KS 66612
(785) 296-1500
http://www.kdheks.gov

KENTUCKY

Kentucky Cabinet for Health Services, Department for Public Health
275 East Main Street
Frankfort, KY 40621
(800) 372-2973
http://chfs.ky.gov

LOUISIANA

Louisiana Department of Health and Hospitals
628 North Font Street
Baton Rouge, LA 70802
(225) 342-9500
http://www.dhh.louisiana.gov

MAINE

Department of Health and Human Services
221 State Street
Augusta, ME 04333
207-287-3707
http://www.maine.gov/dhhs/

MARYLAND

Maryland Department of Health and Mental Hygiene
201 West Preston Street
Baltimore, MD 21201
(410) 767-6500
http:/ /www.dhmh.state.md.us

MASSACHUSETTS

Department of Public Health
One Ashburton Place
Boston, MA 02108
(617) 573-1600
http: //www.mass.gov/dph

MICHIGAN

Michigan Department of Community Health
Capitol View Building
201 Townsend Street
Lansing, MI 48913
(517) 373-3740
http://www.michigan.gov/mdch

MINNESOTA

Minnesota Department of Health
P.O. Box 64975
St. Paul, MN 55164
(651) 201-5000
http://www.health. state.mn.us

MISSISSIPPI

Mississippi State Department of Health
570 East Woodrow Wilson Drive
Jackson, MS 39216

(866) 458-4949
http ://www.msdh.state .ms.us/

MISSOURI

Missouri Department of Health and Senior Services
P.O. Box 570
Jefferson City, MO 65102
(573) 751-6400
http://www.dhss.mo.gov

MONTANA

Department of Public Health & Human Services
111 North Sanders
Helena, MT 59620
(406) 444-5622
http://www.dphhs.mt.gov

NEBRASKA

Nebraska Department of Health and Human Services
301 Centennial Mall South
Lincoln, NE 68509
(402) 471-3121
http://www.hhs.state.ne.us

NEVADA

Nevada State Health Division
4150 Technology Way
Carson City, NV 89706
(866) 767-5038
http://health.nv.gov

NEW HAMPSHIRE

New Hampshire Department of Health and Human Services
Office of Community and Public Health
6 Hazen Drive
Concord, NH 03301
(603) 271-5926
http://www.dhhs.state.nh.us/DHHS

NEW JERSEY

State Department of Health and Senior Services
50 East State Street
Trenton, NJ 08608
(609) 292-9560
http://www.state.nj.us/health

NEW MEXICO

New Mexico Department of Health
1190 South Saint Francis Drive
Santa Fe, NM 87502
(505) 827-2613
http://www.health.state.nm.us/

NEW YORK

New York State Department of Health
Corning Tower
Empire State Plaza
Albany, NY 12237
(866) 881-2809
http://www.health.state.ny.us/

NORTH CAROLINA

Division of Public Health
North Carolina Department of Health and Human Services
5505 Six Forks Road
Raleigh, NC 27609
(971) 673-1222
http://www.ncpublichealth.com

NORTH DAKOTA

North Dakota Department of Health
600 East Boulevard Avenue
Bismarck, ND 58505
(701) 328-2372
http://www.ndhealth.gov/DDH

OHIO

Ohio Department of Health
246 North Main Street
Columbus, OH 43215
http://www.odh.ohio.gov

OKLAHOMA

Oklahoma State Department of Health
1000 Northeast Tenth Street
Oklahoma City, OK 73117
(405) 271-5600
http://www.ok.gov/health

OREGON

Oregon Public Health Division
800 NE Oregon Street
Portland, OR 97232
(971) 673-1222
http://www.oregon.gov/DHS

PENNSYLVANIA

Pennsylvania Department of Health
Health and Welfare Building
7th & Forster Streets
Harrisburg, PA 17120
1-877-724-3258
http://www.dsf.health.state.pa.us/health/site/default.asp

RHODE ISLAND

Rhode Island Department of Health
3 Capitol Hill
Providence, RI 02908
(401) 222-5960
http://www.health.ri.gov

SOUTH CAROLINA

Department of Health and Environmental Control
2600 Bull Street
Columbia, SC 29201
(803) 898-3432
http://www.scdhec.gov

SOUTH DAKOTA

South Dakota Department of Health
600 East Capitol Avenue
Pierre, SD 57501
(605) 773-3361
http://doh.sd.gov

TENNESSEE

Tennessee Department of Health
425 Fifth Avenue North
Cordell HLI1I Building
Third Floor
Nashville, TN 37243
(615) 741-3111
http://health.state.tn.us

TEXAS

Texas Department of State Health
1100 West 49th Street
Austin, TX 78756
(512) 458-7111
http://www.dshs.state.tx

UTAH

Utah Department of Health
P.O. Box 1010
Salt Lake City, UT 84114
(801) 538-6101
http: //health.utah.gov

VERMONT

Vermont Department of Health
108 Cherry Street
P.O. Box 70
Burlington, VT 05402
(802) 863-7200
http://healthvermont.gov

VIRGINIA

Virginia Department of Health
P.O. Box 2448
Richmond, VA 23218-2448
(804) 864-7001
http://www.vdh.state.va.us/

WASHINGTON

Washington State Department of Health
101 Israel Road SE
Tumwater, WA 98501
(800) 525-0127
http://www.doh.wa.gov/

WEST VIRGINIA

West Virginia Bureau of Public Health
350 Capitol Street
Charleston, WV 25301
(304) 558-2971
http://www.wvdhr.org/bph

WISCONSIN

Department of Health Services
1 West Wilson Street
Madison, WI 53702
(608) 266-1865
http://shs.wisconsin.gov

WYOMING

Wyoming Department of Health
401 Hathaway Building
Cheyenne, WY 82002
(307) 777-7656
http://wdh.state.wy.us

APPENDIX III

DIABETES, ULCERS, AND LIVER DISEASE AMONG PERSONS AGES 18 AND OLDER

The presence of diabetes, ulcers, and liver disease varies by gender, age, race, and many different factors, as reflected in this appendix. For example, based on data from 2007, diabetes is most common (20.3 percent) among those ages 65 to 74 years old, while ulcers are most common among those ages 75 years and older (12.6 percent). In considering liver disease by age, it is most common among those ages 65 to 74 years (1.9 percent), followed by those ages 45 to 64 years in age (1.8 percent).

In considering racial differences and the prevalence of diabetes, ulcers, and liver disease, Native Hawaiians and Pacific Islanders have the highest percentage of diabetes (20.6 percent). Individuals of two or more races have the highest rate of ulcers, especially those of both American Indian or Alaska Natives and white racial ancestry (9.8 percent). With regard to race and liver disease, the highest rates were again among those with two or more races, or 5.2 percent among those of both American Indian/Alaska Native and white racial background.

PERCENTAGES OF DIABETES, ULCERS, AND LIVER DISEASE, AMONG PERSONS AGES 18 AND OLDER IN THE UNITED STATES, 2007

Selected Characteristic	Diabetes	Ulcers	Liver disease
Total	7.8	6.5	1.2
Gender			
Male	8.0	6.3	1.1
Female	7.3	6.7	1.2
Age			
18–44 years	2.2	4.2	0.7
45–64 years	10.7	7.4	1.6
65–74 years	20.3	11.0	1.9
75 years and older	17.6	12.6	0.9
Race			
1 race	7.6	6.4	1.1
White	6.8	6.8	1.2
Black or African American	12.3	5.2	0.9
American Indian or Alaska Native	17.2	6.5	Not available
Asian	8.9	3.0	0.9
Native Hawaiian or Other Pacific Islander	20.6	Not available	Not available
2 or more races	10.3	8.0	3.1
Black or African America and white	14.0	Not available	Not available
American Indian or Alaska Native and white	10.5	9.8	5.2

Selected Characteristic	Diabetes	Ulcers	Liver disease
Hispanic or Latino origin and race	11.1	4.9	1.6
Mexican or Mexican American	12.5	5.2	1.7
Not Hispanic or Latino	7.3	6.7	1.1
White, single race	6.4	7.2	1.1
Black or African American, single race	12.5	5.1	0.9
Education			
Less than a high school diploma	13.2	9.2	2.1
High school diploma or GED	9.2	6.7	1.3
Some college	7.8	8.0	1.6
Bachelor's degree or higher	6.4	5.3	0.7
Family income			
Less than $35,000	10.4	8.9	1.9
$35,000 or more	6.5	5.7	0.9
$35,000–$49,999	8.2	7.1	1.4
$50,000–$74,999	7.2	5.8	1.1
$75,000–$99,999	5.9	4.6	0.8
$100,000 or more	4.5	5.2	0.6
Poverty status			
Poor	12.2	9.3	2.5
Near poor	10.6	8.7	1.8
Not poor	6.6	6.1	0.9
Marital status			
Married	7.6	6.0	1.0
Widowed	9.9	7.0	Not available
Divorced or separated	9.2	9.7	2.1
Never married	8.1	5.3	1.3
Living with a partner	6.8	7.6	1.8
Region			
Northeast	6.3	4.9	0.9
Midwest	7.7	7.5	1.2
South	8.3	6.5	1.0
West	7.6	6.4	1.6
Gender and ethnicity			
Hispanic or Latino, male	11.2	4.6	1.1
Hispanic or Latina, female	10.9	5.3	1.9
Not Hispanic or Latino			
White, single race, male	6.8	7.0	1.1
White, single race, female	6.1	7.4	1.2
Black or African American, single race, male	12.2	5.5	1.2
Black or African American, single race, female	12.7	4.9	0.7

Source: Adapted from Pleis, J. R., and J. W. Lucas. *Summary Health Statistics for U.S. Adults.: National Health Interview Survey, 2007.* Hyattsville, Md.: Centers for Disease Control and Prevention, May 2009, 31–32.

APPENDIX IV
FOOD-BORNE ILLNESSES

According to the Centers for Disease Control and Prevention (CDC), at least 250 different food-borne sources causing illness have been identified, and as many as 75 million people in the United States become ill each year from disease-causing substances in food. About 500 people die each year from food-borne diseases; however, many people experience symptoms that they do not report to their doctors, such as nausea and vomiting and diarrhea. Avoiding the mistakes that lead to developing a food-borne illness can reduce the risk for developing these illnesses, such as avoiding the consumption of raw and undercooked meat and poultry and avoiding eating raw or undercooked eggs. This appendix provides common sources of food-borne illnesses, their symptoms, and the bacteria that cause them.

COMMON SOURCES OF FOOD-BORNE ILLNESSES

Sources of illness: Raw and undercooked meat and poultry
Symptoms: Abdominal pain, diarrhea, nausea, and vomiting
Bacteria: *Campylobacter jejuni, E. coli O157:H7, L. monocytogenes, Salmonella*

Sources of illness: Raw foods; unpasteurized milk and dairy products, such as soft cheeses
Symptoms: Nausea, vomiting, fever, abdominal cramps, and diarrhea
Bacteria: *L. monocytogenes, Salmonella, Shigella, Staphylococcus aureus, C. jejuni*

Sources of illness: Raw and undercooked eggs. Raw eggs are often used in foods such as homemade hollandaise sauce, Caesar and other salad dressings, tiramisu, homemade ice cream, homemade mayonnaise, cookie dough, and frostings.
Symptoms: Nausea, vomiting, fever, abdominal cramps and diarrhea
Bacteria: *Salmonella enteriditis*

Sources of illness: Raw and undercooked shell-fish
Symptoms: Chills, fever, and collapse
Bacteria: *Vibrio vulnificus, Vibrio parahaemolyticus*

Sources of illness: Improperly canned goods; smoked or salted fish
Symptoms: Double vision, inability to swallow, difficulty speaking, and inability to breathe. Seek medical help right away if you experience any of these symptoms.
Bacteria: *C. botulinum*

Sources of illness: Fresh or minimally processed produce; contaminated water
Symptoms: Bloody diarrhea, nausea, and vomiting
Bacteria: *E coli O157:H7, L. monocytogenes, Salmonella, Shigella, Yersinia enterocolitica*, viruses and parasites

Source: National Digestive Diseases Information Clearinghouse. *Bacteria and Foodborne Illness.* Bethesda, Md.: National Institutes of Health. May 2007. Available online. URL: http://digestive.niddk.nih.gov/ddiseases/pubs/bacteria/Bacteria_Foodborne.pdf. Accessed January 5, 2010, 5.

APPENDIX V

WEB SITES THAT INCLUDE INFORMATION ON DIGESTIVE DISEASES

American Academy of Allergy, Asthma and Immunology
http://www.aaaai.org

American Association for the Study of Liver Diseases
http://www.aasld.org

American Behçet's Disease Association
http://www.behçets.com

American Cancer Society
http://www.cancer.org

American College of Gastroenterology
http://www.acgi.gi.org

American Diabetes Association (ADA)
http://www.diabetes.org/

American Dietetic Association
http://www.eatright.org

American Gastroenterological Association (AGA)
http://www.gastro.org

American Hemochromatosis Society
http://www.americanhs.org

American Liver Foundation
http://www.liverfoundation.org

American Obesity Association
http://www.obesity.org

American Society for Gastrointestinal Endoscopy
http://www.asge.org

American Society for Parenteral and Enteral Nutrition (ASPEN)
http://www.nutritioncare.org

American Society of Abdominal Surgeons
http://www.abdominalsurg.org

American Society of Bariatric Physicians
http://www.asbs.org

Association of Gastrointestinal Motility Disorders, Inc.
http://www.agmd-gimotility.org

Celiac Disease Foundation
http://www.celiac.org

Celiac Sprue Association
http://www.csaceliacs.org

Centers for Disease Control and Prevention (CDC)
http://www.cdc.gov

Crohn's and Colitis Foundation of America
http://www.ccfa.org

The Cystic Fibrosis Foundation
http://www.cff.org

Digestive Disease National Coalition
http://www.ddnc.org

Food Allergy & Anaphylaxis Network
http://www.foodallergy.org

Food and Drug Administration
http://www.fda.org

Gastro-Intestinal Research Foundation
http://www.girf.org

Gluten Intolerance Group of North America
http://www.gluten.net

Hemochromatosis Foundation, Inc.
http://www.hemochromatosis.org

Hepatitis B Coalition/Immunization Action Coalition
http://www.immunize.org

Hepatitis B Foundation
http://www.hepb.org

Hepatitis Foundation International
http://www.hepfi.org

Hypoglycemia Support Foundation
http://www.hypoglycemia.org

International Foundation for Functional Gastrointestinal Disorders, Inc.
http://www.iffgd.org

Intestinal Disease Foundation
http://www.intestinalfoundation.org

Juvenile Diabetes Research Foundation (JDF)
http://www.jdf.org

National Association of Anorexia Nervosa and Related Disorders
http://www.anad.org

National Association of Nutrition and Aging Service Programs
http://www.nanasp.org

National Clearinghouse for Alcohol and Drug Information
http://www.ncadi.samhsa.gov

National Council on Alcoholism and Drug Dependence
http://www.ncadd.org

National Diabetes Information Clearinghouse
http://www.diabetes.niddk.nih.gov

National Digestive Diseases Information Clearinghouse
http://www.digestive.niddk.nih.gov

National Institute of Allergy and Infectious Diseases
http://www.niaid.nih.gov

National Institute of Diabetes and Digestive and Kidney Diseases
http://www.2niddk.nih.gov

National Institute on Alcohol Abuse and Alcoholism
http://www.niaaa.nih.gov

National Organization for Rare Disorders
http://www.rarediseases.org

North American Society for Pediatric Gastroenterology, Hepatology and Nutrition
http://www.naspghan.org

Oley Foundation
http://www.oley.org

Pancreatic Cancer Action Network
http://www.pancan.org

Pediatric/Adolescent Gastroesophageal Reflux Association (PAGER)
http://www.reflux.org

Scleroderma Foundation
http://www.scleroderma.org

Scleroderma Research Foundation
http://www.srfcure.org

Society for American Gastrointestinal Endoscopic Surgeons
http://www.sages.org

Society for Surgery of the Alimentary Tract
http://www.ssat.com

Transplant Recipient International Organization
http://www.transweb.org

United Network for Organ Sharing
http://www.unos.org

United States Department of Agriculture

Food Safety and Inspection Service
http://www.fsis.usda.gov

Wilson's Disease Association
http://www.wilsonsdisease.org

APPENDIX VI
BODY MASS INDEX (BMI) CHARTS
FOR CHILDREN

Body Mass Index-for-Age Percentiles: Boys, Two to Twenty Years

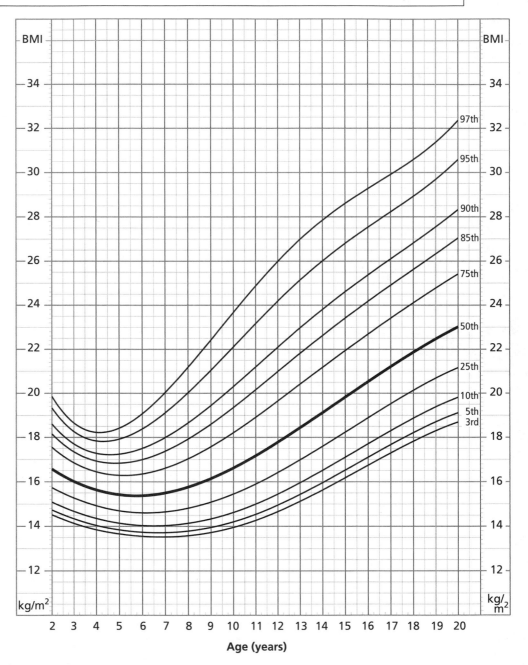

Source: Developed by the National Center for Health Statistics in collaboration with the National Center for Chronic Disease Prevention and Health Promotion (2000).

Body Mass Index-for-Age Percentiles: Girls, Two to Twenty Years

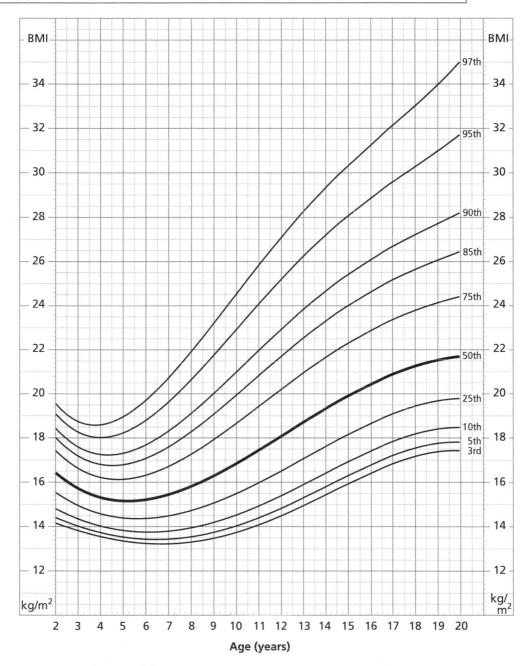

Source: Developed by the National Center for Health Statistics in collaboration with the National Center for Chronic Disease Prevention and Health Promotion (2000).
© Infobase Publishing

CALCULATED BODY MASS INDEX   29 IN.–37 IN. AND 18 LB–26 LB

Height (cm)	Height (in)	Weight kg 8.2 / lb 18	8.4 / 18.5	8.6 / 19	8.8 / 19.5	9.1 / 20	9.3 / 20.5	9.5 / 21	9.8 / 21.5	10.0 / 22	10.2 / 22.5	10.4 / 23	10.7 / 23.5	10.9 / 24	11.1 / 24.5	11.3 / 25	11.6 / 25.5	11.8 / 26
73.7	29	15.0	15.5	15.9	16.3	16.7	17.1	17.6	18.0	18.4	18.8	19.2	19.6	20.1	20.5	20.9	21.3	21.7
74.9	29.5	14.5	14.9	15.3	15.8	16.2	16.6	17.0	17.4	17.8	18.2	18.6	19.0	19.4	19.8	20.2	20.6	21.0
76.2	30	14.1	14.5	14.8	15.2	15.6	16.0	16.4	16.8	17.2	17.6	18.0	18.4	18.7	19.1	19.5	19.9	20.3
77.5	30.5	13.6	14.0	14.4	14.7	15.1	15.5	15.9	16.2	16.6	17.0	17.4	17.8	18.1	18.5	18.9	19.3	19.7
78.7	31	13.2	13.5	13.9	14.3	14.6	15.0	15.4	15.7	16.1	16.5	16.8	17.2	17.6	17.9	18.3	18.7	19.0
80.0	31.5		13.1	13.5	13.8	14.2	14.5	14.9	15.2	15.6	15.9	16.3	16.7	17.0	17.4	17.7	18.1	18.4
81.3	32			13.0	13.4	13.7	14.1	14.4	14.8	15.1	15.4	15.8	16.1	16.5	16.8	17.2	17.5	17.9
82.6	32.5					13.3	13.6	14.0	14.3	14.6	15.0	15.3	15.6	16.0	16.3	16.6	17.0	17.3
83.8	33						13.2	13.6	13.9	14.2	14.5	14.8	15.2	15.5	15.8	16.1	16.5	16.8
85.1	33.5							13.2	13.5	13.8	14.1	14.4	14.7	15.0	15.3	15.7	16.0	16.3
86.4	34								13.1	13.4	13.7	14.0	14.3	14.6	14.9	15.2	15.5	15.8
87.6	34.5										13.3	13.6	13.9	14.2	14.5	14.8	15.1	15.4
88.9	35											13.2	13.5	13.8	14.1	14.3	14.6	14.9
90.2	35.5												13.1	13.4	13.7	13.9	14.2	14.5
91.4	36													13.0	13.3	13.6	13.8	14.1
92.7	36.5														13.2	13.5	13.8	13.7
94.0	37																13.1	13.4

Whenever a child's specific height or weight measurement is not listed, round to the closest number in the table.

CALCULATED BODY MASS INDEX   29 IN.–43 IN. AND 26.5 LB–34.5 LB

Height		Weight (kg)																
		12.0	12.2	12.5	12.7	12.9	13.2	13.4	13.6	13.8	14.1	14.3	14.5	14.7	15.0	15.2	15.4	15.6
cm	in	Weight (lb)																
		26.5	27	27.5	28	28.5	29	29.5	30	30.5	31	31.5	32	32.5	33	33.5	34	34.5
73.7	29	22.2	22.6	23.0	23.4	23.8	24.2	24.7	25.1	25.5	25.9	26.3	26.8	27.2	27.6	28.0	28.4	28.8
74.9	29.5	21.4	21.8	22.2	22.6	23.0	23.4	23.8	24.2	24.6	25.0	25.4	25.9	26.3	26.7	27.1	27.5	27.9
76.2	30	20.7	21.1	21.5	21.9	22.3	22.7	23.0	23.4	23.8	24.2	24.6	25.0	25.4	25.8	26.2	26.6	27.0
77.5	30.5	20.0	20.4	20.8	21.2	21.5	21.9	22.3	22.7	23.1	23.4	23.8	24.2	24.6	24.9	25.3	25.7	26.1
78.7	31	19.4	19.8	20.1	20.5	20.9	21.2	21.6	21.9	22.3	22.7	23.0	23.4	23.8	24.1	24.5	24.9	25.2
80.0	31.5	18.8	19.1	19.5	19.8	20.2	20.5	20.9	21.3	21.6	22.0	22.3	22.7	23.0	23.4	23.7	24.1	24.4
81.3	32	18.2	18.5	18.9	19.2	19.6	19.9	20.3	20.6	20.9	21.3	21.6	22.0	22.3	22.7	23.0	23.3	23.7
82.6	32.5	17.6	18.0	18.3	18.6	19.0	19.3	19.6	20.0	20.3	20.6	21.0	21.3	21.6	22.0	22.3	22.6	23.0
83.8	33	17.1	17.4	17.8	18.1	18.4	18.7	19.0	19.4	19.7	20.0	20.3	20.7	21.0	21.3	21.6	22.0	22.3
85.1	33.5	16.6	16.9	17.2	17.5	17.9	18.2	18.5	18.8	19.1	19.4	19.7	20.0	20.4	20.7	21.0	21.3	21.6
86.4	34	16.1	16.4	16.7	17.0	17.3	17.6	17.9	18.2	18.5	18.9	19.2	19.5	19.8	20.1	20.4	20.7	21.0
87.6	34.5	15.7	15.9	16.2	16.5	16.8	17.1	17.4	17.7	18.0	18.3	18.6	18.9	19.2	19.5	19.8	20.1	20.4
88.9	35	15.2	15.5	15.8	16.1	16.4	16.6	16.9	17.2	17.5	17.8	18.1	18.4	18.7	18.9	19.2	19.5	19.8
90.2	35.5	14.8	15.1	15.3	15.6	15.9	16.2	16.5	16.7	17.0	17.3	17.6	17.9	18.1	18.4	18.7	19.0	19.2
91.4	36	14.4	14.6	14.9	15.2	15.5	15.7	16.0	16.3	16.5	16.8	17.1	17.4	17.6	17.9	18.2	18.4	18.7
92.7	36.5	14.0	14.2	14.5	14.8	15.0	15.3	15.6	15.8	16.1	16.4	16.6	16.9	17.2	17.4	17.7	17.9	18.2
94.0	37	13.6	13.9	14.1	14.4	14.6	14.9	15.2	15.4	15.7	15.9	16.2	16.4	16.7	16.9	17.2	17.5	17.7
95.3	37.5	13.2	13.5	13.7	14.0	14.2	14.5	14.7	15.0	15.2	15.5	15.7	16.0	16.2	16.5	16.7	17.0	17.2
96.5	38		13.1	13.4	13.6	13.9	14.1	14.4	14.6	14.9	15.1	15.3	15.6	15.8	16.1	16.3	16.6	16.8
97.8	38.5			13.0	13.3	13.5	13.8	14.0	14.2	14.5	14.7	14.9	15.2	15.4	15.7	15.9	16.1	16.4
99.1	39					13.2	13.4	13.6	13.9	14.1	14.3	14.6	14.8	15.0	15.3	15.5	15.7	15.9
100.3	39.5						13.1	13.3	13.5	13.7	14.0	14.2	14.4	14.6	14.9	15.1	15.3	15.5
101.6	40								13.2	13.4	13.6	13.8	14.1	14.3	14.5	14.7	14.9	15.2
102.9	40.5									13.1	13.3	13.5	13.7	13.9	14.1	14.4	14.6	14.8
104.1	41											13.2	13.4	13.6	13.8	14.0	14.2	14.4
105.4	41.5												13.1	13.3	13.5	13.7	13.9	14.1
106.7	42														13.2	13.4	13.6	13.8
108.0	42.5															13.0	13.2	13.4
109.2	43																	13.1

Whenever a child's specific height or weight measurement is not listed, round to the closest number in the table.

CALCULATED BODY MASS INDEX 29 IN.–43 IN. AND 35 LB–43 LB

Height		Weight																
cm	in	kg 15.9	16.1	16.3	16.6	16.8	17.0	17.2	17.5	17.7	17.9	18.1	18.4	18.6	18.8	19.1	19.3	19.5
		lb 35	35.5	36	36.5	37	37.5	38	38.5	39	39.5	40	40.5	41	41.5	42	42.5	43
73.7	29	29.3	29.7	30.1	30.5	30.9	31.3	31.8	32.2	32.6	33.0	33.4	33.9	34.3	34.7			
74.9	29.5	28.3	28.7	29.1	29.5	29.9	30.3	30.7	31.1	31.5	31.9	32.3	32.7	33.1	33.5	33.9	34.3	34.7
76.2	30	27.3	27.7	28.1	28.5	28.9	29.3	29.7	30.1	30.5	30.9	31.2	31.6	32.0	32.4	32.8	33.2	33.6
77.5	30.5	26.5	26.8	27.2	27.6	28.0	28.3	28.7	29.1	29.5	29.9	30.2	30.6	31.0	31.4	31.7	32.1	32.5
78.7	31	25.6	26.0	26.3	26.7	27.1	27.4	27.8	28.2	28.5	28.9	29.3	29.6	30.0	30.4	30.7	31.1	31.5
80.0	31.5	24.8	25.2	25.5	25.9	26.2	26.6	26.9	27.3	27.6	28.0	28.3	28.7	29.1	29.4	29.8	30.1	30.5
81.3	32	24.0	24.4	24.7	25.1	25.4	25.7	26.1	26.4	26.8	27.1	27.5	27.8	28.2	28.5	28.8	29.2	29.5
82.6	32.5	23.3	23.6	24.0	24.3	24.6	25.0	25.3	25.6	26.0	26.3	26.6	27.0	27.3	27.6	28.0	28.3	28.6
83.8	33	22.6	22.9	23.2	23.6	23.9	24.2	24.5	24.9	25.2	25.5	25.8	26.1	26.5	26.8	27.1	27.4	27.8
85.1	33.5	21.9	22.2	22.6	22.9	23.2	23.5	23.8	24.1	24.4	24.7	25.1	25.4	25.7	26.0	26.3	26.6	26.9
86.4	34	21.3	21.6	21.9	22.2	22.5	22.8	23.1	23.4	23.7	24.0	24.3	24.6	24.9	25.2	25.5	25.8	26.2
87.6	34.5	20.7	21.0	21.3	21.6	21.9	22.2	22.4	22.7	23.0	23.3	23.6	23.9	24.2	24.5	24.8	25.1	25.4
88.9	35	20.1	20.4	20.7	20.9	21.2	21.5	21.8	22.1	22.4	22.7	23.0	23.2	23.5	23.8	24.1	24.4	24.7
90.2	35.5	19.5	19.8	20.1	20.4	20.6	20.9	21.2	21.5	21.8	22.0	22.3	22.6	22.9	23.2	23.4	23.7	24.0
91.4	36	19.0	19.3	19.5	19.8	20.1	20.3	20.6	20.9	21.2	21.4	21.7	22.0	22.2	22.5	22.8	23.1	23.3
92.7	36.5	18.5	18.7	19.0	19.3	19.5	19.8	20.1	20.3	20.6	20.8	21.1	21.4	21.6	21.9	22.2	22.4	22.7
94.0	37	18.0	18.2	18.5	18.7	19.0	19.3	19.5	19.8	20.0	20.3	20.5	20.8	21.1	21.3	21.6	21.8	22.1
95.3	37.5	17.5	17.7	18.0	18.2	18.5	18.7	19.0	19.2	19.5	19.7	20.0	20.2	20.5	20.7	21.0	21.2	21.5
96.5	38	17.0	17.3	17.5	17.8	18.0	18.3	18.5	18.7	19.0	19.2	19.5	19.7	20.0	20.2	20.4	20.7	20.9
97.8	38.5	16.6	16.8	17.1	17.3	17.6	17.8	18.0	18.3	18.5	18.7	19.0	19.2	19.4	19.7	19.9	20.2	20.4
99.1	39	16.2	16.4	16.6	16.9	17.1	17.3	17.6	17.8	18.0	18.3	18.5	18.7	19.0	19.2	19.4	19.6	19.9
100.3	39.5	15.8	16.0	16.2	16.4	16.7	16.9	17.1	17.3	17.6	17.8	18.0	18.2	18.5	18.7	18.9	19.2	19.4
101.6	40	15.4	15.6	15.8	16.0	16.3	16.5	16.7	16.9	17.1	17.4	17.6	17.8	18.0	18.2	18.5	18.7	18.9
102.9	40.5	15.0	15.2	15.4	15.6	15.9	16.1	16.3	16.5	16.7	16.9	17.1	17.4	17.6	17.8	18.0	18.2	18.4
104.1	41	14.6	14.8	15.1	15.3	15.5	15.7	15.9	16.1	16.3	16.5	16.7	16.9	17.1	17.4	17.6	17.8	18.0
105.4	41.5	14.3	14.5	14.7	14.9	15.1	15.3	15.5	15.7	15.9	16.1	16.3	16.5	16.7	16.9	17.1	17.3	17.6
106.7	42	13.9	14.1	14.3	14.5	14.7	14.9	15.1	15.3	15.5	15.7	15.9	16.1	16.3	16.5	16.7	16.9	17.1
108.0	42.5	13.6	13.8	14.0	14.2	14.4	14.6	14.8	15.0	15.2	15.4	15.6	15.8	16.0	16.2	16.3	16.5	16.7
109.2	43	13.3	13.5	13.7	13.9	14.1	14.3	14.4	14.6	14.8	15.0	15.2	15.4	15.6	15.8	16.0	16.2	16.4

Whenever a child's specific height or weight measurement is not listed, round to the closest number in the table.

CALCULATED BODY MASS INDEX   43.5 IN.–48 IN. AND 35 LB–43 LB

Height		Weight																	
		kg	15.9	16.1	16.3	16.6	16.8	17.0	17.2	17.5	17.7	17.9	18.1	18.4	18.6	18.8	19.1	19.3	19.5
cm	**in**	**lb**	35	35.5	36	36.5	37	37.5	38	38.5	39	39.5	40	40.5	41	41.5	42	42.5	43
110.5	43.5		13.0	13.2	13.4	13.6	13.7	13.9	14.1	14.3	14.5	14.7	14.9	15.0	15.2	15.4	15.6	15.8	16.0
111.8	44				13.1	13.3	13.4	13.6	13.8	14.0	14.2	14.3	14.5	14.7	14.9	15.1	15.3	15.4	15.6
113.0	44.5						13.1	13.3	13.5	13.7	13.8	14.0	14.2	14.4	14.6	14.7	14.9	15.1	15.3
114.3	45							13.0	13.2	13.4	13.5	13.7	13.9	14.1	14.2	14.4	14.6	14.8	14.9
115.6	45.5									13.1	13.2	13.4	13.6	13.8	13.9	14.1	14.3	14.4	14.6
116.8	46											13.1	13.3	13.5	13.6	13.8	14.0	14.1	14.3
118.1	46.5												13.0	13.2	13.3	13.5	13.7	13.8	14.0
119.4	47														13.0	13.2	13.4	13.5	13.7
120.7	47.5																13.1	13.2	13.4
121.9	48																		13.1

Whenever a child's specific height or weight measurement is not listed, round to the closest number in the table.

CALCULATED BODY MASS INDEX   30 IN.–44 IN. AND 43.5 LB–51.5 LB

Height cm	Height in	19.7 kg / 43.5 lb	20.0 / 44	20.2 / 44.5	20.4 / 45	20.6 / 45.5	20.9 / 46	21.1 / 46.5	21.3 / 47	21.5 / 47.5	21.8 / 48	22.0 / 48.5	22.2 / 49	22.5 / 49.5	22.7 / 50	22.9 / 50.5	23.1 / 51	23.4 / 51.5
76.2	30	34.0	34.4	34.8														
77.5	30.5	32.9	33.3	33.6	34.0	34.4	34.8											
78.7	31	31.8	32.2	32.6	32.9	33.3	33.7	34.0	34.4	34.8								
80.0	31.5	30.8	31.2	31.5	31.9	32.2	32.6	32.9	33.3	33.7	34.0	34.4	34.7					
81.3	32	29.9	30.2	30.6	30.9	31.2	31.6	31.9	32.3	32.6	33.0	33.3	33.6	34.0	34.3	34.7		
82.6	32.5	29.0	29.3	29.6	30.0	30.3	30.6	31.0	31.3	31.6	32.0	32.3	32.6	32.9	33.3	33.6	33.9	34.3
83.8	33	28.1	28.4	28.7	29.1	29.4	29.7	30.0	30.3	30.7	31.0	31.3	31.6	32.0	32.3	32.6	32.9	33.2
85.1	33.5	27.3	27.6	27.9	28.2	28.5	28.8	29.1	29.4	29.8	30.1	30.4	30.7	31.0	31.3	31.6	32.0	32.3
86.4	34	26.5	26.8	27.1	27.4	27.7	28.0	28.3	28.6	28.9	29.2	29.5	29.8	30.1	30.4	30.7	31.0	31.3
87.6	34.5	25.7	26.0	26.3	26.6	26.9	27.2	27.5	27.8	28.1	28.4	28.6	28.9	29.2	29.5	29.8	30.1	30.4
88.9	35	25.0	25.3	25.5	25.8	26.1	26.4	26.7	27.0	27.3	27.5	27.8	28.1	28.4	28.7	29.0	29.3	29.6
90.2	35.5	24.3	24.5	24.8	25.1	25.4	25.7	25.9	26.2	26.5	26.8	27.1	27.3	27.6	27.9	28.2	28.5	28.7
91.4	36	23.6	23.9	24.1	24.4	24.7	25.0	25.2	25.5	25.8	26.0	26.3	26.6	26.9	27.1	27.4	27.7	27.9
92.7	36.5	23.0	23.2	23.5	23.7	24.0	24.3	24.5	24.8	25.1	25.3	25.6	25.9	26.1	26.4	26.7	26.9	27.2
94.0	37	22.3	22.6	22.9	23.1	23.4	23.6	23.9	24.1	24.4	24.7	24.9	25.2	25.4	25.7	25.9	26.2	26.4
95.3	37.5	21.7	22.0	22.2	22.5	22.7	23.0	23.2	23.5	23.7	24.0	24.2	24.5	24.7	25.0	25.2	25.5	25.7
96.5	38	21.2	21.4	21.7	21.9	22.2	22.4	22.6	22.9	23.1	23.4	23.6	23.9	24.1	24.3	24.6	24.8	25.1
97.8	38.5	20.6	20.9	21.1	21.3	21.6	21.8	22.1	22.3	22.5	22.8	23.0	23.2	23.5	23.7	24.0	24.2	24.4
99.1	39	20.1	20.3	20.6	20.8	21.0	21.3	21.5	21.7	22.0	22.2	22.4	22.6	22.9	23.1	23.3	23.6	23.8
100.3	39.5	19.6	19.8	20.1	20.3	20.5	20.7	21.0	21.2	21.4	21.6	21.9	22.1	22.3	22.5	22.8	23.0	23.2
101.6	40	19.1	19.3	19.6	19.8	20.0	20.2	20.4	20.7	20.9	21.1	21.3	21.5	21.8	22.0	22.2	22.4	22.6
102.9	40.5	18.6	18.9	19.1	19.3	19.5	19.7	19.9	20.1	20.4	20.6	20.8	21.0	21.2	21.4	21.6	21.9	22.1
104.1	41	18.2	18.4	18.6	18.8	19.0	19.2	19.4	19.7	19.9	20.1	20.3	20.5	20.7	20.9	21.1	21.3	21.5
105.4	41.5	17.8	18.0	18.2	18.4	18.6	18.8	19.0	19.2	19.4	19.6	19.8	20.0	20.2	20.4	20.6	20.8	21.0
106.7	42	17.3	17.5	17.7	17.9	18.1	18.3	18.5	18.7	18.9	19.1	19.3	19.5	19.7	19.9	20.1	20.3	20.5
108.0	42.5	16.9	17.1	17.3	17.5	17.7	17.9	18.1	18.3	18.5	18.7	18.9	19.1	19.3	19.5	19.7	19.9	20.0
109.2	43	16.5	16.7	16.9	17.1	17.3	17.5	17.7	17.9	18.1	18.3	18.4	18.6	18.8	19.0	19.2	19.4	19.6
110.5	43.5	16.2	16.3	16.5	16.7	16.9	17.1	17.3	17.5	17.6	17.8	18.0	18.2	18.4	18.6	18.8	18.9	19.1
111.8	44	15.8	16.0	16.2	16.3	16.5	16.7	16.9	17.1	17.2	17.4	17.6	17.8	18.0	18.2	18.3	18.5	18.7

Whenever a child's specific height or weight measurement is not listed, round to the closest number in the table.

CALCULATED BODY MASS INDEX   44.5 IN.–51 IN. AND 43.5 LB–51.5 LB

Height		Weight																
	kg	19.7	20.0	20.2	20.4	20.6	20.9	21.1	21.3	21.5	21.8	22.0	22.2	22.5	22.7	22.9	23.1	23.4
cm	lb / in	43.5	44	44.5	45	45.5	46	46.5	47	47.5	48	48.5	49	49.5	50	50.5	51	51.5
110.5	43.5	13.0	13.2	13.4	13.6	13.7	13.9	14.1	14.3	14.5	14.7	14.9	15.0	15.2	15.4	15.6	15.8	16.0
113.0	44.5	15.4	15.6	15.8	16.0	16.2	16.3	16.5	16.7	16.9	17.0	17.2	17.4	17.6	17.8	17.9	18.1	18.3
114.3	45	15.1	15.3	15.5	15.6	15.8	16.0	16.1	16.3	16.5	16.7	16.8	17.0	17.2	17.4	17.5	17.7	17.9
115.6	45.5	14.8	14.9	15.1	15.3	15.5	15.6	15.8	16.0	16.1	16.3	16.5	16.6	16.8	17.0	17.2	17.3	17.5
116.8	46	14.5	14.6	14.8	15.0	15.1	15.3	15.5	15.6	15.8	15.9	16.1	16.3	16.4	16.6	16.8	16.9	17.1
118.1	46.5	14.1	14.3	14.5	14.6	14.8	15.0	15.1	15.3	15.4	15.6	15.8	15.9	16.1	16.3	16.4	16.6	16.7
119.4	47	13.8	14.0	14.2	14.3	14.5	14.6	14.8	15.0	15.1	15.3	15.4	15.6	15.8	15.9	16.1	16.2	16.4
120.7	47.5	13.6	13.7	13.9	14.0	14.2	14.3	14.5	14.6	14.8	15.0	15.1	15.3	15.4	15.6	15.7	15.9	16.0
121.9	48	13.3	13.4	13.6	13.7	13.9	14.0	14.2	14.3	14.5	14.6	14.8	15.0	15.1	15.3	15.4	15.6	15.7
124.5	49			13.0	13.2	13.3	13.5	13.6	13.8	13.9	14.1	14.2	14.3	14.5	14.6	14.8	14.9	15.1
127.0	50							13.1	13.2	13.4	13.5	13.6	13.8	13.9	14.1	14.2	14.3	14.5
129.5	51											13.1	13.2	13.4	13.5	13.7	13.8	13.9
132.1	52														13.0	13.1	13.3	13.4

Whenever a child's specific height or weight measurement is not listed, round to the closest number in the table.

CALCULATED BODY MASS INDEX   47 IN.–56 IN. AND 52 LB–60 LB

Weight

Height cm	Height in	23.6	23.8	24.0	24.3	24.5	24.7	24.9	25.2	25.4	25.6	25.9	26.1	26.3	26.5	26.8	27.0	27.2
(kg)	(lb)	52	52.5	53	53.5	54	54.5	55	55.5	56	56.5	57	57.5	58	58.5	59	59.5	60
119.4	47	16.6	16.7	16.9	17.0	17.2	17.3	17.5	17.7	17.8	18.0	18.1	18.3	18.5	18.6	18.8	18.9	19.1
120.7	47.5	16.2	16.4	16.5	16.7	16.8	17.0	17.1	17.3	17.5	17.6	17.8	17.9	18.1	18.2	18.4	18.5	18.7
121.9	48	15.9	16.0	16.2	16.3	16.5	16.6	16.8	16.9	17.1	17.2	17.4	17.5	17.7	17.9	18.0	18.2	18.3
124.5	49	15.2	15.4	15.5	15.7	15.8	16.0	16.1	16.3	16.4	16.5	16.7	16.8	17.0	17.1	17.3	17.4	17.6
127.0	50	14.6	14.8	14.9	15.0	15.2	15.3	15.5	15.6	15.7	15.9	16.0	16.2	16.3	16.5	16.6	16.7	16.9
129.5	51	14.1	14.2	14.3	14.5	14.6	14.7	14.9	15.0	15.1	15.3	15.4	15.5	15.7	15.8	15.9	16.1	16.2
132.1	52	13.5	13.7	13.8	13.9	14.0	14.2	14.3	14.4	14.6	14.7	14.8	15.0	15.1	15.2	15.3	15.5	15.6
134.6	53	13.0	13.1	13.3	13.4	13.5	13.6	13.8	13.9	14.0	14.1	14.3	14.4	14.5	14.6	14.8	14.9	15.0
137.2	54					13.0	13.1	13.3	13.4	13.5	13.6	13.7	13.9	14.0	14.1	14.2	14.3	14.5
139.7	55									13.0	13.1	13.2	13.4	13.5	13.6	13.7	13.8	13.9
142.2	56													13.0	13.1	13.2	13.3	13.5

Whenever a child's specific height or weight measurement is not listed, round to the closest number in the table.

CALCULATED BODY MASS INDEX   35.5 IN.–51 IN. AND 61 LB–77 LB

Height		Weight																
cm	in	kg	27.7	28.1	28.6	29.0	29.5	29.9	30.4	30.8	31.3	31.8	32.2	32.7	33.1	33.6	34.0	34.5	34.9
		lb	61	62	63	64	65	66	67	68	69	70	71	72	73	74	75	76	77
90.2	35.5		34.0	34.6															
91.4	36		33.1	33.6	34.2	34.7													
92.7	36.5		32.2	32.7	33.2	33.8	34.3	34.8											
94.0	37		31.3	31.8	32.4	32.9	33.4	33.9	34.4	34.9									
95.3	37.5		30.5	31.0	31.5	32.0	32.5	33.0	33.5	34.0	34.5	35.0							
96.5	38		29.7	30.2	30.7	31.2	31.6	32.1	32.6	33.1	33.6	34.1	34.6						
97.8	38.5		28.9	29.4	29.9	30.4	30.8	31.3	31.8	32.3	32.7	33.2	33.7	34.2	34.6				
99.1	39		28.2	28.7	29.1	29.6	30.0	30.5	31.0	31.4	31.9	32.4	32.8	33.3	33.7	34.2	34.7		
100.3	39.5		27.5	27.9	28.4	28.8	29.3	29.7	30.2	30.6	31.1	31.5	32.0	32.4	32.9	33.3	33.8	34.2	34.7
101.6	40		26.8	27.2	27.7	28.1	28.6	29.0	29.4	29.9	30.3	30.8	31.2	31.6	32.1	32.5	33.0	33.4	33.8
102.9	40.5		26.1	26.6	27.0	27.4	27.9	28.3	28.7	29.1	29.6	30.0	30.4	30.9	31.3	31.7	32.1	32.6	33.0
104.1	41		25.5	25.9	26.3	26.8	27.2	27.6	28.0	28.4	28.9	29.3	29.7	30.1	30.5	31.0	31.4	31.8	32.2
105.4	41.5		24.9	25.3	25.7	26.1	26.5	26.9	27.4	27.8	28.2	28.6	29.0	29.4	29.8	30.2	30.6	31.0	31.4
106.7	42		24.3	24.7	25.1	25.5	25.9	26.3	26.7	27.1	27.5	27.9	28.3	28.7	29.1	29.5	29.9	30.3	30.7
108.0	42.5		23.7	24.1	24.5	24.9	25.3	25.7	26.1	26.5	26.9	27.2	27.6	28.0	28.4	28.8	29.2	29.6	30.0
109.2	43		23.2	23.6	24.0	24.3	24.7	25.1	25.5	25.9	26.2	26.6	27.0	27.4	27.8	28.1	28.5	28.9	29.3
110.5	43.5		22.7	23.0	23.4	23.8	24.2	24.5	24.9	25.3	25.6	26.0	26.4	26.8	27.1	27.5	27.9	28.2	28.6
111.8	44		22.2	22.5	22.9	23.2	23.6	24.0	24.3	24.7	25.1	25.4	25.8	26.1	26.5	26.9	27.2	27.6	28.0
113.0	44.5		21.7	22.0	22.4	22.7	23.1	23.4	23.8	24.1	24.5	24.9	25.2	25.6	25.9	26.3	26.6	27.0	27.3
114.3	45		21.2	21.5	21.9	22.2	22.6	22.9	23.3	23.6	24.0	24.3	24.7	25.0	25.3	25.7	26.0	26.4	26.7
115.6	45.5		20.7	21.1	21.4	21.7	22.1	22.4	22.8	23.1	23.4	23.8	24.1	24.5	24.8	25.1	25.5	25.8	26.1
116.8	46		20.3	20.6	20.9	21.3	21.6	21.9	22.3	22.6	22.9	23.3	23.6	23.9	24.3	24.6	24.9	25.3	25.6
118.1	46.5		19.8	20.2	20.5	20.8	21.1	21.5	21.8	22.1	22.4	22.8	23.1	23.4	23.7	24.1	24.4	24.7	25.0
119.4	47		19.4	19.7	20.1	20.4	20.7	21.0	21.3	21.6	22.0	22.3	22.6	22.9	23.2	23.6	23.9	24.2	24.5
120.7	47.5		19.0	19.3	19.6	19.9	20.3	20.6	20.9	21.2	21.5	21.8	22.1	22.4	22.7	23.1	23.4	23.7	24.0
121.9	48		18.6	18.9	19.2	19.5	19.8	20.1	20.4	20.8	21.1	21.4	21.7	22.0	22.3	22.6	22.9	23.2	23.5
124.5	49		17.9	18.2	18.4	18.7	19.0	19.3	19.6	19.9	20.2	20.5	20.8	21.1	21.4	21.7	22.0	22.3	22.5
127.0	50		17.2	17.4	17.7	18.0	18.3	18.6	18.8	19.1	19.4	19.7	20.0	20.2	20.5	20.8	21.1	21.4	21.7
129.5	51		16.5	16.8	17.0	17.3	17.6	17.8	18.1	18.4	18.7	18.9	19.2	19.5	19.7	20.0	20.3	20.5	20.8

Whenever a child's specific height or weight measurement is not listed, round to the closest number in the table.

CALCULATED BODY MASS INDEX   52 IN.–64 IN. AND 61 LB–77 LB

Height		Weight																
		kg	27.7	28.1	28.6	29.0	29.5	29.9	30.4	30.8	31.3	31.8	32.2	32.7	33.1	33.6	34.0	34.5	34.9
cm	in	lb	61	62	63	64	65	66	67	68	69	70	71	72	73	74	75	76	77
132.1	52		15.9	16.1	16.4	16.6	16.9	17.2	17.4	17.7	17.9	18.2	18.5	18.7	19.0	19.2	19.5	19.8	20.0
134.6	53		15.3	15.5	15.8	16.0	16.3	16.5	16.8	17.0	17.3	17.5	17.8	18.0	18.3	18.5	18.8	19.0	19.3
137.2	54		14.7	14.9	15.2	15.4	15.7	15.9	16.2	16.4	16.6	16.9	17.1	17.4	17.6	17.8	18.1	18.3	18.6
139.7	55		14.2	14.4	14.6	14.9	15.1	15.3	15.6	15.8	16.0	16.3	16.5	16.7	17.0	17.2	17.4	17.7	17.9
142.2	56		13.7	13.9	14.1	14.3	14.6	14.8	15.0	15.2	15.5	15.7	15.9	16.1	16.4	16.6	16.8	17.0	17.3
144.8	57		13.2	13.4	13.6	13.8	14.1	14.3	14.5	14.7	14.9	15.1	15.4	15.6	15.8	16.0	16.2	16.4	16.7
147.3	58				13.2	13.4	13.6	13.8	14.0	14.2	14.4	14.6	14.8	15.0	15.3	15.5	15.7	15.9	16.1
149.9	59						13.1	13.3	13.5	13.7	13.9	14.1	14.3	14.5	14.7	14.9	15.1	15.3	15.6
152.4	60								13.1	13.3	13.5	13.7	13.9	14.1	14.3	14.5	14.6	14.8	15.0
154.9	61										13.0	13.2	13.4	13.6	13.8	14.0	14.2	14.4	14.5
157.5	62													13.2	13.4	13.5	13.7	13.9	14.1
160.0	63															13.1	13.3	13.5	13.6
162.6	64																	13.0	13.2

Whenever a child's specific height or weight measurement is not listed, round to the closest number in the table.

CALCULATED BODY MASS INDEX   40.5 IN.–60 IN. AND 78 LB–94 LB

Height (cm)	Height (in)	35.4 kg / 78 lb	35.8 / 79	36.3 / 80	36.7 / 81	37.2 / 82	37.6 / 83	38.1 / 84	38.6 / 85	39.0 / 86	39.5 / 87	39.9 / 88	40.4 / 89	40.8 / 90	41.3 / 91	41.7 / 92	42.2 / 93	42.6 / 94
101.6	40	34.3	34.7															
102.9	40.5	33.4	33.9	34.3	34.7													
104.1	41	32.6	33.0	33.5	33.9	34.3	34.7											
105.4	41.5	31.8	32.2	32.7	33.1	33.5	33.9	34.3	34.7									
106.7	42	31.1	31.5	31.9	32.3	32.7	33.1	33.5	33.9	34.3	34.7							
108.0	42.5	30.4	30.8	31.1	31.5	31.9	32.3	32.7	33.1	33.5	33.9	34.3	34.6					
109.2	43	29.7	30.0	30.4	30.8	31.2	31.6	31.9	32.3	32.7	33.1	33.5	33.8	34.2	34.6	35.0		
110.5	43.5	29.0	29.4	29.7	30.1	30.5	30.8	31.2	31.6	32.0	32.3	32.7	33.1	33.4	33.8	34.2	34.6	34.9
111.8	44	28.3	28.7	29.1	29.4	29.8	30.1	30.5	30.9	31.2	31.6	32.0	32.3	32.7	33.0	33.4	33.8	34.1
113.0	44.5	27.7	28.0	28.4	28.8	29.1	29.5	29.8	30.2	30.5	30.9	31.2	31.6	32.0	32.3	32.7	33.0	33.4
114.3	45	27.1	27.4	27.8	28.1	28.5	28.8	29.2	29.5	29.9	30.2	30.6	30.9	31.2	31.6	31.9	32.3	32.6
115.6	45.5	26.5	26.8	27.2	27.5	27.8	28.2	28.5	28.9	29.2	29.5	29.9	30.2	30.6	30.9	31.2	31.6	31.9
116.8	46	25.9	26.2	26.6	26.9	27.2	27.6	27.9	28.2	28.6	28.9	29.2	29.6	29.9	30.2	30.6	30.9	31.2
118.1	46.5	25.4	25.7	26.0	26.3	26.7	27.0	27.3	27.6	28.0	28.3	28.6	28.9	29.3	29.6	29.9	30.2	30.6
119.4	47	24.8	25.1	25.5	25.8	26.1	26.4	26.7	27.1	27.4	27.7	28.0	28.3	28.6	29.0	29.3	29.6	29.9
120.7	47.5	24.3	24.6	24.9	25.2	25.6	25.9	26.2	26.5	26.8	27.1	27.4	27.7	28.0	28.4	28.7	29.0	29.3
121.9	48	23.8	24.1	24.4	24.7	25.0	25.3	25.6	25.9	26.2	26.5	26.9	27.2	27.5	27.8	28.1	28.4	28.7
124.5	49	22.8	23.1	23.4	23.7	24.0	24.3	24.6	24.9	25.2	25.5	25.8	26.1	26.4	26.6	26.9	27.2	27.5
127.0	50	21.9	22.2	22.5	22.8	23.1	23.3	23.6	23.9	24.2	24.5	24.7	25.0	25.3	25.6	25.9	26.2	26.4
129.5	51	21.1	21.4	21.6	21.9	22.2	22.4	22.7	23.0	23.2	23.5	23.8	24.1	24.3	24.6	24.9	25.1	25.4
132.1	52	20.3	20.5	20.8	21.1	21.3	21.6	21.8	22.1	22.4	22.6	22.9	23.1	23.4	23.7	23.9	24.2	24.4
134.6	53	19.5	19.8	20.0	20.3	20.5	20.8	21.0	21.3	21.5	21.8	22.0	22.3	22.5	22.8	23.0	23.3	23.5
137.2	54	18.8	19.0	19.3	19.5	19.8	20.0	20.3	20.5	20.7	21.0	21.2	21.5	21.7	21.9	22.2	22.4	22.7
139.7	55	18.1	18.4	18.6	18.8	19.1	19.3	19.5	19.8	20.0	20.2	20.5	20.7	20.9	21.2	21.4	21.6	21.8
142.2	56	17.5	17.7	17.9	18.2	18.4	18.6	18.8	19.1	19.3	19.5	19.7	20.0	20.2	20.4	20.6	20.8	21.1
144.8	57	16.9	17.1	17.3	17.5	17.7	18.0	18.2	18.4	18.6	18.8	19.0	19.3	19.5	19.7	19.9	20.1	20.3
147.3	58	16.3	16.5	16.7	16.9	17.1	17.3	17.6	17.8	18.0	18.2	18.4	18.6	18.8	19.0	19.2	19.4	19.6
149.9	59	15.8	16.0	16.2	16.4	16.6	16.8	17.0	17.2	17.4	17.6	17.8	18.0	18.2	18.4	18.6	18.8	19.0
152.4	60	15.2	15.4	15.6	15.8	16.0	16.2	16.4	16.6	16.8	17.0	17.2	17.4	17.6	17.8	18.0	18.2	18.4

Whenever a child's specific height or weight measurement is not listed, round to the closest number in the table.

CALCULATED BODY MASS INDEX   61 IN.–71 IN. AND 78 LB–94 LB

Height		Weight																	
cm	in	kg 35.4	35.8	36.3	36.7	37.2	37.6	38.1	38.6	39.0	39.5	39.9	40.4	40.8	41.3	41.7	42.2	42.6
		lb 78	79	80	81	82	83	84	85	86	87	88	89	90	91	92	93	94
154.9	61	14.7	14.9	15.1	15.3	15.5	15.7	15.9	16.1	16.2	16.4	16.6	16.8	17.0	17.2	17.4	17.6	17.8
157.5	62	14.3	14.4	14.6	14.8	15.0	15.2	15.4	15.5	15.7	15.9	16.1	16.3	16.5	16.6	16.8	17.0	17.2
160.0	63	13.8	14.0	14.2	14.3	14.5	14.7	14.9	15.1	15.2	15.4	15.6	15.8	15.9	16.1	16.3	16.5	16.7
162.6	64	13.4	13.6	13.7	13.9	14.1	14.2	14.4	14.6	14.8	14.9	15.1	15.3	15.4	15.6	15.8	16.0	16.1
165.1	65		13.1	13.3	13.5	13.6	13.8	14.0	14.1	14.3	14.5	14.6	14.8	15.0	15.1	15.3	15.5	15.6
167.6	66				13.1	13.2	13.4	13.6	13.7	13.9	14.0	14.2	14.4	14.5	14.7	14.8	15.0	15.2
170.2	67							13.2	13.3	13.5	13.6	13.8	13.9	14.1	14.3	14.4	14.6	14.7
172.7	68									13.1	13.2	13.4	13.5	13.7	13.8	14.0	14.1	14.3
175.3	69												13.1	13.3	13.4	13.6	13.7	13.9
177.8	70														13.1	13.2	13.3	13.5
180.3	71																	13.1

Whenever a child's specific height or weight measurement is not listed, round to the closest number in the table.

CALCULATED BODY MASS INDEX 44 IN.–68 IN. AND 95 LB–112 LB

Height		Weight																
		kg	43.1	43.5	44.0	44.5	44.9	45.4	45.8	46.3	46.7	47.2	47.6	48.1	48.5	49.0	49.4	49.9	50.8
		lb	95	96	97	98	99	100	101	102	103	104	105	106	107	108	109	110	112
cm	in																		
111.8	44		34.5	34.9															
113.0	44.5		33.7	34.1	34.4	34.8													
114.3	45		33.0	33.3	33.7	34.0	34.4	34.7											
115.6	45.5		32.3	32.6	32.9	33.3	33.6	34.0	34.3	34.6	35.0								
116.8	46		31.6	31.9	32.2	32.6	32.9	33.2	33.6	33.9	34.2	34.6	34.9						
118.1	46.5		30.9	31.2	31.5	31.9	32.2	32.5	32.8	33.2	33.5	33.8	34.1	34.5	34.8				
119.4	47		30.2	30.6	30.9	31.2	31.5	31.8	32.1	32.5	32.8	33.1	33.4	33.7	34.1	34.4	34.7		
120.7	47.5		29.6	29.9	30.2	30.5	30.8	31.2	31.5	31.8	32.1	32.4	32.7	33.0	33.3	33.7	34.0	34.3	34.9
121.9	48		29.0	29.3	29.6	29.9	30.2	30.5	30.8	31.1	31.4	31.7	32.0	32.3	32.7	33.0	33.3	33.6	34.2
124.5	49		27.8	28.1	28.4	28.7	29.0	29.3	29.6	29.9	30.2	30.5	30.7	31.0	31.3	31.6	31.9	32.2	32.8
127.0	50		26.7	27.0	27.3	27.6	27.8	28.1	28.4	28.7	29.0	29.2	29.5	29.8	30.1	30.4	30.7	30.9	31.5
129.5	51		25.7	25.9	26.2	26.5	26.8	27.0	27.3	27.6	27.8	28.1	28.4	28.7	28.9	29.2	29.5	29.7	30.3
132.1	52		24.7	25.0	25.2	25.5	25.7	26.0	26.3	26.5	26.8	27.0	27.3	27.6	27.8	28.1	28.3	28.6	29.1
134.6	53		23.8	24.0	24.3	24.5	24.8	25.0	25.3	25.5	25.8	26.0	26.3	26.5	26.8	27.0	27.3	27.5	28.0
137.2	54		22.9	23.1	23.4	23.6	23.9	24.1	24.4	24.6	24.8	25.1	25.3	25.6	25.8	26.0	26.3	26.5	27.0
139.7	55		22.1	22.3	22.5	22.8	23.0	23.2	23.5	23.7	23.9	24.2	24.4	24.6	24.9	25.1	25.3	25.6	26.0
142.2	56		21.3	21.5	21.7	22.0	22.2	22.4	22.6	22.9	23.1	23.3	23.5	23.8	24.0	24.2	24.4	24.7	25.1
144.8	57		20.6	20.8	21.0	21.2	21.4	21.6	21.9	22.1	22.3	22.5	22.7	22.9	23.2	23.4	23.6	23.8	24.2
147.3	58		19.9	20.1	20.3	20.5	20.7	20.9	21.1	21.3	21.5	21.7	21.9	22.2	22.4	22.6	22.8	23.0	23.4
149.9	59		19.2	19.4	19.6	19.8	20.0	20.2	20.4	20.6	20.8	21.0	21.2	21.4	21.6	21.8	22.0	22.2	22.6
152.4	60		18.6	18.7	18.9	19.1	19.3	19.5	19.7	19.9	20.1	20.3	20.5	20.7	20.9	21.1	21.3	21.5	21.9
154.9	61		17.9	18.1	18.3	18.5	18.7	18.9	19.1	19.3	19.5	19.7	19.8	20.0	20.2	20.4	20.6	20.8	21.2
157.5	62		17.4	17.6	17.7	17.9	18.1	18.3	18.5	18.7	18.8	19.0	19.2	19.4	19.6	19.8	19.9	20.1	20.5
160.0	63		16.8	17.0	17.2	17.4	17.5	17.7	17.9	18.1	18.2	18.4	18.6	18.8	19.0	19.1	19.3	19.5	19.8
162.6	64		16.3	16.5	16.6	16.8	17.0	17.2	17.3	17.5	17.7	17.9	18.0	18.2	18.4	18.5	18.7	18.9	19.2
165.1	65		15.8	16.0	16.1	16.3	16.5	16.6	16.8	17.0	17.1	17.3	17.5	17.6	17.8	18.0	18.1	18.3	18.6
167.6	66		15.3	15.5	15.7	15.8	16.0	16.1	16.3	16.5	16.6	16.8	16.9	17.1	17.3	17.4	17.6	17.8	18.1
170.2	67		14.9	15.0	15.2	15.3	15.5	15.7	15.8	16.0	16.1	16.3	16.4	16.6	16.8	16.9	17.1	17.2	17.5
172.7	68		14.4	14.6	14.7	14.9	15.1	15.2	15.4	15.5	15.7	15.8	16.0	16.1	16.3	16.4	16.6	16.7	17.0

Whenever a child's specific height or weight measurement is not listed, round to the closest number in the table.

CALCULATED BODY MASS INDEX   69 IN.–77 IN. AND 95 LB–112 LB

Height		Weight																	
cm	in	kg	43.1	43.5	44.0	44.5	44.9	45.4	45.8	46.3	46.7	47.2	47.6	48.1	48.5	49.0	49.4	49.9	50.8
		lb	95	96	97	98	99	100	101	102	103	104	105	106	107	108	109	110	112
111.8	44		34.5	34.9															
175.3	69		14.0	14.2	14.3	14.5	14.6	14.8	14.9	15.1	15.2	15.4	15.5	15.7	15.8	15.9	16.1	16.2	16.5
177.8	70		13.6	13.8	13.9	14.1	14.2	14.3	14.5	14.6	14.8	14.9	15.1	15.2	15.4	15.5	15.6	15.8	16.1
180.3	71		13.2	13.4	13.5	13.7	13.8	13.9	14.1	14.2	14.4	14.5	14.6	14.8	14.9	15.1	15.2	15.3	15.6
182.9	72			13.0	13.2	13.3	13.4	13.6	13.7	13.8	14.0	14.1	14.2	14.4	14.5	14.6	14.8	14.9	15.2
185.4	73						13.1	13.2	13.3	13.5	13.6	13.7	13.9	14.0	14.1	14.2	14.4	14.5	14.8
188.0	74									13.1	13.2	13.4	13.5	13.6	13.7	13.9	14.0	14.1	14.4
190.5	75												13.1	13.2	13.4	13.5	13.6	13.7	14.0
193.0	76														13.0	13.1	13.3	13.4	13.6
195.6	77																	13.0	13.3

Whenever a child's specific height or weight measurement is not listed, round to the closest number in the table.

CALCULATED BODY MASS INDEX   48 IN.–76 IN. AND 114 LB–146 LB

Weight

Height cm	Height in	kg → lb	51.7 / 114	52.6 / 116	53.5 / 118	54.4 / 120	55.3 / 122	56.2 / 124	57.2 / 126	58.1 / 128	59.0 / 130	59.9 / 132	60.8 / 134	61.7 / 136	62.6 / 138	63.5 / 140	64.4 / 142	65.3 / 144	66.2 / 146
121.9	48		34.8																
124.5	49		33.4	34.0	34.6														
127.0	50		32.1	32.6	33.2	33.7	34.3	34.9											
129.5	51		30.8	31.4	31.9	32.4	33.0	33.5	34.1	34.6									
132.1	52		29.6	30.2	30.7	31.2	31.7	32.2	32.8	33.3	33.8	34.3	34.8						
134.6	53		28.5	29.0	29.5	30.0	30.5	31.0	31.5	32.0	32.5	33.0	33.5	34.0	34.5				
137.2	54		27.5	28.0	28.5	28.9	29.4	29.9	30.4	30.9	31.3	31.8	32.3	32.8	33.3	33.8	34.2	34.7	
139.7	55		26.5	27.0	27.4	27.9	28.4	28.8	29.3	29.7	30.2	30.7	31.1	31.6	32.1	32.5	33.0	33.5	33.9
142.2	56		25.6	26.0	26.5	26.9	27.4	27.8	28.2	28.7	29.1	29.6	30.0	30.5	30.9	31.4	31.8	32.3	32.7
144.8	57		24.7	25.1	25.5	26.0	26.4	26.8	27.3	27.7	28.1	28.6	29.0	29.4	29.9	30.3	30.7	31.2	31.6
147.3	58		23.8	24.2	24.7	25.1	25.5	25.9	26.3	26.8	27.2	27.6	28.0	28.4	28.8	29.3	29.7	30.1	30.5
149.9	59		23.0	23.4	23.8	24.2	24.6	25.0	25.4	25.9	26.3	26.7	27.1	27.5	27.9	28.3	28.7	29.1	29.5
152.4	60		22.3	22.7	23.0	23.4	23.8	24.2	24.6	25.0	25.4	25.8	26.2	26.6	27.0	27.3	27.7	28.1	28.5
154.9	61		21.5	21.9	22.3	22.7	23.1	23.4	23.8	24.2	24.6	24.9	25.3	25.7	26.1	26.5	26.8	27.2	27.6
157.5	62		20.9	21.2	21.6	21.9	22.3	22.7	23.0	23.4	23.8	24.1	24.5	24.9	25.2	25.6	26.0	26.3	26.7
160.0	63		20.2	20.5	20.9	21.3	21.6	22.0	22.3	22.7	23.0	23.4	23.7	24.1	24.4	24.8	25.2	25.5	25.9
162.6	64		19.6	19.9	20.3	20.6	20.9	21.3	21.6	22.0	22.3	22.7	23.0	23.3	23.7	24.0	24.4	24.7	25.1
165.1	65		19.0	19.3	19.6	20.0	20.3	20.6	21.0	21.3	21.6	22.0	22.3	22.6	23.0	23.3	23.6	24.0	24.3
167.6	66		18.4	18.7	19.0	19.4	19.7	20.0	20.3	20.7	21.0	21.3	21.6	22.0	22.3	22.6	22.9	23.2	23.6
170.2	67		17.9	18.2	18.5	18.8	19.1	19.4	19.7	20.0	20.4	20.7	21.0	21.3	21.6	21.9	22.2	22.6	22.9
172.7	68		17.3	17.6	17.9	18.2	18.5	18.9	19.2	19.5	19.8	20.1	20.4	20.7	21.0	21.3	21.6	21.9	22.2
175.3	69		16.8	17.1	17.4	17.7	18.0	18.3	18.6	18.9	19.2	19.5	19.8	20.1	20.4	20.7	21.0	21.3	21.6
177.8	70		16.4	16.6	16.9	17.2	17.5	17.8	18.1	18.4	18.7	18.9	19.2	19.5	19.8	20.1	20.4	20.7	20.9
180.3	71		15.9	16.2	16.5	16.7	17.0	17.3	17.6	17.9	18.1	18.4	18.7	19.0	19.2	19.5	19.8	20.1	20.4
182.9	72		15.5	15.7	16.0	16.3	16.5	16.8	17.1	17.4	17.6	17.9	18.2	18.4	18.7	19.0	19.3	19.5	19.8
185.4	73		15.0	15.3	15.6	15.8	16.1	16.4	16.6	16.9	17.2	17.4	17.7	17.9	18.2	18.5	18.7	19.0	19.3
188.0	74		14.6	14.9	15.2	15.4	15.7	15.9	16.2	16.4	16.7	16.9	17.2	17.5	17.7	18.0	18.2	18.5	18.7
190.5	75		14.2	14.5	14.7	15.0	15.2	15.5	15.7	16.0	16.2	16.5	16.7	17.0	17.2	17.5	17.7	18.0	18.2
193.0	76		13.9	14.1	14.4	14.6	14.9	15.1	15.3	15.6	15.8	16.1	16.3	16.6	16.8	17.0	17.3	17.5	17.8
195.6	77		13.5	13.8	14.0	14.2	14.5	14.7	14.9	15.2	15.4	15.7	15.9	16.1	16.4	16.6	16.8	17.1	17.3
198.1	78		13.2	13.4	13.6	13.9	14.1	14.3	14.6	14.8	15.0	15.3	15.5	15.7	15.9	16.2	16.4	16.6	16.9

Whenever a child's specific height or weight measurement is not listed, round to the closest number in the table.

CALCULATED BODY MASS INDEX   55 IN.–78 IN. AND 148 LB–180 LB

Height		Weight																
		kg	67.1	68.0	68.9	69.9	70.8	71.7	72.6	73.5	74.4	75.3	76.2	77.1	78.0	78.9	79.8	80.7	81.6
cm	in	lb	148	150	152	154	156	158	160	162	164	166	168	170	172	174	176	178	180
139.7	55		34.4	34.9															
142.2	56		33.2	33.6	34.1	34.5	35.0												
144.8	57		32.0	32.5	32.9	33.3	33.8	34.2	34.6										
147.3	58		30.9	31.3	31.8	32.2	32.6	33.0	33.4	33.9	34.3	34.7							
149.9	59		29.9	30.3	30.7	31.1	31.5	31.9	32.3	32.7	33.1	33.5	33.9	34.3	34.7				
152.4	60		28.9	29.3	29.7	30.1	30.5	30.9	31.2	31.6	32.0	32.4	32.8	33.2	33.6	34.0	34.4	34.8	
154.9	61		28.0	28.3	28.7	29.1	29.5	29.9	30.2	30.6	31.0	31.4	31.7	32.1	32.5	32.9	33.3	33.6	34.0
157.5	62		27.1	27.4	27.8	28.2	28.5	28.9	29.3	29.6	30.0	30.4	30.7	31.1	31.5	31.8	32.2	32.6	32.9
160.0	63		26.2	26.6	26.9	27.3	27.6	28.0	28.3	28.7	29.1	29.4	29.8	30.1	30.5	30.8	31.2	31.5	31.9
162.6	64		25.4	25.7	26.1	26.4	26.8	27.1	27.5	27.8	28.2	28.5	28.8	29.2	29.5	29.9	30.2	30.6	30.9
165.1	65		24.6	25.0	25.3	25.6	26.0	26.3	26.6	27.0	27.3	27.6	28.0	28.3	28.6	29.0	29.3	29.6	30.0
167.6	66		23.9	24.2	24.5	24.9	25.2	25.5	25.8	26.1	26.5	26.8	27.1	27.4	27.8	28.1	28.4	28.7	29.1
170.2	67		23.2	23.5	23.8	24.1	24.4	24.7	25.1	25.4	25.7	26.0	26.3	26.6	26.9	27.3	27.6	27.9	28.2
172.7	68		22.5	22.8	23.1	23.4	23.7	24.0	24.3	24.6	24.9	25.2	25.5	25.8	26.2	26.5	26.8	27.1	27.4
175.3	69		21.9	22.2	22.4	22.7	23.0	23.3	23.6	23.9	24.2	24.5	24.8	25.1	25.4	25.7	26.0	26.3	26.6
177.8	70		21.2	21.5	21.8	22.1	22.4	22.7	23.0	23.2	23.5	23.8	24.1	24.4	24.7	25.0	25.3	25.5	25.8
180.3	71		20.6	20.9	21.2	21.5	21.8	22.0	22.3	22.6	22.9	23.2	23.4	23.7	24.0	24.3	24.5	24.8	25.1
182.9	72		20.1	20.3	20.6	20.9	21.2	21.4	21.7	22.0	22.2	22.5	22.8	23.1	23.3	23.6	23.9	24.1	24.4
185.4	73		19.5	19.8	20.1	20.3	20.6	20.8	21.1	21.4	21.6	21.9	22.2	22.4	22.7	23.0	23.2	23.5	23.7
188.0	74		19.0	19.3	19.5	19.8	20.0	20.3	20.5	20.8	21.1	21.3	21.6	21.8	22.1	22.3	22.6	22.9	23.1
190.5	75		18.5	18.7	19.0	19.2	19.5	19.7	20.0	20.2	20.5	20.7	21.0	21.2	21.5	21.7	22.0	22.2	22.5
193.0	76		18.0	18.3	18.5	18.7	19.0	19.2	19.5	19.7	20.0	20.2	20.4	20.7	20.9	21.2	21.4	21.7	21.9
195.6	77		17.6	17.8	18.0	18.3	18.5	18.7	19.0	19.2	19.4	19.7	19.9	20.2	20.4	20.6	20.9	21.1	21.3
198.1	78		17.1	17.3	17.6	17.8	18.0	18.3	18.5	18.7	19.0	19.2	19.4	19.6	19.9	20.1	20.3	20.6	20.8

Whenever a child's specific height or weight measurement is not listed, round to the closest number in the table.

CALCULATED BODY MASS INDEX   61 IN.–78 IN. AND 182 LB–214 LB

Height		Weight																	
cm	in	**kg** 82.6	83.5	84.4	85.3	86.2	87.1	88.0	88.9	89.8	90.7	91.6	92.5	93.4	94.3	95.3	96.2	97.1
		lb 182	184	186	188	190	192	194	196	198	200	202	204	206	208	210	212	214
154.9	61	34.4	34.8															
157.5	62	33.3	33.7	34.0	34.4	34.8												
160.0	63	32.2	32.6	32.9	33.3	33.7	34.0	34.4	34.7									
162.6	64	31.2	31.6	31.9	32.3	32.6	33.0	33.3	33.6	34.0	34.3	34.7						
165.1	65	30.3	30.6	31.0	31.3	31.6	32.0	32.3	32.6	32.9	33.3	33.6	33.9	34.3	34.6	34.9		
167.6	66	29.4	29.7	30.0	30.3	30.7	31.0	31.3	31.6	32.0	32.3	32.6	32.9	33.2	33.6	33.9	34.2	34.5
170.2	67	28.5	28.8	29.1	29.4	29.8	30.1	30.4	30.7	31.0	31.3	31.6	32.0	32.3	32.6	32.9	33.2	33.5
172.7	68	27.7	28.0	28.3	28.6	28.9	29.2	29.5	29.8	30.1	30.4	30.7	31.0	31.3	31.6	31.9	32.2	32.5
175.3	69	26.9	27.2	27.5	27.8	28.1	28.4	28.6	28.9	29.2	29.5	29.8	30.1	30.4	30.7	31.0	31.3	31.6
177.8	70	26.1	26.4	26.7	27.0	27.3	27.5	27.8	28.1	28.4	28.7	29.0	29.3	29.6	29.8	30.1	30.4	30.7
180.3	71	25.4	25.7	25.9	26.2	26.5	26.8	27.1	27.3	27.6	27.9	28.2	28.5	28.7	29.0	29.3	29.6	29.8
182.9	72	24.7	25.0	25.2	25.5	25.8	26.0	26.3	26.6	26.9	27.1	27.4	27.7	27.9	28.2	28.5	28.8	29.0
185.4	73	24.0	24.3	24.5	24.8	25.1	25.3	25.6	25.9	26.1	26.4	26.7	26.9	27.2	27.4	27.7	28.0	28.2
188.0	74	23.4	23.6	23.9	24.1	24.4	24.7	24.9	25.2	25.4	25.7	25.9	26.2	26.4	26.7	27.0	27.2	27.5
190.5	75	22.7	23.0	23.2	23.5	23.7	24.0	24.2	24.5	24.7	25.0	25.2	25.5	25.7	26.0	26.2	26.5	26.7
193.0	76	22.2	22.4	22.6	22.9	23.1	23.4	23.6	23.9	24.1	24.3	24.6	24.8	25.1	25.3	25.6	25.8	26.0
195.6	77	21.6	21.8	22.1	22.3	22.5	22.8	23.0	23.2	23.5	23.7	24.0	24.2	24.4	24.7	24.9	25.1	25.4
198.1	78	21.0	21.3	21.5	21.7	22.0	22.2	22.4	22.6	22.9	23.1	23.3	23.6	23.8	24.0	24.3	24.5	24.7

Whenever a child's specific height or weight measurement is not listed, round to the closest number in the table.

CALCULATED BODY MASS INDEX   66 IN.–78 IN. AND 216 LB–250 LB

Height		Weight																	
cm	in	kg 98.0	98.9	99.8	100.7	101.6	102.5	103.4	104.3	105.2	106.1	107.0	108.0	108.9	109.8	110.7	111.6	112.5	113.4
		lb 216	218	220	222	224	226	228	230	232	234	236	238	240	242	244	246	248	250
167.6	66	34.9																	
170.2	67	33.8	34.1	34.5	34.8														
172.7	68	32.8	33.1	33.5	33.8	34.1	34.4	34.7	35.0										
175.3	69	31.9	32.2	32.5	32.8	33.1	33.4	33.7	34.0	34.3	34.6	34.9							
177.8	70	31.0	31.3	31.6	31.9	32.1	32.4	32.7	33.0	33.3	33.6	33.9	34.1	34.4	34.7				
180.3	71	30.1	30.4	30.7	31.0	31.2	31.5	31.8	32.1	32.4	32.6	32.9	33.2	33.5	33.8	34.0	34.3	34.6	34.9
182.9	72	29.3	29.6	29.8	30.1	30.4	30.7	30.9	31.2	31.5	31.7	32.0	32.3	32.5	32.8	33.1	33.4	33.6	33.9
185.4	73	28.5	28.8	29.0	29.3	29.6	29.8	30.1	30.3	30.6	30.9	31.1	31.4	31.7	31.9	32.2	32.5	32.7	33.0
188.0	74	27.7	28.0	28.2	28.5	28.8	29.0	29.3	29.5	29.8	30.0	30.3	30.6	30.8	31.1	31.3	31.6	31.8	32.1
190.5	75	27.0	27.2	27.5	27.7	28.0	28.2	28.5	28.7	29.0	29.2	29.5	29.7	30.0	30.2	30.5	30.7	31.0	31.2
193.0	76	26.3	26.5	26.8	27.0	27.3	27.5	27.8	28.0	28.2	28.5	28.7	29.0	29.2	29.5	29.7	29.9	30.2	30.4
195.6	77	25.6	25.9	26.1	26.3	26.6	26.8	27.0	27.3	27.5	27.7	28.0	28.2	28.5	28.7	28.9	29.2	29.4	29.6
198.1	78	25.0	25.2	25.4	25.7	25.9	26.1	26.3	26.6	26.8	27.0	27.3	27.5	27.7	28.0	28.2	28.4	28.7	28.9

Whenever a child's specific height or weight measurement is not listed, round to the closest number in the table.

BIBLIOGRAPHY

Abell, T. L., and A. Minocha. "Gastrointestinal Complications of Bariatric Surgery: Diagnosis and Therapy. *American Journal of Medical Science* 331, no. 4 (2006): 214–218.

Adamec, Christine. *Impulse Control Disorders*. New York: Chelsea House, 2008.

Ahmedin, Jemal, et al. "Annual Report to the Nation on the Status of Cancer, 1975–2005, Featuring Trends in Lung Cancer, Tobacco Use, and Tobacco Control." *Journal of the National Cancer Institute* 100, no. 23 (December 3, 2008): 1,672–1,694.

Ahsan Baig, Muhammad, M.D., Abdul Qadir, M.D., and Javeria Rasheed, M.D. "A Review of Eosinophilic Gastroenteritis." *Journal of the National Medical Association* 98, no. 10 (2006): 1,616–1,619.

Allen, Katrina J., M.D., et al. "Iron-Overload-Related Disease in *HFE* Hereditary Hemochromatosis," *New England Journal of Medicine* 358, no. 2 (January 17, 2008): 221–230.

Anand, Preetha, et al. "Cancer is a Preventable Disease that Requires Major Lifestyle Changes." *Pharmaceutical Research* 29, no. 9 (2008): 2,097–2,116.

Andersson, Roland E., M.D., et al. "Appendectomy and Protection against Ulcerative Colitis." *New England Journal of Medicine* 344, no. 11 (March 15, 2001): 808–814.

Angelini, Giampaolo, and Laura Bernardoni. "Management and Treatment of Complications in Diagnostic and Therapeutic Lower Gastrointestinal Tract Endoscopy." In *Intestinal Polyps and Polyposis*, edited by Gian Gaetano Delaini, Tomáš Skřička, and Gianluca Colucci. Milan, Italy: Springer Milan, 2009.

Antman, Karen, M.D., and Yuan Chang, M.D. "Kaposi's Sarcoma." *New England Journal of Medicine* 342, no. 14 (April 6, 2000): 1,027–1,038.

Bacon, Bruce R., M.D., et al. "*HFE* Genotype in Patients with Hemochromotosis and Other Liver Diseases," *Annals of Internal Medicine* 130, no. 12 (June 15, 1999): 953–962.

Bagnardi, Vincenzo, et al. "Alcohol Consumption and the Risk of Cancer." *Alcohol Research e~Health* 25, no. 4 (2001): 263–269.

Bar, Dalsu, M.D., and Sheilia Hoar Zahm. "Epidemiology of Lymphomas." *Current Opinion in Oncology* 12 (2000): 383–394.

Barnes, Patricia M., and Barbara Bloom. "Complementary and Alternative Medicine Use Among Adults and Children: United States, 2007." *National Health Statistics Reports* 18 (December 10, 2008): 1–24.

Belluzzi, Andrea, M.D., et al. "Effect of an Enteric-Coated Fish-Oil Preparation on Relapses in Crohn's Disease." *New England Journal of Medicine* 334, no. 24 (June 13, 1996): 1,557–1,560.

Belmont, John W., M.D., et al. "Congenital Sucrase-Isomaltase Deficiency Presenting with Failure to Thrive, Hypercalcemia, and Nephrocalcinosis." *BMC Pediatrics* 2 (April 2002). Available online. URL: http://www.cdc.gov/tb/publications/faqs/pdfs/qa.pdf. Accessed April 6, 2010.

Berkson, Lindsey. *Healthy Digestion the Natural Way: Preventing and Healing Heartburn, Constipation, Gas, Diarrhea, Inflammatory Bowel and Gallbladder Diseases, Ulcers, Irritable Bowel Syndrome, Food Allergies, and More*. New York: John Wiley & Sons, 2000.

Brolin, Robert E., M.D. "Bariatric Surgery and Long-Term Control of Morbid Obesity." *Journal of the American Medical Association* 288, no. 22 (December 11, 2002): 2,793–2,796.

Brøndum Føkjaer, Jens, et al. "Central Processing of Gut Pain in Diabetes Patients with Gastrointestinal Symptoms." *Diabetes Care* 32, no. 7 (July 2009): 1,274–1,277.

Brown, Robert S., Jr., M.D., et al. "A Survey of Liver Transplantation from Living Adult Donors in the United States." *New England Journal of Medicine* 348, no. 9 (February 27, 2003): 818–825.

Bytzer, Peter, M.D., and Nicholas J. Talley, M.D. "Dyspepsia." *Annals of Internal Medicine* 134, no. 9, part 2 (2001): 815–822.

Cassell, Dana K., and David H. Gleaves, Ph.D. *Obesity and Eating Disorders*. 2d ed. New York: Facts On File, 2000.

Calvert, Paula M., M.D., and Harold Frucht, M.D. "The Genetics of Colorectal Cancer." *Annals of Internal Medicine* 137, no. 7 (2002): 603–612.

Calvo, M. M., et al. "Role of Magnetic Resonance Cholangiopancreatography with Suspected Choledocholithiasis." *Mayo Clinic Proceedings* 77, no. 5 (May 2002): 422–428.

Cavicchi, Maryan, M.D., et al. "Prevalence of Liver Disease and Contributing Factors in Patients Receiving Home Parenteral Nutrition for Permanent Intestinal Failure." *Annals of Internal Medicine* 132, no. 7 (2000): 525–532.

Center for Food Safety and Applied Nutrition. *Safe Handling of Raw Produce and Fresh-Squeezed Fruit and Vegetable Juices.* Food and Drug Administration. Undated. Available online. URL: http://www.cfsan.fda/gov/~dms/prodsafe.html. Accessed June 12, 2008.

Centers for Disease Control and Prevention. "Differences in Prevalence of Obesity among Black, White, and Hispanic Adults—United States, 2006–2008." *Morbidity and Mortality Review* 58, no. 27 (July 17, 2009): 740–744.

———. *U.S. Cancer Statistics: 2004 Incidence and Mortality.* Atlanta, Ga.: Centers for Disease Control and Prevention, 2007.

———. "U.S. Obesity Trends." Available online. URL: http://www.cdc.gov/obesity/data/trends.html. Accessed July 21, 2009.

———. *Travelers' Health: Yellow Book.* Chapter 4, Prevention of Specific Infectious Diseases. Available online. URL: http://wwwn.cdc.gov/travel/yellowBookCh4-Typhoid.aspx. Accessed June 12, 2008.

Chan, Andrew T., M.D., Ogino, Shuji, and Fuchs, Charles, S., M.D. "Aspirin Use and Survival After Diagnosis of Colorectal Cancer." *Journal of the American Medical Association* 302, no. 6 (2009): 649–659.

Chen, Xian-Ming, M.D., et al. "Cryptosporidiosis." *New England Journal of Medicine* 346, no. 2 (May 30, 2002): 1,723–1,731.

Chow, W. H., et al. "Gallstones, Cholecystectomy and Risk of Cancers of the Liver, Biliary Tract and Pancreas." *British Journal of Cancer* 79, nos. 3/4 (1999): 640–644.

Comparato, Giuseppe, et al. "Diverticular Disease in the Elderly." *Digestive Diseases* 25 (2007): 151–159.

Corcoran, Colleen, and Steven Grinspoon, M.D. "Treatments for Wasting in Patients with the Acquired Immunodeficiency Syndrome." *New England Journal of Medicine* 340, no. 22 (June 3, 1999): 1,740–1,750.

Cortese, Aamuele, et al. "Attention-Deficit Hyperactivity Disorder (ADHD) and Obesity: A Systematic Review of the Literature. *Critical Reviews in Food Science and Nutrition* 49 (2008): 524–537.

Cummings, David B., M.D., et al. "Plasma Ghrelin Levels after Diet-Induced Weight Loss or Gastric Bypass Surgery." *New England Journal of Medicine* 346, no. 21 (May 23, 2002): 1,623–1,630.

DeMaria, Eric J., M.D. "Bariatric Surgery for Morbid Obesity." *New England Journal of Medicine* 356, no. 21 (May 24, 2007): 2,176–2,183.

Denshaw-Burke, M.D. et al. "Gallbladder Cancer." eMedicine. Updated June 12, 2008. Available online. URL: http://emedicine.medscape.com/article/278641-overview. Accessed February 6, 2009.

Devon, K.M., et al. "Colorectal Cancer Surgery in Elderly Patients: Presentation, Treatment, and Outcomes." *Diseases of the Colon & Rectum* 52, no. 7 (2009): 1,272–1,277.

Di Franceso, Vincenzo, et al. "The Anorexia of Aging." *Digestive Diseases* 25 (2007): 129–137.

Division of Foodborne, Bacterial and Mycotic Diseases. *Shigellosis.* Available online. URL: http://www.cdc.gov/nczved/dfbmd/disease_listing/shigellosis_gi.html. Downloaded June 13, 2008.

Dixon, John B., Paul E. O'Brien, Julie Playfair, et al. "Adjustable Gastric Banding and Conventional Therapy for Type 2 Diabetes: A Randomized Controlled Trial." *Journal of the American Medical Association* 299, no. 3 (2008): 316–323.

El Mahdy, Christine. *Mummies, Myth and Magic in Ancient Egypt.* New York: Thames and Hudson, 1989.

El-Serag, Hashem B., M.D., John M. Inadomi, M.D., and Kris V. Kowdley, M.D. "Screening for Hereditary Hemochromatosis in Siblings and Children of Affected Parents." *Annals of Internal Medicine* 132, no. 4 (February 15, 2000): 261–269.

Falk, Rodney H., M.D., Raymond L. Comenzo, M.D., and Martha Skinner, M.D. "The Systemic Amyloidoses." *New England Journal of Medicine* 337, no. 13 (September 25, 1997): 898–909.

Fan, S. T., et al. "Early Treatment of Acute Biliary Pancreatitis by Endoscopic Papillotomy." *New England Journal of Medicine* 328, no. 4 (January 28, 1993): 228–232.

Farci, Patrizia, et al. "Treatment of Chronic Hepatitis D with Interferon Alfa-2a." *New England Journal of Medicine* 330, no. 2 (January 13, 1994): 88–94.

Farrell, Richard J,, M.D., and Ciaran P. Kelly, M.D. "Celiac Sprue." *New England Journal of Medicine* 346, no. 3 (January 17, 2002): 180–188.

Farrell, Philip M., M.D., et al. "Early Diagnosis of Cystic Fibrosis through Neonatal Screening Prevents Severe Malnutrition and Improves Long-Term Growth." *Pediatrics* 107, no. 1 (January 2001): 1–13.

Fennell, Diane. "Gastroparesis." Diabetes Self-Management. Available online. URL: http://www.diabetesselfmanagement.com/articles/diabetes-definitions/gastroparesis/print. Accessed July 1, 2009.

Field, Alison B., et al. "Impact of Overweight on the Risk of Developing Common Chronic Diseases during a

10-Year Period." *Archives of Internal Medicine* 161 (July 9, 2001): 1,581–1,586.

Fisher, Richard S., M.D., and Henry P. Parkman, M.D. "Management of Nonulcer Dyspepsia." *New England Journal of Medicine* 339, no. 19 (November 5, 1998): 1,376–1,381.

Flegal, Katherine M., et al. "Prevalence and Trends in Obesity among U.S. Adults, 1999–2000." *Journal of the American Medical Association* 288, no. 14 (October 9, 2002): 1,723–1,727.

Food Safety and Inspection Servce. *Food Safety for Older Adults*. Washington, D.C.: U.S. Department of Agriculture, September 2006.

Gadde, K.M., et al. "Atomoxetine for Weight Reduction in Obese Women: A Preliminary Randomised Controlled Trial." *International Journal of Obesity* 30 (2006): 1,138–1,142.

Gardner, Paula. "Complementary, Holistic, and Integrative Medicine: Chamomile." *Pediatrics in Review* 28, no. 4 (2007): e16–e18.

General Accounting Office. *Dietary Supplements: FDA Should Take Further Actions to Improve Oversight and Consumer Understanding. Report to Congressional Requesters*. Washington, D.C.: General Accounting Office, January 2009.

Ghosh, Subrata, M.D., et al. "Natalizumab for Active Crohn's Disease." *New England Journal of Medicine* 348, no. 1 (January 2, 2003): 24–32.

Gilsen Tsai, Adam, M.D., and Thomas A. Wadden. "Systematic Review: An Evaluation of Major Commercial Weight Loss Programs in the United States." *Annals of Internal Medicine* 142 (2005): 56–66.

Gordon, Benjamin Lee, M.D. *Medieval and Renaissance Medicine*. New York: Philosophical Library, 1959.

Goyal, Raj K., M.D., and Ikuo Hirano, M.D. "The Enteric Nervous System." *New England Journal of Medicine* 334, no. 17 (April 25, 1996): 1,106–1,115.

Gulcan, E., et al. "Increased Frequency of Prediabetes in Patients with Irritable Bowel Syndrome." *American Journal of Medical Sciences* 338, no. 2 (August 2009): 116–119.

Herrine, Steven K., M.D. "Approach to the Patient with Chronic Hepatitis C Virus Infection." *Annals of Internal Medicine* 136, no. 10 (May 21, 2002): 747–757.

Hirschmann, Jan V., M.D. "What Killed Mozart?" *Archives of Internal Medicine* 161 (June 11, 2001): 1,381–1,389.

Horwitz, Brenda J., M.D., and Robert S. Fisher, M.D. "The Irritable Bowel Syndrome." *New England Journal of Medicine* 344 no. 24 (June 14 2001): 1,846–1,850.

Hsu, Chiehwen, et al. "Reducing Liver Cancer Disparities: A Community-Based Hepatitis-B Prevention Program for Asian-American Communities." *Journal of the National Medical Association* 99, no. 8 (2007): 900–907.

Jailwala, Jeegr, M.D., Thomas F. Imperiale, M.D., and Kurt Kroenke, M.D. "Pharmacologic Treatment of the Irritable Bowel Syndrome: A Systematic Review of Randomized, Controlled Trials." *Annals of Internal Medicine* 133, no. 2 (2000): 136–147.

Jay, Melanie, et al. "Physicians' Attitudes about Obesity and Their Associations with Competency and Specialty: A Cross-sectional Study." *BMC Health Services Research* 2009. Available online. URL: http://www.biomedcentrl.com/1472-6963/9/106. Accessed July 19, 2009.

Jemal, Ahmedin, et al. "Cancer Statistics, 2007." *CA: A Cancer Journal for Clinicians* 57 (2007): 43–66.

Jonas, Wayne B., M.D., Ted J. Kaptchuk, and Klaus Linde, M.D. "A Critical Overview of Homeopathy." *Annals of Internal Medicine* 138, no. 5 (2003): 393–399.

Kandel, Joseph, M.D., and Christine Adamec. *The Encyclopedia of Elder Care*. New York: Facts On File, 2008.

Kaplan, Marshall M., M.D. "Primary Biliary Cirrhosis." *New England Journal of Medicine* 335, no. 21 (November 21, 1996): 1,570–1,580.

Key, Timothy J., et al. "Diet, Nutrition and the Prevention of Cancer." *Public Health Nutrition* 7, no. 1A (2004): 187–200.

Khaitan, Leena, M.D., and Michael D. Holzman, M.D. "Laparoscopic Advances in General Surgery." *Journal of the American Medical Association* 287, no. 12 (March 27, 2002): 1,502–1,505.

Khan, Kamran, M.D., et al. "Global Drug-Resistance Patterns and the Management of Latent Tuberculosis Infection in Immigrants to the United States." *New England Journal of Medicine* 347, no. 23 (December 5, 2002): 1,850–1,859.

Khan, Laura Kettel, et al. "Use of Prescription Weight Loss Pills among U.S. Adults in 1996–1998." *Annals of Internal Medicine* 134, no. 4 (2001): 282–286.

Knowles, Michael R., M.D., and Peter R. Dune, M.D. "What Is Cystic Fibrosis?" *New England Journal of Medicine* 347, no. 6 (August 8, 2002): 439–442.

Koch, Christian A., and Gabriel I. Uwaifo. "Are Gastrointestinal Symptoms Related to Diabetes Mellitus and Glycemic Control?" *European Journal of Gastroenterology* 20, no. 9 (2008): 822–825.

Kukka, Christine, "Mutations in the Virus' Surface and Core Proteins Increase Risk of Liver Cancer." *HBV Journal Review* 6, no. 1 (2009): 1.

Kotler, Donald P., M.D. "Cachexia." *Annals of Internal Medicine* 133, no. 8 (2000): 622–634.

Kumar, Shaji, M.D., Michael G. Sarr, M.D., and Patrick S. Kamath, M.D. "Mesenteric Venous Thrombosis." *New*

England Journal of Medicine 345, no. 23 (December 6, 2001): 1,683–1,688.

Lacey, Brian E., M.D., et al. "The Treatment of Diabetic Gastroparesis with Botulinum Toxin Injections of the Pylorus." *Diabetes Care* 27, no. 10 (2004): 2,341–2,347.

Lange, Paul H., M.D., and Christine Adamec. *Prostate Cancer for Dummies.* New York: John Wiley & Sons, 2003.

Langman, Michael J., M.D. "Adverse Upper Gastrointestinal Effects of Rofecoxib Compared with NSAIDs." *Journal of the American Medical Association* 282, no. 20 (November 24, 1999): 1,929–1,933.

Langner, Elke, Stefan Greifenberg, and Joel Gruenwald. "Ginger: History and Use." *Advances in Therapy* 15, no. 1 (January/February 1998): 25–44.

Leitzmann, Michael F., M.D., et al. "Recreational Physical Activity and the Risk of Cholecystectomy in Women." *New England Journal of Medicine* 341, no. 11 (September 9, 1999): 777–784.

Leung, Donald Y. M., M.D., et al. "Effect of Anti-IgE Therapy in Patients with Peanut Allergy." *New England Journal of Medicine* 348, no. 11 (March 13, 2003): 986–993.

Levenstein, Susan, et al. "Stress and Peptic Ulcer Disease." *Journal of the American Medical Association* 281, no. 1 (January 6, 1999): 10–11.

Levi, Jeffrey, et al. *F as in Fat: How Obesity Policies Are Failing in America.* Washington, D.C.: Robert Wood Johnson Foundation, 2009.

Lieberman, David, M.D. "Prevalence of Colon Polyps Detected by Colonoscopy Screening in Asymptomatic Black and White Patients." *Journal of the American Medical Association* 300, no. 12 (September 24, 2008): 1,417–1,422.

Madan, A., and A. Minocha. "Despite High Satisfaction, Majority of Gastro-oesophageal Reflux Disease Patients Continue to Use Proton Pump Inhibitors after Antireflux Surgery." *Alimentary Pharmacology & Therapeutics* 23, no. 5 (2006): 601–605.

Malagelada, Juan-R., M.D. "Gastrointestinal Syndromes Due to Diabetes Mellitus." In *Contemporary Diabetes: Diabetic Neuropathy: Clinical Management*, edited by N. Veves, A. and R. Malik,. 2nd ed., Totowa, N.J.: Human Press, 2007. 433–451.

Mehler, Philip S., M.D. "Diagnosis and Care of Patients with Anorexia Nervosa in Primary Care Settings *Annals of Internal Medicine* 134, no. 11 (June 2001): 1,048–1,059.

Millsten, Rachel A., et al. "Relationships between Body Size Satisfaction and Weight Control Practices among US Adults." *Medscape Journal of Medicine* 10, no. 5 (2008). Available online. URL: http://www.pubmed central.nih.gov/articlerender.fcgi?artaid=2438482. Accessed July 21, 2009.

Minocha, Anil, M.D., et al. "Alterations in Upper Gastrointestinal Motility in *Helicobacter* Pylori-positive Non-ulcer Dyspepsia." *American Journal of Gastroenterology* 89, no. 10, (1994): 1,797–1,800.

Minocha, Anil, M.D., and Srinivasan, Radhika, M.D. "Conscious Sedation: Pearls and Perils." *Digestive Diseases and Sciences* 43, no.8 (August 1998): 1,835–1,844.

Minocha, Anil, M.D. *The Gastroenterology Resident Pocket Survival Guide.* McLean, Va.: International Medical, 1999.

Minocha, Anil, M.D., et al. "*Helicobacterpylori* Is Associated with Alterations in Intestinal Gas Profile among Patients with Nonulcer Dyspepsia." *Digestive Diseases and Sciences* 39, no. 8 (August 1994): 1,613–1,617.

Minocha, Anil, M.D., and Christine Adamec. *How to Stop Heartburn: Simple Ways to Heal Heartburn and Acid Reflux.* New York: John Wiley & Sons, 2001.

Minocha, Anil, M.D., C. A. Racakowski, M.D., and Robert J. Richards, M.D. "Is a History of Tonsillectomy Associated with Decreased Risk of *Helicobacter pylori* Infection?" *Journal of Clinical Gastroenterology* 25, no. 4 (1997): 580–582.

Minocha, Anil, M.D., and David Carroll. *Natural Stomach Care.* New York: Penguin Putnam, 2003.

Minocha, Anil, M.D. "Noncardiac Chest Pain: Where Does It Start?" *Postgraduate Medicine* 100, no. 6 (December 1996): 107–114.

Minocha, Anil, M.D., and David S. Greenbaum, M.D. "Pill-Esophagitis Caused by Nonsteroidal Antiinflammatory Drugs." *American Journal of Gastroenterology* 86, no. 8 (1991): 1,086–1,089.

Minocha, Anil, M.D., et al. "Prevalence of Previous Appendectomy among Patients Needing Gastrointestinal Endoscopy." *Southern Medical Journal* 92, no. 1 (January 1999): 41–43.

Minocha, A., and C. A. Raczkowski. "Role of Appendectomy and Tonsillectomy in Pathogenesis of Ulcerative Colitis." *Digestive Disease Sciences* 42 (1997): 1,567–1,569.

Moawad, Fouad J., Ganesh R. Veerappan, and Roy K. Wong. "Eosinophilic Esophagitis." *Digestive Diseases Science* 54 (2009): 1,818–1,828.

Nahin, Richard L., et al. "Costs of Complementary and Alternative Medicine (CAM) and Frequency of Visits to CAM Practitioners: United States, 2007." *National Health Statistics Report No. 18* (July 30, 2009): 1–15.

National Cancer Institute. *Cancer Trends Progress Report—2007 Update.* Bethesda, Md.: Department of Health and Human Services, December 2007.

————. *What You Need to Know about Cancer of the Colon and Rectum*. Bethesda, Md.: Department of Health and Human Services, May 2006.

National Institute of Diabetes and Digestive and Kidney Diseases. *Hemochromatosis*. Bethesda, Md.: National Institutes of Health, April 2007.

————. *Recent Advances & Emerging Opportunities*. Bethesda, Md.: National Institutes of Health, February 2009.

Newman, Julliana. "Radiographic and Endoscopic Evaluation of the Upper GI Tract." *Radiologic Technology* 69, no. 3 (January/February 1998): 213–227.

Newman, Lee S., et al. "Sarcoidosis." *New England Journal of Medicine* 336, no. 17 (April 24, 1997): 1,224–1,234.

Nishida, T., et al. "Gastroesophageal Refulux DIse Related to Diabetes: Analysis of 241 Cases with Type 2 Diabetes Mellitus." *Journal of Gastroenterology and Hepatology* 19, no. 3 (2004): 258–265.

Noel, Rebecca A., et al. "Increased Risk of Acute Pancreatitis and Biliary Disease Observed in Patients with Type 2 Diabetes." *Diabetes Care* 32, no. 4 (2009): 834–838.

Onken, J. E., et al. "Bromelain Treatment Decreases Secretion of Pro-Inflammatory Cytoknes and Chemokines by Colon Biopsies in Vitro." *Clinical Immunology* 126 (2008): 345–352.

Ostapowicz G., et al. "Results of a Prospective Study of Acute Liver Failure at 17 Tertiary Care Centers in the United States." *Annals of Internal Medicine* 137 (December 2002): 947–954.

Parrish, Carol Lee, and Joyce Green Pastors. "Nutritional Management of Gastroparesis in People with Diabetes." *Diabetes Spectrum* 20, no. 4 (2007): 231–234.

Petit, William, Jr., M.D., and Christine Adamec. *The Encyclopedia of Diabetes*. 2nd ed. New York: Facts On File, 2010.

Petry, Nancy M., et al. "Overweight and Obesity Are Associated with Psychiatric Disorders: Results from the National Epidemiologic Survey on Alcohol and Related Conditions." *Psychosomatic Medicine* 70 (2008): 288–297.

Pleis, J. R., and M. Lethbridge-Çejku. *Summary Health Statistics for U.S. Adults: National Health Interview Survey 2006*. Washington, D.C.: National Center for Health Statistics, 2007.

Podolsky, Daniel K., M.D. "Inflammatory Bowel Disease." *New England Journal of Medicine* 347, no. 6 (August 8, 2002): 417–429.

Puhl, Rebecca M., and Chelsea A. Heuer. "The Stigma of Obesity: A Review and Update." *Obesity* 17, no. 5 (2009): 841–964.

Rabbani, G. H., M.D. "The Search for a Better Oral Rehydration Solution for Cholera." *New England Journal of Medicine* 342, no. 5 (February 3, 2000): 345–347.

Räihh, Ismo, M.D., et al. "Lifestyle, Stress, and Genes in Peptic Ulcer Disease: A Nationwide Twin Cohort Study." *Archives of Internal Medicine* 158 (April 13, 1998): 698–704.

Rao, Patrick M., M.D., et al. "Effect of Computer Tomography of the Appendix on Treatment of Patients and Use of Hospital Resources." *New England Journal of Medicine* 338, no. 3 (January 15, 1998): 141–146.

Ries, L. A. G., et al. eds. *SEER Cancer Statistics Review, 1975–2005*. Bethesda, Md.: National Cancer Institute. Available online. URL: http://seer.cancer.gov/csr/1975_2005/. Based on November 2007 SEER submission, posted to the SEER Web site, 2008. Downloaded February 1, 2009.

Roberts, Lewis R. "Sorafenib in Liver Cancer—Just the Beginning." *New England Journal of Medicine* 359, no. 4 (July 24, 2008): 420–422.

Rockey, Don C., M.D. "Occult Gastrointestinal Bleeding." *New England Journal of Medicine* 341, no. 1 (July 1, 1999): 38–46.

Ruskone-Fourmestraux, A., et al. "Multiple Lymphomatous Polyposis of the Gastrointestinal Tract: Prospective Clinicopathologic Study of 31 Cases." *Gastroenterology* 112, no. 1 (January 1997): 7–16.

Ryan, David R, M.D., Carolyn C. Compton, M.D., and Robert J. Mayer, M.D. "Carcinoma of the Anal Canal." *New England Journal of the Medicine* 342, no.11 (March 16, 2000): 792–800.

Ryan, David P., M.D., and Kevin C. Kain, M.D. "Health Advice and Immunizations for Travelers." *New England Journal of Medicine* 342, no. 23 (June 8, 2000): 1,716–1,725.

Sakane, Tsuyoshi, M.D., et al. "Behçet's Disease." *New England Journal of Medicine* 341, no. 17 (October 21, 1999): 1,284–1,291.

Salam, Gohar A. "Lipoma Excision." *American Family Physician* 65 (March 1, 2002): 901–904, 905.

Salbe, Arline D., et al. "Assessing Risk Factors for Obesity between Childhood and Adolescence. I. Birth Weight, Childhood Adiposity, Parental Obesity, Insulin, and Leptin." *Pediatrics* 110, no. 2 (August 2002): 299–306.

————. "Assessing Risk Factors for Obesity between Childhood and Adolescence. II. Energy Metabolism and Physical Activity." *Pediatrics* 110, no. 2 (August 2002): 307–314.

Seitz, Helmut K., M.D., and Peter Becker, M.D., "Alcohol Metabolism and Cancer Risk," *Alcohol Research & Health* 30, no. 1 (2007): 38–47.

Sherman, Paul W., Erica Holland, and Janet Shellman Sherman. "Allergies: Their Role in Cancer Prevention." *Quarterly Review of Biology* 83, no. 4 (2008): 339–362.

Silviera, Matthew L., et al. "Complications Related to Endoscopic Retrograde Cholangiopancreatography: A Comprehensive Clinical Review." *Journal of Gastrointestinal and Liver Disease* 18, no. 1 (2009): 73–82.

Simon, Gregory E., M.D., et al. "Association between Obesity and Psychiatric Disorders in the US Adult Population." *Archives of General Psychiatry* 64 (2006): 824–830.

Slonim, Alfred E., M.D., et al. "A Preliminary Study of Growth Hormone Therapy for Crohn's Disease." *New England Journal of Medicine* 342, no. 22 (June 1, 2000): 1,633–1,637.

Small, Peter M., M.D., and Paula I. Fujiwara, M.D. "Management of Tuberculosis in the United States." *New England Journal of Medicine* 345, no. 3 (July 19, 2001): 189–200.

Spence, David S., Elizabeth A. Thompson, and S. J. Barron. "Homeopathic Treatment for Chronic Disease: A 6-Year, University-Hospital Outpatient Observational Study." *Journal of Alternative and Complementary Medicine* 11, no. 5 (2005): 793–798.

Spinzi, G. C. "Bowel Care in the Elderly." *Digestive Diseases* 25 (2007): 160–165.

Srinivasan, Radhika, M.D., and Anil Minocha, M.D. "When to Suspect Lactose Intolerance." *Postgraduate Medicine* 104, no. 3 (September 1998): 109–123.

Starzl, Thomas B. "The Contribution of Transplantation to Gastroenterologic Knowledge." In *The Growth of Gastnoenterologic Knowledge During the Twentieth Century.* Philadelphia: Lea & Ferbiger, 1994.

Staud, Roland, M.D., and Christine Adamec. *Fibromyalgia for Dummies.* 2d ed. New York: John Wiley & Sons, 2008.

Steinberg, William, and Scott Tenner. "Acute Pancreatitis." *New England Journal of Medicine* 330, no. 17 (April 28, 1994): 1,198–1,210.

Stern, Robert C., M.D. "The Diagnosis of Cystic Fibrosis." *New England Journal of Medicine* 3,336, no. 7 (February 13, 1997): 487–491.

Stuart, Jon Spechler, M.D. "Barrett's Esophagus." *New England Journal of Medicine* 346, no. 11 (March 14, 2002): 836–842.

Suerbaum, Sebastian, M.D., and Michetti, Pierre, M.D. "*Helicobacter pylori* Infection." *New England Journal of Medicine* 347, no. 15 (October 10, 2002): 1,175–1,186.

Swagerty, Daniel L., Jr., M.D., M.P.H., Anne D. Walling, M.D., and Robert M. Klein. "Lactose Intolerance." *American Family Physician* 65, no. 9 (May 1, 2002): 1,845–1,850.

Swartz, Morton N., M.D. "Whipple's Disease—Past, Present, and Future." *New England Journal of Medicine* 342, no. 9 (March 2, 2000): 648–650.

Tierney, Lawrence M., Jr., M.D., Stephen J. McPhee, M.D., and Maxine A. Papadakis, M.D., eds. *Current Medical Diagnosis and Treatment 2002.* New York: Lange Medical Books, 2002.

Toh, Ban-Hock, Ian R. van Direl, and Paul A. Gleeson. "Pernicious Anemia." *New England Journal of Medicine* 447, no. 20 (November 13, 1997): 1,441–1,448.

U.S. Department of Health and Human Services. *Opportunities and Challenges in Digestive Diseases Research: Recommendations of the National Commission on Digestive Diseases.* Bethesda, Md.: National Institutes of Health, March 2009.

Venook, Alan P., M.D., and Sabrina Selim, M.D. "Cancer of the Gall Bladder." Updated August 19, 2007. Available online. URL: http://www.cancersupportive care.com/gallbladder.html. Downloaded February 6, 2009.

Virnig, Beth A., et al. "A Matter of Race: Early-Versus Late-Stage Cancer Diagnosis." *Health Affairs* 28, no. 1 (January-February 2009): 160–168.

Von Arnim, Ulrike, M.D., et al. "STW 5, a Phytopharmacon for Patients with Functional Dyspepsia: Results of a Multicenter, Placebo-Controlled Double-Blind Study." *American Journal of Gastroenterology* 102, no. 6 (2007): 1,268–1,275.

Walley, Andrew J., Julian E. Asher, and Philippe Froguel. "The Genetic Contribution to Non-Syndromic Human Obesity." *Nature Reviews Genetics* 10 (2009): 431–442.

Yang, Alice L., et al. "Epidemiology of Alcohol-Related Liver and Pancreatic Disease in the United States." *Archives of Internal Medicine* 168, no. 6 (March 24, 2008): 649–656.

Yoon, Young-Hee, and Hsiao-ye Yi. *Surveillance Report #83: Liver Cirrhosis Mortality in the United States, 1970-2005.* National Institute on Alcohol Abuse and Alcoholism. Baltimore, Md.: National Institutes of Health, August 2008.

INDEX

Note: **Boldface** page numbers indicate extensive treatment of a topic. *Italic* page numbers indicate tables.

nonalcoholic steatohepatitis in
214
obesity in 218
oral cancer in 56
pancreatic cancer in 58
sarcoidosis in xx, 246–247
sickle-cell anemia in 29
small intestine, cancer in 58, 252,
252
smokers 253
tuberculosis in 263
ulcers in *101*, 105
African iron overload 164
age xix, 100–103. *See also* elderly
and alternative medicine *13*, 16
and ambulatory visits 100–102,
103
and anemia 29
and appendicitis 35, 100, 130
and BMI 46, *46*
and cancer 55
and celiac disease 65
and colonoscopy 198, *199*
and colorectal cancer 55, 80, 125
and death rates of digestive
diseases 102–103, *103, 104*
and diabetes 100, *101*, 106, 122,
125–126
and digestion 115
and esophageal cancer 56, 140
and exercise 141
and gallstones 154
and hospital discharges 100–102,
103
and liver cancer 57, 191
and liver disease 100, *101*, 122
and pancreatic cancer 231
and small intestine cancer 58
and stomach cancer 257
and ulcerative colitis 269
and ulcers 100, *101*, 122, 272
and Zenker's diverticulum 282
ageusia 259
AIDS. *See* acquired immunodeficiency
syndrome
alactasia 186
alanine aminotransferase 165
albendazole 262
albumin **10–11,** 177
alcohol
breath test for 49, 204
and iron absorption 163
medications interacting with 8,
122–123, *123–125*
in past remedies xxii–xxiii

alcohol abuse and alcoholism xiv,
11–12, 172
acetaminophen use in xviii, 74
and anemia 11, 28, 30, 172
and cancer 60–61
causes of 11
and cirrhosis 11, 73, 74, 82, 172,
189
and colorectal cancer 11, 61, 80,
81, 172
in diabetes 110
diagnosis of 12
in elderly 122–125
and esophageal cancer 11, 61, 140
and esophagitis 141
and liver cancer 172, 191
and magnesium deficiency 197
and Mallory-Weiss syndrome 11,
172, 204–205
medications for 12
and oral cancer 55, 61, 172, 228
and pancreatitis xvii, 11, 129, 172,
233, 234
risk factors of 12, 99
and small intestine cancer 252
smoking and 11, 61, 173, 228
symptoms of 11–12
treatment of 12
and vitamin deficiencies xiv, 11,
172, 274, 275, 278
withdrawal symptoms in 12, 75
and zinc deficiency 172, 283
alcoholic hepatitis 11, 165, 172
Alcoholics Anonymous (AA) 12
Aldactone 36
alendronate 141
aliageusia 259
alkaline phosphatase 192
allergies 54, 137. *See also* food
allergies
alosetron 181–182
alpha-D-galactosidase 155
alpha-fetoprotein (AFP) 191
alpha glucosidase inhibitors 110, 206
alpha thalassemia 30
alpha-3 omega fatty acid 51
alternative medicine xx, 5, **12–25**
for back pain 16, *16*, 38
benefits of 25
for cancer 54
children using 18, 21–22, *21–23*,
24–25
for cirrhosis 75
for constipation 7, 19, 20
cost of 16, *17*

for irritable bowel syndrome 19,
182
medical reasons for 16, *16*
popularity of 16, *18*
problems and risks of 24–25
types of 16, *17, 18*, 22–24
for ulcerative colitis 9, 19, 20
users of *13–15*, 13–16
Amaryl. *See* glimepride
ambulatory visits 100–102, 103
amebiasis **25–26,** 111, 118, 263
American trypanosomiasis 66–67
amino acid supplements 51
aminosalicylates 94, 179, 238
aminotransferase 192
amiodarone 214
Amitiza. *See* lubiprostone
amitriptyline 156
amphetamines 112
ampicillin 188
ampicillin/sulbactam 38
amylase 4, **26,** 115, 153
amyloid 26
amyloidosis **26–27,** 189
anal cancer **27–28**
diagnosis of 27
gender and 27, 28, 99, *100*
prevention of 28
risk factors of 27–28, 61, 87, 172,
253
statistics *xviii*, 27
survival rates for *56*
symptoms of 27
treatment of 27
anal sphincter 254
anal warts. *See* condyloma
acuminatum
Anand, Preetha 54, 58, 61, 62
anaphylaxis 149, 150
Andersson, Roland E. 131
anemia **28–31.** *See also* specific types
alcoholism and 11, 28, 30, 172
and bilirubin levels 44
in blue rubber bleb nevus
syndrome 45
in celiac disease 64, 65
of chronic disease 30
in Crohn's disease 93
diagnosis of 28
in eosinophilic gastroenteritis 136
in familial juvenile polyposis 144
in pregnancy 180
prevention of 29–30
risk factors of 29
symptoms of 28

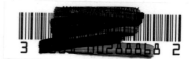